HealthStyles

HealthStyles

Decisions for Living Well

Second Edition

B. E. Pruitt
Texas A & M University

Jane J. Stein
The Stein Group

Allyn and Bacon
Boston • London • Toronto • Sydney • Tokyo • Singapore

Senior Publisher: Joseph E. Burns
Developmental Editor: Mary Kriener
Series Editorial Assistant: Sara Sherlock
Marketing Manager: Richard Muhr
Senior Editorial-Production Administrator: Susan Brown
Composition and Prepress Buyer: Linda Cox
Manufacturing Buyer: Megan Cochran
Cover Administrator: Linda Knowles
Cover Designer: Susan Paradise
Editorial Production and Design Services: Helane Manditch-Prottas
Photo Researcher: Helane Manditch-Prottas
Typographic Services: Dayle Silverman

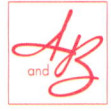

Copyright © 1999 by Allyn & Bacon
A Viacom Company
160 Gould Street
Needham Heights, MA 02494
www.abacon.com

All rights reserved. No part of the material protected by this copyright notice may be reproduced or utilized in any form or by any means, electronic or mechanical, including photocopying, recording, or by any information storage or retrieval system, without written permission from the copyright owner.

Between the time Website information is gathered and published, it is not unusual for some sites to have closed. Also, the transcription of URLs can result in unintended typographical errors. The publisher would appreciate notification of such errors so that they may be corrected in subsequent editions.

A previous edition was published under the title, *Health Styles: Decisions for Living Well*, copyright © 1994 by Harcourt Brace & Company.

Library of Congress Cataloging-in-Publication Data

Pruitt, B. E.
   Healthstyles: decisions for living well/B. E. Pruitt, Jane J. Stein. — 2nd ed.
   Includes bibliographical references and index.
   ISBN 0–205-27229-0
   1. Health.   2. College students—Health and hygiene.   I. Stein, Jane J.   II. Title
RA777.3.P78   1998
613—dc21   98–1450
                                                                                                        CIP

Printed in the United States of America
10 9 8 7 6 5 4 3   VHP   01

Credits begin on page 600, which constitutes a continuation of the copyright page.

Brief Contents

Preface xvii

Part One: Introductory Concepts 1

Chapter 1 Health: Your Personal Responsibility 1
Chapter 2 Assessing Your Health: A Plan for Informed Decision Making 23

Part Two: The Basics of Good Health 47

Chapter 3 Managing Your Mental Health 47
Chapter 4 Coping with Stress 73
Chapter 5 Eating Smart 95
Chapter 6 Maintaining Proper Weight 125
Chapter 7 Keeping Fit 151

Part Three: Controllable Health Risks 177

Chapter 8 Smoking Out Tobacco 177
Chapter 9 Dealing with Drinking 205
Chapter 10 Understanding the Dangers of Drug Use 231
Chapter 11 Recognizing Violent Behavior 263
Chapter 12 Preventing Unintentional Injuries 289

Part Four: Understanding the Disease Process 315

Chapter 13 Reducing the Risk for Chronic Disease 315
Chapter 14 Reducing the Risk for Infectious Disease 351
Chapter 15 Reducing the Risk for Sexually Transmitted Diseases 379

Part Five: Sexuality and Relationships: A Life Span Approach 405

Chapter 16 Sexuality: Developing Healthy Relationships 405
Your Sexual Body: A Primer on Reproductive Anatomy and Physiology 429
Chapter 17 Planning a Family 441
Chapter 18 Aging: Growing Older, Keeping Healthy 475
Chapter 19 Death and Dying 503

Part Six: Participating in a Healthy Community 527

Chapter 20 Living in a Healthy Environment 527
Chapter 21 Making Health Care Decisions 557

Contents

Preface xvii

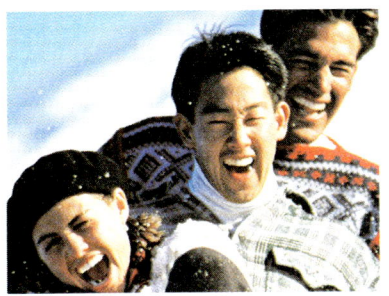

Part 1 Introductory Concepts 1

Chapter 1 Health: Your Personal Responsibility 1

What Is Your HealthStyle? 2

Defining Health 3

Becoming Healthy 5
  Health Knowledge 6
  Health Skills 8
  Health Behavior 10

Establishing a Personal Health Style 12

Prevention: The Best Alternative 14
  Practicing Common Sense 18
  Being Responsible 18

Key Concepts 19
Review Questions 19
Selected Bibliography 19
HealthLinks: Web Sites for Better Health 20
Health Hotlines: Your Personal Responsibility 20

Chapter 2 Assessing Your Health: A Plan for Informed Decision Making 23

What Is Your HealthStyle? 24

Why a Health Assessment? 25
  Problems in Assessing Health 26

Assessing the Health of a Community 27

National Goals for the Year 2000 29

Assessing Your Personal Health 32
  Defining Health Risks: A Look at Your Behavior and Environment 32
  Health Risks: Which Ones Can You Control or Modify? 33
  Health Risk Appraisal: A Measure of Change 34
  Theories about How to Change Health Behavior 34

Assessing, Recording, Changing 36
  Observing Yourself 36
  A Medical Assessment 37
  Keeping Good Health Records 42
  Changing Your Health Behavior 43

Key Concepts 43
Review Questions 44
Selected Bibliography 44
HealthLinks: Web Sites for General Health Information 45
Health Hotlines: Assessing Your Health 45

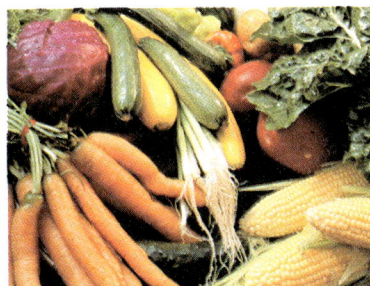

Part 2 The Basics of Good Health 47

Chapter 3 Managing Your Mental Health 47

What Is Your HealthStyle? 48

A Continuum of Well-Being 49
  What Makes a Person Mentally Well? 49
  The Role of Your Emotions 51
  The Benefits of a Good Night's Sleep 52

Who Am I? The Importance of Knowing Yourself 54
  Self-Concept 54
  Self-Esteem 55
  Self-Efficiency 57
  Self-Actualization 58

A Continuum of Mental Dysorganization 58
  From Everyday Problems to Emotionally Crippling Behavior 58

From Being Sad to Depression as a Mental Illness 60
Psychotic Disorders 64

Suicide: A Symptom of Mental Illness 64
Suicide among Teens and Elders 65
How a Suicidal Person Thinks 65
Warning Signs for You to Spot 66

Getting Help for Mental Health Problems 67
When to Call for Help 68

Key Concepts 69
Review Questions 70
Selected Bibliography 70
HealthLinks: Web Sites for Information on Mental Health Issues 70
Health Hotlines: Managing Your Mental Health 71

Chapter 4 Coping with Stress 73

What Is Your HealthStyle? 74

Defining Stress 75
How We React to Stress 75
Stressors: Where Do They Originate? 77
Positive and Negative Stress 77

The Impact of Stress on Health 81
Stress Symptoms Seen in the Physician's Office 81
Research Findings on Stress and the Immune System 81

Stressors of Everyday Living 82
At College 82
At Work 84

Adapting to Stress 85
Coping with Stress 85
Exercise, a Stress Reducer 88
Learning to Relax 89
Cognitive-Behavioral Skills 90

Key Concepts 91
Review Questions 91
Selected Bibliography 92
HealthLinks: Web Sites for a Better Understanding of Stress 92
Health Hotlines: Coping with Stress 93

Chapter 5 Eating Smart 95

What Is Your HealthStyle? 96

What You Need to Eat: The Essential Nutrients 97
Carbohydrates 97
Proteins 99
Fats 100
Vitamins 102
Minerals 103
Water 107

Why Artificial Ingredients Are Added 107

Recommended Dietary Allowances: How Much Do You Need? 109

Eating Styles 112
Eating at Home 112
Fast-Food Living 113
Vegetarian Alternative 113
How Eating Habits Become Unhealthy…and How to Correct Them 119

Selecting and Preparing Healthy Foods 120
How to Read a Food Label 120
Healthful Shopping 121
Preparing Healthy Meals 121

Key Concepts 122
Review Questions 122
Selected Bibliography 122
HealthLinks: Web Sites for a Better Understanding of Nutrition 123
Health Hotlines: Eating Smart 123

Chapter 6 Maintaining Proper Weight 125

What Is Your HealthStyle? 126

How Weight Can Be Harmful to Your Health 127
Problems of Being Overweight 127
Underweight: A Problem Too 128

Assessing Weight 128
Limitations of Height–Weight Tables 129
Measuring Body Fat 131

Why Do Some People Become Obese? 133
Genetic Linkage 134
Eating Behaviors Learned at Home 135

How the Body Stores and Uses Energy 137
The Relationship between Calories and Pounds 137
Fat as Essential, Fat as Excess 139
Your Body's Energy Needs 139
Importance of Exercise 140

Eating Disorders: A Troubled Relationship with Food 141
Athletes and Dancers at High Risk 143

The Reality of Weight Control 143
Controlling Your Weight 144
Dangers of Fad Diets 145
Final Word on Weight Loss 147

Key Concepts 147
Review Questions 148
Selected Bibliography 148
HealthLinks: Web Sites for Maintaining a Healthy Weight 148
Health Hotlines: Maintaining Proper Weight 149

Chapter 7 Keeping Fit 151

What Is Your HealthStyle? 152

Who Is Exercising? 153

The Health Benefits of Exercise 155
  Helping the Heart 156
  Preventing Osteoporosis 158
  Warding Off Infection 160
  Psychological Well-Being 160

The Fitness Triangle 162
  Strength 162
  Flexibility 163
  Endurance and Aerobic Capacity 163

Fitness through Exercise 165
  Measuring Your Heart Rate to Monitor Exercise Intensity 165

Planning and Maintaining a Personal Fitness Program 167
  Three Phases of Exercise: Warm-Up, Conditioning, Cool-Down 168
  Raising Your Safety Consciousness 169
  Patience and Adherence 172
  Tactics for Maintaining a Fitness Program 172

Key Concepts 173
Review Questions 173
Selected Bibliography 174
HealthLinks: Web Sites for Keeping Fit 174
Health Hotlines: Keeping Fit 174

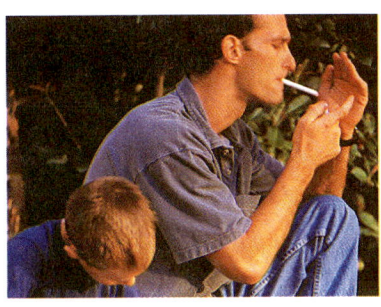

Part 3

Controllable Health Risks

177

Chapter 8 Smoking Out Tobacco 177

What Is Your HealthStyle? 178

Who Smokes? 179

Why People Smoke 181
  Influence from Family and Peers 181
  Advertising Hype 182
  Pleasure and Relaxation 183
  Addiction to Nicotine 183
  Avoiding Tobacco Use 184

The Components of Cigarette Smoke 184
  Nicotine 184
  Tar 185
  Carbon Monoxide 185

Why Smoking Is Dangerous to Your Health 185
  Links to Cancer 186
  Heart Disease and Stroke 188
  Lung Damage 190
  Complications during Pregnancy 190
  Other Health Effects of Smoking 191

Noncigarette Exposure to Tobacco 192
  Passive Smoke: Who Asked for It? 192
  Cigar and Pipe Smoking 193
  The Risks of Smokeless Tobacco 193

Kicking the Habit: How to Stop 195
  Physical Problems of Quitting 195
  Getting Motivated 196
  Cessation Approaches 196

The Changing Climate of Public Acceptance of Tobacco Use 198

Key Concepts 201
Review Questions 202
Selected Bibliography 202
HealthLinks: Web Sites for Preventing Tobacco Use 202
Health Hotlines: Smoking Out Tobacco 203

Chapter 9 Dealing with Drinking 205

What Is Your HealthStyle? 206

Who Drinks: A Picture of Alcohol Consumption 207
  Adult Drinkers 207
  College Student Drinkers 208
  Adolescent Drinkers 209

Why Do People Drink? 209
  Social Reasons 210
  Culture and Tradition 211
  Alcohol Dependence 211

Health Hazards of Alcohol 212
  Central Nervous System Effects 213
  Liver Problems 214
  Fetal Alcohol Syndrome 214
  Drinking and Death 215

Alcoholism as a Disease 218
  Defining Terms 218
  The Role of Genetics and the Environment 219
  Treatment Options 220

Controlling Access to Alcohol 223

Avoiding Problem Drinking 224
  Practice Not Drinking 224
  Pace Your Drinking 224
  Be Aware of the Full-Stomach Factor 225

Don't Mix Alcohol and Drugs 226
Be Socially Assertive 226

Prevention: The Ultimate Answer 227

Key Concepts 227
Review Questions 228
Selected Bibliography 228
HealthLinks: Web Sites for Dealing with Alcohol 229
Health Hotlines: Dealing with Drinking 229

Chapter 10 Understanding the Dangers of Drug Use 231

What Is Your HealthStyle? 232

What the Term *Drug* Means 233

Who Uses Drugs 236
Progression from Cigarettes to Marijuana 236
Why College Students Take Drugs 237
Availability and Legality of Drugs 238

From Drug Use to Drug Abuse 240
Drug Action and Drug Interaction 240

How Drugs Differ 242
By the Way They Are Taken 242
By Their Effects 243
By the Motive of the Abuser 244

The Impact of Drug Abuse 252
The Threat to Public Health 252
The Toll from AIDS 252
Special Concern for the Fetus 253
Drugs in the Workplace 254
Harm Reduction: Preventing Drug Trafficking 254

Treatment Alternatives: The Long Road Back 254
Maintenance Programs 255
Detoxification Programs 255
Therapeutic Communities 255
Other Treatment Modalities 256

Preventing Drug Abuse: Saying No 256

Key Concepts 260
Review Questions 260
Selected Bibliography 260
HealthLinks: Web Sites for Preventing the Illegal Use of Substances 261
Health Hotlines: Understanding the Dangers of Drug Use 261

Chapter 11 Recognizing Violent Behavior 263

What Is Your HealthStyle? 264

The Criminal: Who Commits Acts of Violence? 265

The Victim: Who Is at Risk for Being Assaulted? 266

When and Where Crimes Take Place 267

Homicide: Dying in America 268
Gun Killings 269
The Influence of Drugs 271
The Role of Television 272

Violence at Home and on the Job 273
Domestic Violence 273
When Children Get Hurt 276
Reporting Child Abuse 278
Sexual Harassment: An Abuse of Power 278

The Crime of Rape 280
Defining Rape 281
Attacks by Strangers 283
Acquaintance Rape 283
The Aftermath 284

A Few Words on Violence 285

Key Concepts 285
Review Questions 285
Selected Bibliography 286
HealthLinks: Web Sites for Violence Prevention 286
Health Hotlines: Recognizing Violent Behavior 286

Chapter 12 Preventing Unintentional Injuries 289

What Is Your HealthStyle? 290

Unintentional Injuries: Cause and Effect 291
Why Unintentional Injuries Take Place 291
Profile of an At-Risk Person 292
What Unintentional Injuries Cost Society 293

Safety on the Road 296
Buckling Up 296
Air Bags 298
Motorcycles 299

Recreational Safety 301
Safety Issues for Bicyclists 301
On the Waterfront 302
Diving Safety Tips 303

Safety at Home 303
When a Simple Fall Is Not Simple 304
Up in Smoke 305
Other Burns 306
Poison Alert 307

A Structure for Preventing Unintentional Injuries 308
Take Responsibility 308
Take Preventive Action 309
Be Prepared to Respond 310

Key Concepts 311
Review Questions 311
Selected Bibliography 312

HealthLinks: Web Sites for Preventing Unintentional Injuries 312
Health Hotlines: Preventing Unintentional Injuries 313

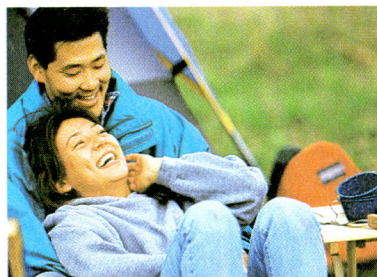

Part 4 Understanding the Disease Process 315

Chapter 13 Reducing the Risk for Chronic Disease 315

What Is Your HealthStyle? 316

Characteristics of Chronic Illness 318
Chronic versus Infectious Diseases 318
Changing Patterns of Mortality 319
Natural History of Chronic Diseases 319
Lifestyle Choices and Disease 319

From the Heart: Cardiovascular Diseases 322
Heart Disease Facts 322
Who Is at Risk? 324
Diagnosing Heart Disease 325
Forms of Heart Diseases 325
Repairing the Heart 327

The Big C: Cancer 330
The Basics of Cancer 330
Who Is at Risk? 332
Types of Cancer 333
Screening for Cancer 336
Self-Tests for Cancer 338
Benefits and Risks of Treatment 339

Smile Please: Dental Disease 341

Living with Chronic Disease 344
Psychological Adjustment 345
The Reality of Pain 346
Concluding Thoughts 346

Key Concepts 346
Review Questions 347
Selected Bibliography 347
HealthLinks: Web Sites for Reducing the Risk of Chronic Disease 348
Health Hotlines: Reducing the Risk for Chronic Diseases 348

Chapter 14 Reducing the Risk for Infectious Disease 351

What Is Your HealthStyle? 352

How Diseases Are Spread 353
Chain of Infection 353
Causes of Infection 355
How Infections Get into Your Body 356
Why Everyone Doesn't Get Sick 357
Nonspecific Lines of Defense 358

Immunity: The Final Line of Defense 359
Active and Passive Immunity 359
A Shot of Protection 360
Disorders of the Immune System 362
Can You Boost Your Own Immunity? 363

Stages of Infectious Disease 363

Common Infectious Diseases 364
Common Cold 364
Influenza 365
Pneumonia 368
Mononucleosis 369
Chronic Fatigue Syndrome 369
Tuberculosis 370
Hepatitis 370
Childhood Diseases 371
Lyme Disease 371
Nosocomial Infections 371
Emerging Diseases 373

Protection Through Prevention 374

Reducing Your Risk for an Infectious Disease 375

Key Concepts 375
Review Questions 376
Selected Bibliography 376
HealthLinks: Web Sites for Reducing Your Risk of Infectious Disease 377
Health Hotlines: Reducing the Risk for Infectious Disease 377

Chapter 15 Reducing the Risk for Sexually Transmitted Diseases 379

What Is Your HealthStyle? 380

What Are STDs? 381
Spread of STDs 382
Prevention and Treatment 383

Viral Diseases 386
HIV Infection and AIDS 386
Papilloma Virus 391
Hepatitis B 392
Genital Herpes 392

Bacterial Diseases 393
　Chlamydia 393
　Gonorrhea 394
　Syphilis 394

Other STDs 395
　Vaginitis 395
　Pubic Lice and Scabies 399

How Do You Know If You Have an STD? 399

Safer Sex 400

Key Concepts 401
Review Questions 401
Selected Bibliography 402
HealthLinks: Web Sites for Reducing the Risk of Sexually Transmitted Diseases 402
Health Hotlines: Reducing the Risk for Sexually Transmitted Diseases 402

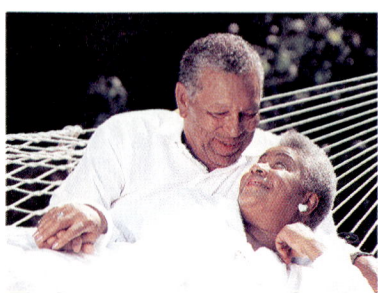

Part 5
Sexuality and Relationships: A Life Span Approach 405

 Chapter 16 Sexuality: Developing Healthy Relationships 405

What Is Your HealthStyle? 406

Points of View about Sexuality 408
　Your Culture 408
　Your Religion 409
　You as an Individual 409
　Your Biology 411
　Your Sexual Orientation 412

Communicating about Sex 413

Love: The Basis of Intimate Relationships 414

Sexual Relationships 417
　Sex Drive 418
　Sexual Pleasuring 418

The Body's Sexual Response 419
　Physiological Changes 419
　Masters and Johnson Four-Stage Model 420
　Psychological Component 421

Sexual Dysfunctions 422
　Male Problems 422
　Female Problems 424
　Therapeutic Interventions 424

Key Concepts 425
Review Questions 425
Selected Bibliography 426
HealthLinks: Web Sites for Developing Healthy Relationships 426
Health Hotlines: Developing Healthy Relationships 426

 Your Sexual Body: A Primer on Reproductive Anatomy and Physiology 429

Reproductive Anatomy and Physiology of the Male 430
　External Organs of the Male Reproductive System 430
　Internal Organs of the Male Reproductive System 431

Reproductive Anatomy and Physiology of the Female 433
　External Organs of the Female Reproductive System 433
　Internal Organs of the Female Reproductive System 434
　The Menstrual Cycle 436

Test Yourself 438

 Chapter 17 Planning a Family 441

What Is Your HealthStyle? 442

The Beginnings of a Family 443

Marriage and Family 444
　Deciding to Have Children 446
　Issues of Infertility 448
　Preconception Care 448

A Healthy Pregnancy 449
　The Importance of Prenatal Care 450
　Testing the Health of the Fetus 452
　Growth by Trimesters 453

Preparing for Childbirth 454
　First-Stage Labor 455
　Second-Stage Labor 455
　Third-Stage Labor 457

Family Planning 458

Birth Control: Assuming Responsibility 459
　The Range of Birth Control Choices 459
　Emergency Contraception 466
　Deciding about Birth Control 466

The Abortion Controversy 467

A Final Word on Planning a Family 470

Key Concepts 471
Review Questions 471

Selected Bibliography 472
HealthLinks: Web Sites Related to Reproductive Sciences 472
Health Hotlines: Planning a Family 472

Chapter 18 Aging: Growing Older, Keeping Healthy 475

What Is Your HealthStyle? 476

Growing Older 477
 Measuring Age 478
 Who Are the Elderly? 478
 Misconceptions about Aging 479
 Psychology of Aging 480
 Caring for an Elderly Parent 482

Aging Body and Mind: Changes that Occur over Time 485
 Health Status 485
 Telltale Signs 485
 Bone Density 486
 The Senses 488
 Sexual Activity 488
 Mental Ability 489
 Living with Alzheimer's Disease 490

Preventable Health Problems 495
 Sadness in Old Age 495
 Medication Abuse 495
 Falls 496

Promoting Healthy Aging 497

Key Concepts 498
Review Questions 499
Selected Bibliography 499
HealthLinks: Web Sites for Healthy Aging 500
Health Hotlines: Aging: Growing Older, Keeping Healthy 500

Chapter 19 Death and Dying 503

What Is Your HealthStyle? 504

The Meaning of Death 505
 The Biological Perspective 506
 The Legal Perspective 507
 The Religious Perspective 507
 Euthanasia 507
 Death as Seen throughout the Life Cycle 512

Dying as a Process 514
 Stages of Dying 514
 Hospice: Comfort for the Dying 515

For Survivors: A Time of Decisions and Bereavement 517
 Decisions about the Body 518
 Planning a Funeral 520
 A Time of Bereavement 520
 Loss as a Creative Force 522

Key Concepts 523
Review Questions 523
Selected Bibliography 524
HealthLinks: Web Sites for Dealing with Death 524
Health Hotlines: Death and Dying 525

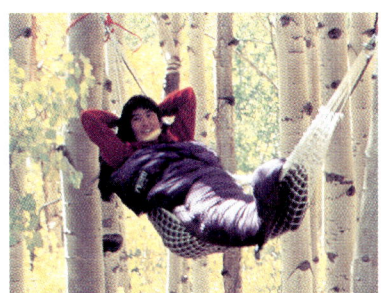

Part 6 Participating in a Healthy Community 527

Chapter 20 Living in a Healthy Environment 527

What Is Your HealthStyle? 528

Environmental Health: How Big Is the Problem? 529
 Identifying Health Effects 529

The Air You Breathe 530
 Why Dirty Air Is Unhealthy 530
 Principal Air Pollutants 532
 The Automobile: King of Air Pollution 535

The Water You Drink 536
 Drinking Safe Water 537
 Sources of Water Pollution 538
 Why Dirty Water Is Unhealthy 538
 Fluoride in the Water: What Does It Really Do? 539

Solid Waste: The Art of Throwing Things Away 540
 Precycling and Recycling Options 541

Health Hazards from Toxic Waste 544

Dangers from Noise 545
 Who Is at Risk? 546
 Physical Damage Caused by Noise 546
 Advice from the Wise 547

Indoor Pollution: Sick Buildings, Sick People 547
 What Are the Risks? 550

Environmental Ethics 551

Key Concepts 553
Review Questions 553
Selected Bibliography 554
HealthLinks: Web Sites for Living in a Healthy Environment 554
Health Hotlines: Living in a Healthy Environment 555

Chapter 21 Making Health Care Decisions 557

What Is Your HealthStyle? 558

Buying Health Care: How Do Consumers Make Decisions? 559
Decision Making and Accurate Health Information 559
Advertising Health Care 561
Health Fraud 562
Your Rights as a Health Care Consumer 563
Filing a Consumer Complaint 564

How to Choose Health Care Providers 565
The Right Physicians for You 565
When You Go to the Hospital 569

Paying for Health Care 569

Health Insurance Terms 571
Traditional Indemnity Plans 571
Managed Care Plans 572
Asking Questions about a Health Plan 574

Drugs as Medicine 575
The Correct Way to Take Medications 576
Sources of Health Information 576

Key Concepts 579
Review Questions 579
Selected Bibliography 580
HealthLinks: Web Sites for Understanding Health Care 580
Health Hotlines: Making Health Care Decisions 580

Glossary 582

Index 592

Feature Boxes

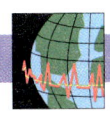
CULTURAL VIEW

A Multifaceted Definition of Health 3
Mormon Lifestyle Leads to Healthier Lives 29
Women and Depression—Greater Risk? 60
Managing Stress through T'ai Chi 88
How to Savor the Flavors Without the Fat 116
How You See Yourself Can Depend on the Culture of the Time 132
Health Problems of Young Women Athletes 159
How One Village Kicked the Habit 196
The French Experience: Does Red Wine Reduce the Risk for Heart Disease? 213
Adolescent Girls Abuse Steroids, Too 251
How Other Countries Get a Grip on Gun Control 270
Researchers Identify Who Drinks and Drives, by Age, Sex, and Ethnic Group 297
Mind–Body Treatments Moving into the Mainstream 342
Heart Disease, Cancer, and Mental Disorders…It May Be a Virus 372
MTV Makes Health Hip 382
Closing the Romance Gap 415
Married, No Kids 444
Domestic Partnership 447
Respect for the Elderly in Japan 480
Religious Traditions about Death 508
The Bicycling City of Groningen, Holland 536
The Chinese Tradition of Acupuncture 567

Foods 138
Starting Out: A Walking Program 166
A Timeline for Self-Treatment of Exercise Injuries 170
Smokeless Tobacco Users: Check Monthly for Early Signs of Disease 194
Why College Students Choose to Drink 210
Speaking Out Against Drinking and Driving 217
At Issue: Should Americans Be Allowed to Smoke Marijuana as Medicine? 239
Perspectives on Solving the Drug Problem: What Will Work 257
How to Avoid Being a Victim of Crime 268
Conflict Resolution 274
First Aid for Burns 305
Smoke Alarm Tips 306
How to Do a Breast Self-Exam 340
Do You Wash Your Hands? 358
How to Cope with a Common Cold 365
Should You Get an AIDS Test? 391
The Proper Use of a Condom 398
Learning How to Say "No" and "Yes" 414
Correct Use of a Male Condom 463
Correct Use of a Female Condom 464
Exercising Your Memory 490
Should Doctors Be Allowed to Help Terminally Ill Patients Commit Suicide? 510
How to Help a Friend 522
Should Pesticides that Cause Cancer in Animals Be Banned from Our Foods? 539
Spotting Health Fraud 563
How to Read a Prescription 577

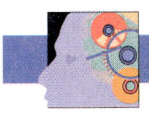
DEVELOPING HEALTH SKILLS

Knowing What to Expect from a Physical Exam 41
Gaining Strength from Solitude 55
Managing Time 86
Stressed Out? Develop a Healthy Style of Talking It Out 87
Eating through the Ages 114
How Not to Gain Weight…When You Eat Low-Fat

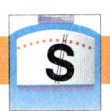
HEALTHWISE CONSUMER

The Butter-Margarine Question 101
Questions to Ask before Going on a Diet 146
The Right Shoe for You 171
Are Low-Tar, Low-Nicotine Cigarettes Safe? 192
The Caffeine High 234
Are Harassing E-Mail Messages Electronic Violations of Stalking Laws? 280

xv

xvi Feature Boxes

What to Look for in Helmet Safety 300
New Treatments for Impotence 423
Should Birth Control Pills Be Sold Over the Counter? 462
Eye Care 487
Multiple Chemical Sensitivity 550
Covering College Students 570

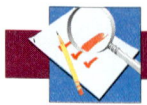
HERE'S LOOKING AT YOU

A Wellness Inventory 16
The Relative Risks in Your Family Tree 38
Your Health Habits 42
How Sleep Deprived Are You? 53
Rating Your Level of Self-Esteem 56
Rating the Stressors in Your Life 78
Testing Your Nutritional Knowledge 110
Are You Hung Up about Your Weight? 136
Are You at Risk for an Eating Disorder? 142
Assessing Your Flexibility 164
The Physical Effects of Smoking 187

How Did You Avoid Smoking This Week? 197
A Self-Assessment of Your Drinking 219
Reacting to Situations: Are You Able to Say No? 258
Are You at Risk for an Unintentional Injury? 294
Detecting an Abusive Relationship 278
How Well Do You Know Your Teeth? 344
Keep Your Immunizations Up-to-Date 361
Should You Believe What You Hear? 387
Are You Ready for a Mature Sexual Relationship? 417
What Is Your Contraceptive Confidence? 468
What's on Your Mind? A Quiz on Aging 492
What Do You Know about Organ Donation? 518
Know Your Recycling 543
What Is Your Best Health Insurance Buy? 572

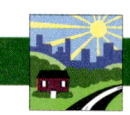
YOUR ENVIRONMENTAL NEIGHBORHOOD

Healthy Places 6
Seasonal Affective Disorder 62
Festive Malaise 80
The Sun and Skin Cancer 336

Preface

Every day, you are involved in making decisions about health—your personal health, the health of your family and friends, and the health of your community. Making such decisions requires having both a sound perspective on health and health behaviors and access to high-quality health information. A healthy lifestyle, something we call *healthstyle*, is a product of healthy decisions followed by skilled actions.

The first edition of *HealthStyles* was written to give perspective to and information about personal-health decision making. This second edition reinforces these messages by encouraging the development of the skills necessary to lead healthy lives—from choosing healthy foods at the local deli to managing social pressures to participate in unhealthy behaviors such as smoking.

In addition to a focus on health skills, the second edition updates important statistics and covers new developments that relate to personal health. New pictures and diagrams illustrate many of the concepts we discuss. Much of the information reprinted from health journals has been updated.

The subject matter of the second edition of *HealthStyles: Decisions for Living Well* remains intentionally conceptual. By "conceptual," we mean that *HealthStyles* focuses on the big ideas rather than the specific details of health. While maintaining currency and accuracy, the material is presented in a nontechnical, journalistic writing style. This approach presents health information in an easily understood fashion.

After completing a course of health study that includes *HealthStyles*, you should be more prepared to face the varied decisions related to your personal health. Some decisions may seem simple (like what to eat for breakfast), while some could be a matter of life and death (like whether or not to use a condom). Also, you should be more skilled at putting into practice what you learn in this book. Health-behavior change is far too complex to be brought about simply by learning some facts. Health-behavior change requires a change in attitude, a change in intention, and a change in perception of "normal" behavior. Health skills, along with health knowledge, are the basic building blocks of a healthy lifestyle.

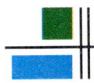 How HealthStyles *Is Organized*

HealthStyles is organized into six parts that address the key areas of personal health. The organization emphasizes the integrated nature of personal health and wellness.

- Part 1: Introductory Concepts presents the basic definitions and concepts of health and well-being that are the foundation of the book. Part 1 introduces the importance of taking responsibility for one's own health, for minimizing risks through prevention, and for developing a plan for informed health decision making.

- Part 2: The Basics of Good Health provides an opportunity to learn about many of the most basic components of a healthy lifestyle, including positive mental health, stress management skills, diet and weight control, and physical fitness.

- Part 3: Controllable Health Risks deals with some risk factors that account for health problems—those we can control. The health threats of smoking, alcohol and drug use, unintentional injuries, and violent behavior are covered in this part of the book.

- Part 4: Understanding the Disease Process addresses chronic, infectious, and sexually transmitted diseases including HIV/AIDS. Prevention and risk reduction of these diseases is a critical component of a positive health style.

- Part 5: Sexuality and Relationships: A Life Span Approach presents a social-health perspective on major stages of life. This part covers the importance of developing healthy relationships, including healthy sexual relationships, with people. Relationships across the life span issues include planning a family, the aging process, dying, and death.

- Part 6: Participating in a Healthy Community deals with environmental health and consumer decisions related to health. This part addresses the health of the community now and for future generations.

The organizational and topical approach to *HealthStyles* was chosen after a thorough examination of the public health threats currently facing people in the United States. A commitment to comprehensive health education, as defined by leading professional health education organizations, accounts for the inclusion of the traditional topics. A recognition of the importance of *Healthy People 2000: National Health Promotion and Disease Prevention Objectives,* accounts for the addition of nontraditional topics. This is particularly the case with Chapter 11, Recognizing Violent Behavior, which discusses violence as a serious public health threat. Chapter 11 focuses on practical guidelines for reducing the risk of being in a violent situation. Also in keeping with *Healthy People 2000, HealthStyles* recognizes the importance of personal health assessment, which is evident in Chapter 2, Assessing Your Health: A Plan for Informed Decision Making, and in many of the pedagogical tools included throughout the book.

Much of the information in *HealthStyles* does not require a full understanding of the human body's biological functions. One exception is human sexuality. We recognize the importance of students knowing human anatomy and physiology to understand sexuality. Accordingly, a special section, "Your Sexual Body: A Primer on Reproductive Anatomy and Physiology" explains the biological functions of the male and female reproductive systems. This section is designed for flexible use in the course and can enhance students' understanding of material presented in other parts of the text relating to sex and sexuality.

Special Features and Learning Aids

The study of health is not a passive encounter with health facts. Therefore, we have written *HealthStyles* to involve the reader in several ways.

Each chapter of *HealthStyles* opens with a **case study** that offers contrasting scenarios of how individuals may face the health-related decision-making process. Most of the cases involve two college students—one who makes a positive health decision while the other does not. A *new* series of questions prompt the reader to analyze the case study to understand the complexity of health-related behavior. These questions preview the concepts and topics discussed throughout each chapter.

Critical Thinking Questions, an important *new* feature, are highlighted at various points throughout each chapter. This feature prompts in-depth thought about some dilemmas and consideration of possible solutions based on information learned in the chapter and from real-life experiences. Every chapter includes at least two Critical Thinking Questions based on *Healthy People 2000*.

In addition, boxes appear throughout the book to highlight, personalize, and otherwise bring special attention to critical, relevant health information. Three of these boxes appear at least once in each chapter.

---

8 | Chapter 1 Health: Your Personal Responsibility

Critical Thinking Question

> Health education is often thought of as a process of information transfer, whether person-to-person (e.g., health educator to students) or via technology (e.g., the Internet). Such a view of health education assumes that the accumulation of health knowledge will lead to healthy behavior. Do you agree with this assumption? Can you present examples in which this assumption does not hold true? How would *you* define health education?

Health Skills

Skills are abilities that can help you achieve tasks. A skill is something you know how to do and feel comfortable doing. Once learned, a skill may become automatic. This is the case when you learn to drive a car safely. When you first start to drive, you have to think about when to signal before making a turn. With practice, however, signaling becomes a task that is done with little thought—it becomes automatic.

Health skills are abilities that can help you achieve good health. They are specific to healthy development or healthy behavior change. As with other skills, they evolve over time and with practice. The better you perform a health skill, the more likely you are to use it.

There are different ways to categorize health skills:

- *Motor skills* involve some physical movement, as in exercising or in brushing and flossing your teeth.
- *Intellectual skills* include decision making, gathering information, and using good judgment.
- *Emotional skills* involve managing stress, dealing with feelings, and using self-control.
- *Social skills* include listening, helping others, and asking for help.

The ability to assess blood pressure provides an example of how these skills interact. It requires (1) the motor skill of using a blood pressure measuring device properly; (2) the intellectual skills of knowing why it is important to know your blood pressure and what you can do if it is too high; (3) the emotional skill of practicing stress reduction as a way to control high blood pressure; and (4) the social skill of asking how to do any of the previous skills (see Figure 1.3).

You use health skills more often than you think you do. In fact, you use them as part of your daily living, learning, working, and playing activities.

LIVING Day-to-day living requires basic health skills. For example, you need to have the basic skill of washing your hands to reduce the spread of infectious diseases. This skill—and the habit of doing it—is usually learned in childhood.

Sleeping is another basic part of living and is an element of health that many people take for granted—until they have trouble sleeping. Relaxation skills can aid in bringing about a good night's sleep. When such skills are applied regularly, a good night's sleep becomes a matter of habit.

health skills Abilities that influence health development, health status, and health maintenance.

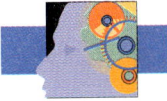

Developing Health Skills boxes focus on the process of developing health-related skills. Education about health skills is not a passive process, but rather an active encounter with the finite behaviors necessary for the maintenance, the restoration, or the improvement of health.

 **Here's Looking at You** boxes offer a series of self-tests that help with self-assessment of attitudes and behaviors and help personalize health information.

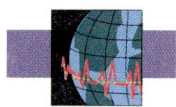 **Cultural View** boxes explore interesting health issues and concepts from a cross-cultural perspective

Other boxes appear at various points in the book in chapters where most applicable.

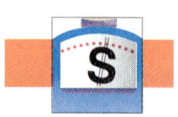 **Healthwise Consumer** boxes examine a wide range of health-related products and services, particularly those relevant to college students.

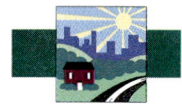 **Your Environmental Neighborhood** boxes examine events and issues specifically related to environmental health.

Several additional learning aids that appear in each chapter are an integral part of *HealthStyles*:

- **Learning Objectives** at the beginning of each chapter—a new feature for the second edition—preview the content of the chapter and serve as a tool for evaluating comprehension once the chapter has been completed.

- A **Running Glossary** defines health terms near text discussion.

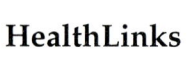 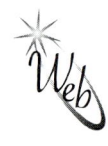

- **HealthLinks** throughout each chapter—another new feature of the second edition—direct students to additional information contained on the World Wide Web. HealthLinks appear within the margin at related sections of the text, as well as at the end of each chapter. These links put students in touch with the latest changes in personal health and wellness.

- A list of **Key Concepts** and a list of **Review Questions** are at the end of each chapter.

- Another new feature, **Health Hotlines,** provides a listing of toll-free telephone numbers for groups and organizations that deal with topics covered in each chapter.

- A **Selected Bibliography** for each chapter is useful for further exploration of the topics discussed.

- At the end of the book is a complete alphabetized **Glossary** of terms defined throughout the text.

Student Supplements

Available with *HealthStyles*, second edition, is a comprehensive set of supplemental materials designed to enhance student learning.

- A **Student Resource Manual** includes a general review of key topics and activities to encourage retention of health concepts. A valuable study tool, it provides learning objectives, critical thinking activities, chapter summaries, key terms, chapter reviews, and practice tests.

- An **Interactive Edition CD-ROM** helps bring the text to life by providing additional information that enhances the learning environment. Video and audio clips help clarify important health concepts, as well as provide updates with changes in personal health and wellness. Activities and practice tests encourage review of key information. Hot links to the Internet connect to all the major health organizations bringing about change in health.
- *Issues in Health: Readings from the Washington Post, Volume 3* is a brief series of timely articles from *The Washington Post* that presents high-interest, topical, and provocative issues related to health.
- *Quick Guide to the Internet* is a brief guide that provides activities and instructions for navigating the Internet for health-related information and material.

Instructor Supplements

The following materials are available to instructors using *HealthStyles*, second edition, to facilitate classroom preparation and enhancement.

- Instructor's Resource Manual
- Test Item File
- Computerized Testing Program (IBM, Mac)
- Digital Image Archive with PowerPoint Presentation
- PowerPoint Presentation for IBM and Mac
- *Total Health: Achieving Your Personal Best* Telecourse Series
- *Images of Health* Laserdisc
- *HealthStyles* Web Site
- Health Transparencies
- AIDS and STDs Slide Set
- Allyn & Bacon Health Video Library

A Word of Thanks

Dozens of health-education experts have contributed to this book through their thoughtful reviews and suggestions over two editions. These reviewers teach health education in colleges and universities across the country. They are at the cutting edge of their profession, and have assured that the contents of *HealthStyles*, second edition, is on the cutting edge as well. We are deeply appreciative of the time they took to comment on this textbook.

Holly Avey
University of Arizona

Judy Baker
East Carolina University

Lori DeWald
Shippensburg University

Richard Hurley
Brigham Young University

Chester Jones
University of Arkansas

Jay Lisk
University of South Carolina–Aiken

David Mason
Northern Illinois

Rusty Pippin
Baylor University

Bruce Ragon
University of North Carolina–Wilmington

Charles Tucker
Valdosta State University

Martin S. Turnauer
Radford University

David Wiley
Southwest Texas State University

Richard Wilson
Western Kentucky University

First edition reviewers include:

Elizabeth Barrington
San Diego Mesa College

Dianne Bartley
Middle Tennessee State University

Bill Beavers
Georgia Institute of Technology

Robert Boyce
University of North Carolina–Charlotte

Karen Camarata
Eastern Kentucky University

Sally Champlin
California State University–Long Beach

Thomas Davis
University of Northern Iowa

Judy Drolet
Southern Illinois University

Kathie C. Garbe
Youngstown State University

Connie Hanson
University of Nebraska at Kearney

Sheila Harbet
California State University–Northridge

Jane Hardell
Palm Beach Community College

Jo Hill
New Mexico State University

Warren McNab
University of Nevada–Las Vegas

Larry Olsen
The Pennsylvania State University

Judy Peel
University of North Carolina–Wilmington

Les Ramsdell
Eastern Kentucky University

Bob Rothstein
Miami-Dade Community College–South Campus

Eugene S. Sobolewski
Clarion University of Pennsylvania

Sondra Wilcox
Middle Tennessee State University

Lynn Wolfe
Georgia Southern College

Charleen Zartman
El Camino College

Words on a piece of paper do not make a book. We are especially grateful to the team at Allyn and Bacon for their work in moving *HealthStyles* into its second edition. Beginning with the editor who brought us aboard, Suzy Spivey, and continued on by Publisher and HPER Editor, Joseph Burns, Senior Development Editor, Mary Kriener, and Production Coordinator, Sue Brown, the professionalism and expertise of this team has been outstanding. A very special thank you to you all. It takes a complete team to pull off such a project, and the team at Allyn and Bacon has been top-notch.

Most of the work on the revision of the second edition of *HealthStyles* was completed while one author was in residence at the University of Newcastle, New South Wales, Australia and the other in Washington, D.C. The revision from "down under" could not have been completed without the support of friends and colleagues, especially Marie and Phil Williams from Newcastle. The hospitality of the University of Newcastle was also key to the successful completion of this revised edition.

The completion of a book demands support and love from all family members. The authors wish to thank Katy and Bob, as well as our children for their love, support, and patience.

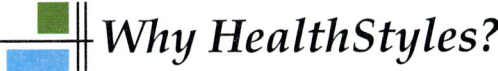 Why HealthStyles?

The subject of health and the knowledge and skills acquired through its study, are personal, relevant, and lifelong. *HealthStyles* is a textbook for the study of health and health behaviors, but it is also much more than that. It is a book to use throughout life for knowledge and skills for living well. Welcome to a study of the most interesting and personally relevant subject in the college catalog.

Buzz Pruitt
College Station, Texas

Jane Stein
Washington, D.C.

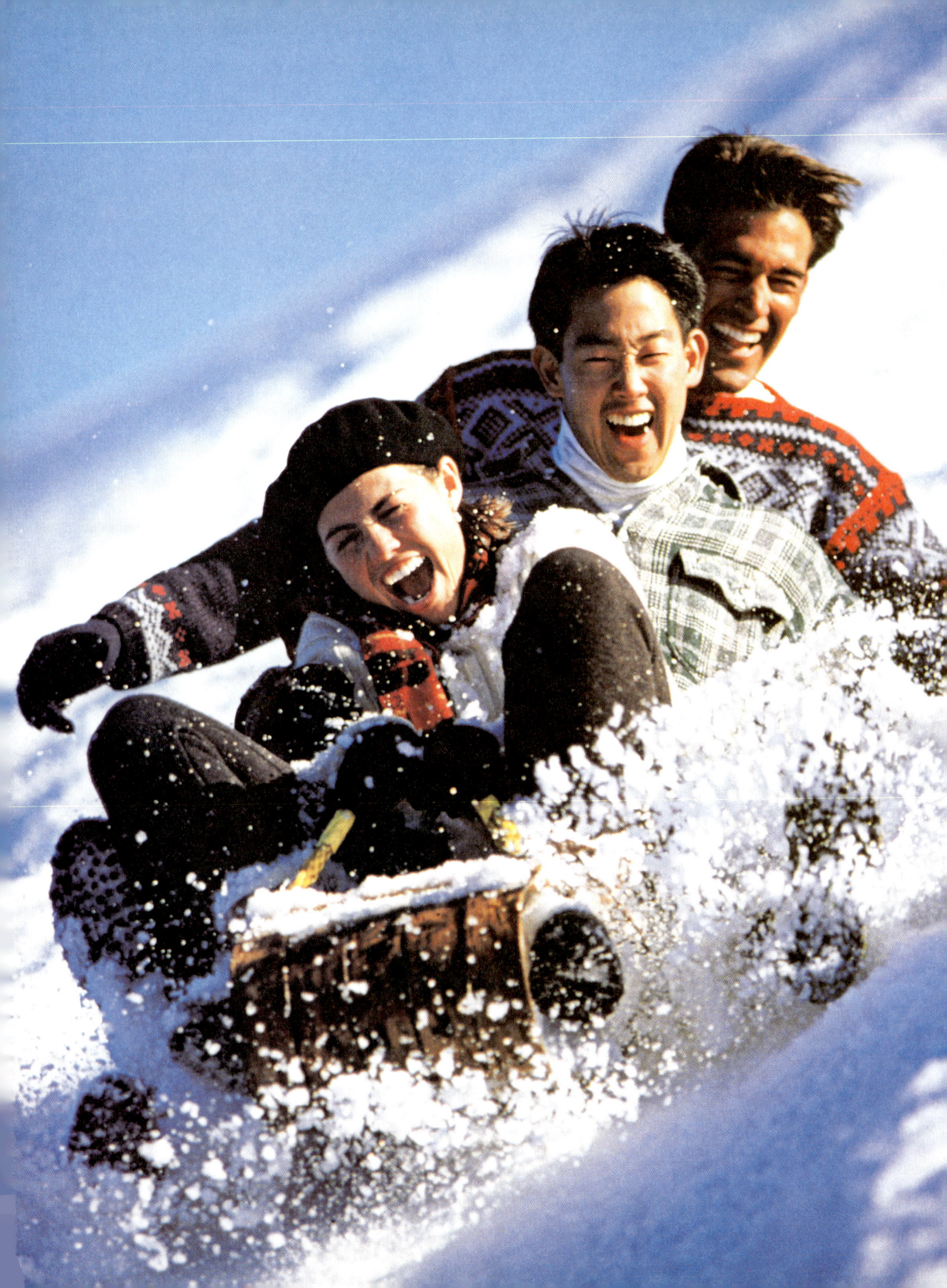

Chapter 1

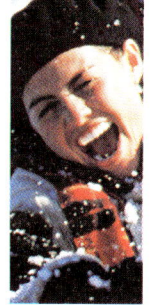
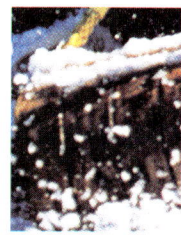
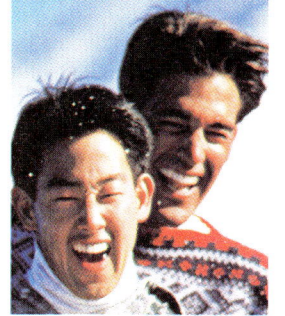

Health

Your Personal Responsibility

Objectives

When you finish reading this chapter, you will be able to:

1. Define health and describe a healthy person.
2. Describe the nature of becoming healthy.
3. Explain the importance of health knowledge to your overall well-being.
4. Explain the importance of health skills to your overall well-being.
5. Differentiate between healthy development and healthy behavior change.
6. Describe the components of health style and factors that influence those components.
7. Understand how health beliefs and health attitudes influence health style.
8. Explain how personal health decisions create a health momentum.
9. Define prevention and explain its importance in your life.
10. Acknowledge that good health practices often come down to common sense.

What Is Your HealthStyle?

Although taking classes and working part-time keep Maria very busy, she still finds time to look after her health. In fact, leading a healthy life is an important priority for her, and she has planned her schedule to make time for an aerobics class three times a week. She usually eats a balanced diet even though she often has to grab food on the run, and she gets the amount of sleep her body needs.

One reason Maria places such a high value on her health is that she knows the consequences of not doing so, including being at greater risk for sickness, feeling fatigued, and not being attentive in class. Maria carries her personal interest in health activities over to the community by volunteering to teach sports to children with disabilities. During the last election season, she worked for a candidate who supported increasing tobacco taxes to help pay for expanded access to health care.

Phil also goes to school and works part-time, but his health style is completely different—by choice. He feels stressed out by the end of the day, and instead of working off tensions with a brisk walk or a game of racquetball, he has a few beers at a local watering hole. He nibbles on chips and nuts before returning to the computer lab to finish his work. The idea of leading a healthier life seems never to occur to him.

How does Phil fare on the community level? Once a year, he joins a group of students to clean up bottles, cans, and other trash on the highway, but he views it more as a party than as something that can affect the health of the community. He votes in almost every election, but so far, he has not taken notice of the increasing number of health-related issues on the ballot or on candidates' agendas.

In Your Opinion

Both Maria and Phil are well-educated and well-read students, but only Maria has made a conscious decision to have a positive health style.

- Why isn't Phil maintaining a positive health style? Could he be afraid of not being able to change well-established habits?
- Could Phil's lack of health skills be a factor in his negative health style?
- Look ahead 10 years. What kind of health style will Maria be leading? What about Phil?
- What steps would you suggest that Phil take to alter his way of living so that he has a healthier lifestyle?

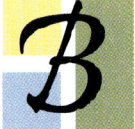

Before you came to class today, did you have breakfast? Did you smoke a cigarette? Did you get seven to eight hours of sleep and wake up feeling alert? Did you work out in the gym or go for a swim or jog?

The answers to these health-related questions are highly personal. Health tends to be a very personal aspect of life. That is why this book and this course of study focus on personal health. During the semester, you will learn that you can significantly influence how healthy you are by what you do and how you relate to the people around you.

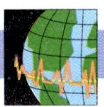

CULTURAL VIEW

A Multifaceted Definition of Health

How broadly can health be defined? Very broadly, the World Health Organization (WHO) decided. According to WHO, the following principles relating to health are basic to the happiness, harmonious relations, and security of all peoples in all countries:

Health is a state of complete physical, mental, and social well-being and not merely the absence of disease or infirmity.

The enjoyment of the highest attainable standard of health is one of the fundamental rights of every human being without distinction of race, religion, political belief, or economic or social condition.

The health of all peoples is fundamental to the attainment of peace and security and depends upon the fullest cooperation of individuals and states.

The achievement of any state in the promotion and protection of health is of value to all.

Unequal development in different countries in the promotion of health and control of disease, especially communicable disease, is a common danger.

Healthy development of the child is of basic importance; the ability to live harmoniously in a changing total environment is essential to such development.

The extension to all peoples of the benefits of medical, psychological, and related knowledge is essential to the fullest attainment of health.

Informed opinion and active cooperation on the part of the public are of the utmost importance in the improvement of the health of the people.

Governments have a responsibility for the health of their peoples which can be fulfilled only by the provision of adequate health and social measures.

Source: Constitution of the World Health Organization. Reprinted by permission.

This textbook is a guide to good health—a guide to things you can do to reduce your risks for disease. *HealthStyles* focuses on you and your abilities as well as on your interaction with the environment and with your community, society, and culture.

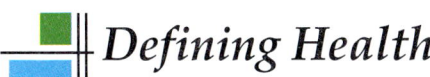

Defining Health

Health is an abstract idea for which there are many definitions. Once, it may have been appropriate to define it simply as the absence of disease. Such a limited definition recognizes health as an end in itself. Obviously, this definition is fraught with problems. Given our modern understanding of the nature of disease, it is highly unlikely that anyone would qualify as healthy under this definition.

Fortunately, the World Health Organization (WHO) recognized this difficulty and provided a multifaceted definition of health. In its founding constitution, adopted in 1946, WHO defined health as "a state of complete physical, mental, and social well-being and not merely the absence of disease or infirmity." This classic definition has become the guidepost for health and health-promotion efforts worldwide. (See the Cultural View box.) By recognizing that health is a measure of well-being, the WHO definition has broadened our understanding of health so that it represents not only an end in itself, but also a means toward that end.

The WHO definition of health is contained in the concept of **holistic health**. In this broad concept, health encompasses physical, mental, emotional, social,

health A state of complete physical, mental, and social well-being; not merely the absence of disease or infirmity.

holistic health The concept of health involving physical, mental, emotional, social, spiritual, and environmental aspects of an individual as well as of the community in which he or she lives.

Chapter 1 Health: Your Personal Responsibility

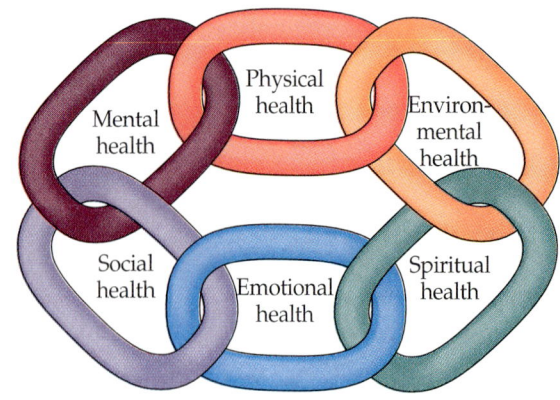

Figure 1.1 Holistic Health. *Holistic health encompasses many aspects of a person's life—physiological, emotional, spiritual, and more. By taking a holistic approach to your health, it means that the whole is greater than the individual parts.*

spiritual, and environmental aspects of an individual as well as of the community in which he or she lives. The word *holistic* is based on the concept that the whole is greater than the sum of its parts (see Figure 1.1).

Even such expansive definitions of health, however, do not take into account the full nature of health and well-being. Most notably missing from the WHO definition or the holistic health concept is the idea of human potential. If health is viewed in terms of potential, everyone can be healthy—and the extent of health is determined not by an externally established standard but by personal potential. This line of thinking has led to the concept of wellness.

Wellness emphasizes your potential and responsibility for health. Physician Halbert Dunn, who coined the term *high-level wellness,* described it as follows:

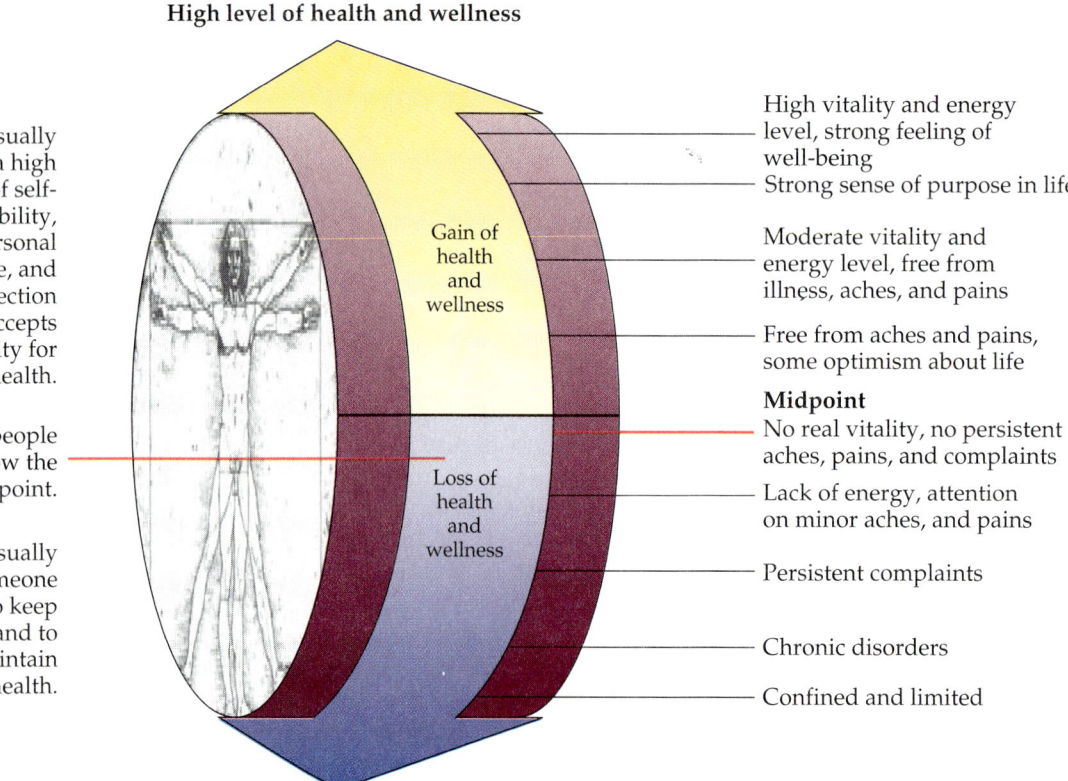

Figure 1.2 The Health and Wellness Continuum. *Wellness is an ongoing process in which you are always moving toward an optimal level of health.*

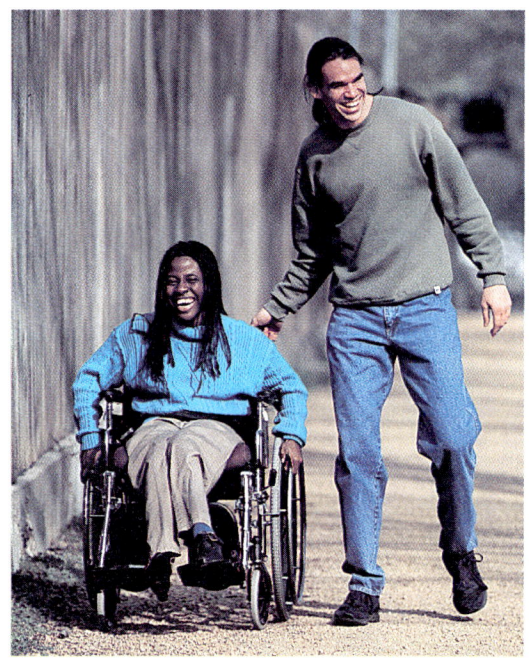

Personal health and wellness are measured individually and ultimately mean reaching your personal best. (Source: © Tony Stone Images/Robert E. Daemmrich)

"You have energy to burn. You tingle with vitality. At times like these, the world is a glorious place." His concept was later portrayed in the form of a continuum. Think of health as a long line of events having premature death at one end and a high level of wellness at the other. An illness/wellness continuum, based on Dunn's original ideas, has been used for decades to illustrate the nature of health, including the potential for a high level of well-being (see Figure 1.2).

Wellness is an ongoing process in which you are always moving either toward or away from the most favorable level of health. According to the wellness model, a person with a physical disability who has good mental health, eats a nutritious diet, and participates competitively in wheelchair tennis tournaments may be healthier—and farther along the illness/wellness continuum—than a person who does not have physical handicaps but who is not as emotionally and physically fit.

HealthLinks
Net Wellness
www.netwellnss.org
Web-based consumer health information service developed as a collaborative of several Ohio universities.

Becoming Healthy

The concept of health is complex, regardless of the definition. So, too, is the process of attaining health—of becoming healthy. There are two ways to view the process of becoming healthy:

1. *You become healthy through developing healthy behaviors.* This assumes that you are healthy and that you move to a stronger position of health by taking health promoting actions.
2. *You become healthy through behavior change.* You may have developed unhealthy behaviors, but you undergo a change in lifestyle or take specific actions that result in a healthier state.

In either case, personal involvement plays a critical role. You will be making decisions that affect your health throughout your life. By now, you have probably developed some good—and some bad—health habits. This book will help you expand your decision-making capabilities to enhance your health.

The process of becoming healthy is influenced by many factors, but significant among them are health knowledge (often expressed in terms of health liter-

wellness A description of health that includes the human potential for a high level of well-being while taking into consideration environmental and personal limitations.

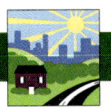

YOUR ENVIRONMENTAL NEIGHBORHOOD

Healthy Places

How healthy is the state in which you live? Here is a ranking of states based on measures that fit with the World Health Organization's definition of health. These measures include lifestyle, disability, disease, mortality, and access to health care.

Lifestyle components that have an impact on health are:

- Prevalence of smoking
- Motor vehicle deaths
- Violent crime (including illegal drug use, murders, rapes, robberies)
- Risk for heart disease (obesity, hypertension, sedentary lifestyle)
- Level of education (graduating from high school in four years)

Disability's effects on daily living include:

- Occupational fatalities
- Limited activity days

The burden that disease places on the overall health of the state's population is measured by:

- Heart disease
- Cancer cases
- Infectious disease, including death certificate data

Mortality is based on traditional death certificate data including:

- Total mortality (age- and race-adjusted)
- Infant mortality
- Premature death (loss of years of productive life due to death before age 65)

Access refers to the availability of health care in the state and includes:

- Unemployment (important because most private health insurance is provided by employers; it is also a measure of ability to pay)
- Adequacy of prenatal care
- Access to primary care
- Support for public health care

The accompanying illustration shows the state health ranking for 1997. Note that there are a number of ties.

Does the ranking for your state surprise you? Why do you think it rated the way it did? Do you think it should be higher or lower on the list? If so, why? On a scale of one to ten, how would you rate your state on the measures listed above?

---

acy), health skills, and health behavior. Together, these components make up your health style.

Health Knowledge

Becoming healthy begins with health knowledge. **Health knowledge** is the accumulation of factual information that influences health decision making. High-quality health knowledge leads to high-quality health decision making. Low-quality health knowledge, alternatively, creates the potential for health-compromising decisions.

Where do you get your health information? From an advertisement in a fashion or sports magazine? A newspaper story? A television program? Your family physician? Or from family myths handed down from generation to generation ("You'll get a cold from wearing wet shoes.")? Do you think your sources of health information are adequate? To make good health decisions, you need accurate and unbiased information.

Health knowledge alone is not enough. You need to be able to use that knowledge—you need to be health literate as well. According to the National

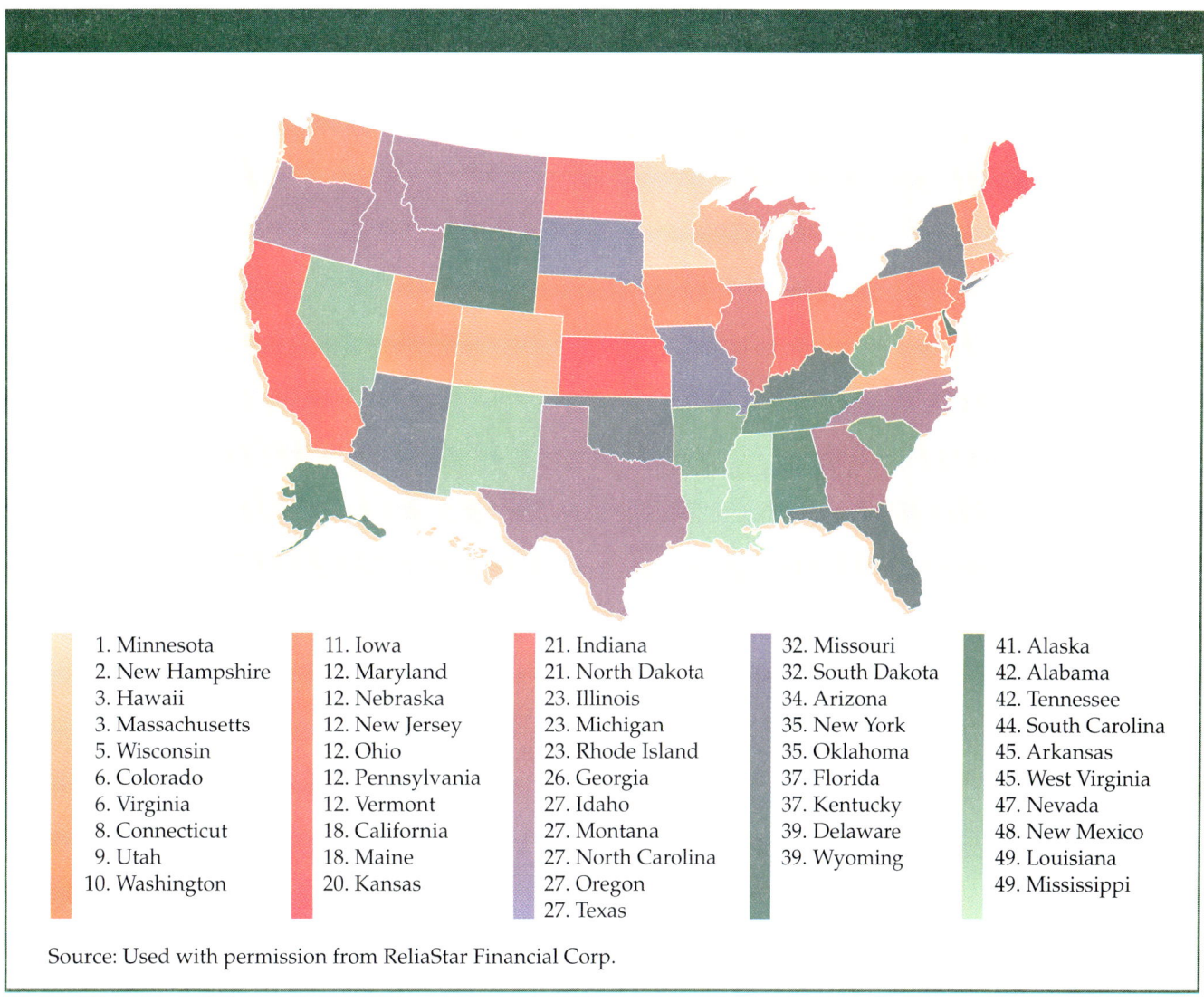

Source: Used with permission from ReliaStar Financial Corp.

1. Minnesota
2. New Hampshire
3. Hawaii
3. Massachusetts
5. Wisconsin
6. Colorado
6. Virginia
8. Connecticut
9. Utah
10. Washington
11. Iowa
12. Maryland
12. Nebraska
12. New Jersey
12. Ohio
12. Pennsylvania
12. Vermont
18. California
18. Maine
20. Kansas
21. Indiana
21. North Dakota
23. Illinois
23. Michigan
23. Rhode Island
26. Georgia
27. Idaho
27. Montana
27. North Carolina
27. Oregon
27. Texas
32. Missouri
32. South Dakota
34. Arizona
35. New York
35. Oklahoma
37. Florida
37. Kentucky
39. Delaware
39. Wyoming
41. Alaska
42. Alabama
42. Tennessee
44. South Carolina
45. Arkansas
45. West Virginia
47. Nevada
48. New Mexico
49. Louisiana
49. Mississippi

Health Education Standards, **health literacy** means being able to get, interpret, and understand basic health information and to use that information in ways that enhance your health—and the health of others.

There are four major components of health literacy:

1. *Critical thinking and problem solving.* Using a variety of sources to get current, credible, and applicable information can help you make sound health-related decisions.
2. *Self-directed learning.* Critical thinking skills can help you gather, analyze, and apply health information to meet your personal needs.
3. *Effective communicating.* There are a wide range of communication approaches—from listening to writing to sharing information on the Internet—that you can use to learn about health issues. With effective communication skills, you can create a climate of understanding and support for others to learn about health.
4. *Being a responsible citizen.* Given your health knowledge, you are in a strong position to help keep yourself, your family and friends, and your community healthy.

health knowledge The accumulation of factual information that influences health decision making.

health literacy The capacity of an individual to get, interpret, and understand basic health information and services and the competence to use such information and services in ways that are health enhancing.

Critical Thinking Question

> Health education is often thought of as a process of information transfer, whether person-to-person (e.g., health educator to students) or via technology (e.g., the Internet). Such a view of health education assumes that the accumulation of health knowledge will lead to healthy behavior. Do you agree with this assumption? Can you present examples in which this assumption does not hold true? How would **you** define health education?

Health Skills

Skills are abilities that can help you achieve tasks. A skill is something you know how to do and feel comfortable doing. Once learned, a skill may become automatic. This is the case when you learn to drive a car safely. When you first start to drive, you have to think about when to signal before making a turn. With practice, however, signaling becomes a task that is done with little thought—it becomes automatic.

Health skills are abilities that can help you achieve good health. They are specific to healthy development or healthy behavior change. As with other skills, they evolve over time and with practice. The better you perform a health skill, the more likely you are to use it.

There are different ways to categorize health skills:

- *Motor skills* involve some physical movement, as in exercising or in brushing and flossing your teeth.
- *Intellectual skills* include decision making, gathering information, and using good judgment.
- *Emotional skills* involve managing stress, dealing with feelings, and using self-control.
- *Social skills* include listening, helping others, and asking for help.

The ability to assess blood pressure provides an example of how these skills interact. It requires (1) the motor skill of using a blood pressure measuring device properly; (2) the intellectual skills of knowing why it is important to know your blood pressure and what you can do if it is too high; (3) the emotional skill of practicing stress reduction as a way to control high blood pressure; and (4) the social skill of asking how to do any of the previous skills (see Figure 1.3).

You use health skills more often than you think you do. In fact, you use them as part of your daily living, learning, working, and playing activities.

LIVING Day-to-day living requires basic health skills. For example, you need to have the basic skill of washing your hands to reduce the spread of infectious diseases. This skill—and the habit of doing it—is usually learned in childhood.

Sleeping is another basic part of living and is an element of health that many people take for granted—until they have trouble sleeping. Relaxation skills can aid in bringing about a good night's sleep. When such skills are applied regularly, a good night's sleep becomes a matter of habit.

---

health skills Abilities that influence health development, health status, and health maintenance.

Motor skills that impact health

brushing and flossing teeth	practicing first aid
exercising	washing hands
practicing basic hygiene	

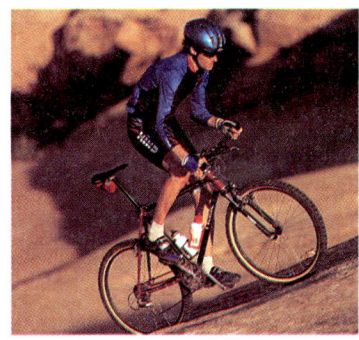

Intellectual skills that impact health

identifying stressors	managing time
reading reports	restructuring environments
reading labels	decision making
setting a goal	setting goals
concentrating on a task	measuring health
gathering information	planning a family
recognizing strengths and weaknesses	planning a diet
analyzing information	practicing safer sex

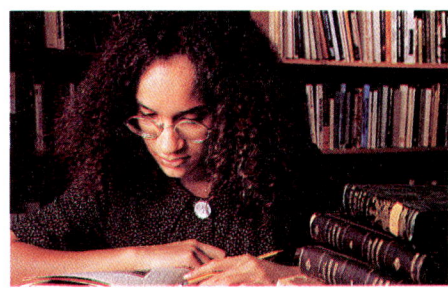

Emotional skills that impact health

dealing with fear	relaxing
expressing affection	responding to failure
rewarding yourself	managing anger
managing emotions	managing stress
using self-control	dealing with pain
coping with stress	

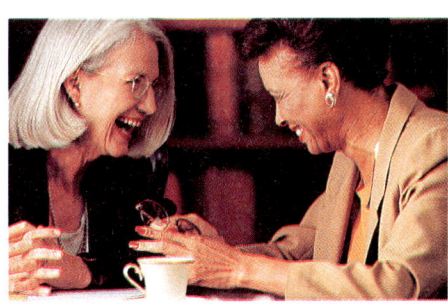

Social skills that impact health

listening	dealing with group pressure
saying thank you	communicating
giving a compliment	active listening
asking for help	giving and receiving criticism
apologizing	negotiating
expressing empathy	resolving conflict
being assertive	working with a group
making a complaint	

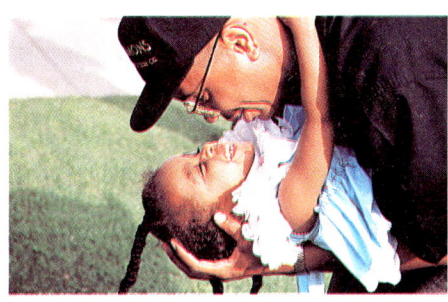

(Source: © Tony Stone Images/Lori Adamski Peek, Mark Lewis, Bruce Ayers, and Mary Kay Denny)

Figure 1.3 A Typology of Health Skills. *There are four major kinds of skills you use to lead a healthy life: motor, intellectual, emotional, and social.*

Day-to-day living also involves having relationships with other people, both social and, at times, romantic. Basic skills of forming and maintaining relationships aid in this aspect of living. Listening skills, for example, are crucial to forming and maintaining all forms of relationships. Failure to listen can lead to the breakup of both social and romantic relationships.

LEARNING Learning involves many skills, including how to evaluate sources of information. This is an especially important skill for health. For example, there is a lot of health-related information on the Internet, but not all of it is based on

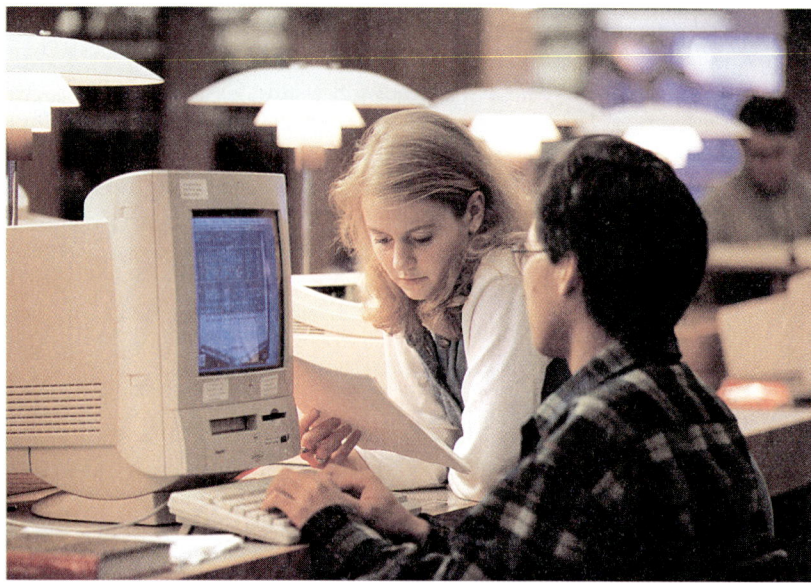

The Internet is a popular place for up-to-date health information. A simple click of a button can put you in touch with the latest in health advances. Check the HealthLinks sites highlighted throughout this book. (Source: © Tony Stone Images/Stewart Cohen)

solid research. It is necessary to determine what is reputable, high-quality information before you can make a high-quality health decision.

Learning also occurs through experience. Sometimes, experiences such as riding a bike safely in traffic, happen daily. Other experiences happen less often, but are very important in terms of safety. For instance, a rip tide is the section of the surf where water naturally returns out to sea from the shore. Failing to recognize a rip tide when swimming in the surf or not knowing how to respond to one can lead to a dangerous situation.

WORKING There are many aspects of work or school that can affect your health. If you don't know how to deal with your emotions, for example, a stressful relationship with your supervisor at work or your lab partner at school can easily get out of hand. By learning how to control your emotions, you will probably be able to relate more effectively with others around you.

PLAYING Playing involves many health skills. By mastering recreational skills, you can participate in a variety of activities, enjoy them better, and reap the health benefits of exercise. For example, knowing how to swim correctly can make swimming a pleasant experience; you will be more likely to swim more often and for longer periods of time.

Health Behavior

health behavior Actions and habits that may lead either to enhancement and protection of a person's health status or to its decline.

preventive behavior Action taken by a person who is essentially healthy in order to remain healthy.

illness behavior Action taken by a person who has reason to believe that he or she is not well.

sick-role behavior Action taken by a person who has been diagnosed as sick.

Health behavior is a complex, interlocked set of actions and reactions to a variety of stimuli. These actions and reactions may lead either to enhancement and protection of your health status or to its decline. There are three basic kinds of health behavior: preventive behavior, illness behavior, and sick-role behavior.

Preventive behavior helps you stay healthy. Examples of preventive behaviors are managing your weight, exercising at least three times a week, not smoking, and keeping your immunizations up-to-date. Preventive behaviors enhance health by reducing your risk for diseases or unintentional injuries.

Illness behavior is what you do when you are not feeling well or have reason to believe you are not well. You respond to bodily signs and symptoms—for example, by taking your temperature or seeking the opinion of someone having health expertise. Your health is enhanced when you engage health professionals in the diagnosis and treatment of an illness or disease. Failure to do so can delay your recovery and, in the case of an infectious disease, inadvertently spread illness.

Sick-role behavior is what you do after you have been diagnosed as sick. These are specific behaviors intended to address the acute nature of the diagnosed illness. An example is taking a drug prescribed by your physician to alleviate symptoms or cure a condition. By following the instructions of your physician, you contribute to your own recovery. By ignoring the instructions—such as by not taking prescription drugs as directed—you may jeopardize your health.

Critical Thinking Question

The medical profession has a good track record in assisting patients with their illness behavior and sick-role behavior. It does not, however, have the same record when it comes to preventive behavior. How would you suggest that the medical profession enhance its role in promoting preventive behaviors?

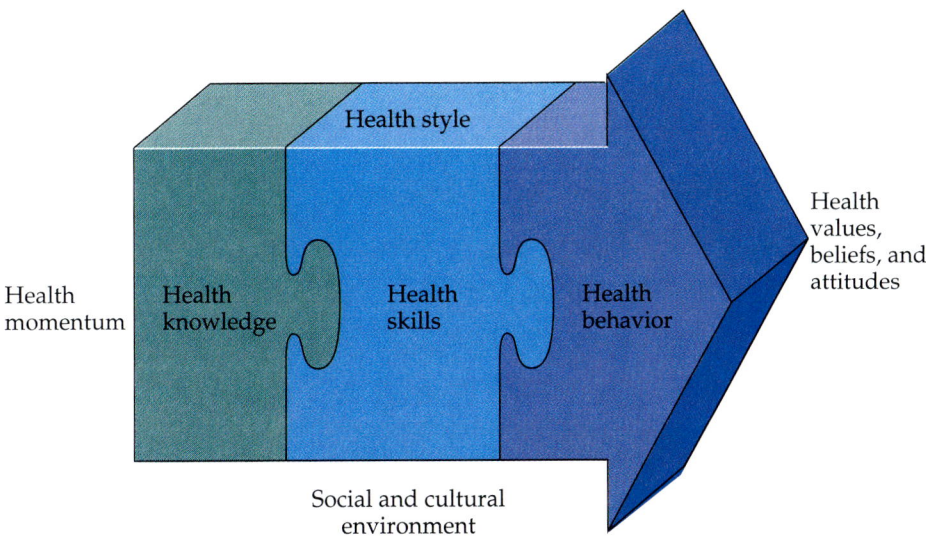

Figure 1.4 Health Style. *Health style is the sum of your health knowledge, health skills, and health behavior.*

Establishing a Personal Health Style

The term *health style* is a shortened version of the two words *healthy* and *lifestyle*. A healthy lifestyle is one type of health style. An unhealthy lifestyle is another type of health style.

Health style is best described as the sum of your health knowledge, your health skills, and your health behavior. Each time you make a choice concerning your health, whether positive or negative, you are contributing to your health style.

Your health style is personal and, at the same time, interpersonal. It is an element of your life over which you can assert much control. It is influenced by (1) the factors that are involved in becoming healthy—health knowledge, health skills, and health behavior; (2) your health-related values; (3) your health-related attitudes and beliefs; (4) your social and cultural environment; and (5) the momentum developed by your health-related decisions and actions.

A value is something that is important to you. A **health value** is something related to health that is important. How prominent is health on your list of personal values? Many college students do not even think about health as a value. Good health is something that most of us are born with, and we think this state of good health will continue for a long time. This thought is at best wishful. People who value good health are more likely to make decisions that promote their health—decisions such as getting the right amount of sleep and eating a healthy diet—than are people who do not think of health as a value.

A **health attitude** is your behavioral intention concerning health. If you intend to exercise, then you are more inclined to do so than if you have no such intention. Likewise, if you intend to drink and then drive, the potential of your having a car crash is greater than if you have no such intention. Health attitudes are usually expressed as either positive or negative—positive if they contribute to good health, negative if they do not contribute to good health.

health style The sum of health knowledge, health skills, and health behavior. Health style is most easily observed in personal health decisions.

health value Something of importance that is related to health.

health attitude A behavioral intention concerning health, usually expressed in positive or negative terms.

health belief A health-related concept thought to be true whether supported by evidence or not.

health momentum A perception of movement toward or away from good health that results from decisions and health behaviors of the past.

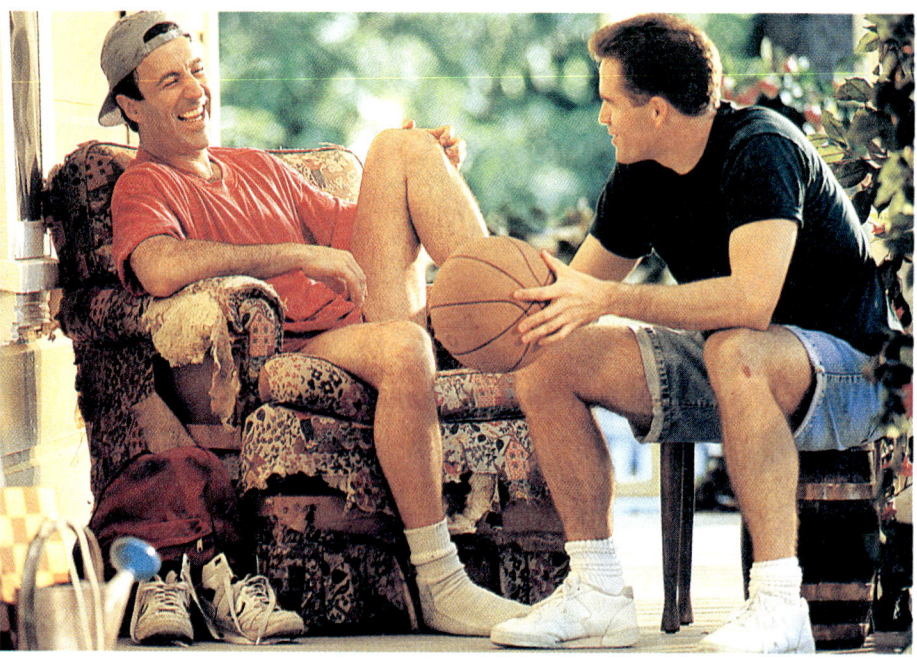

People who have a good social support system generally feel better than those who don't have close friends. (Source: © Tony Stone Images/Bruce Ayres)

Just as your attitudes toward health influence your health style, so do your health beliefs. When you believe something to be true, whether it is true or not, that belief influences your behavior. A **health belief** is something you believe to be true about health. Health beliefs are especially important concerning disease prevention. For example, the extent to which you believe you are susceptible to a disease influences your risk of contracting a disease. One of the problems public health officials are having in combating the AIDS epidemic is convincing people that they are susceptible to the disease. For another example, beliefs about your ability to practice good health behavior effectively ("I can stop smoking") or about what stands in your way ("I can't stop smoking because my roommate smokes") can influence your health style.

Your social and cultural environment also affects your health style. For example, people who have good social support systems report that they feel better than do those who don't have close friends to talk with. This seems to hold true for people of all ages and especially for those with life-threatening illnesses such as AIDS and breast cancer.

Even though your health style is very personal, it can affect others around you just as their health styles can affect you. For example, nearly half of all motor vehicle accidents involve a driver who had been drinking. So if you drink and drive, this health style can affect someone else. For another example, a motorcycle rider not wearing a helmet is more susceptible to serious injury if an accident occurs than one wearing a helmet. Serious injury results in extended medical care, which in turn results in increased medical costs passed on to you by hospitals and other health care providers.

Critical Thinking Question

Motorcyclists who wear helmets are less likely to be seriously injured in an accident than those not wearing helmets. Yet many motorcyclists are opposed to state laws requiring helmets, claiming that they are an infringement on their privacy. Can you justify helmet laws in terms of public health? How do you resolve the infringement question?

A final factor that influences your personal health style is the **health momentum** established by your health-related decisions and behavior. Each time you take an action concerning your health, you are poised to influence the next action you take related to your health. For example, if you always wear a seat belt when you are in a car, you are more likely to wear a helmet when you bike. This is because you have established a momentum for safe health habits on the road. If you have established a momentum for an exercise program, it is likely that you will not smoke because smoking will compromise your aerobic capacity and other aspects of your fitness.

The opposite is also true: One bad habit can lead to another. According to a report from the National Center for Health Statistics, smokers tend to have other bad health habits. A nationwide survey of adults showed that heavy smokers were more likely to skip breakfast, to snack more during the day, to drink more alcohol, and to remain physically less active than nonsmokers. According to a health researcher analyzing the survey data, two possible factors are at work

HealthLinks
National Center for Health Statistics
http://www.cdc.gov/nchswww/nchshome.htm
Definitive reference for vast array of national health statistics.

TABLE 1.1   One Bad Habit Can Lead to Another

A survey of people, 20 years or older, showed that smokers are more likely than nonsmokers to have other unhealthy habits.

	Smoking habit		
Health practice	**Never**	**Former**	**Current**
Never eats breakfast	18.3%	19.0%	37.6%
Heavy drinker*	7.2	11.9	20.1
Sleeps 6 hours or less	20.9	20.0	25.3
Less physically active	17.3	18.1	21.8

*At least 5 drinks on 10 days or more in the past year
Source: National Center for Health Statistics

here. One is that this cluster of bad health habits is associated with a consumption-oriented lifestyle—smoking, drinking, and overeating. The second is that smokers are more prone to risk-taking behaviors and give less attention to healthier practices (see Table 1.1).

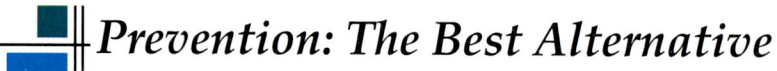 Prevention: The Best Alternative

At the turn of the century, the leading causes of death were infectious diseases. It was a time of great hope, and for most of these diseases, a vaccination or a cure was on the horizon. Today, most of the leading causes of illness and death are not infectious diseases but health-compromising behaviors (see Table 1.2 and Table 1.3). Although the cause of death reported on a death certificate is usually given in terms of disease, the actual cause is often a chosen health behavior. For example, heart disease and cancer are listed as the two leading causes of death for peo-

TABLE 1.2   Nine Leading Causes of Death

All ages	Ages 15–24
1. Heart disease	1. Accidents
2. Cancer	2. Homicide
3. Cerebrovascular diseases, including stroke	3. Suicide
4. Chronic lung disease	4. Cancer
5. Accidents	5. Heart disease
6. Pneumonia/influenza	6. AIDS
7. Diabetes	7. Congenital anomalies
8. AIDS	8. Chronic lung disease
9. Suicide	9. Pneumonia/influenza

Source: National Center for Health Statistics, 1997

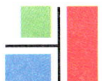

TABLE 1.3   Nine Leading Behavioral Causes of Death

1. Tobacco
2. Diet and activity patterns
3. Alcohol
4. Microbial agents
5. Toxic agents
6. Sexual behavior
7. Firearms
8. Motor vehicles
9. Drug use

Source: Adapted from McGinnis, J. M., and W. H. Foege. "Actual Causes of Death in the United States." *Journal of the American Medical Association* 270, no. 18 (1993): 2207–2212

ple of all age, and as the fourth and fifth leading causes of death for people ages fifteen to twenty-four. For many people, however, smoking is often the actual cause of these two diseases. Diets rich in cholesterol and fats are another actual cause of heart disease.

Compare Table 1.2 and Table 1.3. The two most rapidly growing behavioral causes of death (Table 1.3) are sexual behavior and drug use. Transmission of AIDS, which joined the list of top nine causes of death (Table 1.2) in 1992, is attributed mostly to sexual behavior and drug use. Given that behaviors are often the actual causes of death, the best hope for reducing the number of deaths caused by many diseases lies not in finding cures for them but in changing the behaviors that lead to them in the first place.

Prevention is therefore the best strategy for achieving a healthy future. By following this strategy, you can make health-promoting decisions that reduce

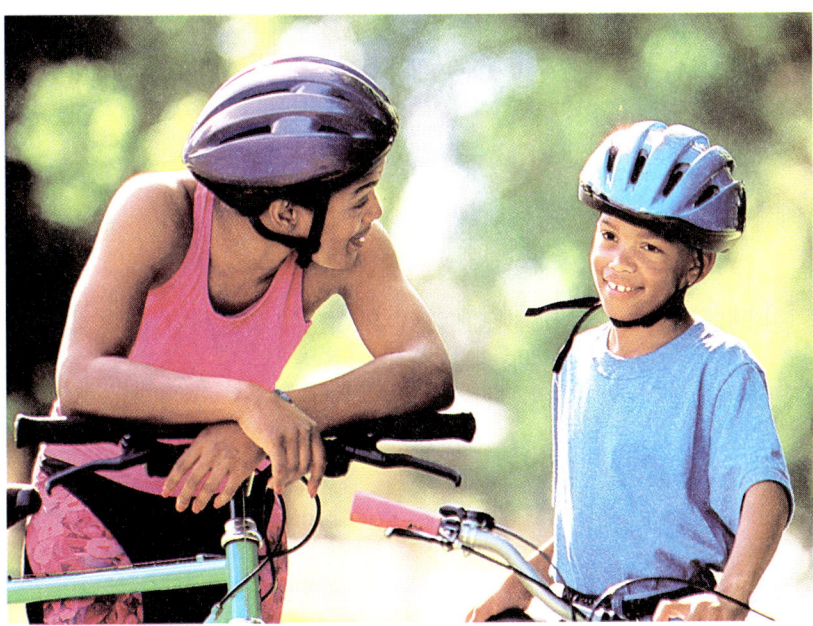

Prevention is the best strategy for achieving a healthy future. For bicyclists, this means wearing a helmet. (Source: © Tony Stone Images/Lori Adamski Peek)

prevention   Taking health-promoting action to reduce the risk of disease or injury.

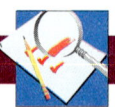

HERE'S LOOKING AT YOU

A Wellness Inventory

Put a check beside each statement that applies to you.

1. **Alcohol Use**
   — I drink fewer than two drinks a day.
   — In the past year, I have not driven an automobile after having more than two drinks.
   — When I'm under stress, I do not drink more.
   — I do not do things when I'm drinking that I later regret
   — I have not experienced any problem because of my drinking in the past.

2. **Tobacco Use**
   — I have never smoked cigarettes.
   — I haven't smoked cigarettes in the past year.
   — I do not use any form of tobacco (pipes, cigars, chewing tobacco).
   — I smoke only low-tar and low-nicotine cigarettes.
   — I smoke less than one pack of cigarettes a day.

3. **Blood Pressure**
   — I have had my blood pressure checked within the last six months.
   — I have never had high blood pressure.
   — I do not currently have high blood pressure.
   — I make a conscious effort to avoid salt in my diet.
   — There is no history of high blood pressure in my family.

4. **Weight/Body Fat**
   — According to height and weight charts, I am in the average range.
   — I have not been on a weight reduction diet in the past year.
   — There is no place on my body that I can pinch an inch of fat.
   — I am satisfied with the way my body looks.
   — None of my family, friends, or health care professionals has ever urged me to lose weight.

5. **Physical Fitness**
   — I do some form of vigorous exercise for at least thirty minutes three times a week or more.
   — My resting pulse is eighty beats a minute or less.
   — I don't get fatigued easily while doing physical work.
   — I engage in some recreational sport such as tennis or swimming on a weekly basis.
   — I would say that my level of physical fitness is higher than most of the people in my age group.

6. **Stress/Anxiety Level**
   — I find it easy to relax.
   — I am able to cope with stressful events as well as or better than most people.
   — I do not have trouble falling asleep or waking up.
   — I rarely feel tense or anxious.
   — I have no trouble completing tasks I have started.

7. **Car Safety**
   — I always use seat belts when I drive.
   — I always use seat belts when I am a passenger.
   — I have not had an automobile accident in the past three years.

(continued)

your risk of acquiring a disease or sustaining an injury. Prevention can be carried out on the personal as well as on the community level.

On the personal level, for example, you can make a decision not to smoke cigarettes and thereby to reduce your risk for a range of illnesses, including cancer, heart disease, stroke, and lung disease. Much can also be done on the community level. Many localities are passing laws that prohibit smoking in an increasing number of public places, including hospitals, office buildings, and bars. State and local taxes on cigarettes are rising in some places, and part of these revenues are used to educate the public—particularly young people—about the health hazards of smoking. And health insurers are taking measures to reward nonsmokers by charging smokers higher premiums. See the Here's Looking at You box to determine whether you have a healthy lifestyle.

- ___ I have not had a speeding ticket or other moving violation for the past three years.
- ___ I never ride with a driver who has had more than two drinks.

8. **Relationships**
   - ___ I am married and living with my spouse.
   - ___ I have a lot of close friends.
   - ___ I am able to share my feelings with my spouse and/or other family members. When I have a problem, I have other people with whom I can talk it over.
   - ___ Given a choice between doing things by myself or with others, I usually choose to do things with others.

9. **Rest/Sleep**
   - ___ I almost always get between seven and nine hours of sleep a night.
   - ___ I wake up few, if any, times during the night.
   - ___ I feel rested and ready to go when I get up in the morning.
   - ___ Most days, I have a lot of energy.
   - ___ Even though I sometimes have a chance, I never take naps during the day.

10. **Life Satisfaction**
    - ___ If I had my life to live over, I wouldn't make all that many changes.
    - ___ I've accomplished most of the things that I've set out to do in my life.
    - ___ I can't think of an area in my life that really disappoints me.
    - ___ I am a happy person.
    - ___ Compared with the people with whom I grew up, I feel I've done as well as or better than most of them with my life.

Scoring:
Record the number of checks (from zero to five) for each area. Then add up the numbers to determine your score.

Area	Subscore
Alcohol use	_____
Tobacco use	_____
Blood pressure	_____
Weight/body fat	_____
Physical fitness	_____
Stress/anxiety level	_____
Car safety	_____
Relationships	_____
Rest/sleep	_____
Life satisfaction	_____

Interpreting Your Score

A score of forty to fifty	Healthier than average lifestyle
A score of twenty-five to thirty-nine	Average lifestyle
A score of zero to twenty-five	Below average: need for improvement
Scores of less than three in any one of the ten areas	Need for improvement in that area

Critical Thinking Question

A familiar saying goes, "An ounce of prevention is worth a pound of cure." This is especially true when most chronic diseases result from chosen behaviors such as smoking cigarettes or eating high-fat foods. What are some of the diseases for which a cure is of no concern and prevention is the only option?

Practicing Common Sense

The practice of preventing detrimental health outcomes and living a positive health style often comes down to common sense. The following are some common-sense suggestions for maintaining a positive health style. In subsequent chapters, you will find a more detailed discussion of each.

Smoking has been identified as the most avoidable cause of death in our society. There is no question that it is dangerous to your health and to the health of those around you. Because of the impact of side-stream smoke that originates from the end of cigarettes, smoking is never simply a personal health decision: What a smoker does can affect the health of others as well. *Common sense suggests that you do not smoke.*

Researchers have found that regular physical activity is related to a reduction of risk for many health threats, including heart disease and hypertension. It is a valuable stress management tool and an important element of weight control and good sleep habits. *Common sense suggests that you exercise on a regular basis.*

Dietary factors have been linked to several health threats, particularly heart disease and cancer of the colon. There is consensus among health professionals that limiting fat consumption reduces health risk. *Common sense suggests that you limit the fat in your diet.*

Alcohol and other drugs have been found to relate to many threats to health, including violent actions, accidents, and some chronic diseases. If alcohol is consumed, it should be taken in moderation and under controlled circumstances that ensure safety. It should not be a means of stress management. *Common sense suggest that you if you drink alcohol, drink wisely.*

Because of AIDS, safer sexual practices have become a matter of life or death. Although use of a condom is considered a highly effective preventive measure, abstinence and monogamy offer the best protection from the health threats of sexual encounters. *Common sense suggests that you practice safer sex.*

By following common sense and good health practices, you can lead a healthy life—and still have fun. The best strategy for a healthy future is prevention—making health-promoting decisions that reduce your risk for acquiring a disease or sustaining an injury. Using common sense and practicing prevention are both elements of being personally responsible for your own health.

Being Responsible

Despite all the advances in medical science—new surgical procedures, wonder drugs, diagnostics that picture the inner workings of your body—your health remains your responsibility. The good news is that acting on this responsibility is not very difficult. As you have just read, for the most part it involves

- common-sense decisions made by a health-literate person;
- the use of health skills that develop with practice; and
- health behaviors that enhance rather than compromise health.

With few exceptions, positive health behaviors are a matter of voluntary action. You choose them; they cannot be forced on you. As you become more knowledgeable about your own health and about the health of others, and more competent in the application of that health knowledge, you will realize that a positive health style offers the best prospect for a healthy, long, happy, and productive life.

Key Concepts

1. According to the World Health Organization, health is "a state of complete physical, mental, and social well-being and not merely the absence of disease or infirmity."
2. Holistic health and wellness are two concepts that expand the definition of health.
3. Wellness emphasizes a person's potential to be healthy in light of disabilities or limitations.
4. An individual who can obtain, interpret, and understand basic health information and services and who possesses the competence to use such information and services is considered health literate.
5. Health skills are abilities that can help you achieve good health. They include motor skills, intellectual skills, emotional skills, and social skills.
6. Health behaviors are actions related to the promotion or maintenance of good health. They include preventive behavior, illness behavior, and sick-role behavior.
7. Your health style is best described as the sum of your personal health decisions, both those that affect you and those that affect others and your community.
8. Health attitudes are behavioral intentions concerning personal health.
9. Health beliefs, whether factual or mythical, influence an individual's health style.
10. The best strategy for a healthy future is prevention—making health-promoting decisions that reduce your risk for acquiring a disease or sustaining an injury.

Review Questions

1. Explain why the absence of disease is an inadequate definition of health.
2. Differentiate between holistic health and wellness.
3. Give examples of healthy development and healthy behavior change.
4. List the three elements of health style.
5. List and explain four characteristics of a health-literate person.
6. Identify four categories of health skills and explain how each impacts health status.
7. Name three types of health behaviors and provide an example of each.
8. Explain how health beliefs and health attitudes influence health style.
9. Describe the role of momentum in maintaining a healthy lifestyle.
10. Explain the saying "an ounce of prevention is worth a pound of cure."

Selected Bibliography

Dunn, H. L. *High Level Wellness.* Arlington, VA: R. W. Beatty, 1961.

McGinnis, J. M., and W. H. Foege. "Actual Causes of Death in the United States." *Journal of the American Medical Association,* 270, no. 18 (1993): 2207–2212.

Health United States, 1996–1997. Hyattsville, MD: U.S. Department of Health and Human Services, National Center for Health Statistics, 1997 (updated annually).

Healthy People 2000: National Health Promotion and Disease Prevention Objectives.

Washington, DC: U.S. Department of Health and Human Services, Public Health Service, 1990.

Healthy People 2000 Review, 1995–1996. Hyattsville, MD: U.S. Department of Health and Human Services, National Center for Health Statistics, 1996.

Prevention Report. Washington, DC: U.S. Department of Health and Human Services, Office of Disease Prevention and Health Promotion (published quarterly).

HealthLinks: Web Sites for Better Health

You can access better health as it relates to this chapter by checking out some of the following sites on the Internet. These and sites identified within the chapter can be accessed directly when you visit the *HealthStyles* Web site located on the Allyn and Bacon homepage at **http://www.abacon.com.**

Health Resources and Services Administration
www.hrsa.dhhs.gov/
Provides a link to news releases and general information on health issues, as well as a listing of employment opportunities and grant funding in the health sciences.

HealthGate
www.healthgate.com
Online source for health, wellness, and biomedical information. Explores health issues from a holistic health perspective.

International Healthy Cities Foundation
www.oneworld.org/cities
Network of interrelated groups dedicated to improving communities and cities and improving the health of the world's population.

Med/Access
www.medaccess.com
An all-encompassing site with information and material on a broad spectrum of topics, all related to healthy living. It also offers a database of hospitals, specialty treatment centers, physicians, and HMOs, just to name a few, as well as overviews of the U.S. health care system.

Health Hotlines: Your Personal Responsibility

Agency for Health Care Policy and Research (AHCPR) Clearinghouse
(800) 359-9295
P.O. Box 8547
Silver Spring, MD 20907-8547

Health Resources and Services Administration, Office of Health Facilities
(800) 492-0359 (within Maryland)
(800) 638-0742 (outside Maryland)
5600 Fishers Lane
Rockville, MD 20857

National Institutes of Health, Division of Public Information
(800) 633-3425
9000 Rockville Pike, Building 1, Room 344
Bethesda, MD 20892-0188

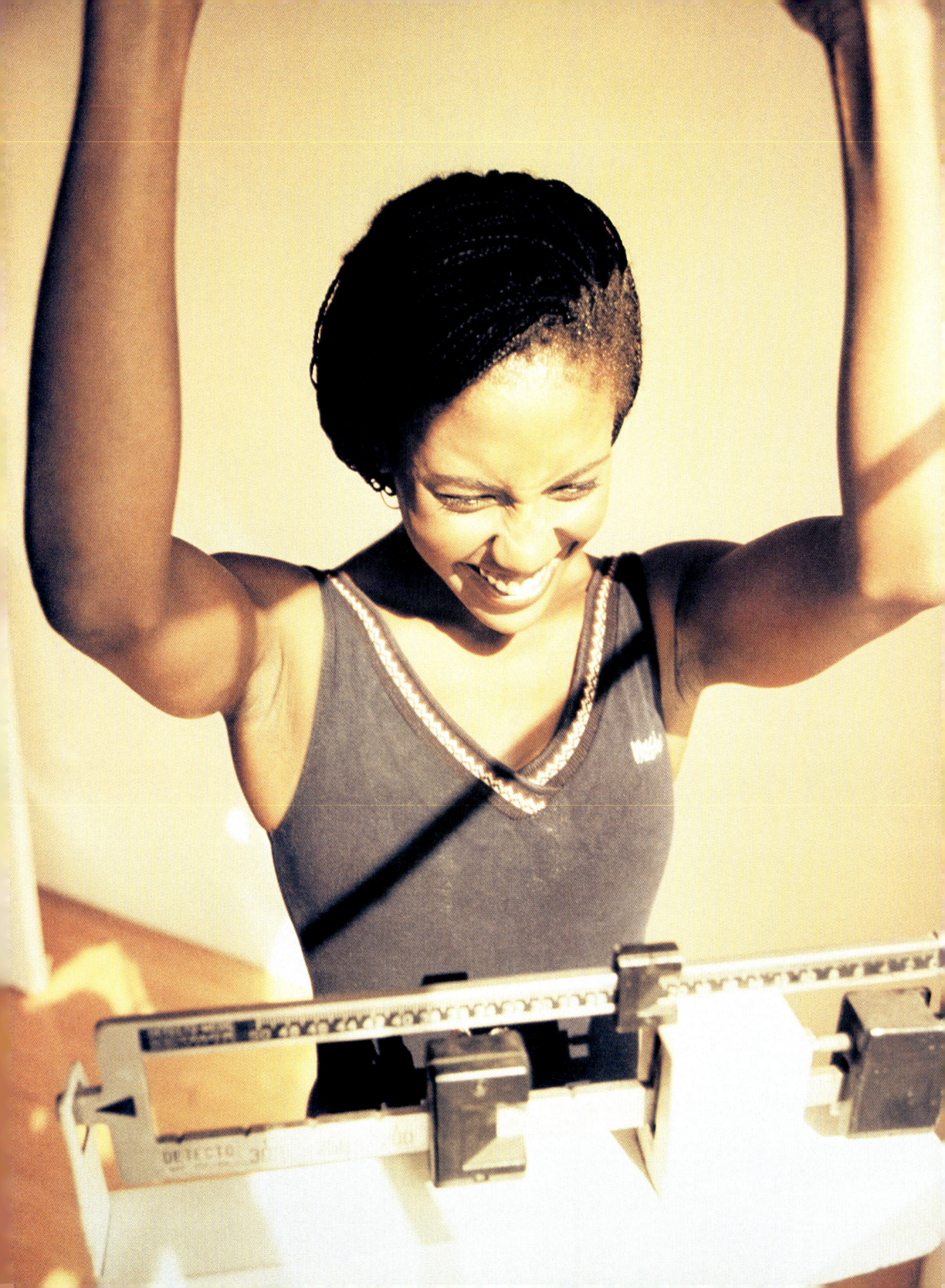

Chapter 2

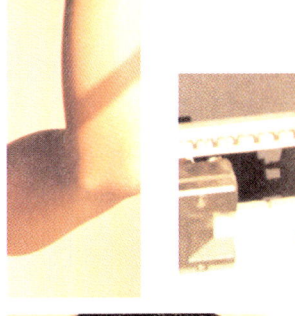

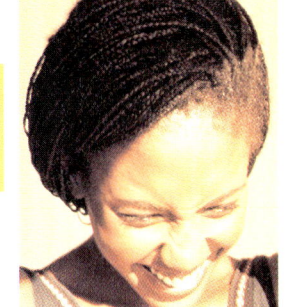

Assessing Your Health

A Plan for Informed Decision Making

Objectives

When you finish reading this chapter, you will be able to:

1. Recognize the value of health assessments to an overall healthy lifestyle.
2. Define *health risk* and understand that some risks are controllable and modifiable and some are not.
3. Examine the wellness inventory, a health risk assessment included in this chapter, and describe its usefulness.
4. Describe the difference between risk age and achievable age.
5. Be aware of the problems associated with laboratory tests, particularly the occurrence of false negatives and false positives.
6. Define *epidemiology* and explain how this area of study has an impact on personal and community health.
7. Differentiate between different types of health data, including morbidity and mortality data.
8. Become familiar with ways of observing yourself and drawing accurate conclusions about your health status from your observations.
9. Understand the value of keeping accurate, up-to-date health records.
10. List several healthy behaviors that may lead to health risk reduction.

What Is Your HealthStyle?

Joe is a good student and is known for his clear thinking and analytical mind in class. But when it comes to himself, Joe is pretty oblivious. When he looks in the mirror either while shaving or after he is dressed, Joe sees an image that he likes: a popular and well-respected student. What he doesn't see is that he is overweight.

During a physical examination, Joe learned that what he did not want to see in the mirror represents a risk factor for heart disease. He also learned that he has high blood pressure. Only after his physician informed him of the relationship of overweight and high blood pressure to heart disease did he begin to focus on his true picture—his health assessment.

Bob, too, checks himself in the mirror every day. But he generally looks for signs of good health—nice skin tone, taut muscles. When he sees signs of bad health habits, such as extra weight due to eating too much or not exercising, Bob knows it is time to tend to his physical and mental health.

He is vigilant for several reasons. He knows that good health habits can put him in a better position to attain a longer and healthier life. He also knows that despite being only twenty-one years old, he is at a higher risk for heart disease than the general population because his father died of a heart attack. Fortunately for Bob, his father's heart disease was likely due to a combination of factors, including smoking, being overweight, and not exercising, in addition to genetics. Clearly, Bob cannot control his genes, but he is determined to control those factors that he can.

In Your Opinion

Joe and Bob look at themselves in the mirror. One of them ignores the risks for heart disease that clearly face him every day; the other acknowledges those risks and works to modify them.

- Why do you think that Joe did not respond to the visual image of himself as overweight?
- What health knowledge did Bob have that prompted his continuous personal health assessment?
- Do you know enough about your health risks that you could control or modify them in a timely fashion?
- Knowing what you do about your health status, what health style changes would you make? It may be interesting to see how you answer this same question at the end of the semester.

How healthy do you feel today? On what information did you base your answer, and how accurate do you think your assessment was? You might be surprised to learn that many people do not assess their own health properly. Studies show that young adults say they suffer more from minor ailments than do people over age sixty-five. Older people have minor ailments, too, but they tend to mention them less in self-assessments.

There are many ways to assess your health accurately. One is by having your physician collect extensive data about you through a battery of tests ranging from analyzing your blood to tracing your heartbeat. A second way is by asking questions about your own health risks. The answer to a question such as "Do I always wear a seat belt?" can provide a good indication of your risk for getting injured if you are involved in an automobile crash.

Your health status today can be an important predictor of your health status in the years ahead. Because change is likely to take place—for better or worse—the information collected today through a **health assessment** also will change—for better or worse. For example, if you decrease the amount of fat in your diet or change your exercise habits and this results in a loss of body weight, you will likely reduce your risk for developing hypertension. Because a health assessment is a measure taken at only one point in time, it is necessary to assess your health and your health risks continually throughout your life.

An assessment provides **baseline data** about health status. A second step, evaluation or interpretation of the data, is necessary if you want to improve your health. An honest evaluation of your baseline data can result in positive health behavior decisions. Conversely, an incorrect interpretation of your baseline data results in inaccurate health knowledge and can lead to poor health-related decisions. Joe thought he looked fine when in fact he was overweight. Bob was better skilled at assessing and interpreting his health status.

Why a Health Assessment?

Health assessment is an analysis of a broad range of measures affecting your health. Some **primary health assessment** procedures are designed to measure a state of well-being in order to prevent disease and are undertaken when no disease is suspected. An example is a blood test to determine your cholesterol level.

Other health assessment procedures are designed to measure the extent of an illness, for example, heart disease, diabetes, or even strep throat. These **secondary health assessments** are used for diagnosing and treating diseases, not for preventing diseases from occurring in the first place. Both primary and secondary health assessments are attempts to define health status and health risks objectively.

Depending on the goal of the assessment, different levels of information are useful, ranging from specific measurements to trends in behavior. If your family physician wants to determine whether to put your mother on medication to lower her blood pressure, the physician needs an accurate and up-to-date measure of her blood pressure levels. But if the physician wants to assess whether your mother is taking risks that might increase her blood pressure, this information comes not from tests but by asking questions such as "Have you been under more stress than usual in recent months?" A "yes" response may increase your mother's risk for high blood pressure.

Critical Thinking Question

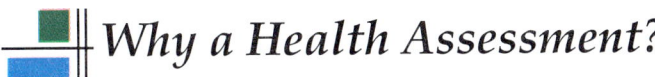

"I am healthy because I *feel* healthy!" This statement was made by a person with extremely high blood pressure. The comment is a subjective health assessment—and totally inaccurate. What other subjective health assessments can you think of that may provide misleading information concerning health status?

health assessment An analysis of a broad range of factors affecting an individual's health.

baseline data Information about health that must be evaluated or interpreted in order to determine health status.

primary health assessment Procedures, usually including identification of risk factors, designed to measure a state of well-being in order to prevent disease.

secondary health assessment Procedures designed to measure the extent of an illness in order to diagnose and treat it.

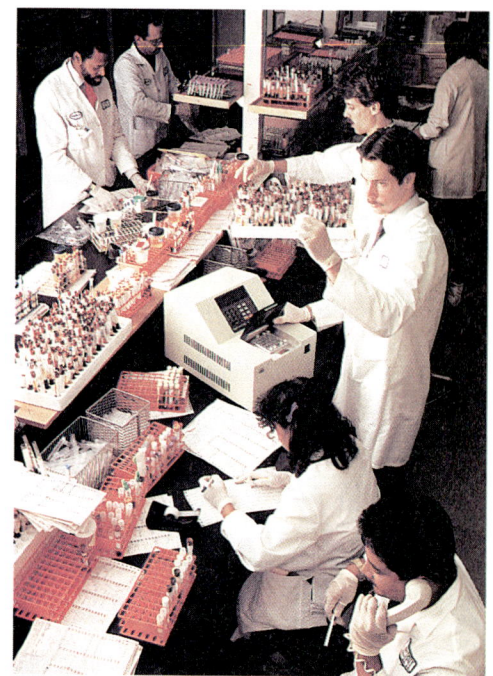

Laboratory tests can provide useful information about your health. Blood samples, for example, can reveal information about your cholesterol level. It is important that the laboratory tests be performed accurately. If there are lab errors, your physician may get an incorrect picture of your health. (Source: © Tony Stone/Tom Tracy)

Problems in Assessing Health

Although it may sound obvious, health assessments are valuable only if they are based on accurate information. Unfortunately, laboratory tests are not always accurate. For example, the Pap test fails to detect cervical cancer or dangerous cell abnormalities up to 40 percent of the time, according to the American College of Obstetricians and Gynecologists. Also, nearly half of all laboratory cholesterol test results vary by 5 percent or more from the correct value, and some of the readings are "highly inaccurate," according to a report from the National Cholesterol Education Program.

A laboratory error can result in a **false negative,** which is when you are told you have no evidence of disease when in fact the opposite is true, or a **false positive,** which is when you are told you have a medical condition when none exists.

Laboratory errors occur for a number of reasons:

- Diet can change blood chemistry enough to cause a false reading on a blood test for cholesterol. For this reason, blood cholesterol tests should be done after you have not eaten for 12 hours.
- Medications can be responsible for false laboratory findings, and a laboratory technician should always ask if you are taking any medication.
- Errors in lab reports can occur because laboratory chemicals lose their potency, test samples are mixed up or misinterpreted, or a machine used in testing is simply inaccurate.

Another source of inaccurate information may be the person being assessed. Information about the risk for contracting sexually transmitted diseases depends on self-report data, usually collected using of a questionnaire about certain behaviors. If a person taking the self-test does not answer accurately because he or she is embarrassed, misunderstands, or does not know how to answer the questions, the usefulness of that questionnaire is significantly compromised. Even though laboratory tests are not perfect, questionnaires and other forms of self-tests allow for far more margin of error.

false negative A test result that indicates no evidence of disease when the disease is present.

false positive A test result that indicates some type of medical condition when none exists.

epidemiology The study of epidemics and the disease process in a population, including factors related to the presence of a disease or health condition.

epidemic The occurrence of disease in a given population at a greater prevalence than would normally be expected.

endemic The persistent presence of a disease in a population.

pandemic The occurrence of a disease that affects virtually an entire population or the entire world.

epidemiologist A person who studies disease in a population.

incidence data Data that provide a precise count of disease cases.

prevalence data Data concerning the existing cases of a specific disease at a certain point in time in a population.

Although medical tests have problems, they still play an important role in measuring your personal health and in helping you stay healthy. There are also ways to measure the health of a community.

Assessing the Health of a Community

Originally, **epidemiology** was the study of epidemics, as the term suggests. An **epidemic** is the occurrence of disease in a given population at a greater prevalence than would normally be expected. The number of cases is less important to the definition of epidemic than is the perceived threat to life or health. AIDS, for example, affects relatively few individuals compared with heart disease or cancer, but because of the seriousness of the disease and the difficulty involved in controlling its spread, AIDS is considered an epidemic.

When a disease is persistently present in a population, it is said to be **endemic.** This is the case with many of the sexually transmitted diseases, such as gonorrhea. When a disease affects virtually an entire population or even the entire world, it is said to be **pandemic.** In some years, influenza is pandemic.

Epidemiology involves far more than the study of epidemics and the distribution of disease in a population. It also includes a study of factors related to the presence of a disease or health condition. For example, these factors can be disease organisms, such as the virus that causes chickenpox; they can be behavior, such as risky sexual activity; or they can be physical entities, such as the automobile (in relation to traffic fatalities).

Epidemiologists, people who study disease in a population, collect information that will be valuable in painting a picture of the impact or importance of that disease. *Incidence* and *prevalence* refer to the number of cases of a disease in a given population during a specific period of time.

Incidence data provide a precise count of new cases of a disease over a specific period of time. For example, the American Cancer Society reports that about 185,000 new cases of breast cancer are detected each year. **Prevalence data**—the total number of cases of a disease at a given point in time—explain the relationship of the incidence to a specific population. The number of new cases of breast cancer suggests that approximately 12 percent of the total population of U.S. women will contract breast cancer in their lifetimes. By monitoring both incidence and prevalence data, researchers can study the extent of a disease in a given population and determine whether it is spreading or slowing down.

Critical Thinking Question

Healthy People 2000 is a large-scale assessment designed to get a picture of the health of the United States (see page 29). Some important health issues could not be included because a lack of available national data would not allow researchers to characterize the problem accurately. Consider the dilemma of the public's right to know of the incidence and prevalence of a disease versus a person's right to privacy. What criteria should be used to determine whether a disease should be reported by the medical profession?

Other important data for epidemiologists include the impact of disease on health. **Morbidity data** are statistical measures of the proportion of a specific population affected by a disease or sickness. For example, currently in the United States, approximately 26 percent of adult males and 20 percent of adult females have high blood pressure. **Mortality data** record the number of deaths by cause (for example, accidents, infant mortality, or AIDS) in a given population. In the United States, lung cancer kills 81 per 100,000 males and 43 per 100,000 females every year. As with incidence and prevalence data, morbidity and mortality data refer to a specific period of time, for example, one year or a lifetime.

Life expectancy is an adaptation of mortality data, and it is often used as a barometer of a nation's health, particularly when it is compared with data from previous years or other countries. For example, the average person may not easily understand the risk for lung cancer death mentioned above (81 per 100,000 males and 43 per 100,000 females) but can understand that he or she can expect to live seventy-four years. By comparing current life expectancy data with those of 1970, a trend can be seen that suggests the success of health care and changes in lifestyle (see Figure 2.1).

Epidemiology takes away much of the mystery of the health status of a community. By carefully monitoring population statistics, epidemiologists are able to paint a clear picture of health behavior, disease, and health risk. In doing so, they provide hints on how to avoid disease, risk, and ultimately death. Thanks to epidemiology, the spread of AIDS has been greatly reduced among homosexuals despite the absence of a vaccine or cure for the disease. Thanks to epidemiology, smoking has been identified as a modifiable risk factor for heart disease, and the prevalence of smoking in the United States continues to decline.

With data on incidence, prevalence, morbidity, mortality, and life expectancy, researchers can study the factors that contribute to people getting sick and dying and how sickness and death might have been prevented. See the Cultural View box to find out what researchers learned about how the Mormons' lifestyle has led to healthier lives.

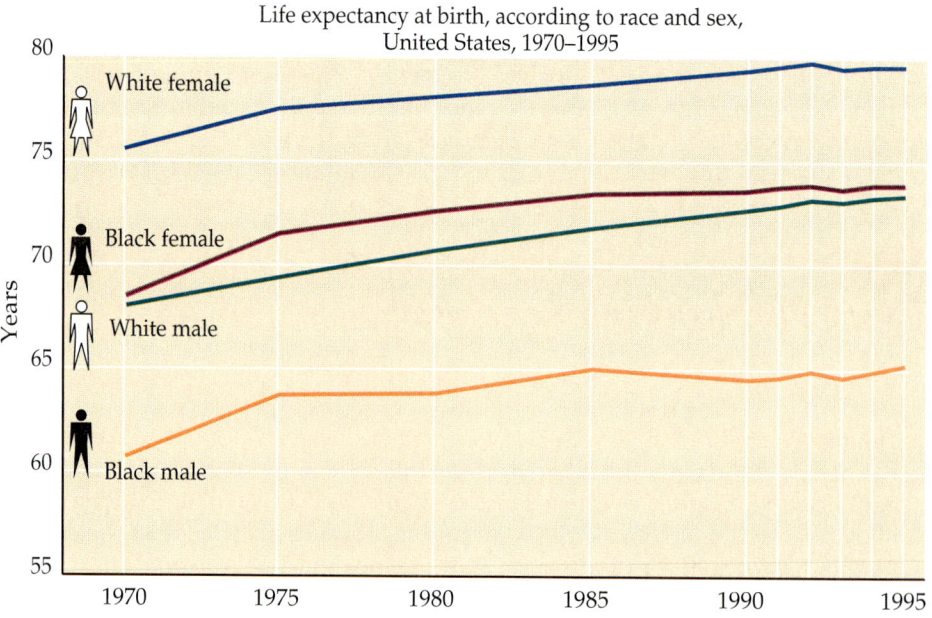

Figure 2.1 Gains in Life Expectancy: Americans Are Living Longer.
If life expectancy is a barometer of a nation's health, how are we doing? (Source: National Center for Health Statistics, National Vital Statistics System, 1997)

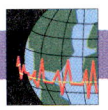

CULTURAL VIEW

Mormon Lifestyle Leads to Healthier Lives

Mormons lead healthy lifestyles and on average live longer. In great part this is due to their adherence to the Word of Wisdom in the Mormon scriptures, which calls for abstinence from wine, strong drink, tobacco, and hot drinks; moderation in eating meat; and eating wholesome foods including fruits and grains.

This plan for healthy living sounds as if it could have been written for a personal health education class in the 1990s, so it may surprise you to learn that it has been a part of the Mormon religion since 1833. In the intervening years, scientific research has shown the soundness of the Mormon approach. In subsequent chapters of *HealthStyles*, you will learn about health hazards associated with alcohol abuse, tobacco, caffeine in coffee and tea (hot drinks), and high-fat meats. You also will learn that a healthy diet includes eating a lot of grains and vegetables.

The Mormons following the Word have had a head start on good health practices, and recent studies have shown just how beneficial this has been. A study of Mormons living in Utah found that they had one-third less cancer than non-Mormons also living in the state. Because they do not smoke, it is not surprising that the incidence of cancers associated with smoking—lung, oral, esophagus, stomach, and bladder—was about one-half that of non-Mormons.

There are some cancers for which Mormons have high incidence rates: skin cancer, lip cancer, and melanoma. But non-Mormons living in Utah also have high rates of these cancers, and researchers speculate they are due in part to genetic and environmental factors. A large percentage of people living in Utah—both Mormons and non-Mormons—are of northern European ancestry and are considered more susceptible to cancers at sites of high sunlight exposure. Utah has a lot of sunlight.

The death rate from cardiovascular disease is also lower for Mormons. Another study found that Utah Mormons had a 35 percent lower death rate for coronary heart disease than the rest of the population. It is believed that this lower death rate is also associated with the fact that Mormons do not smoke. An additional contributing factor is their lower-fat diet, the result of eating only moderate amounts of meat.

Studies of Mormons living out-of-state also show lower mortality rates from cancer and cardiovascular disease. Mortality rates from these conditions are especially low among the more religious Mormons.

Your cultural heritage—the lessons you learned as a child and your family's religious practices—can play an important role in your health and the health of your community. Given the numerous cultures that live side by side in many communities across the country, you can learn much from others that can enrich your life and help you to lead a healthier one.

National Goals for the Year 2000

Healthy People 2000 is an example of a national health assessment process under way in the United States. In 1990, the U.S. Public Health Service established health goals and priorities for Americans that focus on promoting health and preventing disease.

The goals of *Healthy People 2000* are to:

- Increase the span of healthy life for Americans.
- Reduce health disparities among Americans.
- Achieve access to preventive services for all Americans.

To meet these goals, objectives to be achieved by the year 2000 were set in twenty-two priority areas. These twenty-two priority areas are addressed in *HealthStyles*. They are grouped into three broad categories: health promotion,

morbidity data A statistical measurement of the proportion of a specific population affected by a disease or sickness over a specific period of time.

mortality data The number of deaths by disease or sickness in a given population over a specific period of time.

life expectancy The average number of years of life remaining at any given point.

health protection and preventive services. The objectives are to be met through both personal and community efforts. The priority areas are:

Health Promotion

Physical activity and fitness
Nutrition
Tobacco
Alcohol and other drugs
Family planning
Mental health and mental disorders
Violent and abusive behavior
Educational and community-based programs

Health Protection

Unintentional injuries
Occupational safety and health
Environmental health
Food and drug safety
Oral health

Preventive Services

Maternal and infant health
Heart disease and stroke
Cancer
Diabetes and chronic disabling conditions
HIV infection
Sexually transmitted diseases
Immunization and infectious diseases
Clinical preventive services
Surveillance and data systems

These priorities are being monitored with long-term studies of the health behaviors of Americans—health assessments that are combined to paint a picture of the health of a nation. Overall, there have been improvements. As of 1996, 8 percent of the *Healthy People 2000* objectives have been reached or surpassed and progress was made for another 40 percent. For example, more people are exercising and using their seat belts than in the baseline year of 1987. However, there was no change for 3 percent of the objectives and movement went in the wrong direction for 19 percent of them. For example, there are more teenage pregnancies and more overweight people today than in the baseline data. The rest of the objectives showed mixed results or lacked sufficient data to determine progress (see Table 2.1).

Prior to this national health assessment process, it was difficult to track changes in the health behavior of Americans. Data were seldom comparable over time and public health officials were sometimes left with "best guess" assessments. As with personal health assessments, the *Healthy People 2000* process works best when data are collected that are accurate and that present a clear picture of the health of the nation.

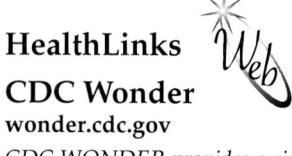

HealthLinks
CDC Wonder
wonder.cdc.gov
CDC WONDER provides a single point of access to a variety of CDC reports, guidelines, and even numeric public health data.

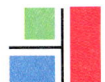

TABLE 2.1 Meeting Selected National Goals for the Year 2000: How Are We Doing? (in percent except where noted)

Objective	Baseline	Update	Target	Progress
Health Promotion				
Years of healthy life	64	63.5	65	Worse
People exercising regularly	22	24	30	Yes
People never exercising	24	24	15	No change
Overweight people	26	34	20	Worse
People with high-fat diets	36	34	30	Yes
People smoking cigarettes	29	26	15	Yes
Youth beginning to smoke	30	30	15	No change
Alcohol-related automobile deaths (per 100,000)	9.8	6.4	5.5	Yes
Alcohol use among youth aged 12–17	25.2	6.0	12.6	Yes
Marijuana use among youth aged 12–17	6.4	4.9	3.2	Yes
Teen pregnancies (per 1,000)	71.1	74.3	50	Worse
Suicides (per 100,000)	11.7	11.6	10.5	Yes
People reporting stress-related health problems	44.2	39.2	35	Yes
Homicides (per 100,000)	8.5	10.6	7.2	Worse
Assault injuries (per 1,000)	9.7	12.7	8.7	Worse
Health Protection				
Unintentional injury deaths (per 100,000)	34.7	29.8	29.3	Yes
Use car safety restraints	42	67	85	Yes
Contraceptive use by women aged 15–44	88.2	90.1	95	Yes
Work-related deaths (per 100,000)	6	5	4	Yes
Work-related injuries (per 100 full-time workers)	7.7	8.4	6.0	Worse
Elevated blood lead level in children (over 25 µg/dL)	234,000	93,000	0	Yes
People with clean air in their communities	49.7	75.1	85	Yes
People in radon-tested homes	5	11	40	Yes
Salmonella outbreaks	77	44	25	Yes
Preventive Services				
Low birthweight babies	6.9	7.3	5	Worse
Mothers with first trimester care	76	80.2	90	Yes
Coronary heart disease deaths (per 100,000)	135	114	100	Yes
Stroke deaths (per 100,000)	30.4	26.7	20.0	Yes
Controlled high blood pressure	11	29	50	Yes
Mean serum cholesterol level (mg/dL)	213	205	200	Yes
Cancer deaths (per 100,000)	134	132	130	Yes
Breast cancer screening (for women over age 50)	25	56	60	Yes
Cervical cancer screening (for women over age 18)	88	94	95	Yes
Fecal occult blood testing (for people over age 50)	27	30	50	Yes
People disabled by chronic conditions	9.4	10.3	8	Worse
Diabetes incidence (per 100,000)	2.9	3.1	2.5	Worse
Gonorrhea infections (per 100,000)	300	168	100	Yes
Syphilis infections (per 100,000)	18.1	8.1	4	Yes
Measles cases	3,396	301	0	Yes
Pneumonia/influenza deaths (per 100,000)	19.9	15.7	15.9	Yes
Immunization levels (for children aged 19–35 months)	54–64	94	90	Yes

Source: U.S. Public Health Service. *Healthy People 2000 Review, 1995–1996*

Assessing Your Personal Health

The health of a nation is determined ultimately by the health of each individual person. How healthy do you think you are? There are several ways to assess your personal health.

A **self-assessment** occurs when an individual collects and interprets his or her own health-related baseline data. Obviously, this is a highly subjective means of health assessment and is often, as illustrated previously in this chapter, inaccurate. A **health risk assessment** is generally done in cooperation with a health educator or health promotion specialist. A health risk assessment can determine your risk of contracting a disease or developing a chronic condition well before the disease or condition shows symptoms. A **medical assessment** is conducted by a medical professional, such as a physician, and focuses on diagnosing whether you have a certain disease or medical condition.

You can learn a lot about your personal health with each kind of assessment. Health risk assessments are discussed in this section; self-assessments and medical assessments are covered later.

Defining Health Risks: A Look at Your Behavior and Environment

A **health risk** refers to the likelihood of having a certain health condition. It is usually defined in terms of behaviors and environment. A person working in a coal mine, for example, is at risk for contracting anthracosis, or black lung disease. This risk is significantly increased if that person smokes cigarettes. In contrast, another person of the same age, sex, and income level who lives and works in a relatively unpolluted community and who does not smoke is not at risk for black lung disease.

The situations that contribute to the risk a person faces are called **risk factors.** Some risk factors are disease-specific. For example, sexually active people who do not use condoms and injecting drug users are at risk for becoming infected with HIV, which causes AIDS. The risk factors are unprotected sex and/or use of unclean needles.

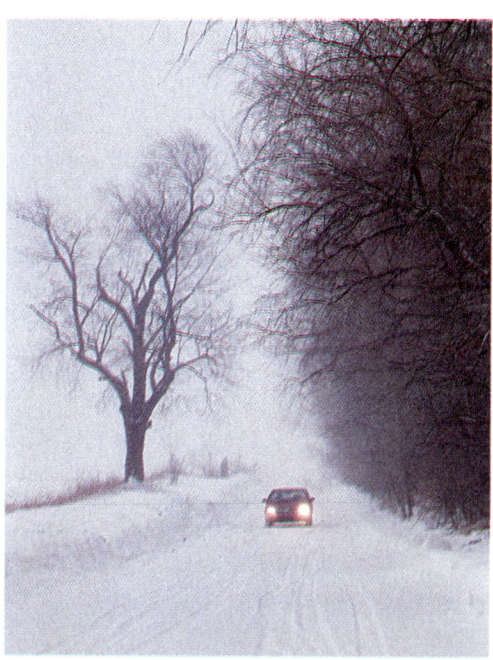

People face numerous risk-factors every day, some more obvious than others. Knowing how to manage risk factors can help reduce your personal risk of injury. (Source: FPG International/© Frank Cezus)

Health Risks: Which Ones Can You Control or Modify?

Risks are not the same for everyone, and not all risks need to be avoided all the time. If you generally follow a healthy diet, there is nothing wrong with occasionally having a one-inch steak smothered with onions sautéed in butter. Although this is an unhealthy load of cholesterol, it will not send you into cardiac arrest if you do it once in a while.

Critical Thinking Question

> Physical activity is recognized as important to the effort to reduce risk for heart disease as well as for other diseases. *Healthy People 2000* suggests that the measure of physical activity be "the sum of all physical activities performed at least thirty minutes per occasion five or more times a week regardless of the intensity." What difficulties are apparent in any attempt to assess physical activity levels according to this standard?

Daily exposure to unavoidable health risks is another matter. Return to the example of the coal miner: merely going to work and breathing puts him or her at risk for black lung disease. Other risk factors over which you may have little control are a family history of heart disease, breast cancer, or diabetes; extreme stress due to a death in the family or job loss; and exposure to violence. Fortunately, many risk factors can be either controlled or modified.

Risk factors considered controllable or modifiable include:

Alcohol use

Blood pressure

Drug abuse

Hours of sleep

Life satisfaction level

Miles driven

Physical activity level

Seat belt use

Strength of social ties

Tobacco use

Risk factors not considered controllable or modifiable include:

Exposure to environmental pollution

Family history of breast cancer

Family history of diabetes

Family history of heart attack

self-assessment An evaluation of health status based on data collected on oneself by oneself.

health risk assessment An assessment to determine the risk for contracting a disease.

medical assessment An evaluation conducted by a medical professional that focuses on identification of the presence or absence of a disease.

health risk The likelihood of developing a certain disease or health condition.

risk factor A condition or habit that puts a person in danger of negative health occurrences.

Having had a hysterectomy

Abnormal Pap smear result

Serious loss or misfortune in the past year

Witnessing or involvement in a violent or potentially violent argument

Health Risk Appraisal: A Measure of Change

Risk factors can be measured in several ways. One of the most common measures is a **health risk appraisal**—a survey instrument that is based on questions about an individual's health history, lifestyle, and medical status. The answers to the questions contained in a health risk appraisal are compared with mortality statistics and epidemiological data to estimate a person's health risks. Originally used by physicians as a way to calculate health-related risks, health risk appraisals are now also used by health educators, fitness personnel, employee groups, and community organizations as a way to stimulate participation in activities aimed at improving health.

Health risk appraisals range from simple questionnaires to elaborate multimedia productions. Their results describe your risk for acquiring a specific disease or dying from it within a defined period of time. Some of the more sophisticated health risk appraisals give feedback not only on your **risk age**—how old you will live to be given the risks you currently have—but also on your **achievable age**—how old you could live to be if you changed certain health behaviors. These feedback reports also include suggestions on how to improve your health behavior.

There are several concerns about the validity of health risk appraisals. They measure behaviors whose predictive importance remains controversial. An example is the role of exercise in reducing the risk for heart disease. They also measure characteristics over which you have no control, including family history of heart disease. Many of the risk factor values are based on data derived from studies involving mostly middle-aged, middle-class, white male subjects, yet their findings are being used to predict the risk of all people—females, African Americans, Hispanics, and members of other ethnic groups—at all ages.

In spite of these drawbacks, health risk appraisals are generally considered to be useful tools in an educational context, and if done correctly, they can help promote good health practices. A number of self-assessments are included throughout the book to help you understand your own health behavior. You would not find these instruments in an elaborate scientific study; they are simply educational tools for you.

Theories about How to Change Health Behaviors

If a high-fat diet is associated with an increased risk for heart disease, why do so many Americans eat fatty food? What causes people to behave in healthy—or unhealthy—ways? There are no easy answers to these and other crucial questions about how people change their health behaviors.

Because we have little real understanding of cause and effect concerning health behavior, health researchers depend on empirically and systematically based theories to explain the way people behave. Following are the leading theories that influence the work of health educators and health promotion professionals today. Some were proposed in the 1930s and 1940s, others more than forty years later. You may want to refer back to these theories as you read the subsequent chapters of *HealthStyles* and attempt to understand why you behave the way you do.

- *Skinner's Theory of Behavior Modification.* In 1938, the behaviorist B. F. Skinner stated his theory that the frequency of a behavior is determined by its consequences, or reinforcement. In terms of health, if a person receives a positive reinforcement for a healthy behavior, he or she is likely to continue practicing that behavior. The same is true for an unhealthy behavior.
- *Maslow's Theory of Human Motivation.* According to psychologist Abraham Maslow, people have five sets of basic needs: physiological, safety, love, esteem, and self-actualization. Motivation for behavior results when any of these needs are not met. Maslow's hierarchy, which he proposed in 1943 and which is discussed in Chapter 3, predicts behavior—including health behavior—according to the nature of unmet needs.
- *Lewin's Field Theory.* Curt Lewin, a field-theory psychologist, suggested in 1948 that behavior results from two sets of forces: driving forces and resisting forces. According to Lewin, for a healthy behavior to develop, the forces pushing toward health must be greater than the forces pushing in an unhealthy direction.
- *Bandura's Social Cognitive Theory.* One of the most widely adopted theories comes from psychologist Albert Bandura, who proposed in 1965 that a person's behaviors are a product of social learning. Social learning results from the approval or disapproval of others felt when behaviors are practiced. Positive reinforcement by others increases the likelihood that those behaviors will occur. The reason his theory has been accepted so widely is that it provides an explanation for vicarious learning—that is, learning that takes place through modeling the behavior of others. For example, teenagers may learn to smoke cigarettes by watching adults smoke and then attempting to "model" the behavior that they observe. An important element of Bandura's theory is self-efficacy, a sense of situational capability that predicts successfully adopting a specific behavior. In other words, if a person believes that he or she is capable of exercising daily, the chances of doing so are good. Also, if a person does not believe that daily exercise is possible, the likelihood of doing so is not good.
- *Becker and Rosenstock's Health Belief Model.* According to this model, proposed by Marshall Becker and Irwin Rosenstock in 1974, health behavior is influenced by (1) a person's perception of susceptibility and/or the severity of a health threat and (2) demographic factors such as socioeconomic status, ethnic background, and age. Cues to action from prompts such as the media are considered important elements in causing behavior to begin. Finally, the likelihood of action related to health is believed to result from a tug between a person's perception of benefits and his or her perception of barriers to behavior.
- *Fishbein and Ajzen's Theory of Reasoned Action and Theory of Planned Behavior.* For Martin Fishbein and Icek Ajzen, attitude, belief, behavioral intention, and behavior are four different constructs, and in 1975 they presented a conceptual framework for studying the relationship between and among them. According to these theorists, a person's intention to behave in a healthy or unhealthy manner is influenced by his or her attitude toward such behavior and beliefs about what other people think he or she should do. Influencing the entire mix is the person's motivation to comply with other factors that affect behavior. Later works have added task self-efficacy to this model.
- *Prochaska and DiClemente's Transtheoretical Model of Behavior Change.* In a relatively new contribution to health behavior theory, psychologists James Prochaska and Carlo DiClemente suggested in 1983 that individual motivation for behavior change occurs in four stages: precontemplation, contemplation, action, and maintenance. A person adopting a healthy practice goes beyond the precontemplation stage, in which the option of this practice (say, starting

health risk appraisal A survey instrument that is based on questions about a person's history, lifestyle, and medical status for the purpose of determining his or her likelihood of developing a health problem.

risk age The age to which a person will probably live given the individual's current risks.

achievable age The age to which a person could live under ideal conditions.

to exercise on a regular basis) has not been considered or is denied, to the contemplation stage, in which the healthy behavior change is given serious consideration, to the action stage, where the new behavior is given a try, and finally to the maintenance stage, in which the behavior becomes part of day-to-day living.

HEALTH SKILLS

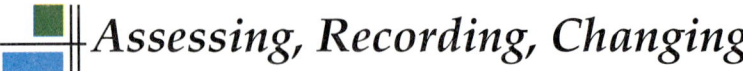

Assessing, Recording, Changing

Health assessment skills are critical to achieving health competence and ultimately maintaining good health. The assessment of your own health begins with your skills of observation and data collection. As important, however, may be your knowledge about when to seek and how to respond to a health assessment expert—a physician, nurse practitioner, or health promotion specialist.

Your health can change from one day to another, even from one second to another. You can be healthy today and suffer from a cold, influenza, or another communicable disease tomorrow. You can be active and able the second before you dive into shallow water and a quadriplegic the next second. Given the range of changes that might occur, it is not possible to know absolutely how healthy you will be at any moment. By conducting periodic assessments and by keeping good health records, you can determine what is normal for you so you can better notice when a change occurs.

Observing Yourself

You can do some of the important health assessments at home by observing your own body. You can assist your physician by providing accurate information about your body temperature, pulse, weight, and overall condition.

Body temperature is a good place to begin, because most people have a thermometer and also have experienced a change in temperature. Body temperature is best measured by placing the thermometer under the tongue or in the armpit or anus. Normal body temperature has long been thought to be 98.6 degrees Fahrenheit, but recent studies indicate that it is 98.2 for adults and between 97.1 and 100 for infants and young children. Even so, some people have a slightly lower body temperature as their norm; others have a slightly higher normal body temperature. In general, women have a higher normal temperature (98.4) than men (98.1). And for everyone, temperature is highest between 4 P.M. and 6 P.M. and lowest at about 6 A.M.

A rise in temperature from your norm is an important sign that you may be sick. Such a rise is commonly called a **fever** and results when internal heat is formed faster than the body can get rid of it. No one fully understands the role of fever, but it is considered to be one way that the body fights illness. According to one theory, the increased heat weakens or kills pathogens. According to another, an infection causes the formation of chemicals in the body called **pyrogens,** a term that means fire makers. In any case, there is no doubt that fever usually means that something may be wrong. There is one exception: Your temperature can rise as a result of exercise—a healthy reason for increased body temperature. After a cooling-down period, it should return to normal.

A drop in body temperature can be a sign of trouble. You can develop **hypothermia,** or a sudden drop in body temperature, from overexposure to cold (as in falling into freezing water) or from overexertion (as in running a marathon).

Your **pulse,** the regular beat in your arteries caused by the contraction of the heart, is another important measure of health that you can observe. The pulse can

fever Above-normal body temperature.

pyrogen A chemical that signals the brain to raise body temperature.

hypothermia A drop in body temperature to subnormal levels; can result in mental confusion, unconsciousness, and death.

pulse The palpable flow of blood in the arteries caused by the regular contraction of the heart.

health history A history of the patient's health as well as of the health of his or her family.

physical examination An examination by a physician that involves inspection, auscultation, and palpation of the body.

auscultation Listening to the sounds made by various body structures.

palpation Touching body parts with the hands.

be felt on the inside of the wrist, in the neck, or over the heart itself. The normal pulse rate, which ranges between sixty and eighty beats per minute (women's rates are at the higher end of this range while men's are at the lower end), has a regular rhythm. An irregular pulse or heart rate may be serious. In adults, a pulse rate greater than 120 beats per minute, taken while resting, is cause to check with a physician.

Changes in body weight are frequently important measures of a change in health. Weight gain that results from poor eating and little or no exercise can lead to greater risk for a variety of diseases, including heart disease. An unexplained weight gain is reason to consult a physician. An unexplained weight loss could indicate the presence of a persistent infection or serious illness. Nearly everyone owns or has access to a scale. It is to your advantage to know your normal weight range and to take notice if it changes, by how much, and over what period of time. This does not mean you should weigh yourself every day or otherwise become obsessed with your weight. A few pounds up or down is normal for most people.

Other parts of your body to observe are your breasts (for females) and testes (for males) for suspicious lumps, your skin for color changes, and your legs or feet for swelling. Not all bodily changes are worrisome or signs of serious illness. Aches, pains, and a slight rise in temperature may be best treated by taking two aspirin or acetaminophen (nonaspirin pain reliever) and resting in bed. Persistently elevated body temperature, severe discomfort, or dramatic changes from the norm such as blood in your urine or feces should lead you to contact your physician immediately.

A Medical Assessment

There are times when it is important to involve a medical professional in your health assessment. A physician is able to give much greater detail to your health assessment and to look for the presence not only of disease risk but also of disease itself. When a physician examines you and assesses your health, he or she looks at three different measures:

- Your health history
- A physical examination
- Laboratory tests

An assessment of your **health history** can often provide clues to disease or discomfort. Your physician needs to know what diseases, injuries, and other health-related experiences you have had. If you have an allergy to penicillin, for example, your physician needs to know that so he or she can choose a different antibiotic when one is needed. Similarly, if you show up at the emergency room with a deep cut on your foot as a result of stepping on a rusty nail, the physician needs to know when you had your last tetanus vaccination and whether you need a booster shot to avoid getting tetanus.

A history of your health should also include a history of your family's health. Has anyone in your immediate family died of heart disease or cancer? Is there a family history of diabetes, obesity, alcoholism, or mental illness? Because some diseases have a genetic link, this information can provide insights into your health as well as into your family's health. For example, an ophthalmologist will ask if your parents have had glaucoma, an eye disease that can result in blindness. If so, you have a higher than usual chance of getting it, so your eyes should be checked regularly. Glaucoma can usually be controlled if it is caught in the early stages (see the Here's Looking at You box).

The **physical examination** involves inspection, **auscultation** (listening), and **palpation** (touching). By inspecting, or looking at, your body, the physi-

HealthLinks

Healthy People 2010
http://web.health.gov/healthypeople/

Link directly into the consortium of health specialists monitoring Healthy People 2000 *objectives and status and developing new objectives for* Healthy People 2010. *Review the latest facts on the nation's health and initiatives.*

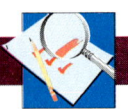

HERE'S LOOKING AT YOU

The Relative Risks in Your Family Tree

For early warning signs of health problems that may lie ahead, most doctors say, study the details of your family's medical past No wonder. More than 3,000 ailments are now known to be inherited, including heart disease, cancer, diabetes, arthritis, Alzheimer's, and even alcoholism, depression, thyroid disease, and schizophrenia. New ones are added to the list every day.

If your own family's health history has gone largely unrecorded, there's no better time than now to get the crucial details down in writing. Here's how to do it:

Getting Started

Using the form (and the sample as a guide), create your own "genogram," or health family tree. Starting with your grandparents, fill in their full names and their dates of birth and death.

Next, add as much as you can about the health of all your close relatives; include chronic ailments, such as ulcers or allergies, as well as major surgeries and causes of death. The more specific the information, the better. Some genetically linked cancers, for example, can be remarkably specific—right down to whether, say, a tumor first appears on the right or left side of the colon.

Dialing for Details

Where memories fail, official records may be useful. Death certificates, for example, typically contain information about the medical cause of death. To locate them, call or write the Division of Vital Records or Division of Statistics in the state where the relative died.

Some hospitals and doctors also keep permanent archives of medical records on microfilm. To get health records for your late Uncle Harvey or Grandma Rose, you'll need a letter of consent from the closest living relative, as well as a copy of the death certificate.

Looking for Patterns

When your genogram is complete, sit down with your family doctor and talk about any obvious patterns that show up. An illness or health condition that appears more than once—especially if it showed up in relatives before age fifty-five—should get special attention. Knowing your predisposition toward a disease makes preventing it easier, either by changing high-risk behaviors or simply by detecting ailments early.

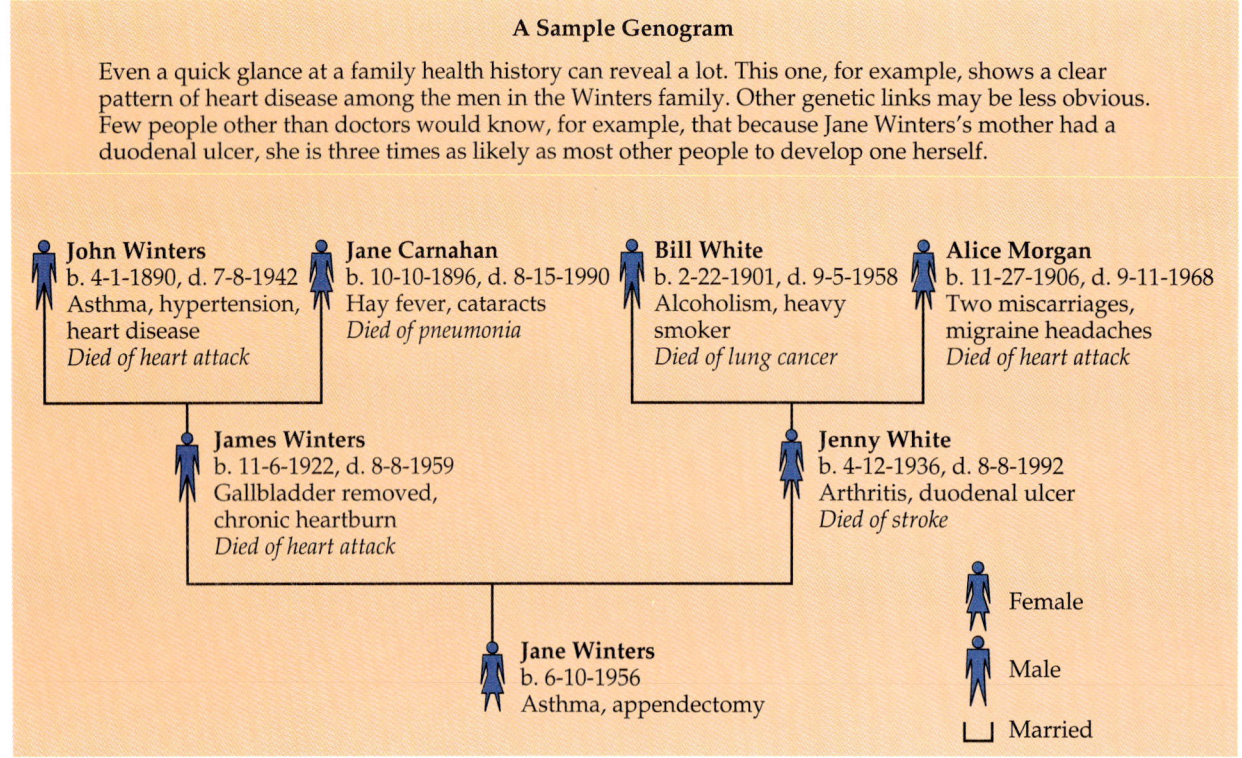

A Sample Genogram

Even a quick glance at a family health history can reveal a lot. This one, for example, shows a clear pattern of heart disease among the men in the Winters family. Other genetic links may be less obvious. Few people other than doctors would know, for example, that because Jane Winters's mother had a duodenal ulcer, she is three times as likely as most other people to develop one herself.

John Winters
b. 4-1-1890, d. 7-8-1942
Asthma, hypertension, heart disease
Died of heart attack

Jane Carnahan
b. 10-10-1896, d. 8-15-1990
Hay fever, cataracts
Died of pneumonia

Bill White
b. 2-22-1901, d. 9-5-1958
Alcoholism, heavy smoker
Died of lung cancer

Alice Morgan
b. 11-27-1906, d. 9-11-1968
Two miscarriages, migraine headaches
Died of heart attack

James Winters
b. 11-6-1922, d. 8-8-1959
Gallbladder removed, chronic heartburn
Died of heart attack

Jenny White
b. 4-12-1936, d. 8-8-1992
Arthritis, duodenal ulcer
Died of stroke

Jane Winters
b. 6-10-1956
Asthma, appendectomy

Female
Male
Married

(Source: "The Relative Risks in Your Family Tree," *Health*, January–February 1997. Reprinted by permission of Time Inc. Health)

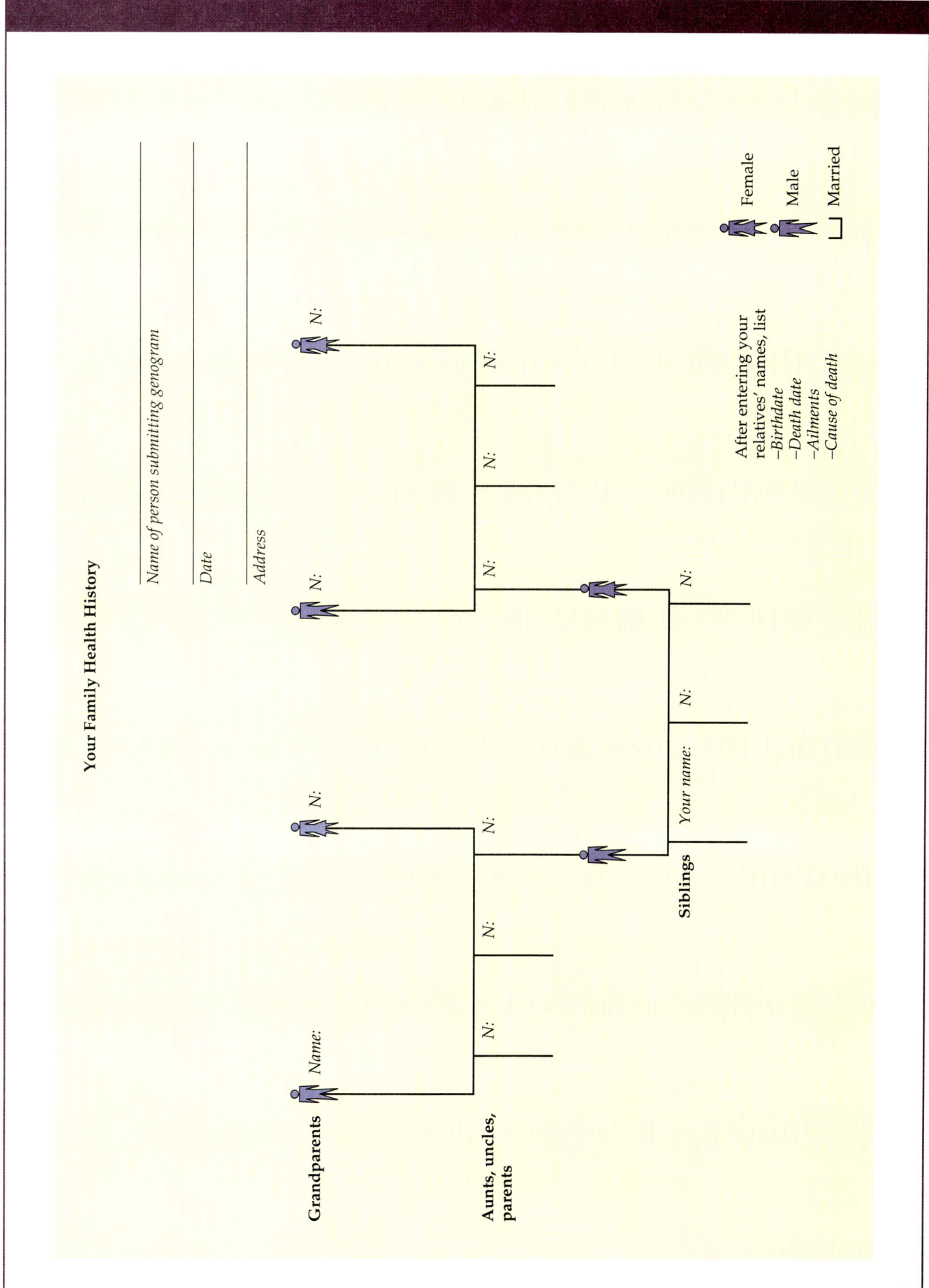

cian can find indications of disease by noting such signs as jaundiced (yellow) skin or extreme overweight. Through his or her trained sense of hearing, a physician listens for abnormalities in the sound of the heart or lungs. Finally, the physician's trained sense of touch permits the examination of body parts for growths and other abnormalities. To aid the physician in this examination, there are tools ranging from the simple flashlight, used to examine the ear canal, to ultrasound machines, used to visually examine a fetus at various stages of pregnancy.

When needed, physicians are assisted in their medical assessment by **laboratory tests,** which involve examining materials taken from the body, such as blood or urine. An automated blood test can analyze up to forty different blood chemicals at once, including cholesterol and glucose. A complete blood count, in addition, can detect disorders such as anemia or chemical or poison reactions. Urinalysis is useful in diagnosing urinary disorders and kidney and liver diseases. Other laboratory tests include throat cultures, used to see whether a bacterial organism such as streptococcus is causing a sore throat; an electrocardiogram, used to evaluate heart rate and to reveal the presence and location of heart damage; and chest X-rays, used to detect abnormalities in patients who have chest symptoms.

Critical Thinking Question

One of the proven means of early detection of breast cancer is a breast self-examination. Mammograms are recommended either every year or every other year for women over age forty and for younger women if there is a family history of breast cancer. Is it possible to conduct too many screening tests? How might breast self-examination actually contribute to the delay in diagnosis and treatment of breast cancer?

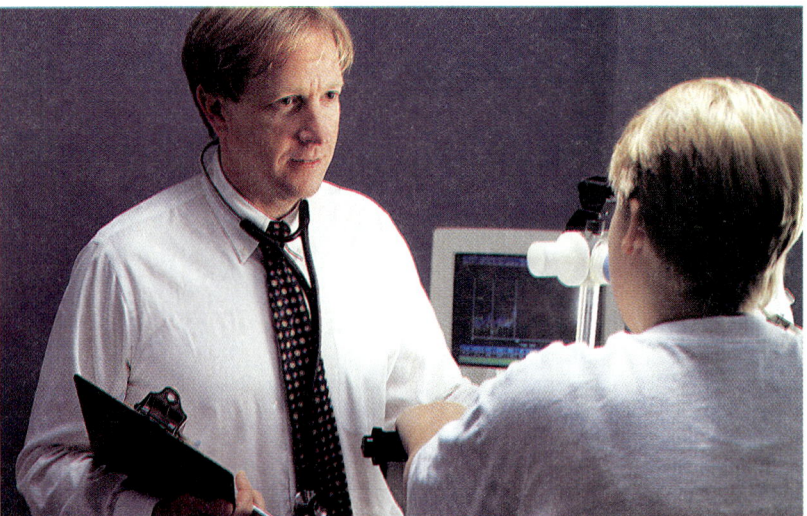

Have you talked with your physician about nutrition, safer sex, and other health-related issues that many college students think about? You can look to your physician for health counseling. (Source: Stock, Boston/©Charles Gupton)

DEVELOPING HEALTH SKILLS

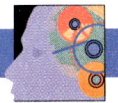

Knowing What to Expect from a Physical Exam

We seldom think of having a physical examination as requiring health skills. But to get the most from a physical examination, you need to apply some basic communication skills.

- Talk clearly and effectively about your wants and needs concerning the examination. Ask questions, expect answers, and probe for information.
- Provide accurate information to your physician. Just because you may have done something embarrassing—for example, having unsafe sex—is no reason to place yourself at risk by withholding information from the physician.
- When you go for a checkup, be sure your physician gives you the following preventive services, which are recommended for men and women ages nineteen to thirty-nine by the U.S. Preventive Services Task Force.

History and Counseling

Dietary intake

Physical activity

Tobacco/alcohol/drug use

Sexual practices

Physical Exam

Height and weight

Blood pressure

Complete oral cavity exam (for people who smoke or chew tobacco)

Clinical breast exam (for females)

Clinical testicular exam (for males)

Complete skin exam (for people with a family history of skin cancer)

Laboratory and Diagnostic Procedures

Blood cholesterol

Urinalysis

Pap smear (for sexually active females)

Testing for HIV and other STDs (for persons seeking treatment for STDs and those with multiple sexual partners)

Mammogram (for women with a family history of breast cancer)

Source: Adapted from the U.S. Preventive Services Task Force

These procedures are necessary to make an accurate diagnosis, but how many of them are needed and how often they should be performed is widely debated. The so-called annual physical examination is a thing of the past. Much depends on your age and health history, but the best advice today from the federal government's *Guide to Clinical Preventive Services* is to have a physical examination to provide baseline data (for example, to record your normal blood pressure, pulse, and cholesterol level) and to have additional examinations only in specific circumstances. Children under age six and adults over age sixty are more likely to get sick, so they should have checkups about once a year even if they do not have any clinical symptoms or other signs of health problems. Adults whose parents, grandparents, or siblings have had heart disease, diabetes, or other conditions also may want to have checkups every year or two.

Most people do not need an annual physical. But when you do have one, you may find that your physician is able to spend time counseling you on the dangers of smoking and alcohol, unsafe sex, and poor eating habits (see the Developing Health Skills box).

laboratory tests Procedures that involve the examination of blood, tissue, and other biologic materials for the diagnosis, prevention, or treatment of disease.

HERE'S LOOKING AT YOU

Your Health Habits

1. List four or five health habits you would like to develop (more sensible eating, regular exercise, coping with stress, etc.).
   a. _____
   b. _____
   c. _____
   d. _____

2. Now, go back and circle the habit you would most like to develop.

3. Turn your wish into a goal. Set target dates for starting toward and reaching that goal.
   _____
   _____
   _____
   _____

4. Helps and hindrances
   What will help you reach your goal? What will stand in the way?

   Helps
   _____
   _____
   _____
   _____

   Hindrances
   _____
   _____
   _____
   _____

5. Action plan:

Who? (name)	Will do what?	Starting when? (date)

6. Write down the names of a few people who will help you reach your goal.

Wellness support system	Signatures (of support people)
Name _____	_____
Name _____	_____
Name _____	_____

7. Evaluation of progress:
   Did I reach my goal? _____
   Did my support system help? _____
   Is it a permanent change? _____
   Do I feel better? _____

Keeping Good Health Records

Health records are important because they are a way to keep track of your health history. Do you know when you had your last vaccination to protect you from getting tetanus? What would you tell the physician if you were to step on a rusty nail? Parents tend to keep health records for their children, but college students are less careful about keeping their own records current.

You should keep your health records easily retrievable in one place. For example, you could keep a copy on a computer and bring it up to date with each new event. Make a note of each diagnosis, the name and telephone number of the physician making the diagnosis, and the treatment taken. Pharmacies keep a record of prescriptions that you have ordered, but most people use more than one pharmacy, so the record in each place is not complete. You should develop your own complete prescription record. This can help in avoiding **drug interactions**—when two drugs or a drug and food taken at the same time produce a bad effect in the body. It is also useful when you want to give an accurate health history to a new physician. Finally, if you travel internationally, it could be important for you to have a complete health history with you in case you get sick. For some countries, you will need evidence of certain vaccinations.

drug interaction An adverse effect on the body that occurs when a drug is taken at the same time as food, vitamins, or another medication.

Changing Your Health Behavior

A health assessment, regardless of its accuracy, is of little value if not acted upon. Once an assessment identifies health risks due to negative health behaviors, a change is called for. Interestingly, health-related behavior change is seldom complex. It usually comes down to a handful of actions that research has consistently found to be very positive contributors to a healthier and longer life. Here is a list of eight good health behaviors. The reason these are so positive is that each serves to reduce risk for a large number of health threats yet involves a small behavioral change.

- Avoid the use of tobacco
- Get seven hours of sleep a night
- Eat breakfast
- Maintain normal body weight
- Drink alcohol in moderation, if at all
- Get exercise on a routine basis
- Practice safer sex
- Wear a seat belt

These good health practices are much like the advice you've heard from your parents. But they are also the result of extensive research by some of the most respected health researchers.

A good way to reduce risk is by increasing good health practices. After a careful examination of personal health habits, a planned strategy for health change is possible. Look at the above list of good behaviors again, and then write on the worksheet in the Here's Looking at You box the three or four health habits you would like to develop.

Key Concepts

1. A health assessment is an analysis of a broad range of measures affecting an individual's health. Because a health assessment is a measure taken at only one point in time, it is necessary to assess your health and your health risks continually throughout your life.
2. Epidemiology is the study of epidemics and the distribution of disease in a population.
3. With data on incidence, prevalence, morbidity, mortality, and life expectancy, researchers can study factors that contribute to people getting sick and dying and how those conditions or deaths might have been prevented.
4. *Healthy People 2000* is a national health assessment procedure undertaken by the U.S. Public Health Service to monitor the health of the United States.
5. The three goals of *Healthy People 2000* are to (1) increase the span of healthy life for Americans, (2) reduce health disparities among Americans, and (3) achieve access to preventive services for all Americans.
6. Health risks are not the same for everyone. Depending on the situation, some are controllable, some can be modified, and some are unavoidable.
7. The health risk appraisal describes an individual's likelihood of dying or of acquiring a specific disease or health condition within a defined period of time.
8. The physical examination done by a physician involves inspection, auscultation, and palpation. Most people do not need an annual physical examination.

9. By keeping good health records, you can determine what is normal for you so you can better notice when a change occurs.
10. Many healthy behaviors, such as avoiding the use of tobacco, maintaining normal body weight, and exercising on a routine basis, serve to reduce the risk for a wide variety of diseases.

Review Questions

1. What are baseline data and how are they used to explain changes in health status?
2. Explain the difference between a primary health assessment and a secondary health assessment.
3. Differentiate between a false positive and a false negative test result.
4. Explain the work of an epidemiologist. How does it contribute to the public's overall health?
5. List the three goals of *Healthy People 2000*.
6. List risk factors that are considered controllable or modifiable. List risk factors that are not considered controllable or modifiable.
7. Give specific examples of skills needed to conduct self-health assessments adequately.
8. List the services you can expect when visiting a physician.
9. Give three reasons for keeping good health records.
10. List eight health behaviors that research has proven to be health enhancing.

Selected Bibliography

Bandura, A. *Social Foundations of Thought and Action: A Social Cognitive Theory.* Englewood Cliffs, NJ: Prentice-Hall, 1986.

Becker, M. H., ed. "The Health Belief Model and Personal Health Behavior." *Health Education Monographs* 2 (Winter 1974): 404–419.

Fishbein, M., and I. Ajzen. *Belief, Attitude, Intention and Behavior: An Introduction to Theory and Research.* Reading, MA: Addison-Wesley, 1975.

Gordis, L., ed. *Epidemiology and Health Risk Assessment.* New York: Oxford University Press, 1988.

Green, L. W., and F. M. Lewis. *Measurement and Evaluation in Health Education and Health Promotion.* Palo Alto, CA: Mayfield, 1986.

Health Risk Appraisal: Methods and Programs, with Annotated Bibliography. Rockville, MD: U.S. Department of Health and Human Services, National Center for Health Services Research and Health Care Technology Assessment, 1986.

Healthy People 2000: National Health Promotion and Disease Prevention Objectives. Washington, DC: U.S. Department of Health and Human Services. Public Health Service, 1990.

Healthy People 2000 Review, 1995-96. Hyattsville, MD: U.S. Department of Health and Human Services, National Center for Health Statistics. 1996.

Lewin, K. *Resolving Social Conflicts.* New York: Holt, Rinehart & Winston, 1948.

Maslow, A. H. "A Theory of Human Motivation." *Psychological Review* 50 (July 1943): 370–376.

Morbidity and Mortality Weekly Report. Centers for Disease Control and Prevention. (published weekly). For example, see "State- and Sex-Specific Prevalence of Selected Characteristics: Behavioral Risk Factor Surveillance System, 1992 and 1993." MMWR 45 (SS-6) (December 27, 1996).

Prochaska, J. I., and C. C. DiClemente. "Transtheoretical Therapy: Toward a More Integrative Model of Change." *Psychotherapy: Theory, Research and Practice* 19 (Fall 1982): 276–288.

Skinner, B. F. *The Behavior of Organisms.* East Norwalk, CT: Appleton & Lange, 1938.

University of California at Berkeley Wellness Letter (published monthly).

Vickery, D. M., and J. F. Fries. *Take Care of Yourself: A Consumer's Guide to Medical Care.* Reading, MA: Addison-Wesley, 1990.

HealthLinks: Web Sites for General Health Information

You can access better health as it relates to this chapter by checking out some of the following sites on the Internet. These and sites identified within the chapter can be accessed directly when you visit the *HealthStyles* Web Site located on the Allyn and Bacon homepage at **http://www.abacon.com.**

CDC National Center for Health Statistics
www.cdc.gov/nchswww/nchshome.htm
Access the latest information in health statistics from the top government agency for health promotion and disease prevention. Obtain fact sheets, news releases, and more.

Office of Disease Prevention and Health Promotion
odphp.osophs.dlihs.gov
A division of the U.S. Department of Health and Human Services, the Office of Disease Prevention and Health Promotion works to strengthen the disease prevention and health promotion priorities of DHHS agencies. Access fact sheets and the latest findings for health promotion for all areas of health ranging from nutrition to consumer health.

Office of Minority Health Research Center (OMH-RC)
www.omhrc.gov/
The OMH-RC serves as a national resource and referral service on minority health issues. The center maintains databases on a wide variety of health topics and facilitates the exchange of information on minority health issues regarding American Indian and Alaskan Native, African American, Asian American and Pacific Islander, and Hispanic populations.

Health Hotlines: Assessing Your Health

National Reference Center for Bioethics Literature
(800) MED-ETHX (633-3849)
Joseph and Rose Kennedy Institute of Ethics
Georgetown University
Washington, DC 20057-1212

People's Medical Society
(800) 624-8773
462 Walnut Street
Allentown, PA 18102

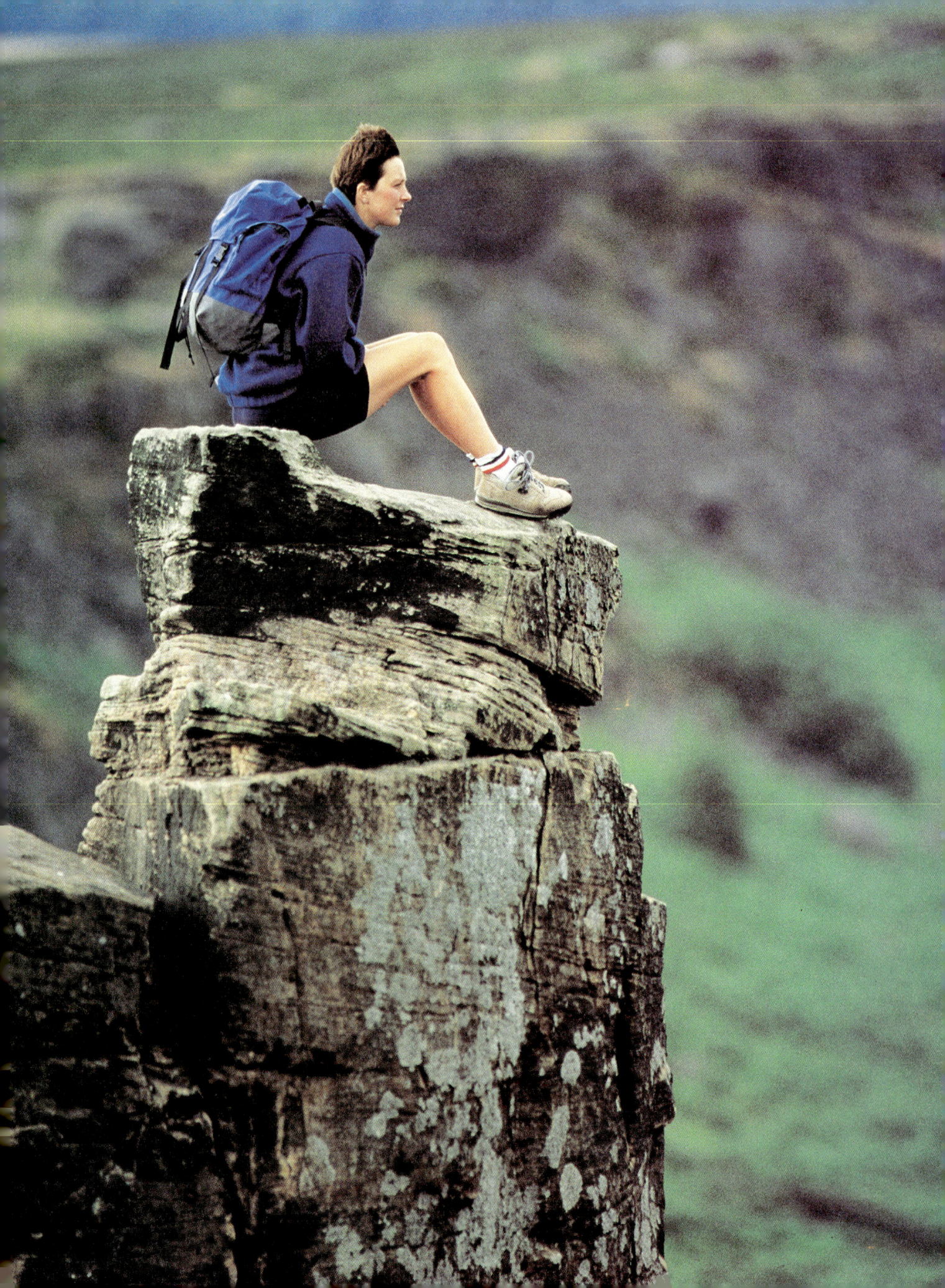

Chapter 3

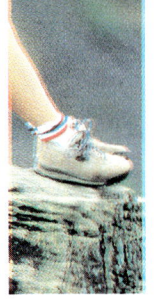
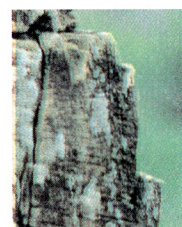
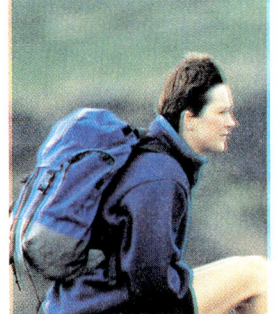

Managing Your Mental Health

Objectives

When you finish reading this chapter, you will be able to:

1. Differentiate between a mentally well and a mentally ill person.
2. Explain what is meant by emotional and social well-being.
3. Identify the role of emotions in a healthy lifestyle and list several normal emotions along with positive and negative ways to express them.
4. Recognize the mental health benefits of sleep.
5. Understand the meanings of the terms *self-concept, self-esteem, self-efficacy,* and *self-actualization.*
6. Recognize a variety of mental illnesses, including anxiety, depression, and schizophrenia.
7. Differentiate between minor depression and major depression.
8. Recognize the characteristics of an individual contemplating suicide.
9. Name a variety of mental health professionals and understand how each addresses emotional problems.
10. Know when to call for help if you suspect that you are experiencing a mental health problem.

What Is Your HealthStyle?

The more she thought about it, the more depressed Elaine became. Her grades began to drop and she was losing sleep over it.

What was happening? Her parents were expecting her to come home from college for the Christmas holiday and she didn't want to go. The holiday season always made her feel blue. Christmas Day was depressing. New Year's Eve was even worse.

Elaine decided to talk about "it" with Marie, her dorm counselor. Marie had helped Elaine work out some other problems. Marie told Elaine that she, too, sometimes felt blue when others were happy. Her solution in that situation was to treat herself to something special to perk herself up. Elaine promised to do the same, and she bought something special for herself. Her trip home turned out far better than she had anticipated. The holidays still weren't fun, but at least she wasn't insufferably sad.

Charles was pleased with how well he did during his first semester at school. His grades were good—A's and B's—and he had made some good friends. But all of a sudden—now that he was ready to go home for the holidays—he came crashing down. He was listless and had no energy or desire to do anything. Charles started cutting classes and not completing his schoolwork.

What had happened? Was there something going on in his life that had upset him? Were the demands he placed on himself realistic? Was he worried about going home and having a fight with his parents?

Charles didn't know the answers to these questions, but, more to the point, he didn't care. He was so depressed when he went home that he didn't return to school. He spoke to his family physician and got a psychiatric referral. Charles stayed in treatment for the next several months, and by the end of the summer, he was ready to go back to school. Charles was in good spirits, but he promised himself that if he got too far down in the dumps again, he would not wait until his depression was out of control before he sought help.

In Your Opinion

Elaine and Charles both faced the preholiday blues, but they handled their problems very differently. Elaine sought answers to her sadness; Charles avoided his problems, at least initially.

- What are the positive steps that both Elaine and Charles took?
- How could Charles have handled his situation differently so that he didn't have to take time off from school?
- Should Charles have sought help earlier than he did? From whom?
- Did Elaine possess a health skill that Charles lacked?
- Think about a recent situation in which you were depressed. What was going on in your life? Did you seek help? Did you work it out yourself? How might you do it differently today?

mental health A state of emotional and social well-being; a state in which an individual is capable of healthy interaction with his or her environment and of enduring the hard times of life, with resilience.

mental illness A disorder or problem of the mind that prevents a person from being productive, adjusting to life, or getting along with other people.

When people ask, "How do you feel?" most often they mean, "How do you feel physically?" How you feel mentally is just as important and is a good indication of your mental health. Mental health, an abstract concept, is usually defined according to normal behavior. What defines normal, as you might expect, remains controversial.

As a healthy college student, you experience a range of emotions. Sometimes you are happy; sometimes you are sad. Sometimes you feel self-confident; sometimes you feel you can't do anything right. Knowing how to deal with your emotions and gaining personal insight and growth from these experiences are two important aspects of good mental health.

Mental health is the ability to negotiate the daily challenges and social interactions of life without experiencing undue emotional or behavioral incapacity. To understand mental health in general—and your mental health in particular—think of yourself as fitting into three systems: a biological system, a psychological system, and a social system. The psychological system is most important when considering mental health. But the relationships among the three systems are so close that the state of your psychological system directly affects the other systems. In other words, how you feel and how you interpret the events around you affect your biological and social well-being. Understanding mental health, therefore, is critical to maintaining an overall healthy life.

A Continuum of Well-Being

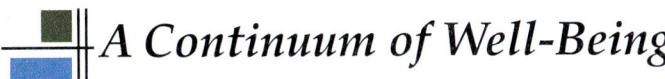

Mental health refers to your emotional and social well-being. Like so many terms in the mental health field, *well-being* suggests an abstract state. In a state of well-being, an individual is capable of (1) healthy interaction with his or her environment and (2) enduring the hard times of life with resilience. The absence of mental well-being is indicated by an inability to interact with the environment and/or a lack of resilience.

Imagine a continuum of mental well-being from mental health to **mental illness.** Most people do not have serious mental or emotional problems and therefore tend to identify with the mentally healthy side of the continuum. This does not mean that, as a mentally well person, you are free from life's stressors. Everyone experiences stress, but those who are mentally healthy are more capable of handling stress with a minimum of difficulty. Everyone experiences important life transitions—going to college, starting a career, getting married or divorced, the death of a loved one. Stressful events present a significant challenge to your mental health. These transitions and the emotions they engender, however, are a part of normal life and are not a cause of pathological disease (see Chapter 4).

The mental illness side of the continuum represents a disorder or problem of the mind that prevents a person from being productive, adjusting to life, or getting along with other people. While most people weather at least one period of minor depression, extreme depression can lead to total incapacitation. Mental health and mental disorders can be affected by numerous factors including (1) genetics; (2) physical abilities, disabilities, or vulnerabilities; and (3) social and environmental conditions and stressors. The details of mental illness are addressed later in the chapter. But first, let us consider the mentally healthy person.

What Makes a Person Mentally Well?

The mentally well person is often referred to as well-adjusted. Note that the word *adjusted* connotes change. A well-adjusted person is not tied to one way of thinking about or doing things or even to maintaining so-called normal behavior. This is because norms change. What is normal today may be abnormal in the near future or may have been abnormal in the past. For example, until 1974, the American Psychiatric Association listed homosexuality among its mental disorders, diseases, and abnormalities. Now homosexuality is recognized as a sexual orientation, not a psychiatric condition subject to treatment.

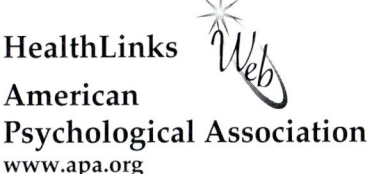

HealthLinks
American Psychological Association
www.apa.org

Includes APA newsletters, links to other sites, information on books, journals, employment, and public, practical, and educational materials.

What characterizes a mentally well-adjusted person? Numerous efforts have been made to define such a person. The following seven qualities might be found on many lists.

A well-adjusted or mentally well person is one who

1. has a positive self-image and good self-esteem;
2. experiences appropriate and stable moods;
3. maintains control of emotions and has the ability to love, feel guilt, and accept remorse;
4. demonstrates flexibility and adaptability in social situations;
5. acknowledges personal strengths and accepts personal limitations;
6. tolerates ambiguity and understands that conflict is normal and that final solutions to problems may not exist; and
7. does not distort reality, consciously or unconsciously.

Critical Thinking Question

In *Healthy People 2000,* the following goal is stated: "Increase to at least 54 percent the proportion of people with major depressive disorders who obtain treatment." Baseline data suggest that only 31 percent of such people currently obtain treatment. These data are based on self-reports. How accurate do you think self-reports are as a means of quantifying people who obtain treatment? What is another way to collect this information?

None of us exhibits these qualities perfectly. We maintain a positive self-image and good self-esteem most of the time. We experience appropriate and stable moods most of the time. We tolerate ambiguity and understand that conflict is normal and that final solutions to problems may not exist most of the time. In other words, we do not live in a continuous state of psychological perfection. Variations and fluctuations of these qualities occur. In fact, it would be highly unusual to find someone who did not experience the natural highs and lows of daily living.

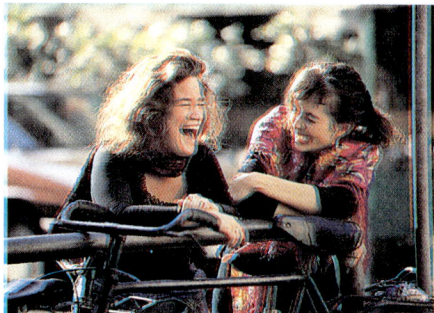
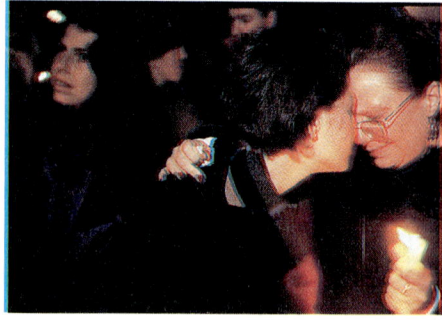

There are countless emotions, such as joy and sorrow. It is mentally healthy to express emotions, but there are healthy and less healthy ways of doing so. (Sources: LEFT, FPG International/ © Stephen Simpson; RIGHT, The Image Works/ © A. Lichtenstein)

The Role of Your Emotions

There are countless emotions, just as there are countless combinations of pigment to form colors of skin. Anger, love, fear, sorrow, and joy are among the most easily identified and expressed emotions. Other emotions that are more difficult to recognize and deal with are guilt and hate. Guilt, for example, is one way for your conscience to distinguish between right and wrong. You can feel guilty over cheating on a test, not helping your roommate clean up the room, or putting off a visit to your grandmother in the nursing home. These are all so-called normal feelings of guilt, but if they build up and are not handled appropriately, they can stifle your enjoyment of living and can cause fears and anxieties that result in debilitating health problems.

It is mentally healthy to express emotions, but there are healthy and less healthy ways of doing so. Consider the emotion of anger. Blowing up at your lab partner because his or her part of the experiment was not completed will not necessarily dissipate your anger. In fact, expressing rage might make you even angrier. Studies conducted at the University of Michigan show that the healthiest people use a reflective style of coping with anger. They put off venting it until they have cooled down. That way, they control their anger rather than letting the emotion control them.

The following are examples of normal emotions that everyone experiences from time to time. In most cases, these emotions do not threaten your health, but the way in which you respond to them may. Responses to emotions can be both positive and negative.

Anger: Anger is a strong feeling of being mad or unhappy. It is usually the result of an event or series of events that did not go as expected or desired.

- \+ A positive response to anger is to go for a walk, count to ten, or just take some time to cool down.
- − A negative response is to punch the wall, break something, drive fast, or drink a great deal of alcohol.

Frustration: Frustration is a feeling of disappointment, usually resulting when a goal has not been or cannot be met.

- \+ A positive response to frustration is to talk with a friend, take some time to think about the problem, and plan a different approach to dealing with it.
- − A negative response is to quit, yell at a good friend, or blame someone else.

Hostility: Hostility is a feeling of intense anger and anxiety, often an aggressive unfriendly attitude.

- \+ A positive response to hostility is to take time to cool down, to talk with a friend or counselor, or simply to walk away from the problem.
- − A negative response is to fight, say abusive words to the source of hostility, or undermine someone's character by talking behind his or her back in an angry manner.

Fear: Fear is a feeling of being frightened and of not knowing what to expect.

- \+ A positive response to fear is to investigate exactly what causes the fear, name the source of the fear, and restructure your environment to eliminate the source.
- − A negative response is to hide from the fear by staying at home, sleeping excessively, or taking drugs.

Love: Love is a strong feeling of affection and/or deep concern for another person. It may involve intimacy and/or commitment.

+ A positive response to love is to feel pleasure at being loved.
− A negative response to love is denial, fear, or extreme emotional anxiety over the possibility of being rejected.

You can survive almost any emotional problem if you have a humorous perspective. This is because a sense of humor is based on the ability to cut loose from your customary mode of thinking. A good sense of humor can also help lighten life's anxieties and relieve stress. Some researchers believe that laughter can also boost the immune system because it promotes the release of protective chemicals in the brain. This is called mind–body healing. An area of research involving mind–body healing is **psychoneuroimmunology,** the study of how the brain affects the immune system.

The Benefits of a Good Night's Sleep

College students are well-known for "all nighters," during which they stay up through the night to study for an exam or to finish—or even to start—a paper due in the morning. Lack of sleep is nothing to brag or laugh about. Sleep is vital to your life and can help you function at optimal levels both physically and mentally.

On the physical side, sleep helps regulate your metabolism and your body's state of equilibrium. On the mental side, it helps restore your ability to be optimistic and to have a high level of energy and self-confidence. To keep your body in balance, more sleep is needed when you are under stress, experience emotional fatigue, or are undertaking an intense intellectual activity such as learning.

Your emotional state greatly affects your sleeping patterns. "I can't sleep" is a common complaint of people experiencing anxiety and depression. Actually, people with anxiety have trouble getting to sleep, whereas people with depression tend to wake too early. In either case, their normal sleeping patterns are disrupted.

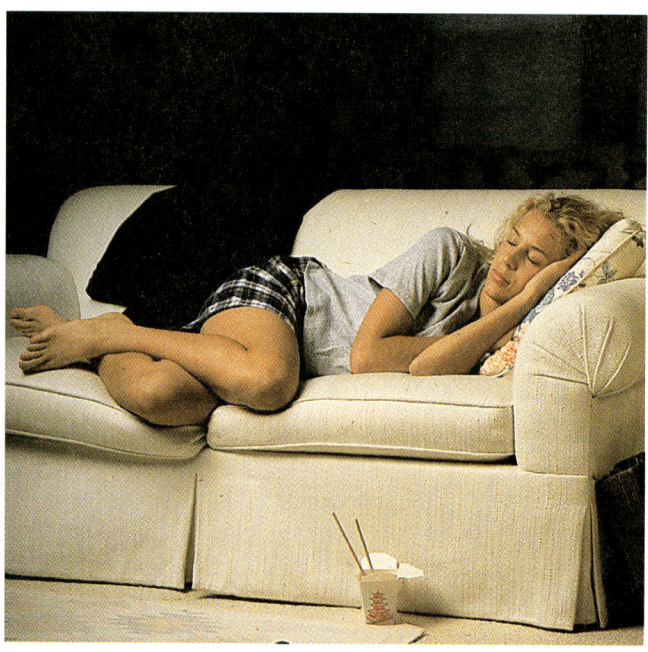

Getting enough sleep is important for your mental health. A catnap in the afternoon can make you feel more alert afterwards, but it is not a substitute for a good night's sleep. (Source: FPG International/© Navaswan)

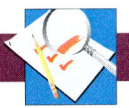

HERE'S LOOKING AT YOU

How Sleep Deprived Are You?

Blame it on the light bulb. Sleep researchers do. Until its invention in 1878, Americans snoozed about nine hours a night, but since then, the average night's sleep has dropped steadily to the current less-than-seven hours. That's not enough. According to the National Commission on Sleep Disorders Research, tens of millions of Americans suffer from a simple lack of sleep that can have grave repercussions—the six-feet-under variety. The National Highway Traffic Safety Administration estimates that as many as 600,000 automobile accidents each year involve driver drowsiness, with about 12,000 resulting in death. Perhaps we need another slogan: "Don't Doze and Drive."

For some, an ideal night's sleep lasts six hours, for others ten. Though catching too few Z's on occasion shouldn't affect your life, night after sleep-deprived night accumulates as a debt. Operate in the red for long enough and tiredness will erode your job performance, relationships, and personality.

So where do you stand? Are you getting enough sleep? Or are you one of many who tries to squeeze as much out of a day as possible? Consider the following:

- Do you ever sleep through your alarm or have difficulty getting up after it's gone off?
- Do you get annoyed by trivial matters as a result of fatigue?
- Do you have difficulty concentrating, or do you find yourself dozing off during the day?
- Do you turn down social events or other activities due to fatigue?
- Do you catch colds or the flu easily?
- Are you needlessly grumpy with your mate or family members because you're tired?
- Do you use caffeine to stay alert during the day or alcohol to help you to relax at night?
- Do you struggle to keep your eyes open when driving at night?
- Are you asleep within five minutes of going to bed?
- Do you wake during the night and find it difficult to fall back to sleep?

If you found yourself answering "yes" to many or most of these questions, you may indeed be getting too little sleep. Try cutting back a little on your busy days. And find a healthy way to unwind at the end of each day—read or watch television. Also, add exercise to your daily routine, although not just before going to bed. Maybe most important, try getting to bed a little earlier each night. If you still find yourself with the same symptoms, your problems may be due to something more serious and you may need to see your doctor.

Source: Adapted from "How Sleep Deprived Are You?" *Health,* September 1993, p. 16. Reprinted by permission of Time Inc. Health

---

For some people, a catnap in the afternoon, lasting about fifteen minutes, offers both physiological and psychological benefits. For example, a catnap can help you digest your food better, and people often report feeling more alert afterwards. Catnaps, however, are not a substitute for a good night's sleep of seven or eight hours, and they do not work for everyone.

Each person has a genetically determined sleep requirement. This level does not change in adulthood. To find out what your sleep requirement is, try going to sleep and waking up at the same time for one month. Then sleep thirty minutes more or less per night and assess whether you feel better or worse during the day. Experiment by adding or subtracting set amounts of sleep until you determine your sleep requirement. It should fall between seven and eight hours per night (see the Here's Looking at You box).

What happens during sleep? Researchers have found several specific stages marking the passage from wakefulness to sleep and back to wakefulness. A peri-

psychoneuroimmunology The study of how the brain affects the immune system.

od of light sleep progresses to deep sleep, with a period of dreaming providing the transition back to light sleep.

During sleep, most people experience periods of what is called rapid eye movement (REM). These movements can be observed beneath closed eyelids. In **REM sleep,** the body is quiet but the mind is active, even hyperactive. Some researchers believe that REM sleep helps you form permanent memories; others believe that this period of active brain waves serves to rid your brain of overstimulation and useless information acquired during the day. REM sleep is the time not only for dreams but also for acceleration of the heart rate and blood flow to the brain. Erections in males and engorgement of the clitoris in females are common. At the same time, skeletal muscles rarely move.

During **non-REM sleep,** in contrast, the body may be active—some people sleepwalk during this period—but the mind is not. In spite of this activity, non-REM sleep is the time when the body does its repair and maintenance work, including cell regeneration.

Although much still needs to be learned about sleep and its functions, few would disagree that sleep plays a role in the maintenance of good mental health. Here is some advice from sleep researchers on how to get a better night's sleep:

- Go to bed and wake up at about the same time each night.
- Exercise regularly, but not just before you go to bed.
- Avoid eating heavy meals two hours before bedtime. Keep nighttime snacks light and easy to digest.
- Stay away from stimulants—coffee, cola drinks, tea, hot cocoa, and chocolate—before you go to bed.
- If you have trouble falling asleep, don't just lie there and become anxious. After thirty minutes, get out of bed, read a book, or do some other restful but productive activity. Try to go to sleep again.
- Don't rely on over-the-counter sleeping aids to help you sleep. They don't always work, and they can have side effects. If you feel you need a sleeping aid more than four days a week or for more than two weeks, consult your physician.

A final point about sleep: Be aware that everyone has sleepless nights on occasion. It is a normal way for the body to adjust to certain situations.

Who Am I? The Importance of Knowing Yourself

Have you ever taken a good look at yourself in the mirror and asked, "Who am I?" The answer is important because who you think you are and what you think of yourself are key indicators of your mental health (see the Developing Health Skills box). Mentally healthy people have an accurate **self-concept** as well as a positive sense of **self-esteem.** They also have a good sense of what they can accomplish (**self-efficacy**) and the ability to fulfill their potential (**self-actualization**).

Self-Concept

Self-concept is how you see yourself. It includes a self-assessment of your strengths and weaknesses. Oliver Cromwell once commissioned a portrait of

rapid eye movement (REM) sleep Sleep during which the eyes flicker back and forth behind closed eyelids; the period of sleep associated with dreaming.

non-REM sleep Sleep during which the eyes are relaxed and not moving; the period of sleep associated with cell regeneration.

self-concept A person's view of himself or herself gained through an assessment of strengths and weaknesses.

self-esteem How a person values himself or herself.

self-efficacy A person's belief that he or she is capable of accomplishing a task or series of tasks under certain conditions.

self-actualization The ability to seek the highest and most idealistic state that can lead to a person's fullest possible development.

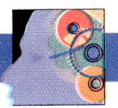

DEVELOPING HEALTH SKILLS

Gaining Strength from Solitude

One way to get to know yourself is through solitude. Being alone gives you a chance to think about yourself and your problems in a concentrated fashion.

Researchers have found that when people are put in isolated environments for even short periods, they are suddenly able to overcome difficulties that have been plaguing them for some time, such as overeating or smoking. Psychologists working on isolation studies conclude that these people mastered their problems because they had the time to sit and think about them.

Most people think of time spent alone as an obstacle to overcome—a void to fill. To gain strength from solitude, think of it instead as an opportunity for self-exploration. Here is some "alone time" advice from experts:

- Keep a journal. Think about yourself and put your thoughts on paper.
- Take on a major project. Instead of buying a bookcase, build one. Instead of reading a poem, write one.
- Develop an interest in something rewarding and intellectually stimulating that you can do by yourself—for example, bird-watch or play the piano.
- Do something that will give you an immediate sense of accomplishment, such as going on a three-mile run or walk, painting the bathroom, or weeding the garden.

The trick to using your solitude effectively is to think of time alone as a luxury instead of a problem.

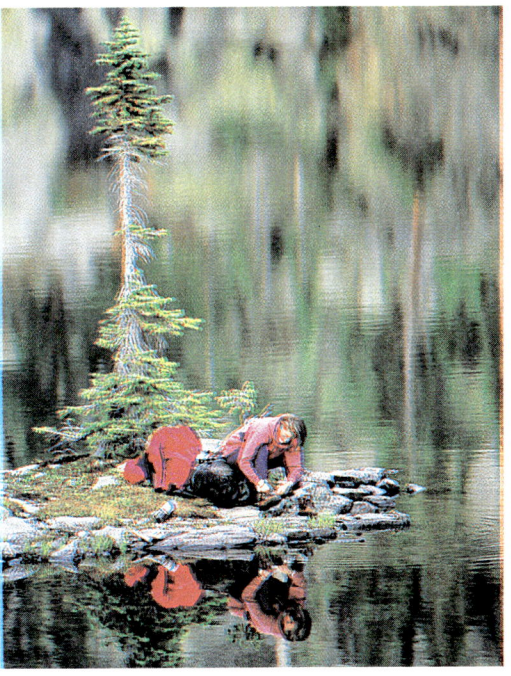

Sometimes it is important to be by yourself. Being alone doesn't necessarily mean being lonely. Solitude can give you time for self-exploration and personal growth. (Source: © Tony Stone Images/Dugald Bremner)

---

himself. When he noticed that the artist was painting the most flattering replica possible, even to the point of leaving out several blemishes, Cromwell said, "Paint me as I am, artist, warts and all!" What Cromwell was seeking was an honest assessment of his physical reality—warts and all.

Acknowledging your less attractive side—for example, a tendency to procrastinate—does not mean that you have to denigrate yourself. A person with an accurate self-concept fully acknowledges who he or she is—warts and all.

Self-Esteem

Self-esteem is how you value yourself. High self-esteem means that you respect yourself and consider yourself worthy. People with high self-esteem recognize their limitations, and they expect to grow and improve themselves. Having a positive sense of self-esteem can contribute to good feelings of competence,

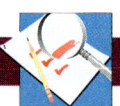

HERE'S LOOKING AT YOU

Rating Your Level of Self-Esteem

This self-esteem scale is designed to assist you in understanding your self-image. Positive attitudes toward "self" are important components of maturation and emotional well-being. Read each statement carefully. Circle the letter in the column that corresponds to your response to each statement.

	Strongly Agree	Agree	Disagree	Strongly Disagree
1. I feel that I'm a person of worth and at least on an equal plane with others.	A	B	C	D
2. I feel that I have a number of good qualities.	A	B	C	D
3. All in all, I am inclined to feel that I am a failure.	D	C	B	A
4. I am able to do things as well as most other people.	A	B	C	D
5. I feel I do not have as much to be proud of as others.	D	C	B	A
6. I take a positive attitude toward myself.	A	B	C	D
7. On the whole, I am satisfied with myself.	A	B	C	D
8. I wish I could have more respect for myself.	D	C	B	A
9. I certainly feel useless at times.	D	C	B	A
10. At times I think I am no good at all.	D	C	B	A

Scoring: To determine your score, first assign a value to each of your answers using the following scale: A = 4 points, B = 3 points, C = 2 points, D = 1 point. Then add up your answers to get your self-esteem score and to see where you fall on the following chart.

Total: _____

40 = Highest self-esteem
35–39 = High self-esteem
30–34 = Above-average self-esteem
20–29 = Below-average self-esteem
less than 20 = Low self-esteem

The higher your score, the more positive your self-esteem. High self-esteem means that individuals respect themselves and consider themselves worthy but do not necessarily consider themselves better than others. They do not feel themselves to be the ultimate in perfection but, on the contrary, recognize their limitations and expect to grow and improve. Self-esteem is the most important variable in regard to human development and maturation. It is the master key that can open the door to the actualization of an individual's human potential.

Source: Robert F. Valois, Sandra K. Kammermann, Kathleen Doyle, & Stafford G. Cox, "Self-Esteem Inventory," pp. 27–28, *Wellness R. S. V. P.*, third edition, 1986, Benjamin/Cummings Publishing Company, Inc., Menlo Park, CA, © 1992 by Valois, Kammerman & Associates and the authors. Used with permission of Valois, Kammerman & Associates and the authors.

worth, and acceptance. It can enhance the formation of meaningful relationships.

Health researchers often link low self-esteem to apathy, anxiety, alcoholism, drug dependence, poor physical health, and lack of accomplishment. In fact, almost every negative health behavior has been linked to some extent to low self-esteem. Without a good sense of self-esteem, you may find it difficult to overcome the fear of rejection or to accept your own limitations or those of others (See the Here's Looking at You box). People who don't have good self-esteem may be especially vulnerable to peer pressures, especially those concerning drug abuse or sexual promiscuity.

Self-Efficacy

If you believe that you can get a job done in an appropriate and timely manner, you have a good sense of self-efficacy. Self-efficacy is more than knowing what to do. It also involves integrating that knowledge into your sense of who you are.

Self-efficacy is one indicator of how you are likely to perform in a specific setting. This sense of self-efficacy is critical to both your mental and physical health. If you believe you can lose weight or stop smoking, you are likely to do so. If you believe you cannot lose weight or stop smoking, your efforts are likely doomed.

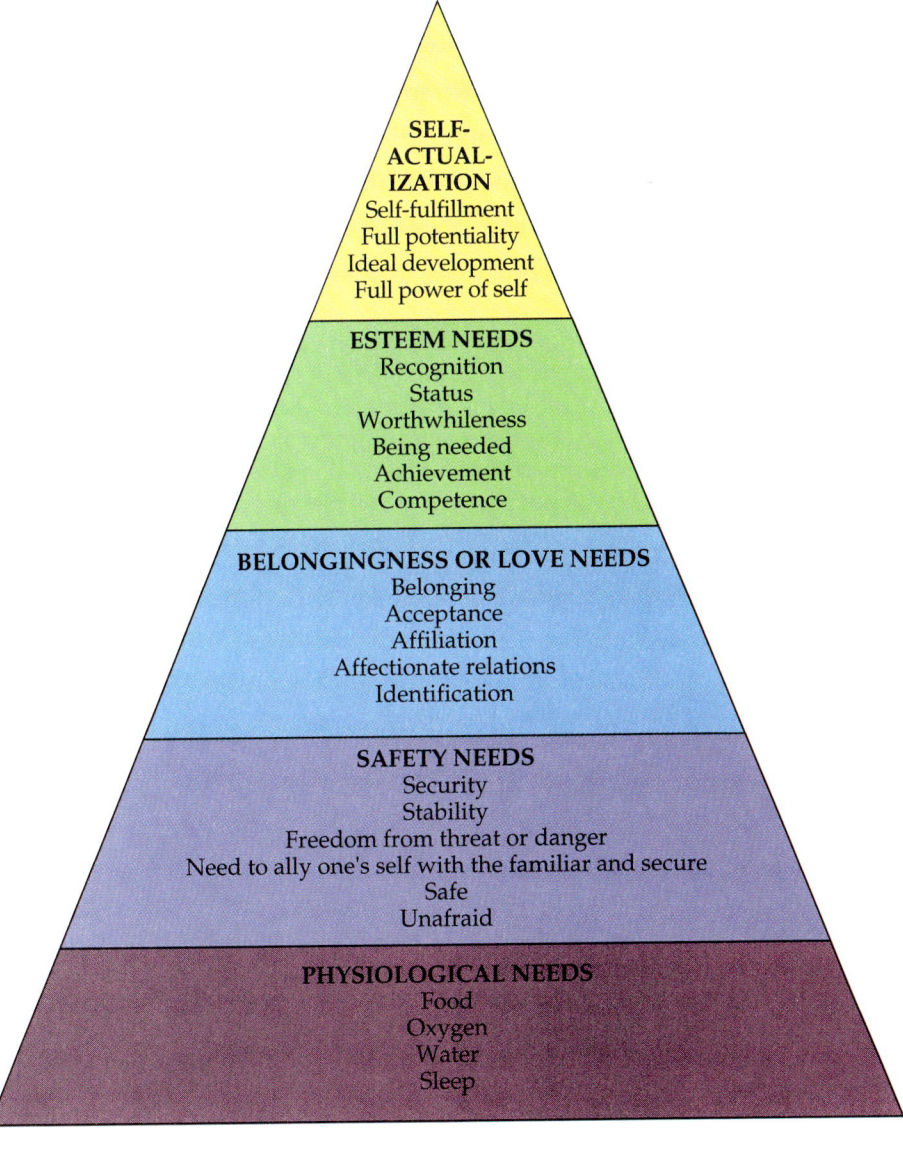

Figure 3.1 Maslow's Hierarchy of Human Needs. *The theory of self-actualization holds that people tend to seek the highest and most idealistic aims that lead to their fullest possible development.*

Self-Actualization

According to the theory of self-actualization formulated by psychologist Abraham Maslow, people tend to seek the highest and most idealistic aims that can lead to their fullest possible development. Maslow has proposed a hierarchy of human needs, and self-actualization is at the top (see Figure 3.1). Once the physiological needs at the bottom have been satisfied, human beings are freed to pursue safety needs, love needs, esteem needs, and, finally, self-actualization.

Self-actualization and good mental health are believed to go hand in hand. Some studies indicate that people who are self-actualizers are likely to be less neurotic. However, Maslow's theory does not lend itself to experimental proof or disproof, so psychologists must take it largely on faith.

A Continuum of Mental Dysorganization

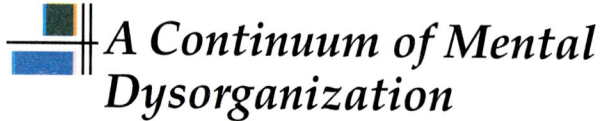

Unfortunately, many people do not live up to their potential because they suffer from mental illness. About one-third of all Americans will have an acute mental illness during their lifetimes, and at any one moment, major mental disorders afflict 16 percent of the nation's population. This in no way suggests that 16 percent of the country is "mad" or "crazy." Such terms, once associated with mental illness, do not fit in with today's concept of mental health and mental illness.

Psychiatrist Karl Menninger coined the word **dysorganization** to describe the difficult and painful experiences someone undergoes in trying to cope with difficult situations in life. According to Menninger, the degree of mental illness a person suffers is in direct proportion to the amount of **dysfunction** present (see Figure 3.2). A person at the first level of dysfunction is what is commonly called nervous; at the second level, neurotic; at the third level, openly aggressive; at the fourth level, psychotic; and at the fifth level, self-destructive. (*Dysorganization* is not the same as *disorganization*. *Dys-* means painful or difficult. In dysorganization, the process of organization or living is painful or difficult. Disorganization connotes a lack of organization, a state of disarray.)

From Everyday Problems to Emotionally Crippling Behavior

Neuroses are the most common type of mental problem. Although neuroses can cause emotional suffering, **neurotic** individuals usually can carry out day-to-day activities. **Anxiety** and **phobia** are examples of neuroses, they are generally viewed as cognitive distortions or unsatisfactory ways of reacting to life situations.

Anxiety is often brought on by an imagined fear of impending danger. Americans experience anxiety more than any other mental health problem (see Figure 3.3). Most anxiety is normal and may play an important role in anticipating situations. For example, the fear of being attacked on a deserted street at night may cause a person to take appropriate actions to avoid such a possibility. You have probably experienced anxiety before taking a final exam. Some of the symptoms you may have had are sweating, dry mouth, heavy breathing, and insomnia. This type of anxiety is in response to a realistic situation.

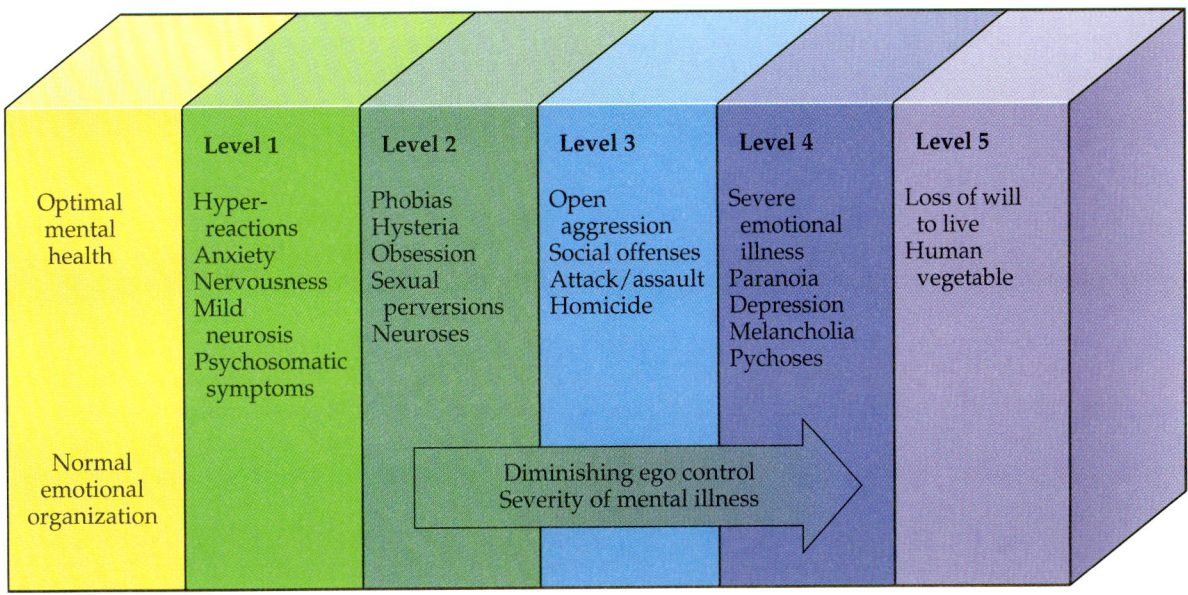

Figure 3.2 A Spectrum of Mental State. *There is a wide range of mental dysfunction. At one end is mild nervousness, which most people experience at one time or another. At the other end is the self-destructive loss of the will to live. Dysorganization is the term that mental health professionals use to describe the difficult and painful experiences someone undergoes in trying to cope with difficult life situations.*

However, some people suffer anxiety over a long period of time and without any apparent cause. A person who has a phobia, for example, has an unreasonable fear of some object or situation. Simple phobias include fear of heights or fear of bees and usually do not interfere with daily activities. Some phobias, however, are more severe and can cause people to lead constricted lives. Because of their irrational fears, some people do not leave the house. Anxiety becomes a serious mental health problem when individuals suffering from it are so emotionally crippled that they cannot continue at school, hold a job, or otherwise lead a satisfying and productive life.

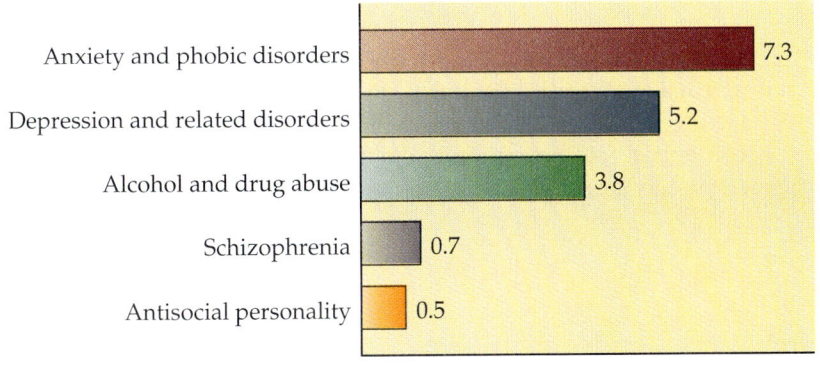

Figure 3.3 The Most Common Mental Health Disorders.
More people experience anxiety than any other mental health problem. Anxiety often stems from an imagined fear of impending danger. (Source: National Institute of Mental Health)

dysorganization Pain or difficulty in the process of organization or living.

dysfunction The inability to function properly.

neuroses Cognitive distortions or unsatisfactory ways of reacting to life situations.

neurotic To display a neurosis.

anxiety A state of apprehension or tension, often accompanied by physiological signs.

phobia An unreasonable fear of some object or situation.

CULTURAL VIEW

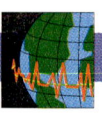

Women and Depression—Greater Risk?

Psychiatrists and psychologists have devoted much thought and study to the issue of gender and depression. Although there is general agreement that numerous factors contribute to a higher rate of depression in women, the nature of those components is a subject of ongoing debate. The commonly acknowledged ones include emotional "hard wiring," developmental experiences, and social conditioning.

These factors are interrelated. Women are considered to be more responsive to signals from others and more reliant on external feedback for their sense of self. They are also more likely than men to repress anger or aggression or to turn those feelings on themselves, rather than to vent them appropriately. Moreover, society expects the "good woman" to subordinate her needs to those of others. All these tendencies contribute to a loss of self-esteem—a central feature of depression.

The stage for depression during adulthood may be set quite early in life. Girls are traditionally taught that reticence and modesty are traits to be cultivated, and they learn to defer to boys in the classroom and in social situations. Being habitually relegated to the background erodes their sense of self-worth. The stresses of adolescence—including the struggle for independence from one's mother, the dawn of awareness of one's sexuality, increased freedom to make one's own decisions, hormonal changes, and, often, a negative body image—can also play a role.

Pregnancy is not associated with an increased risk of depression, but the postpartum period is. About 15 percent of new mothers have symptoms of depression, which may persist for several months. Immediately after childbirth, women who have had major depressive episodes previously are at greater risk for recurrence. When childbirth is experienced as a physical separation from the baby, it may foster feelings of emptiness and depletion; a shift of attention to the baby can bring a sense of abandonment, particularly when the mother's support systems are

(continued)

Critical Thinking Question

Healthy People 2000 established a goal of reducing "the prevalence of mental disorders (exclusive of substance abuse) among adults living in the community to less than 10.7 percent." The latest data suggest that about 16 percent of adults living in the community currently have mental disorders. What strategies would you suggest for achieving this goal?

From Being Sad to Depression as a Mental Illness

minor depression An emotional state in which a person's normal feelings of sadness, guilt, and hopelessness are exaggerated.

Like anxiety, depression is a common disorder experienced by mentally healthy people from time to time. **Minor depression** is a mental state in which feelings of sadness, guilt, and hopelessness are exaggerated. Feeling depressed is so common an emotional state that it would be considered abnormal if you did not, on

inadequate. The roles of hormonal changes and stresses following childbirth are also under study.

Although it was once widely believed that depression was a common consequence of menopause, numerous epidemiologic investigations have failed to demonstrate an increase in the rate of depression at midlife. When the end of fertility comes at the time that one's children are entering adolescence or leaving home, some women experience a sense of loss; in contrast, many others find the release from the possibility of pregnancy to be a liberating experience.

More women than men become depressed late in life, when women often have more risk factors for depression, such as social isolation and bereavement.

It's important to note that depression is often associated with certain medical conditions. It can be precipitated by a stroke, heart attack, or cancer, or by the use of some medications. Because depression can be responsible for memory loss or for difficulty in reasoning, it is often mistakenly identified in older women as dementia or Alzheimer's disease.

Depression can also coexist with another mental illness. It can underlie—or stem from—substance abuse or addiction, eating disorders, or anxiety disorders. In such cases, the clinician usually identifies one disorder as the "primary" condition and treats it first.

Depression is more than the blues. It is not a personal failing, and it is readily treated. If you think you may be suffering from any of the depressive illnesses, it is important to remember that these are conditions that usually do not go away on their own, nor are they alleviated simply by bucking up and adopting a positive attitude. Get help. Seeking treatment for depression is no more a sign of weakness than seeing a doctor for an infection is. With proper therapy you can feel better within weeks.

Source: "Depression", excerpted from the November 1997 issue (pp. 2–4) of the *Harvard Women's Health Watch*, © 1997, President and Fellows of Harvard College

occasion, feel depressed or sad ("I have the blues today."). The breakup of a significant relationship or other traumatic changes involving personal relationships can bring on a brief period of sorrow. Most people rebound from temporary setbacks once the initial sense of loss wears off.

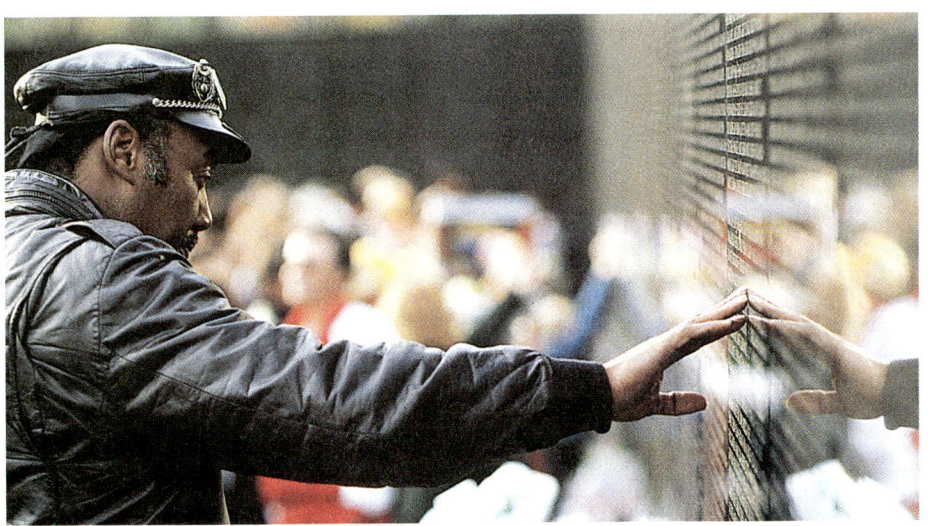

It is normal to be sad and depressed for a brief period of time, especially when you experience a significant loss. But depression can be a serious mental illness when it is accompanied by feelings of helplessness over a long period of time. (Source: © Tony Stone Images/ Paul Merideth)

YOUR ENVIRONMENTAL NEIGHBORHOOD

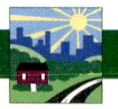

Seasonal Affective Disorder

Although April has been deemed the cruelest month, February may be the SADdest. For many of us in the higher latitudes, seasonal affective disorder (SAD), which recurs in the fall and ends in the spring, has exacted its cumulative toll. Some of its symptoms are typical of depression—sadness, irritability, inability to concentrate, withdrawal into solitude, and loss of interest in life. Other manifestations may include excessive and restless sleep, lethargy during waking hours, increased appetite, carbohydrate craving, and weight gains averaging ten pounds.

Probable Causes

Researchers have associated SAD with a diminished exposure to light and have established that more than 80 percent of patients with SAD are women, most of whom developed their first symptoms while in their twenties. Yet scientists haven't pinpointed the malady's precise mechanism. There are several speculations, most of which relate to melatonin, the hormone thought to play a major role in regulating the body's twenty-four-hour cycle. Melatonin production takes place in the pineal gland, a pea-sized organ buried deep in the brain, and in the photoreceptors of the retina. It is stimulated by darkness and suppressed by light, and thus is present in greater concentrations in the winter.

Many researchers believe that SAD sufferers are either extrasensitive to dim light and manufacture too much of the hormone or are oversensitive to the usual amount that is produced. Others maintain that people with SAD secrete melatonin later in the day than do their unaffected counterparts, disrupting their circadian rhythms. Because most women appear to "outgrow" SAD after menopause, some theorize that it may be related to female hormone levels.

There is also speculation that dopamine—a neurotransmitter, or chemical that ferries signals between nerves and brain cells—may play a role in SAD. Depletion of another neurotransmitter, serotonin, has been implicated in the carbohydrate craving that often accompanies SAD.

Treatment

Whatever SAD's biochemical roots, it can be alleviated with the one thing missing from the winter equation—bright light. Regular exposure to bright light can alleviate the symptoms for up to 80 percent

(continued)

---

major depression Depression that is extreme, more intense, and longer lasting and that usually interferes with daily life; often characterized as a mood or affective disorder.

affective disorder A condition in which moods or emotions become extreme and interfere with daily life.

premenstrual dysphoric disorder A form of depression occurring just prior to menstruation and characterized by fatigue, irritability, mood swings, and physical symptoms such as abdominal bloating, swollen hands or feet, headaches, and tender breasts; a severe form of premenstrual syndrome.

Major depression is when a person experiences the feelings of sadness and hopelessness with such intensity or over such a long period of time that those feelings interfere with normal day-to-day activities. Some people have only one episode of depression in their lifetimes; others slip into depression from time to time. Severe depression takes many forms. Collectively, they are called mood or **affective disorders.** The Cultural View discusses gender differences in depression.

Premenstrual dysphoric disorder (PMDD) is an example of a depressive disorder characterized by feelings of hopelessness, fatigue, mood swings, and other physical symptoms such as bloating, swollen hands or feet, headaches, and tender breasts. This is different from **premenstrual syndrome** (PMS), which has many of the same symptoms but to a much lesser degree. Although as many as 70 percent of menstruating women have some symptoms of PMS, only between 3 percent to 5 percent of women have the most severe form of PMDD. Both are examples of a disorder that involves the biological, as well as the psychological, system.

A form of severe depression, which is characterized by cycles of manic highs and depressive lows, is **manic-depressive illness.** It is also called bipolar disor-

of people with SAD. The simplest solution may be to get to a sunnier climate. The incidence of SAD is almost 10 percent in New Hampshire, but only about 1 percent in Florida.

For those who can't engineer winter getaways, therapy using artificial light may do the trick. During light therapy, the patient sits three feet away from a bank of fluorescent lights mounted on a metal reflector and shielded with a plastic screen. The intensity of light emitted is about 10,000 lux, which is about twenty times brighter than ordinary room light and is designed to approximate dawn. This treatment requires from twenty minutes to two hours of exposure daily and can be undertaken at home. However, it should be done only under the guidance of a qualified health professional.

Light boxes are classified as experimental devices by the U.S. Food and Drug Administration. Therefore, manufacturers are not allowed to market them for the treatment of SAD, and the many different products available are not regulated.

A light box costs anywhere from $300 to $500—an expense that is covered by some, but not all, health plans. Some manufacturers will rent light boxes for a trial period to allow the user to determine whether the therapy is beneficial. Most of the devices are designed to sit on a table or desk; some are portable and lightweight.

Those who respond to light therapy may notice that their moods have improved as soon as two to four days into the course of treatment. The symptoms may disappear completely within a week or two.

A few people have reported side effects from treatment, including irritability, eye strain, headaches, or insomnia. Light therapy is not recommended for people who have photosensitive skin or are taking drugs that increase light sensitivity or for those who have had eye surgery.

SAD can also be treated with antidepressant drugs. Because the standard tricyclics tend to cause drowsiness and increased appetite, the newer selective serotonin reuptake inhibitors (SSRIs), which often have the reverse effects, may be better alternatives. Researchers are also investigating whether a melatonin supplement given at just the right time of day could reset the body's clock. For some patients, a combination of drug treatment and light therapy may be most effective.

Source:"Seasonal Affective Disorder," excerpted from the February 1994 issue (p. 7) of the *Harvard Women's Health Watch,* © 1994, President and Fellows of Harvard College

der. Researchers have found that depression—particularly manic-depressive illness—runs in families. Another form of depression is **seasonal affective disorder,** which is one reason some people get more depressed in the winter. It is believed that the absence of bright daylight causes chemical changes in the brain, which bring on depression (see the Your Environmental Neighborhood box).

The dividing line between sadness and depression is fuzzy, but experts say that you should seek professional help if you have some of the following symptoms for more than two weeks: persistent sadness, feelings of worthlessness or hopelessness, loss of interest or pleasure in daily activities (including sex), inability to concentrate or make decisions, crying a lot, feeling restless or irritable, inability to sleep, and/or suicidal thoughts.

Depression can emerge in early childhood and adolescence, but it usually first appears in young adults—when people are in their early twenties. Although most people with depression are under age forty-five, many elderly people thought to suffer from Alzheimer's disease and other types of **dementia** may instead have treatable depression. Nine out of ten people recover from depression with treatment. Without treatment, depression can last for years and even lead to suicide.

premenstrual syndrome A combination of emotional and physical features which occur before menstruation; characterized by mood changes, discomfort, swelling and tenderness in the breasts, a bloated feeling, headache, and fatigue.

manic-depressive illness A form of depression characterized by cycles of manic highs and depressive lows; also called bipolar disorder.

seasonal affective disorder A form of depression brought on by lack of sufficient daylight.

dementia Mental confusion and loss of brain function that can be caused by disease or old age.

Psychotic Disorders

Psychotic disorders or **psychoses** are mental disorders so serious that they result in loss of touch with reality. Often, psychoses require hospitalization. The most common and disabling psychosis is **schizophrenia.**

Schizophrenia is the word used to describe a complex mental illness in which the person has his or her own view of reality. This view of the world is often very different from the view of normal people. For example, a schizophrenic might see things that do not exist, such as a dead mother, or live in a world without time, dimension, or color. Because of its complexity, few generalizations hold true for all people who are diagnosed as schizophrenic.

Schizophrenia takes two basic forms: acute and chronic. With the onset of delusional symptoms, a person is said to be experiencing acute schizophrenia. Some people may have only one episode in their lives; others have repeated acute episodes and lead relatively normal lives in between. The first symptoms of schizophrenia are often seen in the teens or twenties in men, and in the thirties and early forties in women. These symptoms include **hallucinations** (seeing or hearing things that are not present), delusions (false beliefs despite obvious proof to the contrary), **disordered thinking** (disconnected or incoherent thought processes and speech), and inappropriate affect (showing emotions that are inconsistent with the person's thoughts). Chronic schizophrenics never fully recover normal functioning.

Schizophrenia has no single cause, but it is likely brought on by a combination of factors. Schizophrenia has long been known to run in families, and recently the gene for at least one kind of schizophrenia has been identified. Close relatives of schizophrenics are more likely to develop the disorder than are persons who are not related to a schizophrenic patient. Twin studies provide another indication of a family tie. The development of schizophrenia in both members of a twin pair is more likely among identical twins than among fraternal twins. Researchers are studying other factors as well. For example, brain scans have disclosed that schizophrenics are more likely to have structural brain abnormalities than are normal persons of the same age.

Currently, no single cure exists for schizophrenia, although a review of 2,000 patients' records from first breakdown to old age suggests that 25 percent achieve full recovery, 50 percent recover partially, and 25 percent require lifelong care. Schizophrenia treatments include antipsychotic drugs, shock treatment, psychosocial and behavioral therapy, and skills training. Most patients are treated in halfway houses and group homes, although some chronic schizophrenics require prolonged hospitalization or residential care.

Suicide: A Symptom of Mental Illness

Every year, there are more than 200,000 suicide attempts (an unsuccessful attempt to end one's life) and 30,000 completed suicides. In reality, there are countless more suicides. Suicide is heavily underreported as a result of the social stigma attached to it and the often uncertain circumstances in which it happens. For example, many single-car crashes may be suicides.

The reasons people commit suicide are complex, highly interrelated, and only partially understood. The major causes are psychological, biological, and sociological. Collectively, they contribute to the profile of a suicide.

Suicidologists, specialists who study suicide, report that a cluster of psychological symptoms can be warning signs of depression and possible suicidal behavior. These include a change in behavior, loss of interest in usual activities, weight loss or gain, withdrawal from friends and family, and feelings of hopelessness or guilt. Self-destructive behaviors such as excessive drinking or drug use also indicate an increased risk. According to the National Institute of Mental Health, 15 percent of depressed individuals die by suicide.

In some cases, a family history of suicide suggests a biological component. A study of psychiatric inpatients showed that half of the persons with a family history of suicide had attempted suicide themselves. Researchers also know that people who have committed or attempted suicide tend to have a deficiency of a key chemical messenger in the brain, a neurotransmitter called **serotonin**. Serotonin is associated with the regulation of aggression, mood, and memory.

Social pressures as well can lead a person to commit suicide. The death of a spouse, loss of a job, even eviction from an apartment can be seen as a sign of rejection. Social isolation and family conflict are other factors involved in an increased risk of suicide.

Suicide among Teens and Elders

It has never been easy being a teenager, but spurred by changing social patterns, suicide is becoming an increasing way out of problems for young people. Suicide is the third leading cause of death among people aged fifteen to twenty-four, after unintentional injuries and homicide (see the Cultural View box).

As just one example, more than 60 percent of a group of 380 students attending an academically select public high school in New York City reported having thoughts about killing themselves. Nearly 10 percent reported that they had made at least one actual attempt to kill themselves.

What causes such feelings? According to one psychologist, suicidal teenagers talk about a recurring theme: hopelessness. In growing numbers, adolescents just don't "feel" hopeless; they say, "I am" hopeless. Compounding the problem, as many as 90 percent of suicidal teenagers believe that their parents do not understand them. The teens feel isolated and anonymous.

While adolescent suicide is a focus of media attention, the elderly are quietly taking their lives, too. The elderly comprise only 12 percent of the population but account for about 20 percent of all reported suicides. The most common reason for suicide among the elderly is depression associated with chronic physical ailments. A significant number of elderly suicides likely go unreported. Noncompliance with a drug regimen, refusal to eat, and mixing medications are common ways in which an older person can slip into a nonreported suicide.

How a Suicidal Person Thinks

People who commit suicide act according to their own systems of logic. Suicide, to them, is not an incomprehensible act of self-destruction. Rather, they see death as the only solution to their problems, according to psychologist Edwin Shneidman, founder of the American Association of Suicidology. Based on the hundreds of people with suicidal tendencies whom he has interviewed and the suicide notes and diaries he has read of people who have actually committed suicide, Shneidman has identified ten common characteristics of suicide:

1. *Unendurable psychological pain.* People who commit suicide often feel psychological pain. This pain is so great that it leads the suicidal person to seek escape through death.
2. *Frustrated psychological needs.* Everyone needs security, achievement, trust, and friendship. Likewise, everyone experiences frustration in satisfying these needs. The suicidal person often concludes from such frustration that his or her needs will never be met.

psychoses Mental disorders that can result in a loss of touch with reality.

schizophrenia A complex mental illness in which an individual has a distorted view of reality.

hallucinations The sensation of seeing or hearing things that are not present.

disordered thinking Disconnected or incoherent thought processes and speech.

suicidologist A person who studies suicide.

serotonin A neurotransmitter associated with the regulation of aggression, mood, and memory.

3. *The search for a solution.* Suicide is done for a reason. The suicidal person believes that his or her suicide is a way out of a problem or crisis.
4. *An attempt to end consciousness.* The reason for suicide is to stop awareness of a painful existence. A suicidal person, therefore, seeks to end consciousness and move away from pain.
5. *Helplessness and hopelessness.* Shame, guilt, loss of effectiveness, and frustrated dependency are often cited as reasons for suicide. The suicidal person feels underlying all of these a sense of powerlessness and believes that no one can help with this pain. The only alternative, then, is to commit suicide.
6. *Constriction of options.* Most of the problems of life are highly complex, presenting a variety of options for action and a variety of outcomes. Instead of looking for a range of answers for their problems, suicidal people think of only two alternatives: a total solution or a total cessation.
7. *Ambivalence.* Having ambivalent feelings is common. For example, it is possible both to love and hate your mother. In the case of suicide, ambivalence is a matter of life and death. A suicidal person cuts his or her throat and cries out for help at the same time.
8. *Communication of intent.* About 80 percent of suicidal people give family and friends clear clues about their intention to kill themselves.
9. *Departure.* Running away from home, quitting a job, and abandoning a spouse are all departures. Suicide is the ultimate escape—a plan for a radical, permanent change of scene.
10. *Lifelong coping patterns.* The suicidal person has often established departure as his or her way of coping with difficulty. For example, he or she may have quit a job rather than be fired or walked out of a marriage rather than go through with a divorce. This is a "cut and run" method of solving problems.

Warning Signs for You to Spot

HEALTH SKILLS

Many suicides are preventable—if the clues are seen by others. There are many warning signals that you can watch for in classmates who you think may be suicidal. Here are seven of them:

1. Depression
2. Drop in grades
3. Excessive worrying, especially over grades
4. Social isolation or withdrawal
5. Extreme pessimism
6. Substance abuse
7. Change in normal habits

What can you do if you believe a friend or classmate is suicidal? Here are some tips from psychologists who work with suicidal people.

- Confront the individual with your concerns in this matter. Don't mince words; speak honestly and directly. Ask the person: "Are you thinking about killing yourself?"
- Be a friend. Offer support and a listening ear. Suggest concrete alternative actions.
- Break confidentiality and tell someone else—a close relative, the dorm counselor or resident assistant, or a mental health professional.
- If you are really worried, remove all potentially lethal weapons from that person's house or room. Don't leave him or her alone.

Getting Help for Mental Health Problems

Mild anxiety and depression can be treated over a relatively short period of time through professional counseling and/or stress management techniques (see Chapter 4). College and the years beyond it are among the most unsettling times of life, and nearly half of all visits to psychiatrists are made by people aged twenty-five to forty-four. There are several forms of therapy and types of therapists that you may find helpful at various points in your life.

The following is a list of some of the professionals who are trained specifically to assist with mental health problems:

Psychiatrists. A psychiatrist is a physician who has several years of specialty training in the diagnosis and treatment of mental problems. Psychiatrists understand both the physical and emotional aspects of their patients. Their broad training allows them to use many treatment approaches. Of the mental health professionals, only psychiatrists can prescribe antianxiety drugs, antidepressants, and other drugs. Child psychiatrists specialize in working with children; geriatric psychiatrists specialize in helping the elderly.

Psychologists. The field of psychology covers many specialties, including clinical treatment, testing, community organization, and laboratory research. Psychologists who conduct psychotherapy are generally called clinical psychologists or counseling psychologists. They work in many settings, including private practice, hospitals and clinics, schools, mental health centers, and employee assistance programs. In most states, a licensed psychologist has a doctoral degree in psychology.

Social workers. Some of the tasks that social workers are trained to perform involve individual and group therapy, diagnosis, and referral and consultation for mental health problems. Psychiatric social workers have master's

HealthLinks

National Alliance of the Mentally Ill
www.nami.org/

The latest information and releases about research and care in mental health.

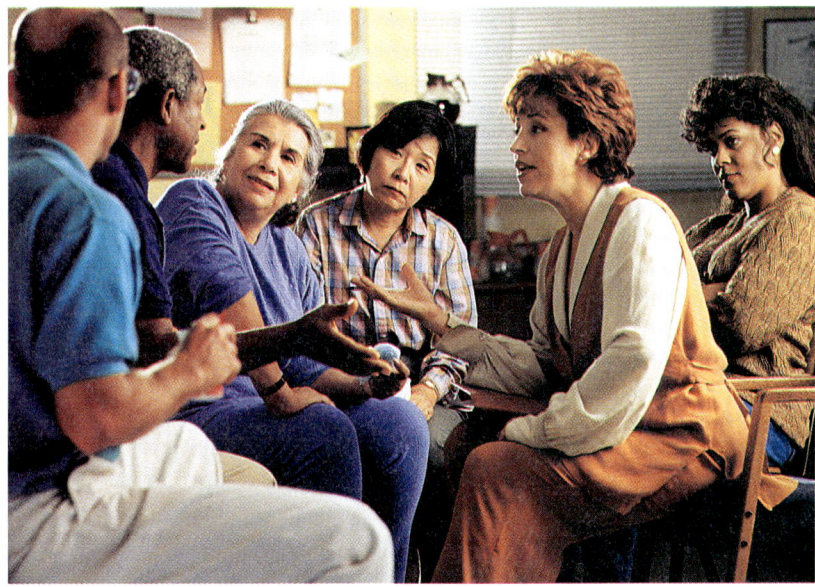

Group therapy has become increasingly popular as members with like issues, guided by the therapist, help each other with problems. (Source: © Tony Stone Images/Bruce Ayers)

degrees in social work and have completed field-placement programs in therapy and consultation.

Mental health counselors. A mental health counselor is trained to help with decision making. Counselors work with individuals and groups in private practice, business, schools, and mental health and other community agencies. A certified clinical mental health counselor has a master's degree and clinical training.

Critical Thinking Question

How accessible are mental health services in your community or on your campus? When considering this question, be sure to differentiate between accessibility and availability. Availability suggests that a service exists in your community or on your campus. Accessibility means that you can get to it. What barriers, both physical and psychological, prevent people from taking advantage of mental health services?

HEALTH SKILLS

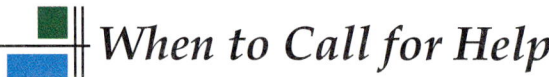

When to Call for Help

Perhaps the most difficult decision concerning mental health is a judgment call—when to call for help. There are several health skills involved in making that decision.

The skill of self-assessment. No one is better equipped to assess your feelings than you. What is your mood? Is it normal? Are you experiencing an unusual amount of anger, depression, anxiety? Have these feelings persisted for too long? Do you need to talk with someone? By assessing yourself, you can help answer the question, "What is the state of my mental health?" The more accurate and honest your self-assessment, the better the chance of getting the right help at the right time.

Decision-making skills. These skills are necessary for you to take action. Because mental problems are a part of normal living, you must decide when the pressures and difficulties of life cross the line from being normal to representing barriers to everyday living. This is most easily accomplished when it is based on a thorough self-understanding of normal emotions and a recognition of extreme emotional distress. Equipped with a thorough self-understanding, you are equipped to make the decision to seek help.

The skill of asking for help. Knowing how to get help is an important skill in tending to your mental health. In its simplest form, calling for help can be asking a friend for advice or seeking someone who will just listen. In a more complex form, it can be arranging for an appointment with a counselor or clinical psychologist.

The following are examples of situations in which you may want to contact a mental health professional for help:

- If you have a problem accepting a new environment
- If a close family member or friend dies
- If you experience financial difficulty
- If you are pregnant (or your girlfriend is) and don't want to have a baby
- If you are fired from a job
- If you experience a personal injury or illness

In some situations help is absolutely necessary. Some examples are:

- If you lose control of your emotions
- If you lose the will to live
- If you can't sleep
- If you have a constant feeling of hopelessness
- If you become dependent on alcohol or drugs
- If you develop an eating disorder
- If you think about suicide

Other situations may occur in which help is absolutely necessary. A brief period during which you lose control of your emotions does not necessarily mean you are having a breakdown or a serious mental upset. But in conjunction with not sleeping well and feeling hopeless, it is an indication of depression. In such a case, professional help is needed.

Calling for help is not a demonstration of weakness. In fact, it may be an important expression of inner strength—of good mental health.

Key Concepts

1. Mental health refers to an individual's emotional and social well-being.
2. There are countless emotions, such as anger, love, fear, and joy. These emotions occur at different levels of intensity.
3. It is mentally healthy to express emotions, but there are healthy and less healthy ways of doing so.
4. Self-concept, self-esteem, and self-efficacy are all elements of knowing oneself—self-assessment.
5. Neuroses are the most frequent type of mental disorder. They can cause emotional suffering, but most people who have neuroses can carry out day-to-day activities.
6. Some anxiety is normal and may play an important role in anticipating situations. Anxiety sustained over a long period of time, however, may result in physical symptoms such as muscle tension and back and neck pain.
7. It is common to feel sad and depressed from time to time, but depression becomes a mental illness when it is experienced with such intensity and over such a long period of time that it interferes with normal day-to-day activities.
8. Psychoses are mental disorders that are so serious as to result in loss of touch with reality. Schizophrenia is the most common and disabling psychosis.

9. Every year, there are more than 200,000 suicide attempts, and 30,000 are completed. Suicide is the third leading cause of death among people aged fifteen to twenty-four years old.
10. Many types of professionals are trained specifically to assist with mental health problems, including psychologists, psychiatrists, and counselors.

■ Review Questions

1. Differentiate between mental health and mental illness.
2. Explain the concept of "normal" as it is used to define both mental health and mental illness.
3. List seven characteristics of a mentally healthy (well-adjusted) individual.
4. Explain what is meant by "a good night's sleep," and explain the health implications of a lack of sleep.
5. Describe the similarities and differences between the following elements of knowing yourself: self-concept, self-esteem, self-efficacy, self-actualization.
6. Define neurosis and give examples of this mental problem.
7. Explain how depression is both normal and abnormal, and differentiate between simply feeling sad and being clinically depressed.
8. Describe the symptoms of schizophrenia.
9. List the warning signs that suggest that an individual is contemplating suicide.
10. Differentiate between each of the following mental health professionals: psychiatrist, psychologist, social worker, mental health counselor.

■ Selected Bibliography

Diagnostic and Statistical Manual of Mental Disorders (4th ed., rev.). Washington, DC: American Psychiatric Association, 1994.

Johnson, J. E., and E. B. Zechmeister. *Critical Thinking: A Foundational Approach.* Pacific Grove, CA: Brooks/Cole, 1992.

Kessler, R., et al. "Lifetime and 12-Month Prevalence of DSM-IIIR Psychiatric Disorders in the U.S." *Archives of General Psychiatry* 51 (1994): 8–19.

Kime, R. E. *Wellness: Mental Health.* Guilford, CT: Dushkin, 1992.

Maslow, A. H. *Motivation and Personality* (3rd ed.). New York: Harper & Row, 1987.

Mental Health, United States, 1996. Rockville, MD: 1996. U.S. Department of Health and Human Services, Substance Abuse and Mental Health Administration.

Reiger, D. A., et al. "The De Facto U.S. Mental and Addictive Disorders Service Systems." *Archives of General Psychiatry* 50 (1993): 85–94.

■ HealthLinks: Web Sites for Information on Mental Health Issues

You can access better health as it relates to this chapter by checking out some of the following sites on the Internet. These and sites identified within the chapter can be accessed directly when you visit the *HealthStyles* Web Site located on the Allyn and Bacon home page at **http://www.abacon.com**.

National Institute of Mental Health
www.nimh.nih.gov
General information on mental disorders, diagnosis, and treatment, as well as the latest research in the field.

National Mental Health Association
www.worldcorp.com/dc-online/nmha/index.html
The nation's only citizen volunteer advocacy organization dedicated to improving mental health of all individuals and achieving victory over mental illness.

Health Hotlines: Managing Your Mental Health

National Alliance for the Mentally Ill
(800) 950-6264
200 North Glebe Road, Suite 1015
Arlington, VA 22203-3754

National Institute of Mental Health, Depression Awareness
(800) 421-4211
1401 Peachtree Street
Atlanta, GA 30309

National Mental Health Association Information Center
(800) 969-6642
1021 Prince Street
Alexandria, VA 22314-2971

National Mental Health Consumer Self-Help Clearinghouse
(800) 553-4539
1211 Chestnut Street
Philadelphia, PA 1910

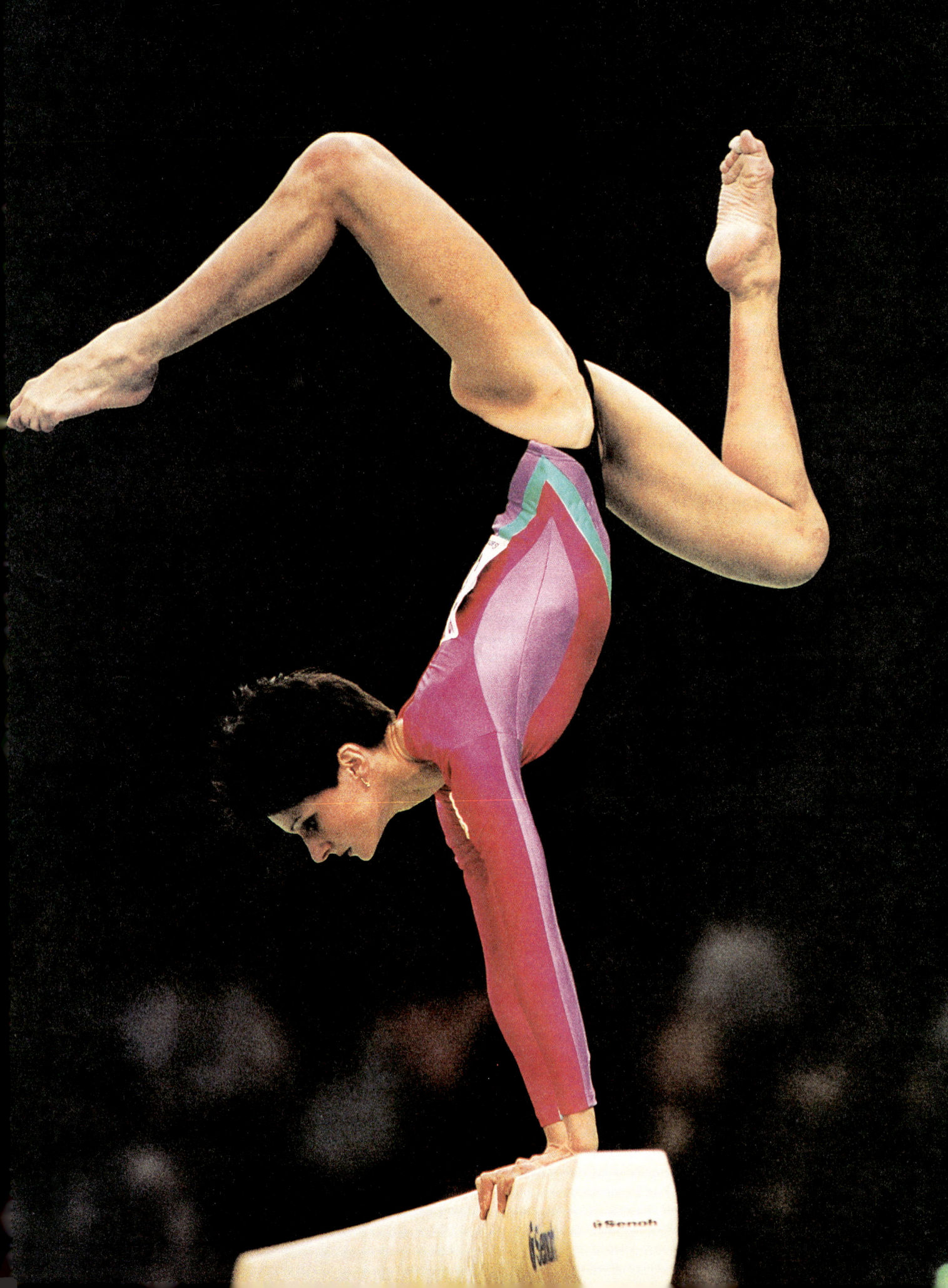

Chapter 4

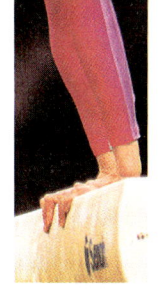
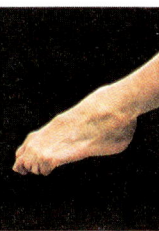
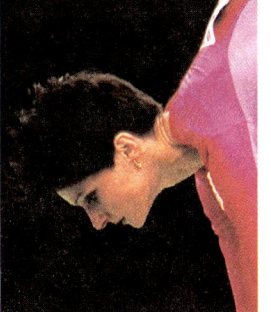

Coping with Stress

Objectives

When you finish reading this chapter, you will be able to:

1. Define *stress* and recognize it as a part of your daily life.
2. List several common stressors and the origin of each.
3. Differentiate between primary stressors and secondary stressors and explain the effect of each.
4. Understand that stress results from a reaction to events, not from the events themselves.
5. Differentiate between distress and eustress.
6. Recognize the scientific connection between too much stress and the incidence of disease.
7. Describe sources of stress in college life and in the work environment.
8. Develop skills of coping with stress, including changing the perception of stressors, managing time, and managing emotion.
9. Recognize that exercise is an effective stress-management practice.
10. Practice relaxation skills, including progressive muscle relaxation and meditation.

What Is Your HealthStyle?

George knew it would be a bad day. It started out wrong as soon as he woke up and saw that it was raining hard. Traffic would be backed up, and he hated getting stuck like that. In fact, George was right. There was a tie-up, and he arrived late for class—and fuming. George was still angry at lunch time, when he gulped down a sandwich and a cup of black coffee before rushing off to the library. Later, he took two aspirins for his "stress" headache, which he said he knew was coming. This is George's way of coping with things out of his control—getting angry and letting the daily hassles of life fester and bother him for hours.

When Juan woke up and saw that it was raining hard, he got dressed quickly, ate breakfast, and began driving to school early. He knew from experience that he was likely to get caught in a traffic jam, and he had a lot to get done in the library and didn't want to lose any time. He also knew how stressful it could be sitting in a car that was going nowhere. But Juan had his way of dealing with this, too—books on tape, which allowed him to use the "dead" time productively, and more important, enjoyably. He arrived at school feeling good and on time to get his work done.

Juan usually handles stress well. Instead of getting angry at things, such as the traffic, he tries to find ways to deal positively with frustrating situations that are out of his control.

In Your Opinion

George and Juan faced the same stressor—the promise of a long line of slow-moving traffic. From the start, George mismanaged his stress, while Juan managed his situation well.

- What steps did George take that started him on his downward spiral?
- At what point could he have reversed the situation?
- What health skills did Juan possess that George did not?
- What message do you get from Juan's way of handling stress?
- What would you have done in this situation?

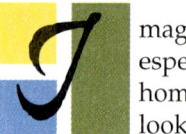

Imagine life without stress. It might sound like a good thing to you, especially when you are facing the pressures of exams, conflicts at home or at work, or daily hassles such as running to catch a bus or looking for a parking space.

In reality, there is no such thing as a stress-free life. However, there are positive and negative stressors and positive and negative ways of coping with them. Low levels of stress can act as motivators. For example, the stress of having done poorly on a test can prompt you to study and do well on the final exam. But too much stress and poor coping strategies can be harmful to your health and can lead to a wide range of conditions, including migraine headaches, rashes, ulcers, anxiety, depression, and heart disease.

Some stressors can be avoided or the impact of them made less taxing. You can drop a course that is too difficult or be tutored so that you keep up with the class. Other stressors, such as the sickness or death of a loved one, are totally unavoidable. Stress, whether avoidable or unavoidable, and how you deal with it can have a significant impact on your health.

Defining Stress

Stress is a perception of an external situation or event taking place in your life that can result in an internal response such as nervous tension, an upset stomach, or other physical or psychological symptoms. The **stress response** is a series of events within the body that involves chemicals, hormones, and neural impulses. The stress response is caused by **stressors,** specific events that disrupt equilibrium and initiate this complex biochemical response. Stress is highly individualized, and what one person perceives as stressful may be thought of as highly stimulating and not at all stressful by another. This is why Hans Selye described stress as the "nonspecific response of the body to any demand."

How We React to Stress

The grandfather of stress research, University of Montreal biologist Hans Selye, developed a theoretical basis for the stress response in 1956. Selye theorized that, in what he called the **general adaptation syndrome (GAS),** there are three distinct phases to the body's reaction to stress: alarm reaction, resistance, and exhaustion (see Figure 4.1).

The first stage of the general adaptation syndrome is shock, or an **alarm reaction** to the stressful situation. The body mobilizes its forces to meet the threatening situation. It is like a call to arms. Muscles tighten, particularly those in the

HealthLinks

American Psychological Association Help Center
helping.apa.org/stress3.html
Identifies and discusses six myths about stress.

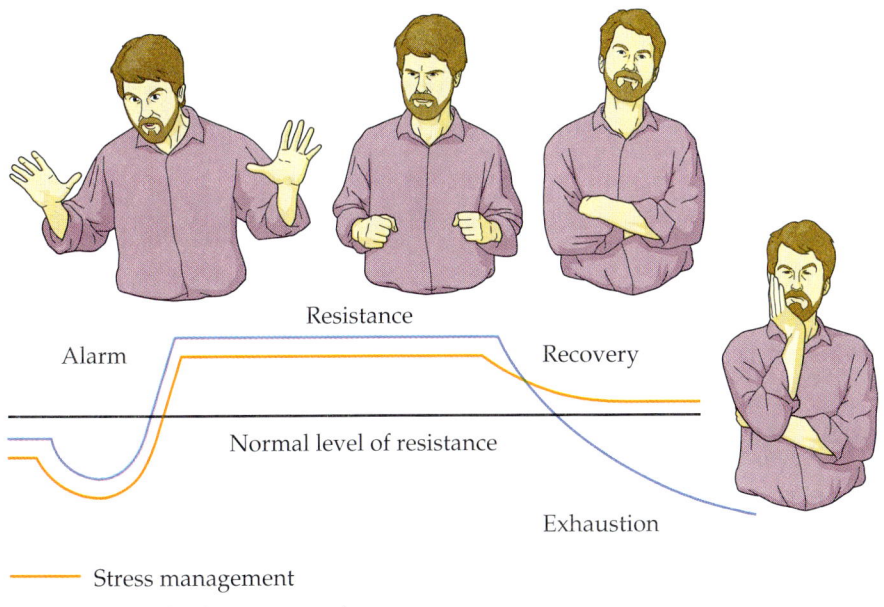

Figure 4.1 **The General Adaptation Syndrome.** *The three stages of the general adaptation syndrome are alarm, resistance, and exhaustion. Most people go through the first two stages as a way of adapting to everyday stressors.*

stress A reaction of the body and mind to the mental and emotional strain placed upon them.

stress response A series of events, caused by stressors, within the body that involves chemicals, hormones, and neural impulses.

stressor A specific event that disrupts equilibrium and initiates complex biochemical responses.

general adaptation syndrome (GAS) The theory proposed by Hans Selye in which there are three distinct phases to the body's reaction to stress: alarm reaction, resistance, and exhaustion.

alarm reaction The first stage of the general adaptation syndrome; the body mobilizes its forces to meet a threatening situation.

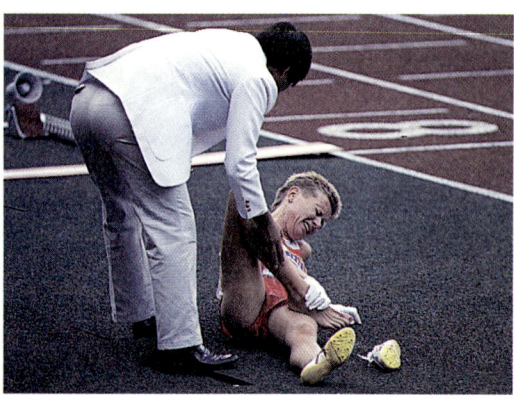

1. Physical stressors: strenuous physical activity, hunger, thirst, pain, cold, lack of sleep, illness, injury, temporary disability. (Source: The Image Works/© Bob Daemmrich)

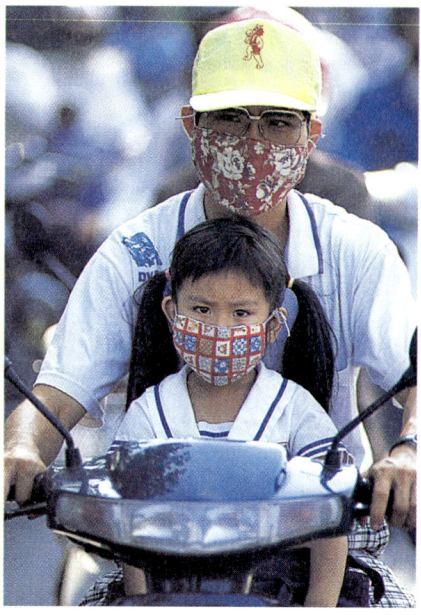

2. Environmental stressors: polluted air and water, extremes in temperature, noise, crowding and overpopulation, lack of privacy, natural disasters, exposure to radiation. (Source: The Image Works/© F. Hoffmann)

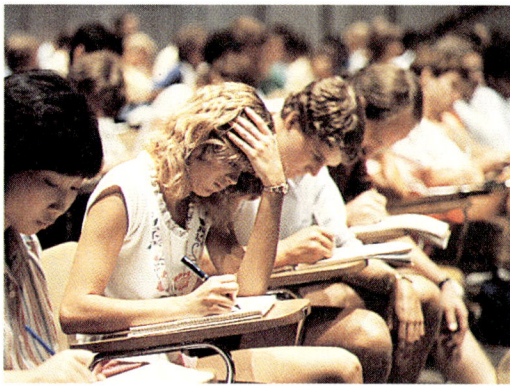

3. Psychological stressors: test taking, academic failure, boredom, graduation from college, frustration, anger, guilt, worry, anxiety, marriage, loss of a friend, vacation, threats to self-esteem, death of a relative, extreme joy, excitement in anticipation of an event. (Source: The Image Works/©Bob Daemmrich)

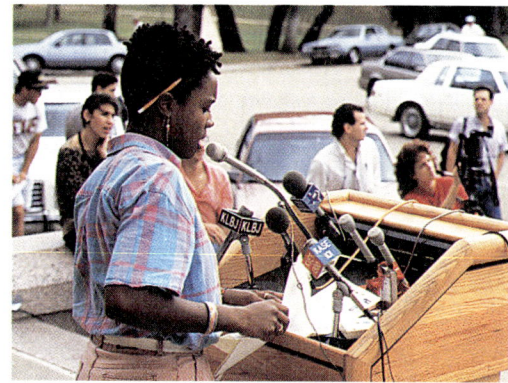

4. Social stressors: racial and religious prejudice, sexual harassment, underemployment and unemployment, public speaking, a class reunion, isolation. (Source: The Image Works/©Bob Daemmrich)

Figure 4.2 Sources of Stress.

face and neck. Lactate, a substance formed when muscles contract, appears in the blood. Adrenaline and noradrenaline, the hormones that speed up heartbeat and constrict blood vessels, are also secreted into the bloodstream. Blood pressure rises, breathing accelerates, blood sugar increases, and so does general alertness. The full force of physical and mental resources of the individual is brought to bear on the stress-producing situation.

The next stage of adaptation is called **resistance.** At this point, calming chemicals are produced, and the body relaxes and returns to its normal state after the immediate threat has disappeared. Most people go through these first two stages time and time again, and they become a way of adapting to the conflicts of everyday life.

However, sometimes there are so many stressors that a person cannot react to them. When stress is persistent and chronic, the body may not have a chance to restore itself to a state of equilibrium, or its prestressed state. When this happens, a person enters the **exhaustion** stage. It is in this stage that you are more susceptible to illness and disease.

Stressors: Where Do They Originate?

Some stressors are obvious and are related to a specific event, such as writing a major research paper or being evaluated for your work performance. Others are hidden, such as worrying about your finances or the health of your parents. A **primary stressor** (the assignment of a research paper) initiates the stress response. A **secondary stressor** (worry) keeps the stress response activated.

There are four basic sources of stress in society today. The examples listed in Figure 4.2 illustrate the kinds of situations that can trigger stress.

Critical Thinking Question

> To what extent should public health policy be used to control stressful environments? For example, should a government agency monitor stress levels at worksites? Should employers be held responsible for stress-related illnesses that are caused by stress on the job? After all, it is not the environment but rather the reaction to the environment that produces stress.

Positive and Negative Stress

The effects of stress appear to be the same for happy, positive experiences as for negative ones. This is why when medical researchers Thomas Holmes and Richard Rahe devised their list of major stressors, they put seemingly positive experiences as well as negative events near the top. For example, both getting married and the death of a parent are high on the list. The following student life-change rating scale is adapted from the original Holmes-Rahe Social Readjustment Rating Scale (SRRS) (see the Here's Looking at You box). Research suggests that people with high stress scores on evaluations such as this tend to be more vulnerable to illness.

Special terms differentiate between bad stress (distress) and good stress (eustress). **Distress** is the type of stress that brings about negative mental or physical responses. After experiencing distress, people are often wound up and have trouble relaxing or calming down. Examples of events that cause distress are exams, trouble with relatives, and burnout at school or work, as well as major life events such as family celebrations, loss of a job, separation from family and moving (see the Your Environmental Neighborhood box).

In addition, the minor daily hassles of life can wear a person down by over-stimulating the body. Some of these hassles might be concern about weight and

resistance The second stage of the general adaptation syndrome; the body relaxes and returns to its normal state after the immediate threat has disappeared.

exhaustion The final stage of the general adaptation syndrome; it occurs when the body does not have a chance to restore itself to a state of equilibrium.

primary stressor Something that initiates the stress response.

secondary stressor An additional stressor that continues the stress response.

distress The type of stress that brings about negative mental or physical responses, also known as bad stress.

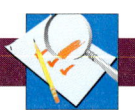

HERE'S LOOKING AT YOU

Rating the Stressors in Your Life

Stress can play a powerful role in your life. Often, when we think of personal stressors, we think of major events or even catastrophes. But even little daily things can bring about stress when added together. Use the following scale to test your stress level. Consider each of the following events and, in Column A, indicate the number of times you have experienced each one during the last twelve months.

Column A		Life-change event	Column B	Column C
_____	1.	Entered college	50	_____
_____	2.	Married	77	_____
_____	3.	Trouble with your boss	38	_____
_____	4.	Hold a job while attending school	43	_____
_____	5.	Experienced the death of a spouse	87	_____
_____	6.	Major change in sleeping habits	34	_____
_____	7.	Experienced the death of a close family member	77	_____
_____	8.	Major change in eating habits	30	_____
_____	9.	Change in or choice of major field of study	41	_____
_____	10.	Revision of personal habits	45	_____
_____	11.	Experienced the death of a close friend	68	_____
_____	12.	Found guilty of minor violations of the law	22	_____
_____	13.	Had an outstanding personal achievement	40	_____
_____	14.	Experienced pregnancy, or fathered a pregnancy	68	_____
_____	15.	Major change in health or behavior of family member	56	_____
_____	16.	Had sexual difficulties	58	_____
_____	17.	Had trouble with in-laws	42	_____
_____	18.	Major change in number of family get-togethers	26	_____
_____	19.	Major change in financial state	53	_____
_____	20.	Gained a new family member	50	_____
_____	21.	Change in residence or living conditions	42	_____
_____	22.	Major conflict or change in values	50	_____
_____	23.	Major change in church activities	36	_____

(continued)

overall appearance, health of a family member, inflation, too many things to do, misplacing or losing things, and fear of crime.

Another aspect of distress is **burnout.** This is the relative term used to describe what happens to people who work hard with few or no tangible results. They become frustrated, depressed, thwarted, tired, and burned out. For example, it is common for young school teachers to experience burnout. The intensity of the job, the long hours working both in the classroom and at home preparing plans and correcting papers, and the difficulties of classroom management can lead to feelings of frustration about an inability to accomplish all that is desired. Although burnout is most associated with the workplace, it happens to college students as well.

In contrast to bad stress, or distress, **eustress** is the type of stress that is a healthy part of daily living. After experiencing eustress, people are able to relax and enjoy a feeling of peacefulness and calm. Examples of events that cause

_	24.	Marital reconciliation with your mate	58	_
_	25.	Fired from work	62	_
_	26.	Were divorced	76	_
_	27.	Changed to a different line of work	50	_
_	28.	Major change in number of arguments with spouse	50	_
_	29.	Major change in responsibilities at work	47	_
_	30.	Had your spouse begin or cease work outside the home	41	_
_	31.	Major change in working hours or conditions	42	_
_	32.	Marital separation from mate	74	_
_	33.	Major change in type and/or amount of recreation	37	_
_	34.	Major change in use of drugs	52	_
_	35.	Took on a mortgage or loan of less than $10,000	52	_
_	36.	Major personal injury or illness	65	_
_	37.	Major change in use of alcohol	46	_
_	38.	Major change in social activities	43	_
_	39.	Major change in amount of participation in school activities	38	_
_	40.	Major change in amount of independence and responsibility	49	_
_	41.	Took a trip or a vacation	33	_
_	42.	Engaged to be married	54	_
_	43.	Changed to a new school	50	_
_	44.	Changed dating habits	41	_
_	45.	Trouble with school administration	44	_
_	46.	Broke or had broken a marital engagement or steady relationship	60	_
_	47.	Major change in self-concept or self-awareness	57	_
			Total	_

To find your score on this scale, multiply the number under Column B by the number in Column A and place it in Column C. Finally, total Column C. If your score totals 1,435 or higher, you are in the "high" category for developing an illness. If your total is 347 or less, you fall into the "low" category. The "medium" score is 890.

Source: Reprinted with permission of Elsevier Science Inc. from M.T. Mark et al., "The Influence of Recent Life Experiences on the Health of College Freshmen," *Journal of Psychosomatic Research* 19: 87–98, 1975

eustress are the excitement of a vacation, the accomplishment of an outstanding personal achievement, and the stimulus of an exciting classroom or workplace experience. Eustress can help you channel nervous energy into a better performance.

Not only are there two kinds of stress, but also there are at least two personality types that relate to stress. In 1974, Drs. Meyer Friedman and Ray Rosenman identified these personalities as Type A and Type B. The **Type A personality** is described as being excessively competitive, aggressive, driven, and impatient. Someone with this personality would find it extremely stressful to be stuck in a traffic jam or to wait in a supermarket or bank line. The **Type B personality,** in contrast, is described as being more relaxed and patient. There is some indication that Type A's tend to be more prone to heart disease. However, this finding is controversial because of the influence on Type A's of other risk factors associated with coronary disease, including age, sex, family history, and occupation.

burnout The emotional exhaustion caused by the stresses of work and other responsibilities.

eustress The type of stress that is a healthy part of daily living; it can result in the ability to relax and enjoy a feeling of peacefulness and calm.

Type A personality A person who is excessively competitive, aggressive, driven, and impatient.

Type B personality A person who is more relaxed and patient than one who has a Type A personality.

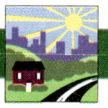

YOUR ENVIRONMENTAL NEIGHBORHOOD

Festive Malaise

One sure sign that the Christmas season has begun is the annual crop of articles about holiday depression, which appear as reliably as department store Santas and fruitcakes. This has led to the widespread belief that the holidays breed serious emotional troubles, and even that the suicide rate is likely to peak around December 25. Are the holidays "public health hazards"?

No, according to Dr. James Hillard of the University of Cincinnati, who a few years back examined these assumptions about holiday misery and found that suicides do not occur more frequently during the weeks before Christmas, nor are people more likely to suffer from severe depression (as measured by hospital admissions for psychiatric problems). In fact, December has a comparatively low rate of suicides and other psychiatric emergencies. The suicide rate usually does not begin to rise until January and then peaks in April or May.

Why is there this gap between belief and reality? Two common by-products of holiday celebrations are indeed stress and anxiety. People tend to spend more than they can afford, eat and drink too much, and disrupt their normal patterns of sleep, exercise, and work. Those without close friends may see their problems worsening around Christmas. "Festive malaise," as one study termed it, may arise from the conflict between our idea of what the holiday *should* be and its reality. And certainly some people do have a severe emotional crisis then, though there aren't enough of them to show up in the official statistics. Even for the relatively well adjusted, life is frenetic—the shops are mobbed and traffic is snarled. On top of all that, many people, especially in northern states, suffer from seasonal affective disorder (SAD) due in large part to the lack of sunlight during the short days this time of year.

But the holiday season can have plenty of benevolent effects to counteract these negatives. People tend to mobilize their coping mechanisms—that is, they are able to rely on increased social support, within the family and outside it. Thus if serious psychological problems emerge, it's likely to be after the holidays. In addition, all those magazine articles about Christmas depression may serve a purpose. As Hillard wrote, "Belief in Christmas depression syndrome gives people permission not to feel euphoric" when all other signals turn euphoria into a civic duty.

Source: "Festive Malaise," reprinted with permission from the *University of California at Berkeley Wellness Letter*, December 1993, p. 7. © Health Letter Associates, 1993. To order a one year subscription, call 800/829–9170

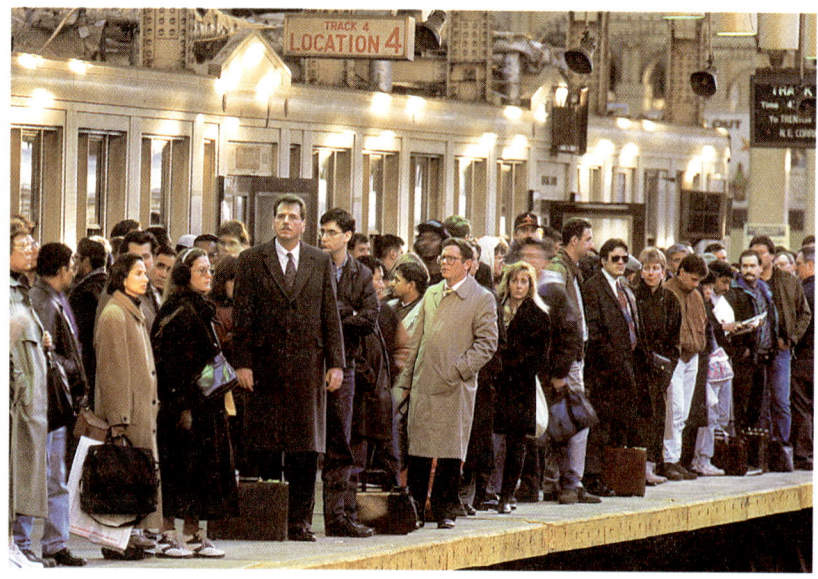

People with Type A personality are described as being competitive, driven, and impatient. For Type A's waiting for a train can be very stressful. (Source: © Tony Stone Images/© Don Spiro)

Overall, smoking and high cholesterol predict coronary disease among Type As more strongly than does personality.

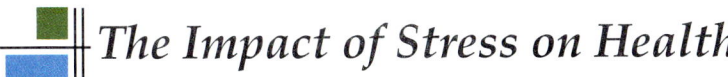 The Impact of Stress on Health

The primary reason that it is important to understand the underlying source of stress and to come to grips with it is that there is a well-established scientific connection between too much stress and the incidence of disease. Research has demonstrated a relationship between stress and several biochemical changes such as changes in adrenaline levels and in cholesterol and triglyceride levels. Physiological effects of stress have been documented as well, including increased heart rate, blood pressure, and muscle tension. Finally, psychological responses to stress have been documented, including anxiety and depression.

Surveys persistently show that stress-related disorders account for a significantly high number of visits to primary care physicians. Typical of these symptoms are irritability, insomnia, heart palpitations, migraine headaches, stomach aches, and skin rashes. Although these are not life-threatening conditions, they should not be discounted, because if they continue and build up, they can cause more serious problems.

Stress Symptoms Seen in the Physician's Office

One of the most common reasons for going to a physician is stress. Some of the stress-related symptoms that bring people to a physician's office are listed here in three categories:

1. *Health effects:* Asthma, amenorrhea, back pains, chest pains, diarrhea, dizziness, heart palpitations, heartburn, headaches, hives, insomnia, loss of sexual interest, nightmares, psychosomatic disorders, skin rashes, ulcers, and weakness.
2. *Subjective effects:* Anxiety, apathy, boredom, depression, fatigue, frustration, guilt, irritability, inability to make decisions, moodiness, nervousness, and tension.
3. *Behavioral effects:* Being accident prone, drug taking, emotional outbursts, excessive eating and drinking, impulsive behavior, lack of concentration, loss of appetite, nervous laughter, restlessness, and trembling.

Clearly, you don't go to the physician to complain about the fact that you are having difficulty making decisions or that you are bored and restless. But if these problems are coupled with other symptoms—perhaps weight loss or gain or a skin rash—your physician may diagnose a stress-related disorder.

Research Findings on Stress and the Immune System

Several recent studies have found that stress can result in a weakening of the immune system. One study demonstrated that the level of important immune system cells in the body measurably decreased among a group of medical students in response to the stress of taking final exams. These cells are important in fighting diseases ranging from the common cold to cancer. According to researchers at the Ohio State University College of Medicine, the activity levels of the students' immune cells were significantly lower than the levels recorded one month earlier, when the students were not taking exams.

People who are stressed by assuming long-term caregiving responsibilities for an ailing spouse do not mount as good an immune response after getting a flu shot as do other people, according to a recent study. Moreover, researchers at Ohio State found that caregivers show no significant psychological or immunological improvement up to three years after the death of their spouses.

Other studies show that bereavement can adversely affect the immune system. A psychologist at the University of California, Los Angeles, found an acceleration in immune system failure among men infected with HIV when their lovers died of AIDS.

Researchers at the University of California, San Francisco, found a correlation between positive psychological characteristics—low levels of tension, depression, fatigue, and anger—and increased numbers of disease-fighting immune system cells in patients with AIDS. Of the 104 patients studied, those who coped better with the distress associated with their illness and were assertive had higher numbers of such cells. It is possible, the researchers concluded from both California studies, that adaptive coping styles might modify the course of immunologically related diseases such as AIDS.

Stressors of Everyday Living

Stress is a part of every phase of life, starting from the moment of birth—and even before. Prenatal heart rates have been found to increase and decrease in response to the mother's listening to various forms of music. This suggests that a fetus senses the stress levels of the mother. Predictable stresses occur at different stages throughout life. For children, the first day of school is a classic example of a stress experience. For young adults, the rite of passage from the world of college to the world of work is a predictable period of stress. And for older adults, retiring from work can be extremely stressful.

At College

The transition from high school to college presents numerous potentially stressful demands. Prominent among stressors are

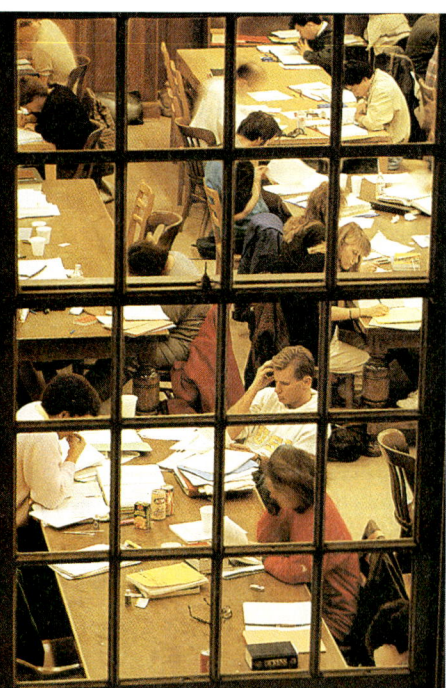

The stress of taking final exams can lower immune cells, which are necessary for fighting diseases such as the common cold. (Source: © Tony Stone/Phil Schofield)

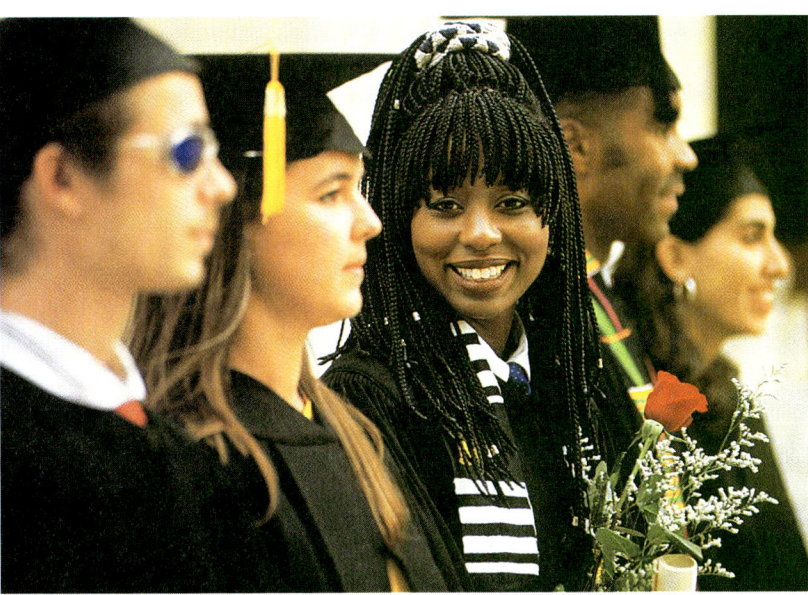

College includes many stressors—including graduating, leaving close friends, and even the excitement of heading out into the "real" world. Coping involves dealing constructively with stress. (Source: FPG International/ © Telegraph Colour Library)

- leaving your parents, siblings, and friends—perhaps for the first time;
- making a new network of friends;
- assuming responsibility for yourself, including buying clothes and balancing a budget;
- making decisions about drugs and alcohol and sexual behavior;
- facing new intellectual challenges; and
- juggling the pressures and time constraints of working while going to school.

What happens to the mental and physical health of college students as a result of these multiple demands? Suicide is the third leading cause of death among college students, and drug abuse and sex-related problems, as well as outbreaks of influenza and mononucleosis, are prevalent on college campuses. In another indication of how stressful college life is, many students drop out before earning a degree.

One of the reasons that college life is so stressful is that many of the decisions that students make can have long-term consequences. Choosing a major, for example, can be especially stressful because this decision affects a student's course selection for the remainder of college life. The same decision may also amount to a career choice. A decision about whether to study abroad for a semester or to take a year off from school could likewise have a ripple effect on other life decisions.

Not all college students go to school directly from high school. An increasing number of college students have worked for a while. Some go to school and work in the evenings or work in the day and go to school at night. Still others have worked long enough to have retired. Older students face some of the same stressors as younger students. After all, both groups are embarking on a new experience. But older students especially face the stress of fear of failure: Will I be able to do the work? How can I keep up with younger people? Can I successfully juggle school with the other parts of my life—my children, my job, my spouse, my sick parents?

Another group of students facing multiple pressures are married graduate students. About one-half of graduate students in the United States are married.

Problems tend to arise when course or dissertation work drags on longer than either partner had originally expected or when the supporting spouse becomes resentful. These problems are less acute when both partners are at graduate school at the same time, but then they face other stresses such as having little time to spend together and limited financial resources.

At Work

Stress in the workplace is pervasive. A Blue Cross–Blue Shield survey of a broad cross-section of workers in two midwestern states found that five out of six workers at all levels of employment—from the assembly line to the executive suite—complained that job stress was a major factor resulting in anxiety, depression, colds, asthma, chest pains, and difficulty in breathing.

In contrast to the stereotype of a high-pressured executive having a heart attack, in reality, a receptionist or junior assistant is more prone to get sick, according to researchers at the University of Southern California. What these nonexecutives have in common—and what makes their jobs particularly stressful—is a lack of control over their work. Apparently, they have trouble dealing satisfactorily with time pressures and heavy workloads. In this context, executive and professional jobs are considered less stressful because they include greater control.

Bus drivers are a prime example of workers who are under stress and who have little flexibility on the job. They often start their shifts behind schedule and have to rush to catch up with an unrealistic timetable that they did not set. They face traffic jams, broken lights, potholes, and arguments with passengers. Studies of bus drivers worldwide show that they have higher than average incidences of high blood pressure, musculoskeletal disorders, and gastrointestinal problems.

Critical Thinking Question

> Noise is a stressor for some workers. Think of how stressful it is to hear the noise of a jackhammer or an ambulance siren when you are walking down the street. Now think of how you might react if you were exposed to such high noise levels throughout your work day. *Healthy People 2000* includes the goal of reducing to no more than 15 percent the proportion of workers exposed to average daily noise levels above eighty-five decibels—the noise level of a gas-powered or electric lawnmower. Currently, nearly 20 percent of workers are exposed regularly to such levels. How might we accomplish this goal of noise reduction? To what extent would it reduce worksite stress?

personality hardiness   A state of resiliency due to clear self-concept.

coping   An adaptation to stress.

fight-or-flight reaction   The body's reaction to stress in which it becomes physically ready to resist or fight a stressor or to run from it.

defense mechanisms   Coping strategies by which people defend themselves against negative emotions.

As more and more women enter the workplace, two patterns are emerging that relate to stress. One is that an increasing number of women in middle- to high-level jobs are demonstrating Type A behavior and previously male-associated disorders such as coronary heart disease. Women in clerical jobs are also experiencing high levels of stress because they are working in positions in which they have little control and cannot express themselves. A recent National Heart,

Lung and Blood Institute study showed a 100 percent increase in heart attacks among secretaries, typists, clerks, and bookkeepers compared with women who do not work outside the home.

Chronic stress affects employers as well in terms of absenteeism due to stress-related illness, high turnover, poor productivity, high accident rates, low morale, antagonism at work, and job dissatisfaction. In fact, according to the American Institute of Stress, American business pays an estimated $75 billion to $100 billion a year for these effects of stress.

What is the key to getting sick—or staying healthy—on a stressful job? A University of Chicago researcher studied 200 executives over a three and one-half year period when the company was undergoing major corporate changes. Half of the executives took ill, whereas the other half stayed well. Why? It is hypothesized that the group that stayed well had **personality hardiness**—that is, they had a clear sense of who they were. They looked at the tensions on the job and saw them as challenges, not threats. In a word, they felt they were in "control."

As for the relationship between hardiness and health, the group of 100 executives who were well at the time of the study stayed well during the next two years. They developed only half as many symptoms of illness as a control group of less hardy people.

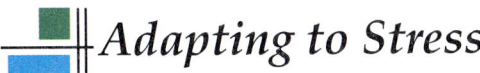

Adapting to Stress

HEALTH SKILLS

Although there will always be some stress in your life, that does not mean you cannot do anything about it. In fact, the best medicine for stress appears to be learning how to adapt to or cope with stress.

Coping is adaptation to stress. In primitive times, coping with stress meant little more than exercising the basic **fight-or-flight reaction** to threatening situations. For example, if a tiger threatened a primitive man, he would either stand and fight (and do so with added strength and cunning brought about by the stress reactions described by the general adaptation syndrome) or run from the threat (also with the added strength and cunning brought about by the stress reaction).

Today, we are not threatened by tigers. Threats come instead from difficult working situations, unexpected bills, and disappointing news. Although survival is still at issue, it is not as much the survival of an individual or the species as maintaining self-esteem in stressful situations. The fight-or-flight response still works well in some cases, as do **defense mechanisms** such as avoidance and denial. These responses, however, are usually effective only for the short term. In our complex society, more adaptive methods of coping are necessary for a long-term adaptation to stress. Fleeing or denying a stress situation might be very useful in diminishing the acute pain of an unhappy event, but it does not help you deal with the source of the stress over the long run.

Coping with Stress

There are several ways you can effectively minimize the negative effects of everyday stress, whether it is in school, on the job, or at home. One preventive action is to make sure that you take good care of your physical health. You do this by eating nutritiously, exercising, not smoking or using drugs, and getting an adequate amount of sleep. You will find tips on how to develop good health habits in the related chapters in this textbook. Being in good physical health can help your body fight the negative health effects that can accompany stress.

DEVELOPING HEALTH SKILLS

Managing Time

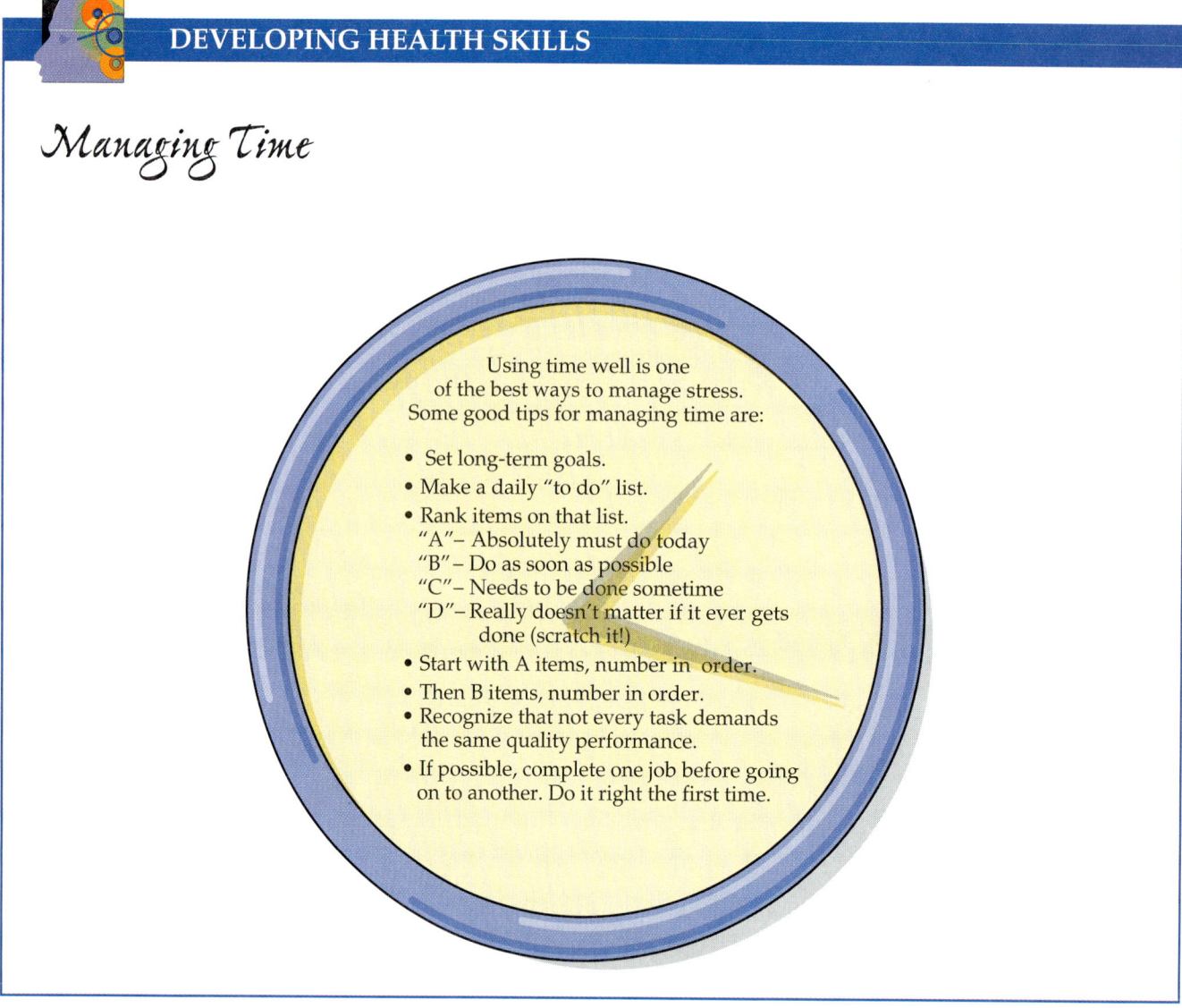

Using time well is one of the best ways to manage stress. Some good tips for managing time are:

- Set long-term goals.
- Make a daily "to do" list.
- Rank items on that list.
  "A"– Absolutely must do today
  "B"– Do as soon as possible
  "C"– Needs to be done sometime
  "D"– Really doesn't matter if it ever gets done (scratch it!)
- Start with A items, number in order.
- Then B items, number in order.
- Recognize that not every task demands the same quality performance.
- If possible, complete one job before going on to another. Do it right the first time.

Another preventive way to deal with stress is to recognize it so that you can begin to manage it effectively. Stress researchers call this process **stressor identification**. Once you identify a stressor, it is possible to develop coping strategies.

There are many things you can do to deal constructively with stressors. Collectively, these are called **coping skills,** and they fall into one of three categories: changing perception, managing time, and managing emotion.

1. *Changing perception.* This involves changing the way you perceive and define a stressful event. One way to do this is by improving communications so that you can better understand the nature of the stressor and how it occurred. Another is to remove yourself from the stressor by depersonalizing it. Remember, for example, that an accident that causes a traffic tie-up doesn't occur just to harass you. Similarly, if someone gets angry at you, it might be because he or she is distressed over something that has nothing to do with you.

2. *Managing time.* By setting personal priorities, you can control the stressors in your life rather than allow them to control you. In addition to preventing stressors from building up, time management can lead to changes in behav-

stressor identification The recognition of stress in order to begin effective management.

coping skills Strategies used to deal constructively with stressors.

DEVELOPING HEALTH SKILLS

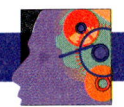

Stressed Out? Develop a Health Style of Talking It Out

The stage of life between eighteen and thirty-five years of age is often described as a time when men and women focus on developing lasting friendships and marriage or other long-term partnerships. During these crucial years, the critical choice between intimacy and isolation is often made. Simon and Garfunkel sang about this struggle: "If I'd never loved,/I never would have cried…/I am a rock/I am an island/And the rock feels no pain/and an island never cries."

Although developing relationships that allow you to talk to someone intimately has many rewards, one benefit that is overlooked is the link between close communication and good health. Researchers have found that people with the highest immunity to the common cold are honeymooners. Apparently, the intimacy of a honeymoon encourages the immune system to fight infection.

Some people, for whatever reason, have difficulty talking openly about their feelings. If they choose isolation instead of intimacy, they are in danger of heightening their stress level. Research indicates that such lonely people are much more vulnerable to developing illnesses of every sort, from the common cold to life-threatening diseases such as cancer. In fact, some cancer specialists believe there is a cancer-prone personality. The person with such a personality tends to be very resentful and has a lot of self-pity, a poor self-image, and little ability to develop and keep meaningful long-term relationships.

There is no denying it. Open communication takes courage. Allowing another person to really know and understand how you think and feel can be frightening at best, but the consequences—both psychologically and physically—are well worth the risk. So the next time you feel stressed, seek out someone you feel close enough to talk to. You will find out that it is not only a health behavior that will reduce your current stress, but also a health style that will benefit you throughout your lifetime.

Source: Lyrics from "I Am a Rock." Copyright © 1965 Paul Simon. Used by permission of the publisher, Paul Simon Music

ior that better meet your personal needs and enhance your sense of self-esteem and general well-being (see the Developing Health Skills box).

3. *Managing emotion.* The emotional aspects of stress—whether they be happy or sad—need to be managed. If you are angry about something, it is usually better to recognize that anger and express it rather than to suppress it. Once an emotion is honestly labeled, actions can be undertaken to release it. In the case of anger, this might mean laughing it off, talking it out, seeking support or solace from another person, or in some cases crying.

Critical Thinking Question

Healthy People 2000 lists a goal of decreasing "to no more than 5 percent the proportion of people aged 18 and older who report experiencing significant levels of stress who do not take steps to reduce or control their stress." Currently 35 percent of adults report experiencing significant levels of stress. What can you do to contribute to the accomplishment of this goal? Should the goal be accomplished, how would it affect disease prevalence data?

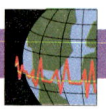

CULTURAL VIEW

Managing Stress through T'ai Chi

Chi (pronounced CHEE) is a Chinese term representing the life force; t'ai chi is a form of exercise that regulates this energy to improve balance, strength, and flexibility. The Chinese have been practicing t'ai chi for thousands of years as a way to live in harmony and balance with the world. Today, groups of thousands of people gather in various parts of Beijing, Shanghai, and other Chinese cities to practice t'ai chi in the early morning hours before work. Even visits to American cities with large Chinese populations provide an opportunity to witness this ancient martial art. An early morning stroll through parks in or near San Francisco's Chinatown district or Boston's Public Garden provide passers-by with a basic demonstration of t'ai chi.

What motivates practitioners of t'ai chi are both the physical and psychological benefits of this ancient form of exercise. Studies show that people who practice t'ai chi have a marked decrease in their resting heart rate and stress hormones for the rest of the day, and feel less physical tension, fatigue, anxiety, and anger than those who do not practice t'ai chi. This holds true for beginners of the technique as well as long-time practitioners.

Even though it is a branch of martial arts, t'ai chi is well known for its calming experience. In fact, it is often called a "moving meditation." With the proper training, t'ai chi teaches you how to live in harmony with aggression, fear, and other stressors, rather than fight them. As one instructor said, "t'ai chi teaches you how to be relaxed in all aspects of your life and how to stay relaxed in the face of stress."

Using more than 100 positions or movements, t'ai chi embraces four basic philosophical concepts:

- Finding comfort in solitude
- Returning to the joys of childhood, such as embracing laughter and play
- Moving with the flow of nature, as exemplified by a ping pong ball in water—when you push it under water, it always pops back up with little or no energy
- Acknowledging failure as the first step to success.

T'ai chi classes are offered at many colleges and at Y's and other community programs. Before signing up, make sure the instructor's philosophy is similar to yours. Some instructors focus on t'ai chi as a form of martial arts; others teach it as a form of meditation; others emphasize health and fitness. The key is finding the right class for your needs.

Most coping skills also involve **interpersonal skills** because many stress-producing situations involve relations with other people. Interpersonal skills include getting help from others, sharing feelings, effective communication, conflict resolution, active listening, assertiveness, and team building. These skills help to build a network of personal support that can be used to manage the stress in your life and help you cope competently (see the Developing Health Skills box). Conflict resolution is discussed in further detail in Chapter 11, as a way to deal with feelings that could escalate into violent encounters.

A strong social support system of family and friends not only can help you in times of stress but also can lower your risk for serious illness. One reason for this, according to researchers, is that social relationships can facilitate health-promoting behaviors such as proper sleep, diet, exercise, or seeking appropriate medical care when needed.

Exercise, a Stress Reducer

There is evidence that exercise functions as a stress reducer. Most people report that they "feel good" or "feel better" following vigorous exercise. It may well be that exercise reduces stress through an individual's increased sense of well-being or by simply providing a "time out" (see the Cultural View box).

Depending on your lifestyle, there are many ways to exercise to reduce stress. For people who like to jog, a run before or after school can be an excellent way to get the day's stressors under control. This can be attributed to a release of tension or the so-called runner's high (which is thought to result from the release of brain hormones called endorphins). Walking can also have a soothing effect on emotions. It can provide an excellent opportunity to clearly contemplate and solve problems. Conversely, a walk can distract you from your problems and give your mind a rest so that when you return you can better tackle the problems at hand (see Chapter 7). Researchers are also finding that exercising the spirit—for example, by volunteering—can make people feel good physically and emotionally and can reduce their levels of stress.

Learning to Relax

Relaxation is another way to reduce stress. The following are examples of two different kinds of relaxation exercises that have been used to reduce stress. You might want to try one.

PROGRESSIVE MUSCLE RELAXATION Relaxation and muscle tension are incompatible. Therefore, reducing muscle tension leads to a reduction in anxiety and stress levels. The relaxation technique described here involves focusing attention on muscle activity, learning to identify even small amounts of tension in a muscle group, and practicing releasing tension from the muscle.

Here's how to do it. Make a tight fist with one of your hands for several seconds. Focus on the tension; become aware of it. Gradually ease the tension. Feel the relaxation rising up your arm and slowly spreading over your entire body.

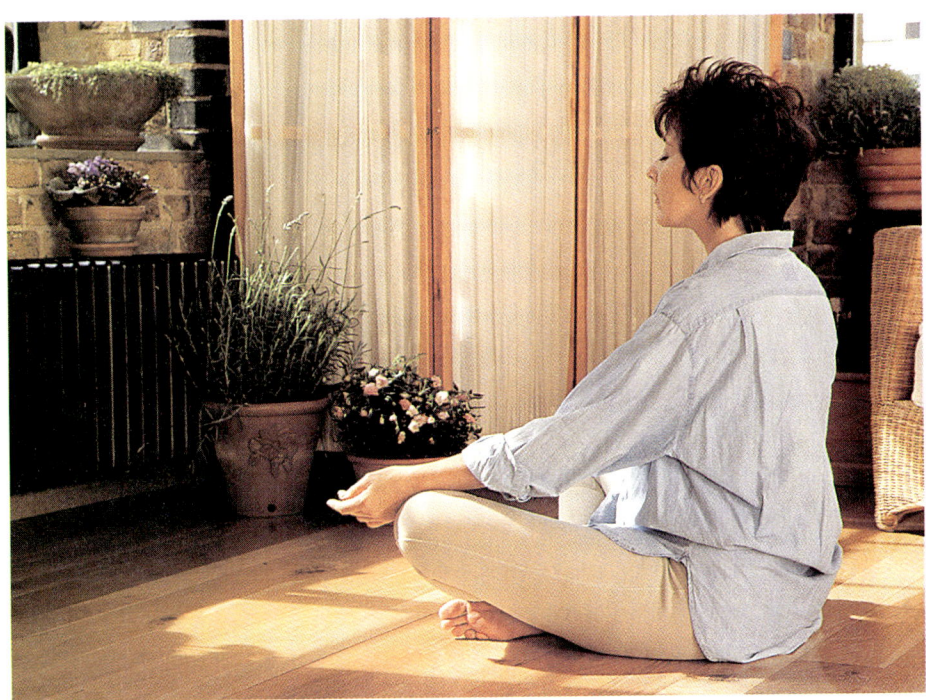

One way to relax and reduce your stress levels is by practicing yoga. This requires learning special relaxation skills. (Source: FPG International/© Telegraph Colour Library)

interpersonal skills The techniques involved in relating to other people.

Close your eyes and rest. Repeat the tensing and relaxing process with the muscles in your midsection, holding each muscle tight for five to ten seconds. Tense your arm, raise your shoulders, tighten your stomach muscles, calves, and feet. Lastly, furrow your brow, close your eyes tightly and clench your jaw. Always remember to relax each muscle for at least fifteen seconds before tensing the next muscle.

The progressive muscle relaxation process is one of the easiest stress management skills, but like all health skills, it takes practice. Don't judge its success by the first time you attempt it.

MEDITATION Meditation takes many forms. In its simplest form, it amounts to little more than calm thinking. You can try this form of meditation, also referred to as breathing relaxation. Relax quietly with your eyes closed and focus on your breathing. Each time you inhale, fill your lower abdomen with air first and allow your stomach to expand upward until your chest is full of air. Exhale at half the rate that you inhaled, slowly and completely, each time thinking about the world *calm*. Stretch out the word so that it becomes *caaaaalllllmmmmm*. If thoughts arise or your attention wanders, simply focus on your breathing.

A popular form of meditation is known as transcendental meditation (TM), a component of yoga made popular by the Maharishi Mahesh Yogi. Transcendental meditation involves sitting upright in a comfortable position in a quiet place, with eyes closed, and mentally repeating a secret mantra (a word or sound) while maintaining a passive mental attitude. Unlike breathing relaxation, transcendental meditation requires considerable practice.

All forms of meditation are believed to invoke a relaxation response. Research literature on the effectiveness of meditation as a stress-management technique consistently supports this method of stress management.

Critical Thinking Question

> Despite reports of effectiveness, meditation is not widely practiced. To what extent could this be the result of its association with religion? To what extent could this be the result of simple lack of appropriate health skills?

HealthLinks
Medical Basis of Stress
www.teachhealth.com

Special excerpts from a publication by two practitioners in stress reduction work.

stress inoculation A cognitive-behavioral stress management program involving education, rehearsal, and application of stress-management techniques.

Cognitive-Behavioral Skills

It is possible to manage stress by protecting yourself from the impact of potentially stressful situations through cognitive-behavioral skills. A common form of cognitive-behavioral skills training, often provided in worksite settings, is **stress inoculation.** This technique involves three stages:

1. The education stage involves learning how you have responded in the past to stressful experiences.
2. The rehearsal stage involves learning coping skills and stress-reduction techniques, such as problem solving and relaxation.
3. The application stage involves practicing the skills under simulated conditions in a classroom.

Even though stress inoculation requires training, you can use the principles to manage some stress situations. Suppose you have a stressed relationship with your roommate. Following the stress inoculation approach, make a list of the ways you have responded to that relationship, including negative ones, such as screaming at him or her and leaving the room, slamming the door on the way out. Then make a list of more positive skills that you have learned in this chapter. Practice using those skills with your roommate.

A final word: Positive and negative stressors are everyday experiences. It is not the existence of stressors but how you respond to them that is important for your overall health. A healthy response to stressors begins with an overall healthy approach to living. "Take good care of yourself!" is good advice because people who lead healthier lives also do a better job of managing the normal stress of day-to-day living.

Key Concepts

1. Stress is a perception of an external situation that brings about an internal response.
2. A stressor is an event or circumstance that brings about stress.
3. According to the classic theory of stress, the general adaptation syndrome, there are three distinct phases to the body's reaction to stress: alarm reaction, resistance, and exhaustion.
4. Stressors can be psychological, physical, environmental, social, or a combination of two or more of these.
5. Not all stress is bad. Harmful stress is referred to as distress and may result in serious health problems. The good kind of stress is called eustress and is considered an important aspect of healthy living.
6. Stress-related reasons account for a high percentage of all visits to primary care physicians.
7. Being in good physical condition can help your body fight the negative health effects that can accompany stress.
8. Coping involves dealing constructively with stress.
9. Coping skills fall under one of three categories: changing perception, managing time, and managing emotion.
10. Physical exercise and relaxation techniques can reduce levels of stress. Relaxation techniques include breathing relaxation, muscle relaxation, and visualization relaxation.

Review Questions

1. Define stress using Hans Selye's general adaptation syndrome theory.
2. List four types of stressors and give examples of each.
3. Differentiate between eustress and distress.
4. Describe the impact of stress on physical health.
5. Cite examples of stressors that occur in the college environment, at home, and at work.
6. Describe the fight-or-flight reaction. How does it help and/or hinder daily living?

7. Name three coping skills that are useful in dealing with the normal stress of daily living.
8. Describe the role of exercise in stress management.
9. Explain how volunteering can serve as a stress management strategy.
10. Explain the processes of progressive muscle relaxation, meditation, and cognitive-behavioral skills development as each relates to stress reduction.

■ Selected Bibliography

Carlin, P. "Treat the Body, Heal the Mind." *Health* (January/February 1996): 73–78.
Cottrell, R. R. *Wellness: Stress Management.* Guilford, CT: Dushkin, 1992.
Goldberger, L., and S. Breznitz. *Handbook of Stress: Theoretical and Clinical Aspects.* New York: The Free Press, 1986.
"Healthy Lives: A New View of Stress." *University of California at Berkeley Wellness Letter* (June 1990): 4–5.
Holmes, T. H., and R. H. Rahe. "The Social Readjustment Scale." *Journal of Psychosomatic Research* 11 (1967): 213–218.
Lazarus, R. S. *Psychological Stress and the Coping Process.* New York: McGraw-Hill, 1966.
Murphy, L. R. "Stress Management in Work Settings: A Critical Review of the Health Effects." *American Journal of Health Promotion* 11, no. 2 (1996):112–135.
Rosenman, R. H., and M. Friedman. "Neurogenic Factors in Pathogenesis of Coronary Heart Disease." *Medical Clinics of North America* 58 (1967): 269–276.
Selye, H. "The General Adaptation Syndrome and Diseases of Adaptation." *Journal of Clinical Endocrinology* 6 (1946): 217–230.
Selye, H. *Stress without Distress.* New York: Signet, 1974.

■ HealthLinks: Web Sites for a Better Understanding of Stress

You can access better health as it relates to this chapter by checking out some of the following sites on the Internet. These and sites identified within the chapter can be accessed directly when you visit the *HealthStyles* Web Site located on the Allyn and Bacon homepage at **http://www.abacon.com.**

Center for Anxiety and Stress Treatment
stressrelease.com
Provides resources and services regarding a broad range of stress-related topics.

National Center for Post-Traumatic Stress Disease
www.dartmouth.edu/dms/ptsd
Research and education on PTSD, offering a variety of links to fact sheets and help sites from around the world.

Health Hotlines: Coping with Stress

American Institute of Stress
(800) 24-RELAX (247-3529)
124 Park Avenue
Yonkers, NY 10703

Association for Applied Psychophysiology and Biofeedback
(800) 477-8892
10200 West 44th Street, Suite 304
Wheat Ridge, CO 80033

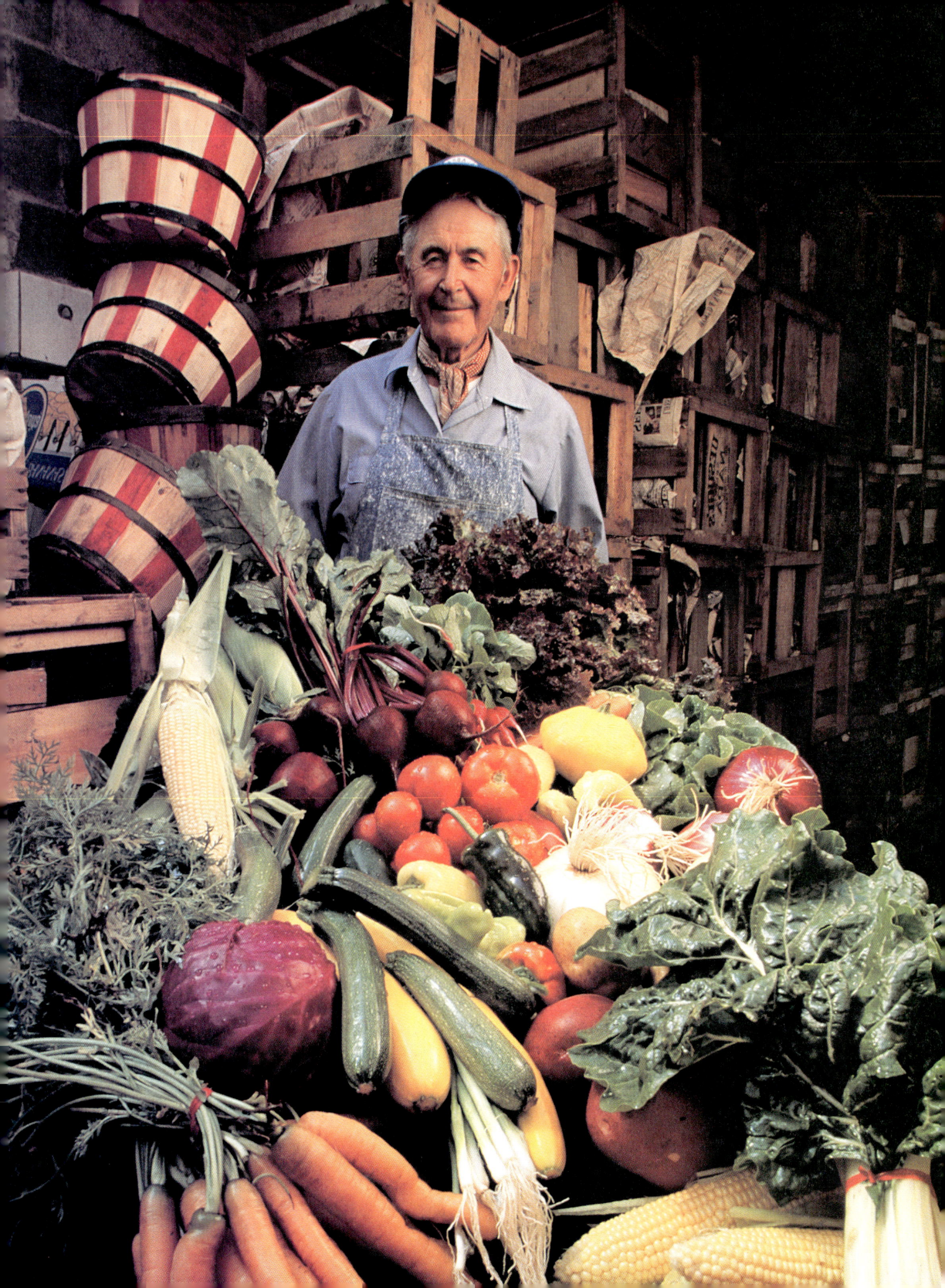

Chapter 5

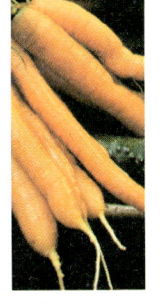
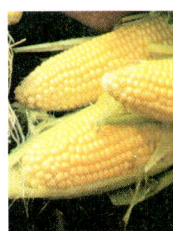
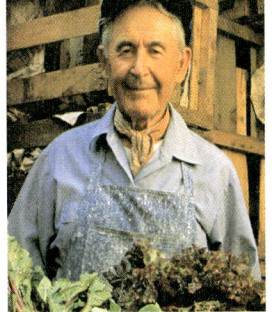

Eating Smart

Objectives

When you finish reading this chapter, you will be able to:

1. List the essential nutrients that make up food.
2. Describe the primary sources for each nutrient and give examples of how each contributes to overall health.
3. Know the difference between a complete protein and an incomplete protein.
4. Explain how blood cholesterol is affected by diet.
5. Identify the types of food additives and explain how each contributes to the quality of food.
6. Explain the purpose and function of the recommended dietary allowances (RDAs) published by the Food and Nutrition Board of the National Academy of Science.
7. Describe several eating styles and cite examples of how each contributes or detracts from overall health.
8. Identify common eating habits that present a threat to the health of college students.
9. Read a food label and understand how it describes the nutritional value of a food.
10. Explain how food preparation both enhances and detracts from the quality of food.

What Is Your HealthStyle?

Fred was rushing out to his first class of the day. He was running late, as usual, but stopped by the cafeteria for his breakfast—a cup of coffee. His lunch usually isn't nutritious either—a candy bar or two and a can of soda.

By dinnertime, Fred is starved and eats whatever the main course is in the cafeteria—beef tacos, chicken casserole, meat loaf with sauce. Two or three times a week, he goes to a fast-food place for dinner with friends for hamburgers and french fries, pizza, submarine sandwiches, or deep-fried chicken. Fred's daily diet is high in cholesterol and fats, low in essential vitamins and minerals, and almost nonexistent in fruits and vegetables.

Now consider what Antonio eats. He, too, has an early morning class, but gets up in time to have breakfast in the cafeteria. He drinks a glass of juice while going through the line, then selects a low-sugar cold cereal with skim milk. Sometimes he has a bran muffin or whole wheat toast with jam.

For lunch, Antonio usually gets something from the salad bar. He goes heavy on the vegetables—tomatoes, cucumbers, radishes, lettuce, beans—and lighter on cholesterol-rich foods such as sliced eggs and cheese. He bypasses the artificial, high-sodium bacon bits and the creamy salad dressings. If there is fresh fruit, he might take a piece or two for a mid-afternoon snack.

For dinner, he chooses fish or chicken when it is offered in the cafeteria—and asks for a serving without the rich sauce it always seems to be swimming in. Just like Fred, Antonio and his friends go out to fast-food places a few nights a week but he orders broiled fish, not fried chicken sandwiches. And if he orders pizza, his "extras" are vegetables—onions, mushrooms, peppers, and tomatoes—not sausage, meatballs, and cheese.

In Your Opinion

Fred and Antonio have two different nutritional health styles.

- What do you think of Fred's food choices?
- What can he do to eat more nutritiously while on the run?
- What health skills does Antonio use that Fred does not use?
- Why is Antonio's diet healthier? Why does it lead to a health style of more nutritious eating?
- How do you rate your nutritional health style?

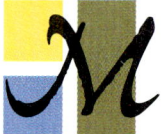

Most Americans are not smart eaters. We eat too much fat and too little fiber, consume excesses of salt, sugar, and meat and do not get enough of all the essential vitamins and minerals from our diets.

Because of these nutritional habits and other dietary and lifestyle factors, there has been an increase in the incidence of diet-related diseases, such as heart disease, obesity, and certain cancers. The good news is that you can do something about it. Nutritionists are finding out that in some cases, the effects of these diseases can be reversed or slowed down considerably just by a change in diet.

By developing the skills of food selection and preparation, you can break many unhealthy habits.

The choices are vast—an elegant four-course meal in a fine restaurant, dinner at the student cafeteria, grabbing a bite on the run. No matter what your pace of life or taste in food, your diet can be healthy—or unhealthy. It depends on what you choose to eat and how you choose to prepare it. Because there is no such thing as a food instinct in humans—eating is a learned behavior—it requires skill to have a good diet. With a better understanding of nutritional needs, and healthy ways to meet those needs, your choices can become smarter choices that benefit your health now and in the future.

What You Need to Eat: The Essential Nutrients

A recent survey by the U.S. Department of Agriculture showed that many people are consciously changing their diets. Nutritionists, however, caution that as a society, we have a long way to go.

- The good news is that Americans are eating more poultry and less red meat than they were ten years ago. Poultry is low in saturated fats; red meat is high.
- The bad news is that people are eating more cheese—in part because of the increasing demand for pizza and other take-out foods. Cheese is often high in saturated fats.

Lowering your fat intake with one kind of food and raising it with another does not lead to a balanced and healthy diet. Whether you are a red meat eater or a vegetarian, you have to know what you need to eat to stay healthy.

Such an understanding begins with knowing the basic structure of foods. All foods are composed of chemical compounds. The body's digestive system breaks down the complex compounds into substances that the body can use for building tissue and creating energy. The basic chemical compounds that make up food are generally referred to as **nutrients** and are specifically called carbohydrates, proteins, fats, vitamins, minerals, and water. (Although water contains no nutritious value, it is essential for life; therefore it is presented with the other chemical compounds necessary for life.)

Carbohydrates

Carbohydrates are made up of sugars and starches. Sugars such as table sugar (sucrose), honey, and corn syrup are **simple carbohydrates** and contain molecules made of only one or two sugar units. Starches found in whole grains, fruits, and vegetables are **complex carbohydrates;** chemically, they are composed of chains of many sugar units.

Carbohydrates represent the body's primary source of energy. According to the U.S. Department of Agriculture's *Dietary Guidelines for Americans*, about 50 percent of your calories should come from complex carbohydrates and about 10 percent from refined sugars. This is because there is a big difference between getting energy from sugar (simple carbohydrates) and from starches (complex carbohydrates). Energy derived from simple carbohydrates, such as those found in a candy bar, lasts only a short period of time. Energy from complex carbohydrates, such as those found in an apple, lasts for a longer period of time. Unfortunately, most people's diets are high in sugar and fat and low in starches.

nutrients The basic chemical compounds that make up food.

carbohydrate Nutrients made of sugars and starches; the body's primary source of energy.

simple carbohydrate A basic nutritional compound made of short chains of simple sugars that are broken down quickly in the body.

complex carbohydrate A basic nutritional component made of long chains of simple sugars that are slowly broken down in the body.

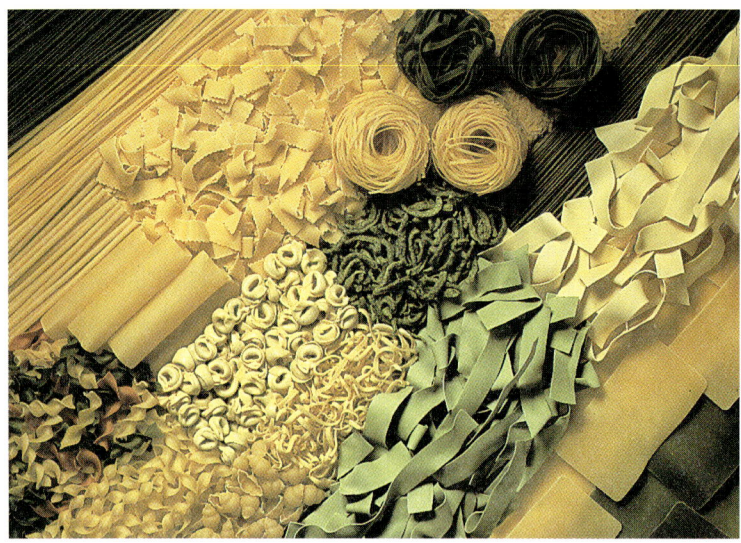

Pasta is a good source of carbohydrates. About 60 percent of your daily calories should come from carbohydrates. (Source: © Tony Stone Images)

Sugar is often found in desserts and soft drinks, but it is also in processed foods including breakfast cereals, canned soups, and prepared main dishes. Although sugar supplies energy, or calories, foods high in sugar provide few nutrients. This is why high-sugar foods are called **empty calories.** Eating too much sugar can fill you up and keep you from eating nutritious food; it can also contribute to tooth decay and excess weight.

Starches are a better way to get carbohydrates. In addition to providing energy, they are a source of many vitamins and minerals. You find them in grain products such as bread, pasta, rice, and cereal and in vegetables such as potatoes, peas, and beans. Many people think that starchy foods are fattening. Actually, eating starchy foods can be a low-calorie way to fill up with good nutrients. What is fattening are the additions, such as butter and sour cream heaped into a baked potato or cream cheese smeared on a bagel.

Fiber is a complex carbohydrate. Starchy vegetables and whole grain breads and cereals are rich in fiber. Fiber plays a particularly important role in the digestive system. **Dietary fiber** cannot be broken down by human digestive enzymes, so it passes down the intestinal tract and contributes bulk to the stool. It binds to water in the digestive process and aids in moving your bowels, producing softer, bulkier stools and more rapid movement of wastes through the intestines. Easy bowel movements are normal for people who consistently choose a high-fiber diet.

A diet that is high in fiber and low in fat may reduce the risk of cancer. Studies show that cancer of the large bowel (**colon cancer**) is very common in economically developed countries such as the United States, Canada, and Western Europe. In contrast, colon cancer is relatively rare in less developed areas of Africa, where the diet consists of high-fiber, unprocessed plant foods. (Other factors in the African diet have to be considered, including the fact that it is also usually low in fat and animal protein.) The possible benefits of fiber for heart disease, diabetes, and obesity are also being studied.

Given this scientific uncertainty, how much fiber should your diet include? The National Cancer Institute recommends eating between twenty and thirty grams a day—considerably more than the average of eleven grams that Americans consume. The old adage, "an apple a day keeps the doctor away," might

empty calories High caloric foods that contain sugar but few nutrients.

starches White, tasteless substances found in potatoes, rice, corn, wheat, and other vegetable products.

fiber A complex carbohydrate that is indigestible by humans.

dietary fiber Food that cannot be broken down by digestive enzymes. It passes down the intestinal tract and contributes to more rapid movement of wastes through the intestines.

colon cancer Cancer of the large bowel.

protein A group of complex compounds containing amino acids that are essential for growth and repair of tissue.

amino acids A class of organic compounds that are the building blocks of proteins.

prove to have a scientific basis, at least as far as the apple's fiber content is concerned (see Figure 5.1).

Proteins

Proteins are the building blocks of the body. They provide the structural framework for the skin, hair, nails, cartilage, tendons, and muscles. They provide an important structural part of the bones and are essential for growth as well as maintenance, regulation of body processes, and replacement of body cells. In fact, they are a vital part of every cell.

Proteins are made up of over twenty **amino acids**. Most of these amino acids can be made, or synthesized, by the body. Nine amino acids cannot be synthesized yet are considered essential for health, so they must be consumed every day to ensure an adequate protein supply. A second reason that proteins must be consumed every day is that, unlike other nutrients such as fat, proteins are not stored. They are used up by the body to make structures such as muscles in a matter of hours. The *Dietary Guidelines* recommends that 12 percent of calories consumed in the diet come from protein.

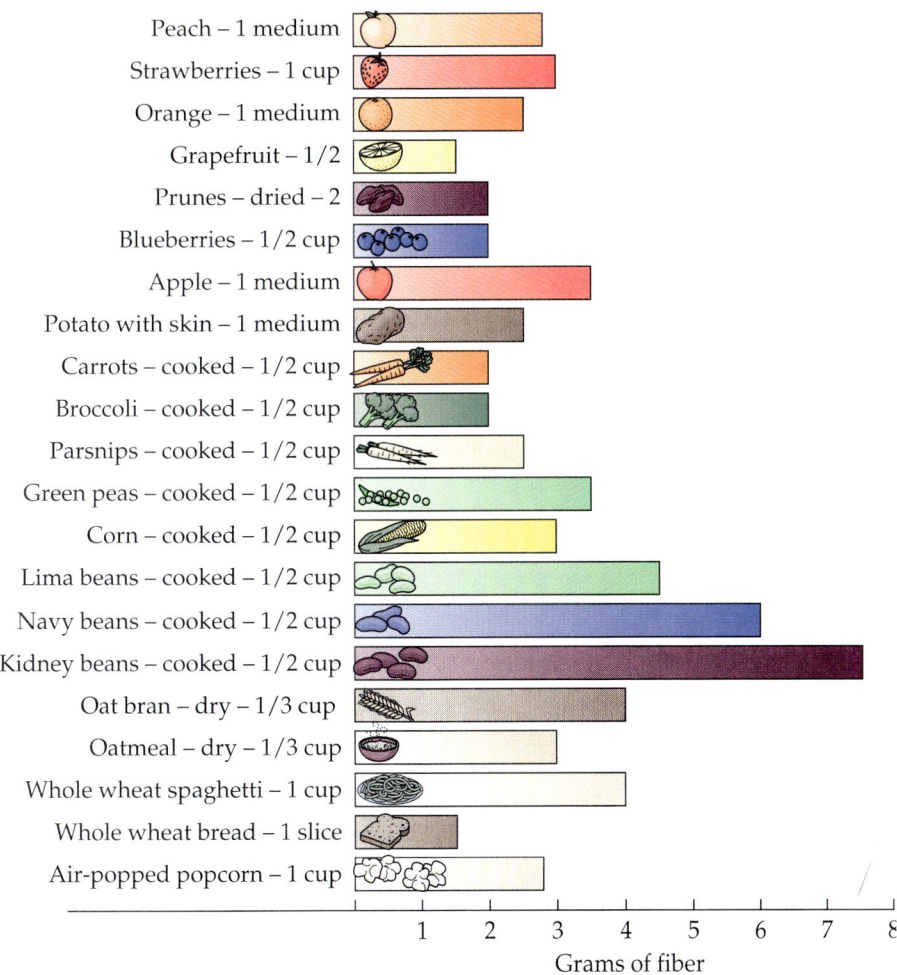

Figure 5.1 Foods with Fiber. *Fiber is found in fruits, vegetables, beans, and grains. This chart lists foods that are good sources of fiber.*

A **complete protein** in food is one that contains all nine of the essential amino acids in amounts that correspond to human needs or amounts needed to make body protein. Complete proteins are found in animal products such as eggs, meat, milk, poultry, fish, and cheese. Unfortunately, many of these sources of protein are also high in fat and cholesterol.

An **incomplete protein** is one in which one or more of the essential amino acids are missing or in short supply relative to the need for protein synthesis. Plants contain incomplete proteins and are divided into three groups: grains, legumes (starchy peas, beans, and lentils), and vegetables. Foods from the grain group must be combined with foods from the legume or vegetable group to form a complete protein. Examples are beans and rice, a bean burrito, or a bean tostada. Any legume plus any grain, or legumes plus nuts and seeds, will give you a complete protein. The concept of **complementary protein relationships** is especially important to **vegetarians,** who must continually combine nonanimal sources of protein to ensure adequate complete protein intake.

Fats

Fats are the most concentrated source of energy in your diet. They also add flavor to foods and are essential for the body's absorption of fat-soluble vitamins (A, D, E, and K). Fatty substances in the body, which are called lipids, also provide insulation from temperature extremes.

There are different kinds of dietary fat. **Saturated fats** are found in animal products such as meat, eggs, milk, and dairy products and in palm oil and coconut oil, which come from plants. This is the type of fat that is deposited along the walls of your arteries. The accumulation of this fat is a contributing factor to diseases of the cardiovascular system such as high blood pressure and heart attack. Because of this, the *Dietary Guidelines* recommends that saturated fats account for less than 10 percent of your total caloric intake.

Unsaturated fats are either polyunsaturated or monounsaturated. Both types of unsaturated fats can lower body cholesterol. Examples of **polyunsaturated fat** are corn oil, soybean oil, and cottonseed oil. Some fish are also sources of polyunsaturated fat. **Monounsaturated fats** are found in peanut oil, olive oil, and canola oil. Although beef fat, lard, and chicken fat have quite a bit of monounsaturated fat, they are also very high in saturated fat. Less than 10 percent of your total daily calories should come from polyunsaturated fat and a little more than 10 percent from monounsaturated fat.

Cholesterol is a fat-like substance that is manufactured by the liver and is necessary for certain bodily processes, including the formation of sex hormones, vitamin D, and bile. Cholesterol is also taken into the body when you eat animal products such as meat, milk, eggs, and dairy foods. Plant foods do not contain cholesterol.

Cholesterol in the body circulates in the blood stream. Eating a diet high in saturated fats causes blood cholesterol levels to rise because once saturated fats enter the body they are not easily used up. Conversely, substituting unsaturated fats for saturated fats can cause blood cholesterol levels to drop. Total cholesterol should be below 200 milligrams per 100 milliliters of blood serum, according to the National Cholesterol Education Program of the National Heart, Lung and Blood Institute. Above that puts you at higher risk for heart disease. You can have too much cholesterol in your blood because your liver overproduces it—a genetically determined factor—and/or because you eat too many foods that contain saturated fat or cholesterol.

High density lipoproteins (HDLs) and **low density lipoproteins (LDLs)** transport cholesterol through the body to cells. HDLs are called the "good guys" because they carry cholesterol in the bloodstream to the liver, where it is used to

---

complete protein A protein containing all nine essential amino acids.

incomplete protein A protein in which one or more of the essential amino acids is missing.

complementary protein relationship The idea that two or more foods, none of which when taken alone would provide a complete protein, can be combined at a meal resulting in a complete protein.

vegetarian A person who follows a diet consisting of no meat, chicken, or fish; all nutrition is obtained from vegetables, fruits, and grains. Some vegetarians eat dairy products.

saturated fat The type of fat that has all hydrogen sites occupied and is usually solid at room temperature; usually comes from animal sources and is thought to encourage plaque build-up.

polyunsaturated fat The type of fat that has several hydrogens available to bind and is soft at room temperature; usually comes from plant or fish sources.

monounsaturated fat The type of fat that has one hydrogen available to bond and is liquid at room temperature; usually comes from plant or fish sources.

cholesterol A white, crystalline substance found especially in animal fats, blood, nerve tissue, and bile; in excessive amounts, a factor in atherosclerosis.

high density lipoproteins (HDLs) A fatty substance that is the type of cholesterol that is considered good and that prevents atherosclerosis.

low density lipoproteins (LDLs) A fatty substance that is the type of cholesterol that is considered bad and that promotes atherosclerosis.

atherosclerosis Hardening of the arteries due to a buildup of fatty plaque.

plaque A buildup of cholesterol in the arteries, which over time can restrict blood flow.

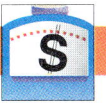

HEALTHWISE CONSUMER

The Butter-Margarine Question

Many people switched to using margarine instead of butter as a way to reduce their intake of saturated fats. Now researchers are questioning how healthy a choice stick margarine is, even though it has far less saturated fat than butter. On a list of ingredients in margarine you are likely to find liquid soybean, corn, or another liquid oil, and partially hydrogenated oil. What do these do? In order to turn an unsaturated fat such as soybean oil into margarine, a process called hydrogenation is used. By adding hydrogen to a liquid oil, the consistency is changed to a solid form. What you get with margarine is a product that contains both saturated and unsaturated fat. Moreover, during the processing, trans fat acids are formed, causing an increase in the LDLs (the bad cholesterol) and a decrease in the HDLs (the good cholesterol). Regular stick margarine is typically about 17 percent trans fat, and researchers now believe that trans fat is the worst type of fat.

A recent study by researchers of more than 80,000 female nurses who were followed for 14 years showed that those who had the highest intake of trans fats had a 53 percent greater risk of having a heart attack than those at the low end of trans fat consumption. The researchers, who were from the Harvard School of Public Health and Brigham and Women's Hospital in Boston, also found that consumption of total fat made no difference to the heart. Women who had the largest consumption of total fat (46 percent of calories) had no greater risk of heart attack than those who had the lowest consumption of total fat (29 percent of calories).

So what should you use? "You can't protect your heart by substituting butter for margarine or margarine for butter," says Dr. Frank Hu, co-author of the nurses study. One solution is to use vegetable oils for cooking and baking. Another is to drip olive oil on your bread rather than spreading on either butter or margarine.

Butter or margarine makes corn taste great. But is it good for you? (Source: © Tony Stone Images/George Kamper)

produce bile. LDLs are called the "bad guys" because they pick up the excess cholesterol and deposit it in the walls of the arteries. If there is a rough spot in an artery, the lipoprotein carrying the fat may get stuck there. When the protein dissolves, the cholesterol is left in the artery. This buildup of cholesterol is called **plaque**. If this process continues for years, it causes **atherosclerosis**, hardening of the arteries.

Plaque causes narrowing of the vessels, which results in reduced blood flow and can cause heart disease. If this occurs in the arteries feeding the heart muscle, a heart attack may occur.

Researchers believe that a healthy blood cholesterol ratio should be one HDL to three LDLs. The best way to lower your cholesterol overall and at the same

HealthLinks
U.S. Department of Agriculture (USDA)
www.nalusda.gov/fnic/dga/dga95/cover.html

A full discussion of the USDA Dietary Guidelines for Americans.

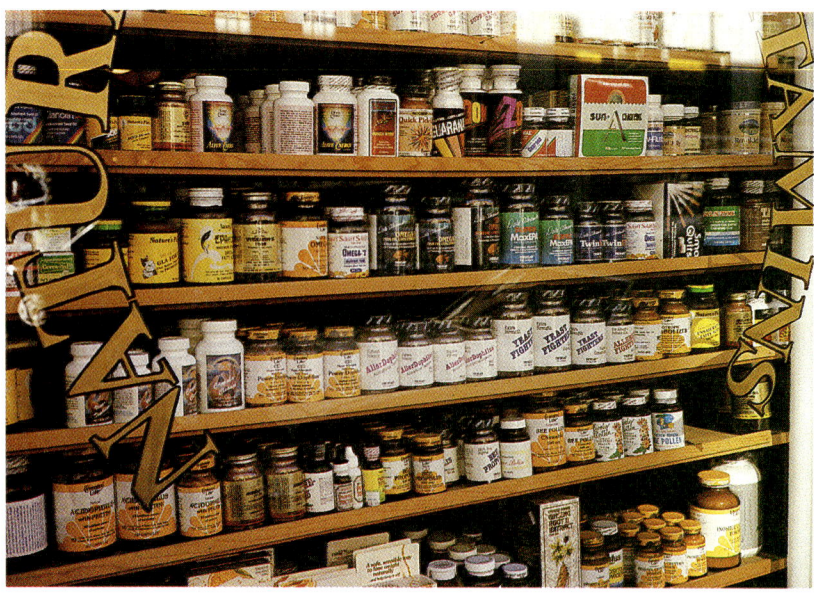

Vitamins, minerals, and other dietary supplements line the shelves of drug and health food stores. The best source of nutrients for you, however, is in the food that you eat—not supplements from bottles. (Source: The Image Works/© T. Shumsky)

time raise the number of HDLs is through diet, aerobic exercise, and not smoking. In some cases, drug therapy is needed to bring the total cholesterol level down. This is particularly true for people with a genetic predisposition to high cholesterol. Given the complexities of cholesterol, only your physician can tell which is the best way to keep your cholesterol levels in check.

Vitamins

Vitamins are the tools used by the body to process food. They do not supply energy, but they help release it from carbohydrates, proteins, and fats. They occur in foods as either fat-soluble or water-soluble substances. In general, the **fat-soluble vitamins** (A, D, E, and K) are stored by the body's fat cells. The **water-soluble vitamins** (the B vitamins and vitamin C) are not stored by the body, and amounts not used by the body are excreted in urine. This is why water-soluble vitamins must be consumed daily. The B vitamins include thiamine, riboflavin, niacin, pyridoxine (B_6), cyanocobalamin (B_{12}), folic acid, pantothenic acid, and biotin. Table 5.1 describes the effects and sources of eleven major vitamins and lists the amount you need.

According to the Food and Drug Administration (FDA), Americans spend $3 billion a year on vitamins and minerals. Who are the buyers of these products? Nearly 40 percent of the public, according to the FDA, purchase vitamin and mineral supplements. Such expenditures are often a waste of money. Taking large doses of vitamin C has never been proven effective for curing conditions ranging from cancer to the common cold. Because vitamin C is a water-soluble vitamin, what is not used by the body is excreted in the urine, so there are few harmful effects to taking it. This is not the case with all vitamins. Taking large amounts of fat-soluble vitamins A and D, which are stored in the body, can lead to toxicity, serious illness, and even death.

In special circumstances, some people need to take supplemental vitamins. Included in this group are pregnant women and nursing mothers; strict vegetarians; the elderly who do not eat balanced meals; and people recovering from

fat-soluble vitamins Those vitamins that are transported and stored by the body's fat cells; examples are vitamins A, D, E, and K.

water-soluble vitamins Those vitamins not stored in the body, with excesses excreted in the urine; examples are B-complex vitamins, and vitamin C.

trace minerals Minerals that are essential for proper growth and functioning but are needed in very small amounts.

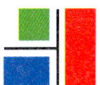

TABLE 5.1   How Vitamins Help You

Vitamin	What it does	Sources	Recommended Dietary Allowance*
A	Maintains skin and eyes; is needed for normal growth of bones and teeth, and for good night vision	Milk, liver, fish, eggs, butter, green and yellow vegetables, cheese	5,000 International Units
B_1	Helps in normal metabolism of carbohydrates; helps in the release of energy from food	Meat, whole-grain cereals, nuts, soybeans, peas, potatoes, and most vegetables and fruits	1.5 milligrams
B_2	Helps the body cells use oxygen; assists in repair of tissue and healthy skin, maintains nervous tissue	Milk, cheese, liver, fish, poultry, yeast, fruits, lean meats	1.7 milligrams
Niacin	Is needed for cell metabolism of carbohydrates; helps maintain healthy skin	Liver, yeast, lean meat, enriched breads and cereals	20 milligrams
B_{12}	Is essential for red blood cell development; helps proper function of nervous system	Eggs, meat, milk, milk products	6 micrograms
K	Is essential for normal blood clotting	Leafy vegetables; made by intestinal bacteria	No official RDA
Biotin	Maintains the circulatory system and maintains healthy skin	Eggs, liver, kidney, most fresh vegetables; available in a great variety of foods	0.3 milligram
Folic acid	Essential in the production of red blood cells	Green leafy vegetables, yeast, meat, liver	0.4 milligram
C	Essential for growth and maintenance of bones and teeth; needed for tissue metabolism and wound healing	Citrus fruits, tomatoes, raw cabbage, potatoes, strawberries, green peppers, cantaloupe, other vegetables	60 milligrams
D	Essential for calcium and phosphorus metabolism	Fish liver oils, fortified milk, eggs, tuna, salmon, sunlight on the skin	400 International Units
E	Helps maintain heart and skeletal muscles and may help maintain the reproductive system	Whole-grain cereals, lettuce, vegetable oils	30 milligrams

*For ages 4 and older.

major wounds such as burns or from specific vitamin deficiency diseases, malabsorption, or prolonged illness. Most healthy people, however, do not need supplements. The best sources of vitamins are found in foods.

Minerals

Minerals form healthy bones and teeth, regulate body functioning, and help nerves and muscles react normally. Minerals are divided into two categories: major and trace. Major minerals are needed in the diet in amounts of 100 milligrams or more per day. Other minerals are essential to healthy living but are needed in smaller amounts and are referred to as **trace minerals.**

Major minerals	Trace minerals
Calcium	Chromium
Chloride	Cobalt
Magnesium	Copper
Phosphorus	Fluoride
Potassium	Iodine
Sodium	Iron
Sulfur	Manganese
	Molybdenum
	Selenium
	Zinc

As with vitamins, daily needs can generally be met by eating a balanced diet. Milk products and vegetables are particularly important sources of minerals. Some groups of people have difficulty meeting their needs for certain minerals in their diet. For example, iron is often limited in the diets of children under four years old and women up to age fifity. Supplements are often recommended in these instances, particularly for pregnant women and those who are breast feeding.

Many diets are also not sufficient in calcium, a mineral important for building strong bones and teeth in growing children and for helping maintain the bones of adults. A condition that may be related to calcium intake throughout life is osteoporosis. **Osteoporosis** is a disorder in which bone density decreases and bones are more likely to break. The risk for osteoporosis is greater for women than for men, especially after women experience menopause. Many health researchers believe that adequate calcium in the diet or calcium added as supplements may help prevent or slow osteoporosis.

Dairy products are usually the first calcium-rich foods that come to mind, but these can be high in fat content. Surprisingly, about half of the daily needs for calcium can come from nondairy food. For a list of good sources of calcium and the amount a serving of each contains, see Figure 5.2.

Figure 5.2 Foods Rich in Calcium. *Recognizing that most Americans do not get enough calcium to promote bone growth, in 1997, the Institute of Medicine upped the daily calcium-intake recommendation. College students ages 19 to 30 should consume 1,000 milligrams (mg) of calcium a day, and those under age 19 need 1,300 mg, according to new dietary recommendations. Here's how you can get the calcium you need.*

Calcium (mg)	Food product
400	Yogurt, plain, low-fat, 1 cup
370	Sardines, with bones, 3 oz.
300	Milk, all types, 1 cup
290	Orange juice, enriched, 1 cup
270	Swiss cheese, 1 oz.
250	Pizza, 1 slice, 4 oz.
225	Salmon, with bones, 3 oz.
200	Turnip greens, 1 cup cooked
175	Ice cream or ice milk, 1 cup
150	Cottage cheese, 1 cup
150–250	Cereal, fortified, 3/4 cup
140	Baked beans, canned, 1 cup
115	Tofu, 2 oz.
70	Broccoli, 1 cup cooked

Calcium supplements can pose problems, such as kidney damage in susceptible people, so getting calcium from your diet is the preferred way, according to most nutritionists. The calcium supplement issue is further complicated because some nutritionists say it is not possible to truly know what an adequate calcium intake is. This is because it is believed that the body can compensate for lowered calcium in the blood by cutting down on the amount of calcium that is excreted in the stool and urine. This, in turn, could increase the amount of calcium the body absorbs from dietary intake. One nondietary way to prevent or retard the onset of osteoporosis is through weight-bearing exercise, such as walking or biking.

Since most people reach their peak bone mass by the time they are thirty years old, it is important to begin to take actions earlier in life to retard the progress of or prevent the disease. You can read more about preventing osteoporosis through exercise in Chapter 7 and the effects of it later in life in Chapter 18.

Sodium is a puzzling mineral. It is essential to health and at the same time it can cause health problems—at least in the amounts consumed by most people. It is the only mineral that is too abundant in most American diets.

Sodium draws water into the body's blood vessels and therefore helps maintain normal blood volume and blood pressure. It is also needed for the normal function of nerves and muscles. The body needs only a small amount of sodium to carry out these functions—perhaps as little as 500 milligrams per day. The daily average currently consumed—5,000 to 7,000 milligrams—far exceeds this. Between 2,000 and 2,500 milligrams a day is a good target for healthy people.

High sodium intake is of concern because it may be linked with **hypertension** (high blood pressure), a condition that affects about one quarter of the population and leads to higher risk for stroke, heart attack, and kidney failure.

Critical Thinking Question

An objective in *Healthy People 2000* is to "Decrease salt and sodium intake so at least 80 percent of people avoid using salt at the table, and at least 40 percent of adults regularly purchase foods modified or lower in sodium." What strategies do you think public health officials should undertake to bring about the successful accomplishment of this objective? Currently, 56 percent of adults avoid using salt at the table and 19 percent buy reduced-salt products. To what extent is the barrier to this objective a lack of health knowledge, health skills, and health values?

The direct relationship between sodium and hypertension is not well understood. Studies show that population groups that consume a lot of sodium tend to have a high incidence of hypertension, whereas those groups that consume little sodium have a low incidence. Salt consumption is high in northern Japan—about twenty to twenty-five grams per day—and so is the prevalence of hypertension. In contrast, the Luo tribe in Kenya have a diet that is low in sodium; they also have a low incidence of hypertension. When Luos migrate to urban areas and switch to a higher-sodium diet, their incidence of hypertension goes up. Researchers are cautious about blaming sodium alone because other factors may

osteoporosis A disorder in which bone density decreases, making the bones more likely to break.

hypertension A chronic disease better known as high blood pressure.

be involved. For example, rural diets often include large amounts of fresh vegetables that are rich in potassium, a mineral that may protect against hypertension.

Even though some people may never have health problems because of high sodium intake, nutritionists recommend that everyone be cautious about eating foods that contain a great deal of sodium. Virtually everything you eat contains *some* sodium. It is found naturally in foods—and even in the water supply. But most of the sodium in our diet comes from that added to foods as a preservative and as a way to enhance taste. Foods that are particularly high in sodium include cured and processed meats, canned vegetables, dairy products—especially many cheeses—and many bread and bakery products. You should beware also of the high sodium levels in condiments, sauces, and seasonings such as onion salt, meat tenderizer, soy sauce, barbecue sauce, ketchup, mustard, pickles, and relish. Review Table 5.2, and compare the recommended daily sodium intake of 2,000 to 2,500 milligrams to what you may typically consume each day from this list.

TABLE 5.2   Where's the Salt

Food groups	Sodium, mg
Bread, cereal, rice, and pasta	
Cooked cereal, rice, pasta, unsalted, 1/2 cup	Trace
Ready-to-eat cereal, 1 oz.	100–360
Bread, 1 slice	110–175
Vegetable	
Vegetables, fresh or frozen, cooked without salt, 1/2 cup	Less than 70
Vegetables, canned or frozen with sauce, 1/2 cup	140–460
Tomato juice, canned, 3/4 cup	660
Vegetable soup, canned, 1 cup	820
Fruit	
Fruit, fresh, frozen, canned, 1/2 cup	Trace
Milk, yogurt, and cheese	
Milk, 1 cup	120
Yogurt, 8 oz.	160
Natural cheeses, 1-1/2 oz.	110–450
Processed cheeses, 2 oz.	800
Meat, poultry, fish, dry beans, eggs, and nuts	
Fresh meat, poultry, fish, 3 oz.	Less than 90
Tuna, canned, water pack, 3 oz.	300
Bologna, 2 oz.	580
Ham, lean roasted, 3 oz.	1,020
Other	
Salad dressing, 1 tbsp.	75–220
Ketchup, mustard, steak sauce, 1 tbsp.	130–230
Soy sauce, 1 tbsp.	1,030
Salt, 1 tsp.	2,000
Dill pickle, 1 medium	930
Potato chips, salted, 1 oz.	130
Corn chips, salted, 1 oz.	235
Peanuts, roasted in oil, salted, 1 oz.	120

Source: U.S. Department of Agriculture

dehydration An abnormal loss of water.

food additive Any substance used in producing, processing, treating, packaging, transporting, or storing food to enhance food, enrich food, or lengthen its grocery store shelf life.

The salt habit is just that—a habit. People who have high-sodium diets crave salt because their tastes are used to it. But like any habit, it can be broken, and after cutting back for several weeks, the craving—or even the desire—for salt disappears.

To start breaking the salt habit:

- Sprinkle herbs and spices, rather than salt, on food to heighten the flavor.
- Select foods that are naturally lower in sodium.
- Have an apple or some peeled carrots as a snack instead of salted peanuts or potato chips.

Water

Often called the forgotten nutrient, water is essential to life. Without it, you could live only about one week. About 65 to 70 percent of your body weight is made up of water in the form of blood, saliva, sweat, urine, cellular fluids, and digestive enzymes. In all these various forms, water helps transport nutrients, remove wastes, and regulate body temperature.

Water carries nutrients along the digestive path and to the cells. First, it does this by liquefying food and moving it through the stomach, small intestine, and large intestine. When the food is absorbed into the blood, water plays an important role by regulating the concentration of nutrients on both sides of the cell walls.

Water needs vary, depending on the climate and a person's activity level. In a cold climate, the demand by the body for water is less than in a warm climate. An active person's demand for water is much greater than a sedentary person's demand. Also, more water is needed at higher altitudes than at lower altitudes. Bodily water is lost through perspiration and respiration.

There are many ways to get liquid from your diet. The most obvious source is a glass of water. Most authorities agree that six to eight glasses of water per day provide an adequate supply to the average adult. Other healthy beverages are skim or low-fat milk and fruit juices. In addition, many fruits and vegetables are excellent sources of water.

Conditions such as high fever, nausea, or diarrhea may result in an abnormal loss of water called **dehydration.** Extended periods of dehydration resulting in as much as a 10 percent reduction in intracellular water concentration may lead to death.

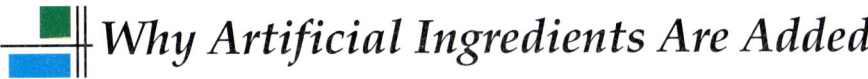

Why Artificial Ingredients Are Added

There is an alphabet soup of chemicals—BHT, BHA, MSG, and as many as 3,000 other compounds—added to many of the foods you buy at the supermarket. In one sense, food additives are not new. For thousands of years, salt has been used as a meat preservative.

Food additives serve a number of functions, including making foods more attractive, enhancing their taste or quality, and ensuring that they last longer in storage. Under the Food, Drug and Cosmetic Act, the term **food additive** is defined as any substance that "results or may be reasonably expected to result—directly or indirectly—in its becoming a component or otherwise affecting the characteristics of any food." Anything used in producing, processing, treating, packaging, transporting, or storing food is included in the definition of a food additive.

There are five broad types of additives. In decreasing order of their contribution to health, they are nutrients, preservatives, processing aids, flavorings, and colorings.

HealthLinks

U.S. Food and Drug Administration (FDA)
www.fda.gov

Provides information for consumers and professionals in the areas of food safety, supplements, and medical devices and links to other sources of nutrition and food information.

NUTRIENTS Vitamins and minerals are used to increase the nutritional value of a food. This is referred to as fortification. Fortification provides nutrients lacking in the diet—for example, by adding vitamins A and D to milk—or replaces nutrients lost in processing, particularly in bread products. The added vitamins are chemically identical to those that were removed in processing.

PRESERVATIVES A variety of chemicals are used to preserve foods. BHT (butylated hydroxytoluene) and BHA (butylated hydroxyanisole), for example, are used to keep fats from turning rancid in vegetable oils, potato chips, cereals, and other convenience foods. Nitrates and nitrites are used as meat preservatives. Many food manufacturers are finding the same preservative effects in natural substances such as ascorbic acid, citric acid, and vitamin E.

PROCESSING AIDS Emulsifiers such as lecithin, mono- and diglycerides, and polysorbate keep particles evenly mixed and homogeneous. Stabilizers and thickeners, including gums, gelatin, pectin, cellulose, and starch, improve consistency and provide desired texture. In addition, agents such as citric acid, acetic acid, alkalis, and buffers control the acidity or alkalinity of foods, which also affects texture and taste.

FLAVORINGS The most commonly used additives—sugar, salt, and corn syrup—give food a more agreeable flavor. They are added to candies, baked goods, soft drinks, and many processed foods. Some of these appear in their natural form, such as simple sugar, whereas others are artificial, such as aspartame. Other flavor enhancers include monosodium glutamate (MSG), hydrolyzed vegetable protein, and malt.

COLORINGS Artificial colors are perhaps the most controversial additives. They provide no nutrients, and their safety is under continuing review. The primary concern about artificial dyes is the fear of their carcinogenic effect. Many dyes have been banned by the FDA, including Red No. 2, which was once the

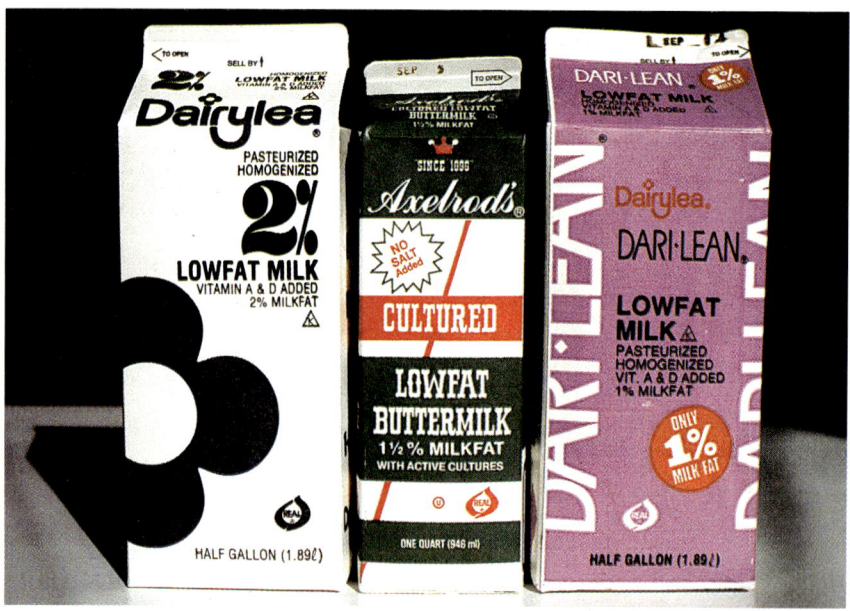

Vitamins A and D are added to milk as a way to fortify some of the nutrients lacking in the normal diet. (Source: Photo Researchers, Inc./© Art Attack)

most widely used food coloring in the United States. Only Yellow No. 5 must be listed by name on a food label because many people are allergic to it. Food colorings also come from natural sources such as carotene, caramel, and fruit juice.

You may be concerned about the possible carcinogenic or allergic effects of additives. Nitrates and nitrites are known to promote cancer in laboratory animals but continue to be used in food processing. Some studies have shown that BHA and BHT cause cancer in rats, whereas other studies have found that they may actually prevent cancer in some circumstances. BHA and BHT remain in processed foods, as well as in raw and cooked meat-based toppings for pizza and meatballs. Sulfites cause breathing difficulties, wheezing, hives, diarrhea, vomiting, and even death in people allergic to them, yet they are used in many packaged foods and some seafood to retard spoilage. Although only a fraction of the public is allergic to sulfites, the reactions are severe enough that the FDA now requires that sulfites be included in the ingredients listed on the labels of packaged foods that contain them. With all these problems, why do these additives remain in foods? Because their benefits are still believed to outweigh their risks.

To limit your intake of additives, eat mainly fresh or minimally processed foods. This makes good overall nutritional sense. Highly processed food—cookies, candy, and soda—is low in nutrients and high not only in artificial coloring and other additives but also in calories, sugars, fats, and sodium. Eating a variety of foods reduces your exposure to any one additive, a smart choice if that additive turns out to pose long-term risks.

Recommended Dietary Allowances: How Much Do You Need?

It is easy to be overwhelmed by the idea of the number of nutrients found in food. To simplify things, the Food and Nutrition Board of the National Academy of Science publishes **recommended dietary allowances (RDAs).** RDAs are guidelines for the average amounts of some of the essential nutrients to be consumed by healthy individuals over a period of time. Notice that additives are not found in the list of essential nutrients. That is because they are not essential to a healthy diet. There are RDAs for vitamins, minerals, protein, and energy (calories). In general, the RDAs are set at a value greater than the needs of most people. This is because the body does not utilize some nutrients as efficiently as others. For example, the recommendation for iron is based on the understanding that the body absorbs only about 10 percent of the iron eaten.

Keep in mind that the RDAs are not quotas that have to be met every single day in order to avoid health risks and that nutrients are needed in various amounts depending on your age, gender, size, health, and level of activity. But the longer you deviate from the RDAs, the more you risk incurring health problems. Consuming less than 70 percent of the RDAs on a regular basis is a cause for concern. Look at the RDAs for vitamins in Table 5.1. To test your overall nutrition knowledge, see the Here's Looking at You box.

You may have heard of the four food groups. For years, nutritionists used these groups to measure what has been called a balanced diet. *Balanced* referred to the amount of nutrient intake based on the following groupings: the meat group (meat, poultry, fish); the milk group (milk, yogurt, cheese); the fruits and vegetables group (fruits and vegetables); and the bread group (bread, cereal, rice). This convenient grouping of foods was a very successful marketing device for the meat and milk products industries. But the four food groups did not accurately measure nutritional balance in a diet. In fact, with what we know about nutrition today, the emphasis on meat and milk could be considered unhealthy.

recommended dietary allowances (RDAs) Guidelines for the average amounts of some of the essential nutrients to be consumed by healthy individuals over a period of time.

HERE'S LOOKING AT YOU

Testing Your Nutritional Knowledge

What should you do to have a nutritionally adequate diet and at the same time reduce the incidence of disease? According to the most recent dietary guidelines of the U.S. Department of Health and Human Services and Department of Agriculture, the best advice is to

- Eat a variety of foods
- Maintain a healthy weight
- Choose a diet low in fat, saturated fat, and cholesterol
- Choose a diet containing plenty of vegetables, fruits, and grain products
- Use sugar only in moderation
- Use sodium only in moderation
- Drink alcoholic beverages in moderation if you do so

The following test consists of twenty statements about eating patterns based on the *Dietary Guidelines for Americans*. Put a check to show whether you think each statement is true or false. If you don't know whether a statement is true or false, put a check under don't know.

	True	False	Don't know
1. One way for people to increase the amount of fiber in their diets is to eat more fruit.	( )	( )	( )
2. Cooking chicken without the skin reduces its fat content.	( )	( )	( )
3. Flavorings such as soy sauce, mustard, and garlic salt are good low-sodium substitutes for table salt.	( )	( )	( )
4. Most cheeses are high in salt.	( )	( )	( )
5. Hot dogs are a good source of protein.	( )	( )	( )
6. Broiled foods have more fat than fried foods.	( )	( )	( )
7. A breaded pork chop has more fat than a broiled pork chop.	( )	( )	( )
8. Chicken nuggets are much lower in fat than a hamburger.	( )	( )	( )
9. Foods that are low in cholesterol are naturally low in fat.	( )	( )	( )

(continued)

Critical Thinking Question

The four food groups were, at one time, our best guide to proper nutrition. This guide was successfully used by the meat and milk products industries to increase sales. The six-part Food Guide Pyramid now replaces the four food groups. How might different food industries take advantage of this new guide to nutrition? What industries stand to gain the most from the new guide? What industries will be harmed?

In the early 1990s, a more accurate device—the Food Guide Pyramid—was developed for the *Dietary Guidelines for Americans*. It is a general guide of what to eat daily. It recommends that you eat a variety of six different kinds of foods to get the nutrients you need and the right amount of calories to maintain proper

	True	False	Don't know
10. Butter and margarine have about the same amount of cholesterol.	( )	( )	( )
11. Pizza is high in fat.	( )	( )	( )
12. Dry cooked beans are a good source of fiber.	( )	( )	( )
13. Expensive brands of ice cream usually have less fat than the cheaper brands.	( )	( )	( )
14. Most people should eat fewer starchy foods, such as bread and potatoes.	( )	( )	( )
15. Eating a lot of salt may increase a person's chance of developing high blood pressure.	( )	( )	( )
16. Eating starchy foods, such as crackers, between meals increases a person's chance of developing tooth decay.	( )	( )	( )
17. Drinking a lot of alcohol interferes with the body's ability to use vitamins and minerals.	( )	( )	( )
18. Being overweight does not affect a person's chance of developing coronary heart disease.	( )	( )	( )
19. Diets that are very low in calories can cause serious health problems.	( )	( )	( )
20. Most people should take a multivitamin every day.	( )	( )	( )

Scoring

Item No.	Answer	Item No.	Answer	Item No.	Answer
1	T	8	F	15	T
2	T	9	F	16	T
3	F	10	F	17	T
4	T	11	T	18	F
5	F	12	T	19	T
6	F	13	F	20	F
7	T	14	F		

Source: U.S. Public Health Service

weight. The Food Guide Pyramid is a little more complicated than the four food groups model, but it is based on scientifically arrived at guidelines, not on business interests.

Look at the illustration of the Food Guide Pyramid in Figure 5.3. Notice how the meat and milk groups of food receive a much smaller emphasis than do breads and cereals. Also notice what is meant by a serving size. Some of the serving sizes are smaller than what you might usually eat. For example, many people eat a cup or more of pasta in a meal, which, according to the Food Guide Pyramid, is equal to two or more servings.

One way to understand how big a serving size is with reasonable accuracy is to compare it visually to something common. Consider the following serving sizes:

- 1 ounce of meat = matchbook
- 3 ounces of meat = bar of soap
- 8 ounces of meat = tennis ball
- 1 cup of vegetables or fruit = your fist
- 1 cup of dry cereal = large handful
- 1 teaspoon of butter or margarine = tip of your thumb
- 1/2 cup of cooked pasta = scoop of ice cream

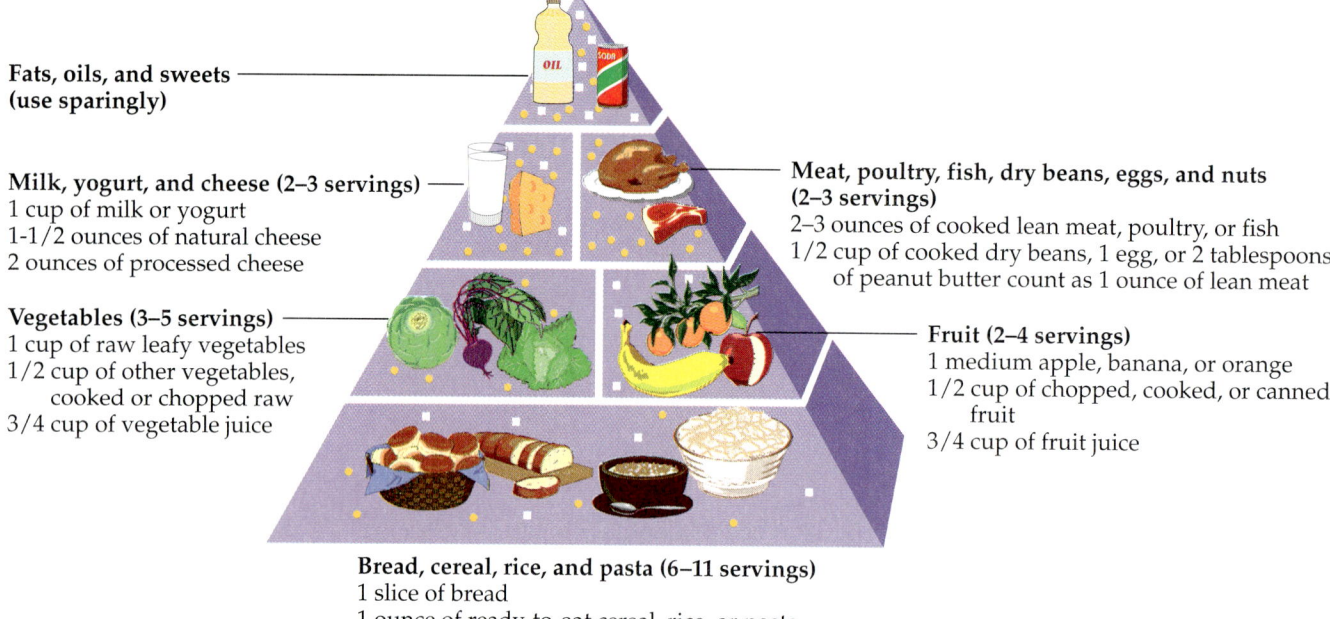

Fats, oils, and sweets (use sparingly)

Milk, yogurt, and cheese (2–3 servings)
1 cup of milk or yogurt
1-1/2 ounces of natural cheese
2 ounces of processed cheese

Meat, poultry, fish, dry beans, eggs, and nuts (2–3 servings)
2–3 ounces of cooked lean meat, poultry, or fish
1/2 cup of cooked dry beans, 1 egg, or 2 tablespoons of peanut butter count as 1 ounce of lean meat

Vegetables (3–5 servings)
1 cup of raw leafy vegetables
1/2 cup of other vegetables, cooked or chopped raw
3/4 cup of vegetable juice

Fruit (2–4 servings)
1 medium apple, banana, or orange
1/2 cup of chopped, cooked, or canned fruit
3/4 cup of fruit juice

Bread, cereal, rice, and pasta (6–11 servings)
1 slice of bread
1 ounce of ready-to-eat cereal, rice, or pasta

*Some foods fit into more than one category. Starchy vegetables such as potatoes, corn, sweet potatoes, and taro (poi) can be counted as servings in the grain products instead of as vegetables. Dry beans, peas, and lentils are in the meat group but can be counted as servings of vegetables instead. These crossover foods can be counted as servings from either one or the other group but not from both.

Figure 5.3 The Food Guide Pyramid. *The Food Guide Pyramid is a general guide of what to eat each day. It recommends that you eat a variety of foods to get the nutrients you need and the right amount of calories necessary to maintain a healthy weight. The pyramid focuses on fats because most American diets are too high in fat. (Source: U.S. Department of Agriculture,* Dietary Guidelines for Americans)

Eating Styles

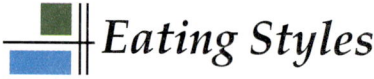

The fast pace of today's lifestyle has led to eating patterns that often present health problems. For the college student, breakfast is often skipped or consists of coffee and sweet rolls, and lunch may be only a large soft drink. Snacks often take the place of missed meals. Most college students are eating on their own for the first time and have no parents around to remind—or nag—them to eat a balanced diet.

Throughout the life cycle, special nutritional needs must be met. Teenagers are growing rapidly, undergo hormonal changes, and often have high levels of physical activity. Pregnant women and nursing mothers have obvious additional nutritional requirements. As people get older, adjustments generally need to be made in eating habits. Part of this is due to a natural slowing of the metabolic processes. Another reason is that most people tend to exercise less as they age. More sedentary people need to eat less food. Specific adjustments, such as low-salt or low-fat diets, may be prescribed by a physician due to a particular risk factor.

Runners, bikers, swimmers, volleyball and basketball players, and weekend athletes of any age need extra calories to accommodate their high-intensity exercise needs. However, athletes do not need extra protein and, despite what some advertising suggests, should avoid protein drinks as a source of energy. The Developing Health Skills box describes the special, age-related nutritional needs and concerns of each of the five stages in the life span.

Eating at Home

Most people learn their eating behaviors around the family table. African Americans and Hispanics, for example, are more likely to have a lifelong habit of eating fruits and vegetables than are whites. However, whites eat vegetables cooked in fat to a lesser degree than do the other two ethnic groups. The type of food prepared, the atmosphere in which it was consumed, and the amount of food eaten quite often can be traced to past experiences.

Historically, many of the foods consumed at home had an ethnic tie. Today, eating styles are far more alike than different. You do not have to be Jewish to eat bagels and cream cheese. Fresh tortillas are in supermarkets across the country. And more than 95 percent of Americans say they eat pizza often—both at home and in restaurants.

Another aspect of life that is changing is dinner as a relaxed family affair including time for communication. Increasingly, family dinners are eaten at fast food places, and when they are eaten at home, they are often consumed while the family watches a television show. Around the world, American-type fast food establishments are changing traditional eating habits.

Fast-Food Living

People all over the world are eating out in restaurants more than they have ever done before. The National Restaurant Association estimates that more than 45 billion meals are eaten in restaurants and cafeterias in the United States each year. This means that on the average, each person eats out almost 200 times a year.

Two of every five dollars spent on eating out goes to fast food restaurants. For the most part, consumers are willing to pay for this convenience even though they most often do not get good nutritional value for their money. Fast food hamburgers, fried chicken, and milk shakes are usually high in fats, salt, and sugar.

Not all fast food is synonymous with junk food. Some fast foods are healthy, depending on the ingredients and how they are cooked. A grilled chicken sandwich or a salad with a light vinaigrette, for example, are on the top of the list of a group of health experts. To help health-conscious customers, more and more restaurants are providing nutritional information on their menus. Read the Cultural View box to learn how to savor flavors without fat when you go out for ethnic food, and review Figure 5.4 the next time you are going to order out from a deli.

Vegetarian Alternative

The vegetarian diet has gained popularity in recent years, particularly among college students. There have always been vegetarians who, for religious or ethical reasons, choose not to eat meat. But now people are choosing a vegetarian diet on health grounds alone.

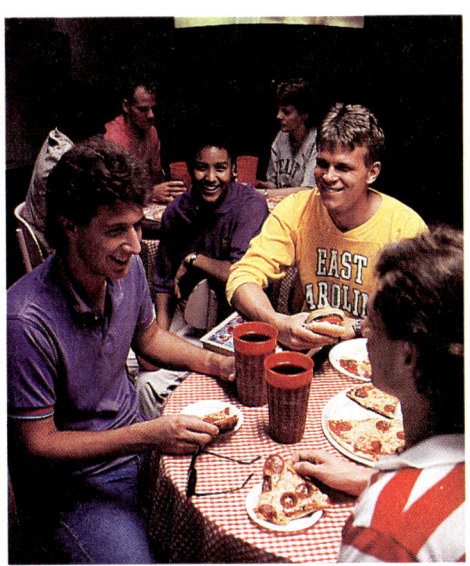

Pizza is a favorite fast food for college students, but it can be high in saturated fat if you go heavy on the cheese, sausage, and pepperoni. Ask for mushrooms, green peppers, or other vegetable toppings, instead. (Source: Tony Stone Images/© Charles Gupton)

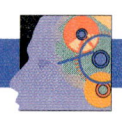

DEVELOPING HEALTH SKILLS

Eating through the Ages

Take it from a former Surgeon General: Not many Americans of any age are undernourished. For most, he says, the problem is overeating; not surprisingly, obesity is a health concern for Americans from the age of six months to sixty years. Beyond that, he says, most Americans do have trouble striking an ideal balance among the foods they choose. During life's five stages, that imbalance—typically in the direction of too much fat—can lead to various health worries, including long-term risks for heart disease, cancer, stroke, and diabetes. Compared to these big threats, vitamins and minerals seem like a minor issue. All the same, there are some special age-related eating problems worth protecting against.

	Special Conditions	May Be Low	What To Do
Infants and Toddlers Humans grow fastest in the first year of life, more than doubling their weight in the first twelve months. Metabolism races: Babies' hearts beat 120 to 140 times a minute, almost twice as fast as adults'. Most babies are very good at demanding nourishment, but sometimes parents overdo their response.	Tooth decay (toddlers)	Fluoride Vitamin D Iron	From birth to four months, most infants get all the nutrients they need in breast milk or iron-fortified formulas. After that, up to age two, the only common worries are obesity and tooth decay, especially if teeth are bathed in juice or milk when bottles are given as pacifiers. Parents should resist offering food for comfort or as a reward. Regular meals and snacks will help thwart impulsive eating. Weaned infants should be fed baby foods with no extra fat and sugar, then switched gradually to the family's diet. (It's easiest to detect allergies if foods are added one at a time.)
Children Lifelong eating habits are shaped in childhood, making it the perfect time for parents to accustom their kids to healthful meals—whether or not the foods served become favorites. Children's tastes and appetites will swing wildly as their growth speeds up and slows down.	Iron-deficiency anemia Tooth decay	Iron Zinc	If the everyday fare includes skim or low-fat milk, lean meats, whole grains, fish, beans, and plenty of fruits and vegetables, kids will get enough iron and zinc. But it's up to parents to select those foods and then set consistent times for meals and snacks. Beyond that, children should be given freedom to decide whether to eat what they're served, and how much. They seem to prefer vegetables slightly undercooked and not served in a jumble. For snacks, keep fruit, muffins, whole-grain crackers, and low-fat yogurt—and hold back on the tooth-rotting sweets.

(continued)

Teenagers Girls' adolescent growth spurt is over around age fifteen. For boys, it winds down by nineteen. An active fifteen-year-old boy may eat fully twice as much as his twin sister does. While both girls and boys need relatively high amounts of calcium and iron, boys are more likely to get enough because they eat so much, while girls are often dieting.	Iron-deficiency anemia Anorexia and bulimia	Calcium Iron Vitamin A Vitamin C	Teenagers may skip meals, wolf fast foods, and snack constantly, but they can still be well-nourished if the kitchen is stocked with easy-to-grab foods, such as broiled chicken, fresh fruit, low-fat yogurt and milk, whole-grain breads, and popcorn. By appealing to teenagers' concerns about their looks, parents can promote regular exercise and rational eating—the best ways around the starvation disorders anorexia and bulimia, which bedevil one percent of teenage girls.
Adults Young and middle-aged adults often violate their own better judgment at mealtime in the face of hectic family lives and demanding jobs. Chronic diseases don't usually strike people when they're twenty or thirty, but a poor diet can increase their likelihood later on.	Iron-deficiency anemia	Vitamin B_6 Calcium Iron Vitamin E Folacin Zinc Magnesium	To make meals nutritious and fast, keep it simple: Stir-fry some vegetables with lean meat or tofu. Or make a batch of spaghetti sauce on the weekend to eat during the week. If you must rely on convenience foods, check the labels for the ones with the least fat, cholesterol, and salt. And if you often eat in restaurants, order salad and vegetables with your entree and then go easy on the dressing and butter. By steering clear of highly processed foods and favoring fresh ones, you're more likely to get all the nutrients you need. Pregnant women may need to take iron and folacin.
Elderly In old age, metabolism slows, bones thin, the senses of smell and taste weaken, and stomach enzymes diminish. Chronic diseases can strike, depending on lifelong health habits and inherited tendencies. And drugs, especially in combination, may keep the body from properly absorbing nutrients.	Osteoporosis Indigestion, heartburn, constipation	Calcium Iron Zinc Folacin Vitamin B_6 Magnesium	Older people in good health should probably keep on with their current diet and exercise routines. One way to beat a sluggish metabolism is to get moving in any way you can. The more active you are, the more calories you can afford and the more vitamins and minerals you'll get with them. For those who don't exercise, a daily multiple vitamin and mineral supplement may be in order. Eating fiber-rich foods, such as whole grains, fruits, and vegetables, and drinking plenty of milk, juice, or water each day can offset the need to take laxatives.

Source: "Eating through the Ages," researched by Patricia Long, *Hippocrates,* May–June 1989. Reprinted by permission of Time Inc. Health

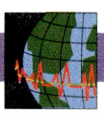

CULTURAL VIEW

How to Savor the Flavors without the Fat

Eating out should be an exotic adventure—not a guilt-ridden misadventure. Is the Korean specialty *gul jun* going to show up on your thighs next week? Is Indonesian *opor ayam* going to stick your arteries with the bill? Here's a guide to the ins and outs of fifteen popular ethnic menus.

	Fine any time	**Go easy on**
Cajun	Red beans and rice (without sausage); greens, meaning kale, mustard greens, or okra; cornbread; shrimp creole (in a tomato sauce over rice); jambalaya or gumbo (order the poultry or seafood versions); blackened fish (heavily seasoned and cooked quickly with very little oil); boiled seafood dishes.	Hush puppies (fried cornbread); dirty rice (fried rice with fatty meats); sausage dishes including *boudin* or *andouille*; rich soups or stews like bisque (cream broth) and *etouffé* (lots of butter); batter-fried seafoods.
Caribbean	Black bean soup or pepper pot (spicy vegetable and pork soup); vegetables like callalo (similar to spinach), okra; jerk meats (spicy marinade, usually grilled); curried chicken; seafood in fruit sauces like lime-garlic prawns, shrimp with garlic and papaya, or red snapper in bananas and rum.	Conch fritters (fried); soups made with cream, like yam bisque, or coconut, such as hot banana soup; fish poached in coconut milk.
Chinese	Hot-and-sour or wonton soup; steamed dumplings; steamed or braised whole fish or scallops with black bean sauce; chicken or eggplant steamed or braised; stir-fried dishes (ask the cook to go easy on the oil or to use broth instead); dishes made with sliced meat rather than diced (often hides a fatty cut).	Fried egg rolls and dumplings; sesame noodles; fried rice; Peking duck; anything "crispy" or "batter-coated" (both terms indicate deep-frying); dishes heavy on nuts, such as *kung pao* chicken.
Eastern European	Rice-stuffed cabbage or peppers; borscht or fruit soups (if possible, made with yogurt instead of cream); knishes (pastry filled with spinach, kasha, or mushrooms); Russian herring salad; poached fish; pierogi or piroshki (pastry filled with meat or vegetables) without sour cream, preferably steamed or boiled instead of fried.	Goulash and *paprikache* (made with cream and fatty cuts of meat); blintzes (lots of cheese); schnitzel (meat breaded, fried, and covered with cream sauce); sausages like kielbasa.
French	*Salade niçoise*, spinach salad (sans bacon); consommé and other stock-based soups; stews like bouillabaisse or ratatouille; poached or steamed fish or seafood; seared or oven-roasted scallops or salmon; dishes with sauces labeled *coulis,* vegetable puree, or reduction; roast chicken.	Cassoulet and gratins (made with a lot of cheese or egg); dishes heavy with eggs, such as quenelles and soufflés; hollandaise, beurre blanc, and other dairy-based sauces; fatty meats such as sweetbreads, duck, and pâté.
Greek	*Torato* (cold soup with eggplant, peppers, and yogurt); grilled fish or octopus; skewered and grilled vegetables and meat dishes, such as souvlaki and shish kebab; grilled lamb chops or roast leg or braised shanks; fish baked with *plaki* sauce.	*Taramasalata* (creamy fish roe dip); meats in *augolemono* (egg-based lemon sauce); *bourekakia* (cheese-stuffed pastry); moussaka and *pastitsio* (casseroles made with eggs and cheese); *skordalia* (almond-garlic sauce).
Indian	Baked breads like *chapati, nan, kuicha;* lentil soups like mulligatawny or *dal rasam;* chicken or fish prepared in tandoori-, *tikka-, vindaloo-,* or *masala*-style; yogurt-based curries.	Fried appetizers like *samosas* and *pakoras* or fried breads such as *poori* and *paratha;* any dishes called *kandhari, malai,* and *korma* (lots of cream or coconut).

(continued)

Indonesian	*Rijsttafel:* rice served with a variety of small dishes, such as *ayam panggang* (grilled chicken), *ayam kalasan* (fried chicken), and *gado-gado* (vegetables—ask for the peanut sauce on the side).	Coconut milk-based dishes like the chicken and nutmeg *opor ayam* or the beef and lemon grass *kalio daging;* fried dishes like *dendeng putri manis* (steak) or *ayam goreng kalasan* (chicken).
Italian	Vegetable antipasto (roasted peppers and zucchini, grilled mushrooms, caponata); salads such as *panzanella* (with tomatoes and bread); pasta with tomato- or wine-based sauce; linguine with clam sauce; *pasta e fagioli* (shells and beans); *ribollito,* the thick vegetarian stew; grilled game, veal, and fish; chicken cacciatore; snapper in *cartoccio* (baked in parchment); marinated calamari.	Meat and cheese antipasto; *fritto misto* (the "fried mixed" seafood, meat, or vegetable platter); cannelloni, lasagne, and other cheese-filled pasta; pesto and pasta with cream sauces, including carbonara and *alfredo;* risotto (heavy with butter and cheese); cheesy eggplant or veal parmigiana; veal *piccata* and marsala.
Japanese	Miso soup; yakitori (broiled chicken); *sunomono* (cucumber salad); teriyaki; *yosenabe,* a seafood and vegetable stew; *shabu-shabu,* a variety of vegetables and meats boiled in broth; sashimi and sushi.	Tempura or anything else under the heading of *agemono* (deep-fried); sukiyaki; egg dishes such as *oyako-donburi.*
Korean	Soups like the bean paste and vegetable *doen jang chi gae* or the seafood and tofu *kang doen jang;* pickled vegetables called *kimchi; nang myon* dishes featuring cold buckwheat noodles in a spicy sauce with vegetables or poultry; barbecued meats like *bul go ki* (beef) are good—order lean cuts like sirloin.	Egg drop soups like *duck kuk;* barbecued ribs, *kal bi;* panfried fish dishes like *gul jun* or *sang sun jun.*
Mexican/ Southwestern	Mesquite-grilled chicken, seafood, or lean cuts of beef or pork, especially with fresh salsa; fajitas or tacos *al carbon,* especially seafood (hold the sour cream); bean or vegetable burritos; soft tacos.	Tortilla chips and nachos; guacamole; fried dishes such as chimichangas, hard-shell tacos, *flautas, taquitos;* tamales, quesadillas, cheese enchiladas, and chile *con queso;* dishes with *poblano* aioli (chile mayonnaise) or cilantro pesto (nuts and oil); refried beans (ask for whole ones).
Middle Eastern	*Hummus* (mashed chick-peas); *baba ghanoush* (mashed eggplant); pita bread; *ful medames* (fava beans and chick-peas); any of the salads, such as tabouleh or *fattoush;* lentil soup; rice pilaf; shish kebab; kibbe (baked meat with wheat, onions, and pine nuts); kofta (grilled ground beef with parsley and onions).	*Saganaki* (contains fried cheese and butter); falafel (deep fried); *kasseri* (cheese and butter casserole).
Spanish	*Tapas*—Spanish appetizers, such as *chicharron de gallina* (chicken in lemon and pepper sauce), *escabeche* (fish marinated in wine vinegar), gazpacho (a cold soup); or for entreés, paella, a sort of rice stew with vegetables and seafood, pork, or chicken; fish or chicken baked in *picada* (sweet and sour) sauce.	*Aceitunas* (olives); *jamon serrano* (fatty ham); *tortilla española* (potato and onion omelette); *chorizo salteado* (pork sausage in oil).
Thai	Lemon grass soups like *tom yum koong* (shrimp and chili paste); *pad thai* (stir-fried noodles and sprouts); sautéed ginger beef or chicken (request a light touch with oil).	Coconut-based soups and curries, peanut sauce, deep-fried dishes like royal tofu and hot Thai catfish.

Source: John Hastings, "World's Fare: How to Savor the Flavors without the Fat," *Health,* September 1994, pp. 44–45. Reprinted by permission of Time Inc. Health

True vegetarians, also called **vegans,** have no meat, chicken, fish, or any milk products in their diet. They get all of their protein from vegetables, fruits, and grains. **Lactovegetarians** eat dairy products but no other animal products. Another variation of vegetarians is **ovolactovegetarians,** who eat eggs as well as dairy products.

Selecting a healthy vegetarian diet is far more complicated than just deciding not to eat meat or animal products. Because vegetarians do not eat animal products, which are a source of complete protein, they must combine the incomplete proteins in plant foods to get the proper amount of all essential amino acids. This is important at all times, but especially during periods of rapid growth such as childhood and adolescence and during pregnancy. Vegetarians also must make sure they get enough minerals such as calcium and iron and must guard against long-term vitamin B_{12} deficiency, which can cause mild, and if untreated, irreversible nerve damage. Holding to a strict vegetarian diet can be a healthy way to live, but it requires a specific health skill based

■ **Figure 5.4 Your Fast-Food Sandwich Guide.** *This sandwich guide gives you the calorie count and fat, cholesterol, and sodium levels for what falls between the bread. It also gives this information for the bread. (Source: U.S. Department of Agriculture)*

Use this guide to compare and to choose sandwich ingredients that are lower in calories, fat, cholesterol, and sodium.

Food	Approximate amount per serving			
	Calories	Fat (grams)	Cholesterol (milligrams)	Sodium (milligrams)
Breads:				
2 slices whole wheat	140	2	0	360
1 pita bread, 6 1/2 inches in diameter	165	1	0	339
1 croissant, 4 1/2 by 4 by 1 3/4 inches thick	235	12	13	452
Fillings:				
2 ounces home-cooked lean roast beef	110	4	46	37
2 ounces deli roast beef	145	9	47	234
2 ounces lean, boiled ham	75	3	27	815
1 slice (1 ounce) bologna	90	8	16	289
1 slice (1 ounce) processed American cheese	105	9	27	406
2 tablespoons peanut butter	190	16	0	150
1/4 cup tuna salad[1]	95	5	7	206
Sandwich Add-ons:				
1 teaspoon butter	35	4	10	39
1 teaspoon margarine	35	4	0	51
1 teaspoon prepared mustard	5	trace	0	63
1 teaspoon mayonnaise	35	4	3	26
1 teaspoon sweet pickle relish	5	trace	0	36

1. Tuna salad made with light tuna packed in oil, and mayonnaise-type salad dressing.

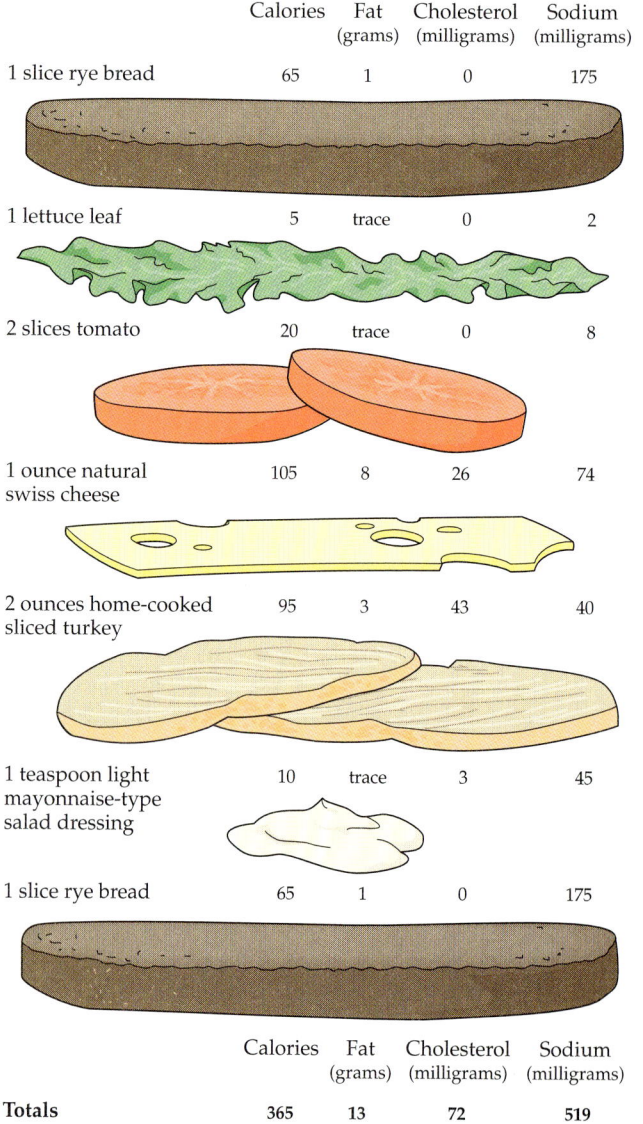

	Calories	Fat (grams)	Cholesterol (milligrams)	Sodium (milligrams)
1 slice rye bread	65	1	0	175
1 lettuce leaf	5	trace	0	2
2 slices tomato	20	trace	0	8
1 ounce natural swiss cheese	105	8	26	74
2 ounces home-cooked sliced turkey	95	3	43	40
1 teaspoon light mayonnaise-type salad dressing	10	trace	3	45
1 slice rye bread	65	1	0	175
Totals	365	13	72	519

on a good understanding of the principles of nutrition and on giving considerable attention to one's daily diet.

A vegetarian diet can meet all nutritional needs, according to the American Dietetic Association. The key—as with any other diet—is to eat a wide variety of foods and to limit your intake of sweets and fatty foods.

Vegetarian diets are usually lower in fat than a traditional diet, but even so, vegetarians can decrease fat consumption by substituting fruit juices or water for oil in recipes and by using soy lecithin sprays instead of oil when sautéing. Vegetarians do not really have to be concerned about cholesterol, since only animal products contain it. But coconut and palm oil are high in saturated fat and may raise your cholesterol.

For a balanced diet, vegetarians should eat:

Foods	Suggested Daily Serving
Breads, cereals, rice, and pasta	6 or more
Vegetables	4 or more
Legumes and other meat substitutes	2 to 3
Fruits	3 or more
Dairy products	Optional—up to 3
Eggs	Optional—3 to 4 a week

How Eating Habits Become Unhealthy... and How to Correct Them

For the most part, eating is a healthy activity. But some eating habits, if repeated for long enough, become very unhealthy. Three such habits are skipping meals, eating too many snacks, and taking too many vitamins.

Skipping meals. Unfortunately, many college students skip meals. How many times have you heard your classmates say, "I don't want to gain weight," or, "I'm simply too busy to eat." Breakfast seems to be the most frequently missed meal of the day. Some studies have suggested that missing breakfast can affect your concentration as well as your overall health. In addition, most people who skip breakfast tend to substitute a less nutritious, midmorning snack because they feel hungry. Another common habit is to skip dinner. Whether in order to write a paper or to reduce your intake of calories, skipping dinner is not a good idea. Eat nutritious meals on a regular schedule. You will find that you are better equipped to meet the demands of school or work and that you will be less hungry for snacks.

Eating too many snacks. Most commercial snack foods are high in fat, sugar, or salt and have few healthy nutrients. Apart from not making much of a contribution to your dietary needs, as outlined by the Food Guide Pyramid, they may lead to overweight, dental caries (cavities), and other health problems. Occasional snacking is fine, especially when you need extra energy, but don't overdo it. Snacks of yogurt, vegetables, fruits, unsalted nuts, whole grain rolls, or crackers are tasty, healthy, and nutritious alternatives.

Taking too many vitamins. "I know I don't have a good diet, so I'll make up for it by taking vitamins." This mistake in logic is made by many college students. As you read earlier, vitamins serve to help other nutrients (proteins, carbohydrates, fats, and minerals) function effectively and efficiently. Vitamins do not replace the need for other nutrients. It is a mistake to attempt to rectify a poor diet by taking vitamin supplements. In fact, a real health hazard can result. Taking too many vitamins can cause toxicity, illness, and, in extreme cases, even death. If you eat a healthy diet, vitamin supplements are usually not necessary. If in doubt, ask a doctor for an opinion.

vegan Vegetarians who do not eat any food of animal origin.

lactovegetarians Vegetarians whose diet includes dairy products but no other animal products.

ovolactovegetarians Vegetarians whose diet includes eggs as well as dairy products.

HEALTH SKILLS

Selecting and Preparing Healthy Foods

Selecting foods based on their nutritional content can be a daunting task. After all, there are so many nutrients in so many different foods. Yet shoppers always want good value for their money; this increasingly means that they want good nutritional value, not just a bargain. A Food Marketing Institute survey reported that more than 95 percent of shoppers rate the quality of fruits, vegetables, and meats and having a wide selection of foods as important factors in their choice of a supermarket.

By knowing the meaning of a few key terms, you can make your food selection easier—and, by making the right selections, you can make your diet more healthy. Here are several terms you should know when shopping for food:

Processed food. Food that has been cooked, frozen, or otherwise treated to preserve it for a period of time or to improve its taste is referred to as processed food. Processing often destroys many of the nutrients, such as vitamins, normally found in foods.

Vitamin enriched food. Vitamin enriched food tries to make up for the vitamins destroyed by processing. Sometimes it contains supplemental vitamins—that is, vitamins that are not naturally found in the food.

Organically grown food. Food grown without the use of pesticides or fertilizers is referred to as organically grown. There is likely little difference in the nutritional quality of such food, but there is an assurance that additives and certain contaminants are not present.

Fat-free food. To comply with FDA regulations, any food labeled "fat-free" must contain less than half a gram of fat per serving.

Low-fat food. To comply with FDA regulations, any food labeled "low-fat" must contain three grams of fat or less per serving.

Light food. To comply with FDA regulations, any food labeled "light" must have less than half the fat or at least one-third fewer calories than the regular version of the food.

Lower, reduced, or less fat food. To comply with FDA regulations, any food labeled "lower fat," "reduced fat," or "less fat" must contain 25 percent less fat than a regular version of the product or some other logical reference food.

Reading a Food Label

Food labels have become popular reading. A nationwide survey found that about four out of five adults "pay attention" to ingredient lists and that two out of three say that they use the list to avoid or limit consumption of certain items.

Food labels list ingredients in order of their prominence by weight, from the greatest to the least. This lets you know that a product is high in sugar when the label lists sugar or other sweeteners first or lists several sugars. Similarly, a product is likely to be salty if sodium-based products—salt, onion salt, MSG, baking soda—are high on the list.

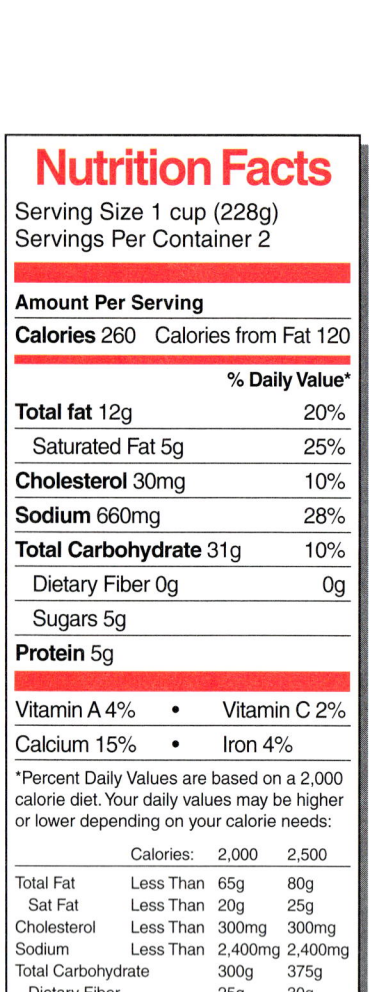

Figure 5.5 The Food Label. *The ingredients on a food label are listed in order of their prominence by weight, from the greatest to the least. The label also gives nutrition information, including levels of sodium, fat, cholesterol, fiber, and other nutrients.*

Critical Thinking Question

An objective of *Healthy People 2000* states: "Increase to at least 85 percent the proportion of people aged 18 and older who use food labels to make nutritious food selections." Sixty-six percent of shoppers say they review food labels. Eating habits begin early. How can public health educators, parents, and others teach children to use food wisely?

There is also nutrition information on the labels of all packaged goods. This information, required by the federal government, includes the amount per serving and the percent daily value of sodium, total fat (including saturated fat), cholesterol, proteins, total carbohydrates (including dietary fiber and sugars), vitamins, and minerals. In addition, the label lists the number of servings per container and number of calories per serving. Fresh meat, poultry, fish, and produce are not required to have nutritional labels. Look at the label in Figure 5.5. How can it help you the next time you shop at the supermarket?

Healthful Shopping

HEALTH SKILLS

When you enter a supermarket, the first thing you see are rows and rows of canned, frozen, and packaged goods. These products are usually located in the center of the store. Look along the walls for foods that have not been highly processed: meats, poultry, and fish; vegetables and fruits; and milk and dairy products. Increasingly, supermarkets are installing salad bars. These, like the other low-process foods, are located near the walls. The foods near the walls require careful handling and refrigeration and have rapid turnover. The foods in the center of the store can generally stay on the shelf for months or even years.

What does a healthy shopper do? Shop along the walls for foods that have undergone little processing and have high nutritional value. Shop throughout the store to find more highly processed foods that may be needed to complement a healthy diet.

Critical Thinking Question

> Good nutrition might be made much simpler if tighter controls were placed on the food industries. Why, for example, do we continue to produce masses of junk food despite the clear understanding that such food products are not nutritious? How do you think we can best balance the freedom to choose with what is in the best interest of the public's health?

Preparing Healthy Meals

HEALTH SKILLS

You don't have to be a gourmet chef to know how to prepare healthy foods. Even the healthiest of foods, such as a baked potato, can be made unhealthy by adding things to it, such as butter or sour cream. Here are some common sense skills for preparing healthy meals:

- Serve as much unprocessed food as possible.
- Bake, steam, or broil food. Don't fry it.
- Baste roasted food with tomato juice or broth in place of oil or butter.
- Have a variety of colors on the plate—green (spinach), red (beef), yellow (corn), black (beans), brown (bread), beige (chicken), white (rice). This helps assure that there is a full range of nutrients in the meal.

In fact, pay attention to how food is presented. Healthier foods actually look and smell delicious. Spend a little extra time and make the meal look attractive—for example, add fresh orange slices to a chicken or pork dish. You will enjoy eating healthy food if it looks good.

Key Concepts

1. A diet that is high in fiber and low in fat may reduce the risk of cancer.
2. Proteins are the building blocks of the body and are essential for growth, maintenance, and replacement of body cells.
3. Fats are the most concentrated source of energy in your diet. Fats are found in saturated and unsaturated forms.
4. Vitamins are the tools used by the body to process food. They do not supply energy, but they help release it from carbohydrates, proteins, and fats. Minerals form healthy bones and teeth and help nerves and muscles react normally.
5. About 60 to 70 percent of the body is made up of water. Without drinking it, you could live only about one week.
6. RDAs (recommended dietary allowances) are guidelines for the average amounts of some essential nutrients to be consumed by healthy individuals over a period of time.
7. Vegetarians need to combine vegetables, grains, and fruits in careful amounts to ensure adequate, complete protein consumption.
8. Three common eating habits that are unhealthy are skipping meals, eating too many snacks, and taking too many vitamins.
9. The ingredients on a food label are listed in order of their prominence by weight, from the greatest to the least.
10. When shopping for food at a grocery store, look along the walls for the unprocessed foods. The center of the store is where you will find the more processed foods.

Review Questions

1. List six nutrients found in food and describe the primary function of each.
2. Differentiate between the RDAs and the Dietary Guidelines for Americans.
3. Describe how consumption of fat can actually lower blood cholesterol.
4. Describe the health hazards of taking high doses of vitamin supplements.
5. What is the difference between major minerals and trace minerals?
6. List several natural sources of sodium and explain why it is usually not necessary to add salt to meet the daily requirement for sodium.
7. List five categories of preservatives and describe the function of each.
8. Identify three common eating habits that can lead to unhealthy results.
9. Explain why one ingredient on the food label is listed before another.
10. Describe how food preparation can enhance—or lessen—the nutritional quality of food.

Selected Bibliography

Diet and Health: Implications for Reducing Chronic Disease Risk. Washington, DC: National Academy Press, 1991.

Dietary Guidelines for Americans. Washington, DC: U.S. Department of Agriculture and Department of Health and Human Services, 1995.

FDA Consumer. Food and Drug Administration (published monthly).

Food Guide Pyramid. Hyattsville, MD: U.S. Department of Agriculture, Human Nutrition Information Service, 1992.

Levine, B.S. "Most Frequently Asked Questions about Water." *Nutrition Today* 31, (September/October 1996): 209–210.

Recommended Dietary Allowances (10th ed.). Washington, DC: National Academy Press, 1989.

"The Facts about Fats." *Consumer Reports* (June 1995): 389–393.

Tufts University Diet and Nutrition Letter (published monthly).

HealthLinks: Web Sites for a Better Understanding of Nutrition

You can access better health as it relates to this chapter by checking out some of the following sites on the Internet. These and sites identified within the chapter can be accessed directly when you visit the *HealthStyles* Web Site located on the Allyn and Bacon homepage at **http://www.abacon.com.**

American Dietetic Association (ADA)
www.eatright.org
Provides information on a full range of dietary topics, including sports nutrition, healthful cooking, and nutritional eating. Also links to scientific publications and provides information on scholarships and public meetings.

International Food Information Council
ificinfo.health.org
The International Food Information Council (IFIC) Foundation provides sound, scientific information on food safety and nutrition to journalists, health professionals, educators, government officials, and consumers.

Health Hotlines: Eating Smart

Food Allergy Network
(800) 929-4040
10400 Eaton Place, Suite 107
Fairfax, VA 22030-2208

National Center for Nutrition and Dietetics
American Dietetic Association
(800) 366-1655
216 West Jackson Boulevard
Chicago, IL 60606-6995

Nutrition Information Center
(800) 231-DIET (231-3438)
University of Alabama at Birmingham
Webb Building, Room 447, UAB Station
Birmingham, AL 35294

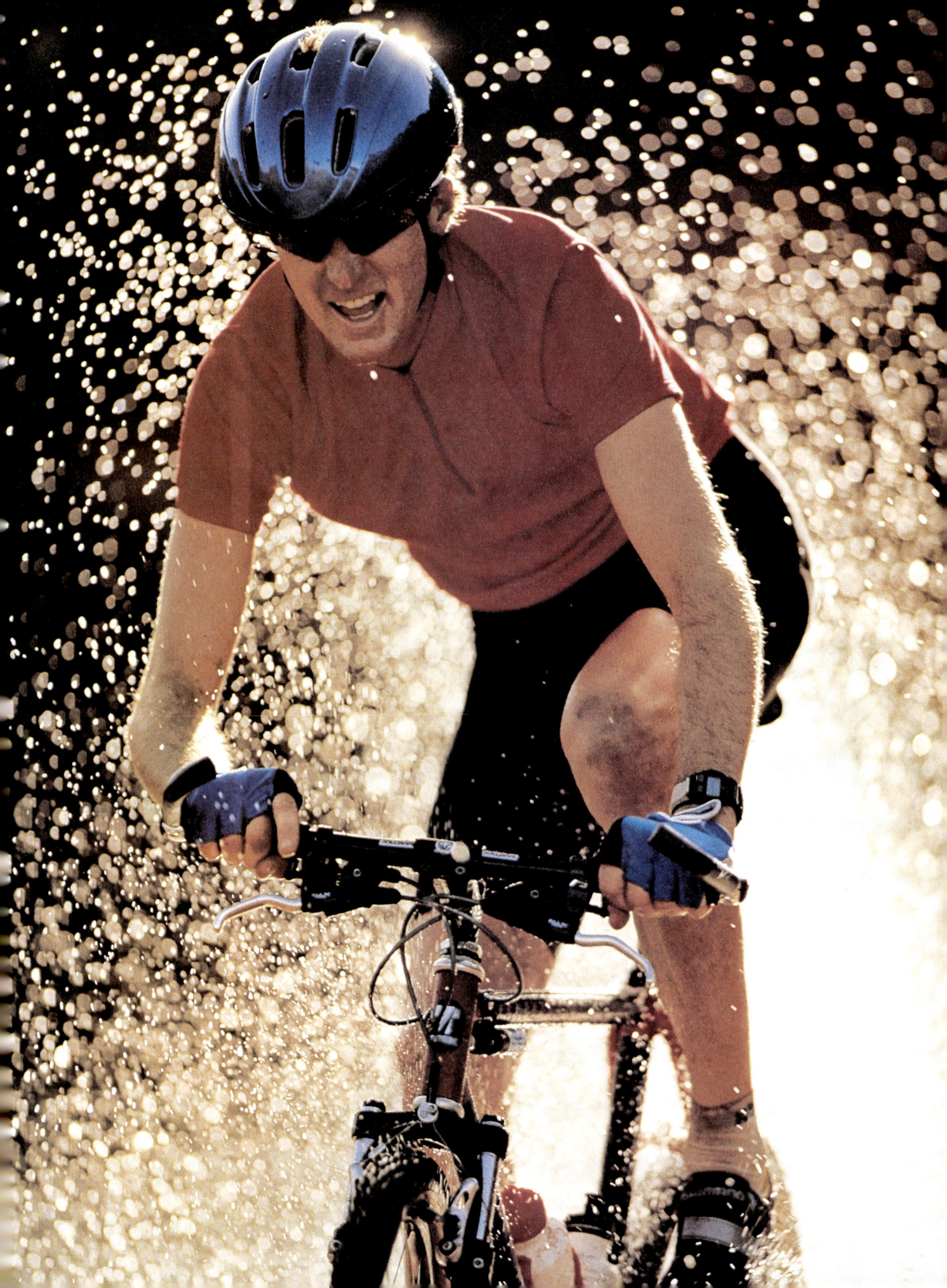

Chapter 6

Maintaining Proper Weight

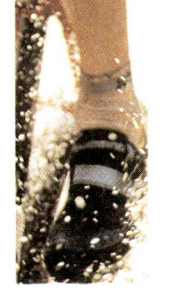
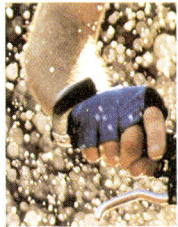
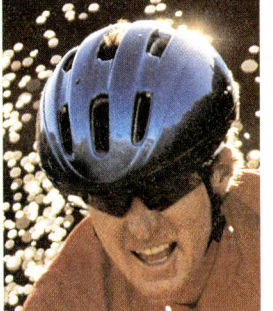

Objectives

When you finish reading this chapter, you will be able to:

1. Explain the benefits of maintaining normal weight and the health risks associated with overweight.
2. Describe the health risks of underweight.
3. Accurately assess your body weight as well as approximate your body mass.
4. Explain why some people become overweight more easily than others.
5. Describe how eating behaviors influence body composition and how eating behaviors are learned.
6. Explain why fat in the diet is essential for health and why excess fat leads to health risks.
7. Explain the relationship between exercise and weight control.
8. Understand the nature of anorexia and bulimia, two eating disorders that are potentially fatal.
9. Describe ways to control your weight and maintain health.
10. Identify fad diets and describe how they can be harmful to your health.

What Is Your HealthStyle?

Sarah has had a weight problem most of her life. When she was in grade school, the children called her fatso, and she bought her clothes in the chubby girls department. As an adult, she shops for clothes designed for "larger sized women." Yet when Sarah looks through the fashion magazines, she desperately wants to look like the thin models.

How desperately? Enough to go on diet after diet. She thought she had won the last diet battle after spending a few weeks on a liquid diet and dropping twenty pounds. But as soon as she went back to eating solid foods, nearly all the weight came back.

Sarah does not know how to say no to food or yes to exercise. She claims she doesn't have time for exercise, but because she has led a sedentary, "fat girl's" life, she is afraid that she will be clumsy in an aerobics class.

Kisha has also had a long-time battle with weight. Although she wasn't taunted as a "fatty" as a child, she was always saying, "I just want to lose a few pounds." Instead, she gained the standard "freshman fifteen" pounds in college. She, like Sarah, went on numerous quick weight loss diets, but she always put the weight back on.

Her last diet, however, *really* was her last diet because it became a lifelong diet. She lost twenty pounds—and has kept them off for nearly two years. To do this, Kisha changed her eating habits—including what she eats, when she eats, and how much she eats. She also exercises regularly. What motivated Kisha to lose weight was her physician, who warned her of the health implications of the high cholesterol levels he found in her blood, which resulted from a rich diet and lack of exercise. Her other motivation was her overweight uncle, who had had a minor heart attack.

In Your Opinion

Sarah and Kisha are both fighting the same problem, but one is winning the battle, the other is losing it.

- Why was Sarah so unsuccessful in losing weight permanently? What was wrong with her attitude?
- What behavior was she trying to change?
- What are the reasons behind Kisha's success story?
- What conscious decisions did Kisha make concerning weight loss?
- What steps would you take if you wanted to lose weight?

One of the first announcements made when a baby is born is "… and she weighs seven pounds, three ounces." Children learn early to make jokes about body weight and to label at least one classmate "fatso" and another "skin and bones." And for adults, scores of greeting cards poke fun at the person who has a weight problem.

Having a weight problem—and this can mean being underweight as well as being overweight—is not a laughing matter. It can contribute to heart disease, diabetes, cancer, and many other unhealthy conditions.

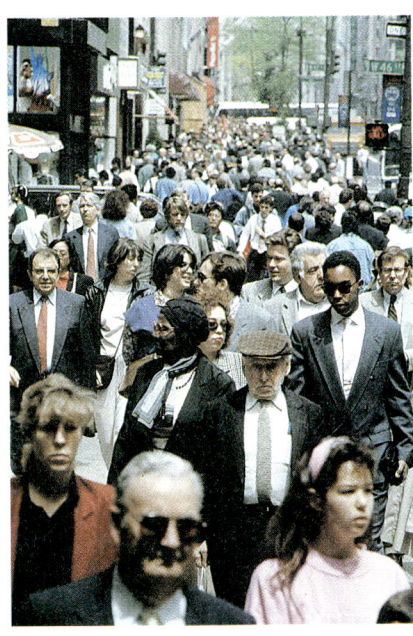

At any given point, 20 percent of the population is on a diet, although not all need to be. People who are overweight are more likely to have health problems, such as hypertension and heart disease. (Source: © Tony Stone Images/Jim Pickerell)

Weight—or more precisely the inability to maintain proper weight—is a serious public health problem in the United States. According to the Centers for Disease Control and Prevention (CDC), nearly one in three American adults is overweight. In addition to those who are seriously overweight, millions more want to lose a few pounds. As a result, the country is swept with diet mania. At any given time, at least 20 percent of the population is on some kind of weight-loss program. In spite of this obsession with weight, the prevalence of overweight has actually increased in recent years and the proportion of overweight adults who use exercise and dieting to lose weight has decreased.

How Weight Can Be Harmful to Your Health

Concerns about being overweight are based on more than vanity. Too much weight is harmful to your health and may significantly increase your risk for hypertension, cancer, stroke, heart disease, and adult-onset diabetes, which together account for about 70 percent of U.S. deaths.

Obesity is not a synonym for overweight. Obesity refers to **adiposity,** a surplus of body fat. The health problems related to obesity do not occur until surplus body fat reaches a level that produces overweight in excess of 20 percent above the desirable body weight. **Overweight,** on the other hand, refers to a simple excess of body weight relative to a specified standard for height. Neither term involves accurate measurements, but health researchers recognize that extremes of overweight or obesity indicate greater risk for a number of health problems.

Problems of Being Overweight

Obese people aged twenty to forty suffer hypertension five times more frequently than do peers who are not obese. Obese people are also twice as likely to have elevated blood cholesterol levels, a key risk factor for heart disease and stroke, and three times more likely to develop adult-onset diabetes.

The Framingham (Massachusetts) Heart Disease Epidemiology Study has been looking at the health of men and women between the ages of thirty and

obesity An excessive amount of body weight relative to body fat.

adiposity A surplus of body fat.

overweight An excess of body weight relative to a specified standard for height and age.

sixty for more than fifty years. This highly respected study reported that the risk for suffering from **angina** rises significantly as weight rises. Angina is chest pain resulting from a lack of blood supply to the heart.

The Framingham Study also reported that the chance of sudden death from heart attack is more than three times as great for people who are 20 percent overweight. Other studies show that regardless of smoking habits, obese men have a higher chance of dying from cancer of the colon, rectum, and prostate, and obese women have a higher chance of dying from cancer of the gallbladder, breast, uterus, and ovaries.

Some overweight people may be at greater risk than others, depending on where the fat is. Research shows that people who tend to have their fat concentrated in the waist and abdomen rather than in the thighs and buttocks are more prone to high blood pressure, diabetes, early heart disease, and certain types of cancer.

There is also a relationship between weight and the length of a hospital stay, according to a study reported in the *American Journal of Public Health*. Researchers studying records of patients hospitalized at the Brigham and Women's Hospital in Boston for total knee replacement and total hip replacement found that those who were extremely overweight had average hospital stays 35 percent longer (28.9 days versus 21.5 days) than patients of normal weight. At the other end of the weight spectrum, patients who were extremely **underweight** had average lengths of stay that were 40 percent longer (30.1 days versus 21.5 days).

Among the reasons that obese patients might stay in the hospital longer are prolonged anesthesia time, greater likelihood of pulmonary infections, increased incidence of postoperative wound infections, and/or a longer recovery period. As for those who are considerably underweight, having a low amount of body fat can interfere with the immune system; underweight patients might have a slower response to treatment and therefore a longer hospital stay.

Underweight: A Problem Too

In many respects, underweight represents as serious a health threat as obesity. Low birthweight is a leading cause of infant death. Two thirds of babies born weighing less than five and a half pounds die at birth, and those who survive are twenty times more likely to die before they are a year old. Low body weight is implicated in **amenorrhea,** the abnormal absence or suppression of menstruation, and may affect the ability of women to conceive. In addition, underweight women are at a higher risk for gaining too little weight during pregnancy, which can affect their infant's birth weight. Thin smokers are at a higher risk for developing a serious disease and dying from it than are smokers of average weight. Even thin men and women who are well have higher mortality rates than do well men and women of average weight. Taken to an extreme and if left untreated, compulsive eating behaviors directed toward achieving excessivly low body weights, behaviors typical of disorders such as **anorexia nervosa** and **bulimia,** may become life-threatening conditions. We will discuss eating disorders later in this chapter.

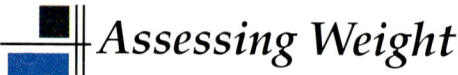

Assessing Weight

Accurately assessing your body weight is a health skill that you will use your entire life. It is not as simple as stepping on a bathroom scale and reading from the dial. A simple measure of weight, although informative, is not very important from a health perspective. It becomes important, however, in relation to other factors such as age, height, body type, and level of exercise (see the Cultural View box). For example, it is not necessarily unhealthy to weigh 170 pounds. It depends on who weighs that 170 pounds. For a 5-foot-tall woman, 170 pounds would be considered obese and thus unhealthy. For a 6-foot-tall man, 170 pounds might be considered ideal.

The most common measure of appropriate body weight is a height–weight chart, such as the one featured in Table 6.1. Weight ranges are given because people of the same height may have different amounts of body fat, muscle, and bone. The higher weights apply to people who have more muscle and bone and generally apply to men. The lower weights generally apply to women. Because there is a wide range of weight for each height, it could be unhealthy for someone normally at the lower end of the range to gain enough weight to be at the higher end.

The farther you are above the healthy weight range for your height, the higher your weight-related risk. Weights slightly below the range may be healthy for some people, but they could be the result of health problems, especially when weight loss is unintentional. See where your weight falls on the chart for people of your height.

Limitations of Height–Weight Tables

Height–weight tables provide only guidelines, not accurate information. But over the years these guidelines have provided valuable insights to large segments of the population who would otherwise be unaware of their weight-related

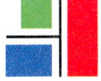

TABLE 6.1 What You Should Weigh Based on Your Height

Height	Weight (in pounds)
4'10"	91–119
4'11"	94–124
5'0"	97–128
5'1"	101–132
5'2"	104–137
5'3"	107–141
5'4"	111–146
5'5"	114–150
5'6"	118–155
5'7"	121–160
5'8"	125–164
5'9"	129–169
5'10"	132–174
5'11"	136–179
6'0"	140–184
6'1"	144–189
6'2"	148–195
6'3"	152–200
6'4"	156–205
6'5"	160–211
6'6"	164–216

Source: U.S. Department of Agriculture, 1997

angina Chest pain resulting from a lack of blood supply to the heart.

underweight Less body weight relative to a specified standard for height and age.

amenorrhea An abnormal absence or suppression of menstruation.

anorexia nervosa An eating disorder characterized by starvation behavior brought on by a preoccupation with thinness.

bulimia An eating disorder characterized by the extreme behavior of binge eating and vomiting.

Chapter 6 Maintaining Proper Weight

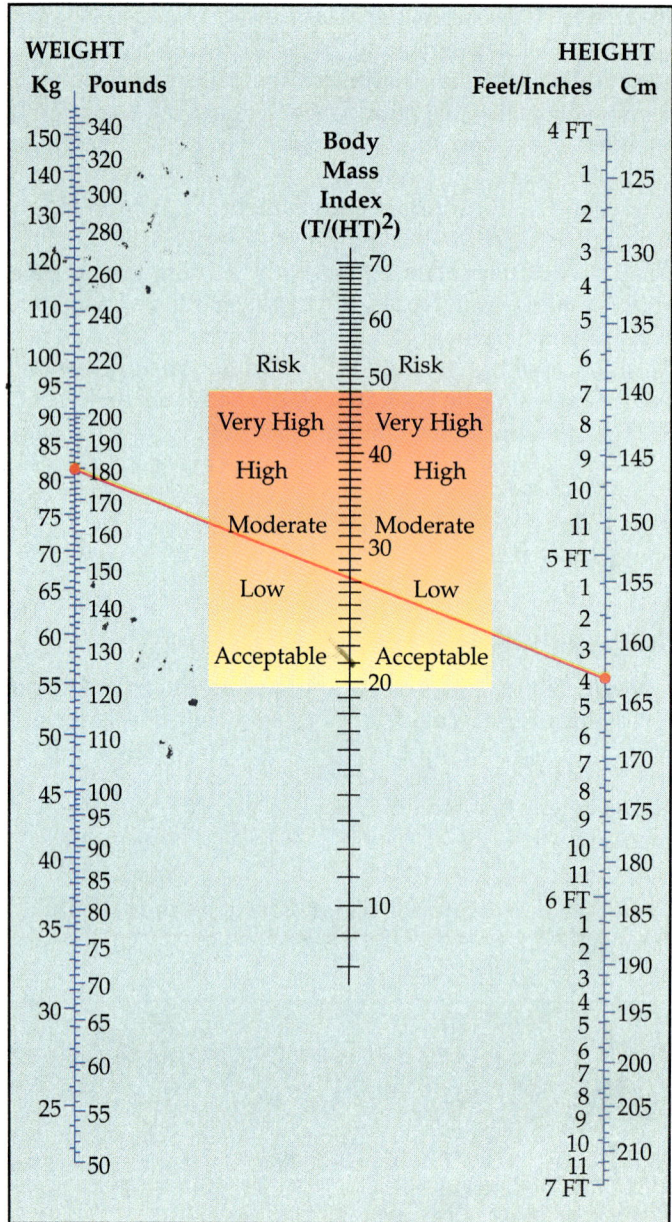

Figure 6.1 What You Should Weigh Based on Your Body Mass Index. *(Source: Rebecca J. Donatelle and Lorraine G. Davis,* Access to Health, *5th ed., p. 259 (Figure 10.1). Copyright © 1998 by Allyn & Bacon. Reprinted by permission of Allyn & Bacon)*

risk level. Experts caution against relying too much on height–weight tables alone for the following reasons:

- The tables are not applicable to the entire population, particularly to some ethnic groups.
- They ignore other risk factors, such as smoking, lack of activity, and genetics.
- They do not measure the degree of obesity or distribution of fat in the body.

A **body mass index (BMI)** is a far more accurate indicator of weight-related risk level because it is an easy way to compare the fatness of people of different heights. Use the following formula to calculate your BMI:

$$\text{BMI} = \frac{\text{Weight in kilograms}}{\text{Height in meters}^2}$$

Instructions:

Multiply your weight in pounds by .45 to get kilograms. Convert your height to inches and multiply this number by .0254 to get meters. Multiply your height in meters by itself. Divide this number into your weight in kilograms.

A study of 115,000 women nurses, which was conducted recently by researchers at the Brigham and Women's Hospital and Harvard Medical School and published in the *New England Journal of Medicine,* found that women with BMIs below 19 had the lowest risk of death:

- Between 19 and 24.9, the risk was 20 percent higher.
- Between 25 and 26.9, it was 30 percent higher.
- Between 27 and 28.9, it was 60 percent higher.
- Over 29, it was doubled.

In general, desirable body mass for women is 21.5; obesity (20 percent overweight) for women begins at approximately 27, and serious obesity (40 percent overweight) begins at 30. For men, desirable body mass is 22; obesity begins at approximately 28, and serious obesity begins at 31.

What is your BMI? Are you in the safe zone? Are you moving toward the high-risk area? Figure 6.1 shows weights that qualify for low BMI scores.

Measuring Body Fat

The most accurate way to measure the health risks of body weight is to determine how much fat tissue you have. There are three ways to do this.

The first is a **pinch test,** in which a technician uses special skin-fold calipers to pinch layers of fat at specific body sites. This provides a fairly accurate measure of your percentage of body fat. However, there are some drawbacks. To get a reliable skin-fold measurement, the person taking it must be skilled in the proper procedures. Usually, three or more measurements are taken to ensure accuracy. Even then, technicians may miss the correct sites for measurement. Also, the method does not account for inherited variations in fat distribution.

Underwater weighing, or hydrostatic immersion, is a more accurate way to measure percentage of body fat. It involves total submersion in a swimming pool or special tank. After the person being weighed exhales as much air as possible, body density is measured and the percentage of body fat is calculated. This calculation process does not correct for age and body type and can result in as much as 5 percent error, depending on how much air is exhaled.

Another way to measure fat is a technique called **bioelectrical impedance.** With small electrodes attached to a person's wrists and ankles, a weak electrical current is used to measure the body's water content. The water content information is used to calculate the percentage of body fat. Only fat-free tissues contain water. The results can vary, depending on how much food a person has recently eaten and how hydrated or dehydrated the person is.

body mass index (BMI) A numerical representation of the relationship of height and weight that correlates positively with measures of body composition such as underwater weighing and the pinch test.

pinch test A test that uses special skin-fold calipers to pinch layers of fat at specific body sites; a measure of body fat.

underwater weighing A test of body fat that weighs a person underwater to determine body composition.

bioelectrical impedance A test that uses a weak electrical current to measure the body's fat content.

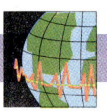

CULTURAL VIEW

How You See Yourself Can Depend on the Culture of the Time

What is the ideal body shape? It depends on where you live—and when. Seventeenth-century painters such as Peter Paul Rubens preferred the full-bodied, voluptuous female. Today, angular, muscular bodies for both men and women are seen as "perfect." These values are not based on health but rather are related to clothing styles, role models, and other artificial standards. No matter what the time period, cultural norms greatly influence a person's perception of what is overweight and underweight.

Teenagers are particularly sensitive to prevailing cultural tastes regarding physical appearance. In a survey of more than 1,000 high school students, 63 percent of the girls and 16 percent of the boys reported that they were on weight-reducing regimens. The most popular methods of weight reduction were exercise, decreasing calories, omitting snacks, and skipping meals. A closer look at the dieters indicated that most of the girls trying to lose weight were already at a normal weight. Moreover, 18 percent of underweight girls were dieting, too. Because there was no obvious physical need to lose weight, the driving force behind the dieting must have been psychological, social, or both.

Overweight girls had a truer perception of their needs. Nearly all of them were trying to lose weight. In contrast, only half of the overweight boys were reducing.

What about weight gain? Twenty-eight percent of the boys and nine percent of the girls were actively working to put on pounds. They did this by eating more foods, particularly those higher in calories and protein.

The typical boy who wanted to gain weight and the typical girl who wanted to lose weight were similar in that both were likely to be of normal weight to begin with. What they were doing, however, was modifying their weight so that they conformed to culturally popular ideals of a thin girl and a muscular boy.

It is time for Americans to make peace with their bodies. If you are a large-framed person who is within the healthy weight range—and who is active and continues to eat in a healthy manner—you do not have to worry about your weight. Perhaps you should play up the parts of your body that you do like. Get a haircut or wear clothes that go well with your complexion. Remember, most people—thin or fat—are not happy with some part of their bodies.

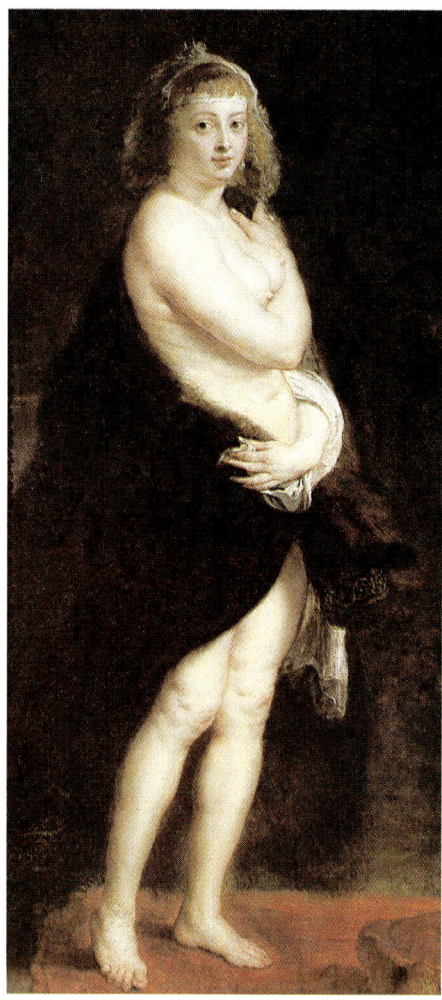

Seventeenth-century painters liked to portray full-bodied figures. What is in vogue today? (Source: Courtesy Erich Lessing/Art Resource, NY. The Furlet (Helene Fourment) by Peter Paul Rubens (1577–1640). Kunsthistorisches Museum, Vienna, Austria. Used with permission.)

Critical Thinking Question

The bathroom scale is a common means of monitoring body weight, yet many weight management experts consider it your worst enemy. Why might this be? How "healthy" is this tool for weight assessment?

The most common way of determining weight, however, is not scientific at all but may be as effective for most people. It involves simply looking in the mirror. If you appear overweight and feel overweight, you may indeed be overweight. A major drawback of this observation method of weight assessment is that it is difficult for some people to assess their own weight accurately by visual observation. In fact, one of the characteristics of anorexia nervosa is an unrealistic perception of a need to lose weight. Before beginning weight-control strategies, you should confirm your weight through other measurements. Regardless of the measurement technique applied, the assessment of weight is an important first step in the weight-control process.

Critical Thinking Question

In *Healthy People 2000*, the following objective is listed: "Reduce overweight to a prevalence of no more than 20 percent among people ages 20 and older and not more than 15 percent among adolescents ages 12 to 19." Data show that 34 percent of people over age 20 and 21 percent of teenagers were overweight in 1992. If we were to reach this objective, what are the implications for society? Would there be economic impact? Would there be a public health impact? What would these impacts be?

Why Do Some People Become Obese?

"I just look at food and I gain weight." How many times have you heard someone say that? Of course, that doesn't actually happen. It just seems so. But the fact remains that some people can eat enormous amounts of food and maintain a constant body composition and weight whereas others who have similar characteristics—for example, the same sex, age, height, and basic body build—gain weight even when they eat small amounts of food.

Why is this so? There are a number of endocrine-related diseases such as **hypothyroidism** (not having enough thyroid activity) and some forms of diabetes that may be responsible for obesity. But for the most part, the tendency to be overweight appears to be related to heredity, eating behavior, and exercise patterns.

hypothyroidism Not enough thyroid activity.

Genetic Linkage

Obesity is known to run in families, but the cause—genetics or environment—has long been debated. Two studies by researchers at the University of Pennsylvania found evidence in favor of a genetic cause.

One study looked at nearly 4,000 sets of twins—one half were identical, the other half nonidentical. Identical twins are genetically the same, whereas nonidentical twins are not. The sample was drawn from a registry of twins born between 1917 and 1927 who served in the armed forces in World War II or in Korea. The identical sets of twins were twice as likely as the nonidentical twins to show the same degree of obesity at the time they entered the armed services. This shared tendency toward obesity was still there when they were measured again twenty-five years later.

Another study looked at a sample of 540 adopted Danish men and women, dividing them into four groups: thin, median weight, overweight, and obese. When the researchers compared the adoptees to their biological parents, a clear relation was noted between their BMIs. However, no such relationship was found between the adoptive parents and the adoptees. This suggests that childhood family environment alone may have little or no effect on body weight.

In 1994, researchers at Rockefeller University found a gene that is thought to be responsible for at least some types of obesity in mice—and possibly in humans. The gene, which acts only in fat cells, normally controls appetite by sending a message to the brain that there is enough fat in the body. When the gene malfunctions, however, it fools the brain into thinking that there is not enough fat and that more food is needed. This discovery supports the theory that some people are destined to be overweight.

Other scientific theories about a genetic trigger for obesity point toward:

- A susceptibility to form fat cells
- A deficiency in one or more hormones, which leads a person to overeat
- A low activity level of the **vagus nerve,** which runs between the posterior part of the brain stem and the stomach. (This means that it takes more food in your stomach to give your brain the message that you are full.)

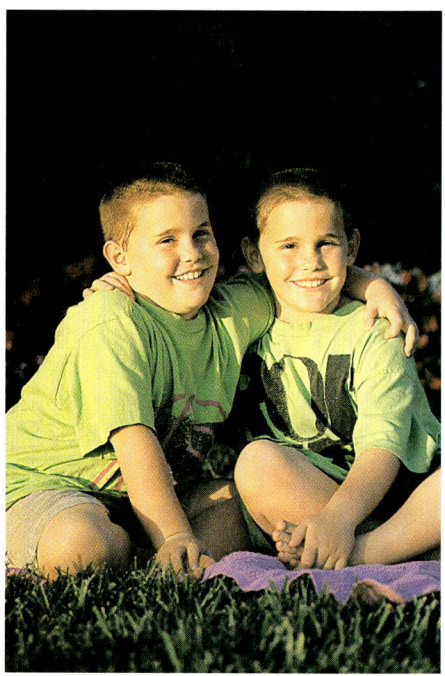

There is a genetic susceptibility to obesity, but not all family members—even identical twins—show the same degree of it. (Source: FPG International/© Dennie Cody)

If overweight or obesity runs in your family, these research findings do not mean that you should give up trying to control your weight. People who have a genetic susceptibility to fatness can lose weight and stay slim, but they have to work hard at it by maintaining a high level of physical activity and watching what they eat.

Some researchers believe that each person has a particular weight at which his or her body functions normally. This is called a **set point.** According to the set point theory, people who lose weight will return to their set points once they begin eating in response to hunger. Fortunately, a person's set point can change, so overweight people are not locked into their current body weights. Again, exercise plays a role. When an inactive person starts to exercise regularly, his or her set point will decrease.

Eating Behaviors Learned at Home

Eating behaviors established in childhood and reinforced throughout life can lead to an overweight condition. For example, childhood obesity is influenced by a number of factors, including parents' weight, age, marital status, socioeconomic class, and race.

A study of eighteen infants, half from obese mothers and half from thin mothers, found that by the time the infants from obese mothers were one year old, most were showing signs of an overweight condition. The researchers determined that at three months of age, the infants from very fat mothers were burning nearly 21 percent fewer calories than the infants from very thin mothers, even though no signs of overweight were observable. The infants of obese mothers were also less active than infants of thin mothers. Researchers can only speculate whether such inactivity was the result of modeling behavior or triggered by some genetic code.

Family traditions also play an important role. Scarcity of food at one time in a family's history—perhaps during the Depression or World War II—may make a "clean plate and full belly" particularly important for generations afterwards. Many families have eating rituals, such as a big breakfast on the weekends, eating together in front of the television, or having a snack just before going to bed.

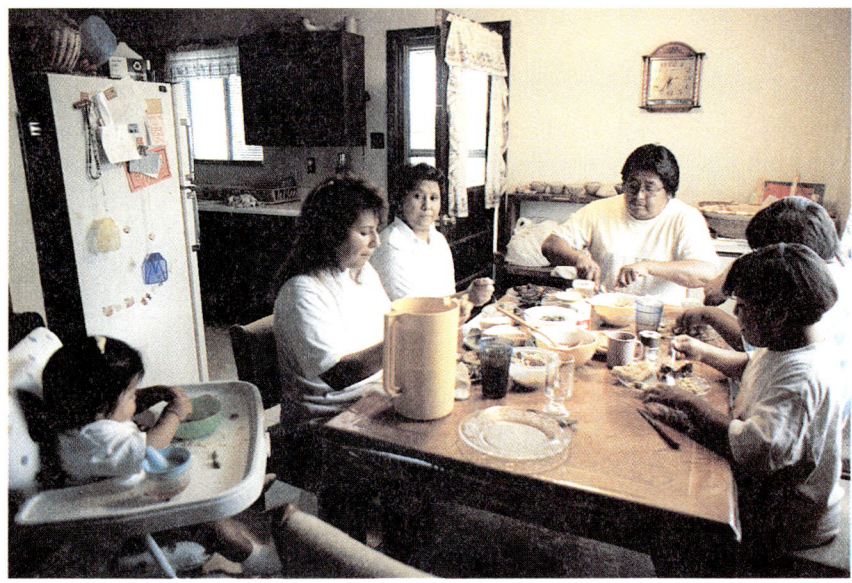

Family traditions can play an important role in maintaining proper weight. Sitting down together for a healthy and well-balanced dinner promotes healthy habits in children. (Source: The Image Works/© Nita Winter)

vagus nerve The nerve that runs between the posterior part of the brain stem and the stomach and gives your brain the message that you are full.

set point A particular weight at which a person's body functions normally.

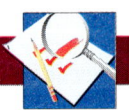

HERE'S LOOKING AT YOU

Are You Hung Up about Your Weight?

Eat when you're hungry, stop when you're full, and choose foods that are good for you. Oh, and while you're at it, learn to love your body, whatever its shape or size. If only it were so simple. But experts say that until we learn to respect our natural hunger signals and to accept the way we look, we'll never be able to kick the dieting habit. To find out how close you are to that healthy goal, pick up a pencil and circle true or false for each of the following statements.

My life would be better if only I could lose some weight.	True or False
I often eat when I am upset, depressed, anxious, or angry as a way of feeling better.	True or False
I tend to overeat in social situations.	True or False
I avoid mirrors.	True or False
I keep eating even when I'm full.	True or False
If I ate whenever I wanted to, I would get very fat.	True or False
I choose clothes that hide the size of my body.	True or False
I often feel guilty after I eat.	True or False
I'm afraid to have even a taste of dessert because I might lose control and eat too much.	True or False
I have tried many diets.	True or False
I prefer to make love in the dark because I'm embarrassed about my body.	True or False
I eat even when I don't feel hungry.	True or False
I compare my body unfavorably with those of others.	True or False
I eat normally when I'm with friends; when I'm by myself I tend to pig out.	True or False
I think about food nearly all the time.	True or False
I'm embarrassed about the fact that I like to eat.	True or False

Total number of trues _____

Five or fewer true

Congratualtions. You're in tune with your hunger, and you've resisted the pressures—cultural or otherwise—that make so many people dissatisfied with their bodies.

Six or more true

You probably realize that your relationship with food and your view of your body are somewhat troubled. Try to ease up on yourself and take steps to relearn a more natural way of eating.

Source: "Are You Hung Up about Your Weight?" *Health,* April 1997, p. 61. Reprinted by permission of Time Inc. Health

---

Cultural influences also affect a family's eating habits, including the selection and preparation of food. For instance, deep fat cooking is a popular feature of many classic southern recipes.

Television advertisers spend considerable money promoting high-calorie foods such as beer and hamburgers but give less attention to healthier, low-calorie alternatives. There is little doubt that television ads affect food choice. Television provides yet another link to being overweight. It is speculated that the number of hours spent watching television contributes to obesity because watching requires no energy. Therefore, the more a person—particularly a child—

watches television, the greater the risk of obesity. More to the point, a sedentary lifestyle is not conducive to expending calories. If you lead a sedentary life yet continue to consume a high-calorie diet, becoming overweight is highly likely.

Critical Thinking Question

Healthy People 2000 seeks to "Increase to at least 75 percent the proportion of the Nation's schools that provide nutrition education from preschool to 12th grade, preferably as part of comprehensive school health education." Sixty percent of schools have such a program. Why is nutrition education an important strategy for achieving weight-control objectives?

There are also unconscious and emotional reasons for eating. For example, some people try to eat their way out of loneliness, boredom, or stress. This does not help the underlying problem and can result in unwanted weight gain. An important health skill is learning how to be in tune with your hunger. This involves respecting your natural hunger instincts and accepting the way you look (see the Here's Looking at You box).

How the Body Stores and Uses Energy

Food is the body's source of energy. As you learned in Chapter 5, some sources of energy are more nutritious than others. Table sugar, for example, is an energy source that is virtually devoid of nutrition.

The body uses energy for basic functions such as breathing, blood circulation, and growth. When the amount of food consumed is not burned in the performance of these normal bodily processes, it is stored for future use in the form of fat. When the body needs more energy than the amount provided by food, it uses the energy stored in fat tissue.

The Relationship between Calories and Pounds

Fattening foods do not make you fat. What makes you fat is eating more calories than your body needs. A calorie, to a scientist, is the heat required to raise the temperature of 1 gram of water 1 degree Celsius. To a nutritionist, however, a **calorie** is a unit measuring the energy produced by food when oxidized in the body. A simple way to measure how many calories your body needs is to multiply your desirable weight by eighteen if you are a man and by sixteen if you are a woman. This means that a woman weighing 125 pounds uses up about 2,000 calories a day (125 × 16). Be cautious, however, because the number of calories each person needs depends on several factors in addition to gender, including age, body frame, and, of course, exercise or activity level.

As strange as it may seem, a high-carbohydrate meal consisting of spaghetti and tomato sauce could contain fewer calories than a steak dinner. Carbohydrates and proteins contain approximately four calories per gram; fat contains approximately nine calories per gram. Moreover, you can fill up with calories from carbohydrates quicker than you can with calories from fat. A two-ounce

calorie A unit measuring the energy produced by food when oxidized in the body.

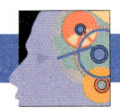

DEVELOPING HEALTH SKILLS

How Not to Gain Weight...When You Eat Low-fat Foods

Almost every day another low-fat food appears on supermarket shelves. So why aren't Americans getting thinner? It may be human nature: many people seem to feel that it's okay to eat more since they're making low-fat choices. In other words, a person who would normally eat six Oreos might eat a whole box of fat-free cookies—which adds up to less fat, sure, but more calories. To test how a low-fat or nonfat label affects food intake, Barbara Rolls, professor of nutrition at Penn State University, gave 48 women (healthy and not currently dieting) three indistinguishable raspberry flavored yogurts:

Yogurt (per cup)	Fat (grams)	Calories
1 High-fat, high-calorie	18	240
2 Low-fat, high-calorie	2	240
3 Low-fat, low-calorie	2	105

The women ate about a cup and a half of one of the yogurts 30 minutes before lunch; on the next two days, they ate one of the two other types of yogurt before lunch. For half the women, the yogurt was labeled simply "high-fat" or "low-fat"; the others ate unlabeled yogurt. The result: When the women ate the yogurts labeled "low-fat" they consumed significantly more calories during the subsequent lunch and dinner than they did after eating the yogurt labeled "high-fat." When the yogurts weren't labeled for fat content, these differences did not occur.

That's a classic dieting scenario. People eat low-fat foods, pat themselves on the back, and feel they can indulge. Some even think they can eat unlimited amounts of a food if it's low in fat. Low-fat foods *can* help promote weight loss—but only if they are also low in calories, are eaten in "normal" portions, and don't serve as a license to overeat later. It seems obvious, but many people just don't get it: if they don't cut down on calories (and/or exercise more) over the course of the day, they won't lose weight.

Source: "How Not to Gain Weight When You Eat Low-Fat Foods," reprinted with permission from the *University of California at Berkeley Wellness Letter,* April 1997. © Health Letter Associates, 1997. To order a one year subscription, call 800/829-9170.

piece of a chocolate bar has the same number of calories as three medium-sized bananas that together weigh more than a pound.

Two recent studies dramatically illustrate the relationship between carbohydrates and fat and weight gain. In one study conducted in a Vermont prison, a group of male prisoners had difficulty gaining weight on a high-carbohydrate, low-fat diet despite an enormous caloric intake. A second group gained weight easily on a low-carbohydrate, high-fat diet. In another study, a group of men were fed 2,000 calories of carbohydrates at one meal. When tested ten hours later, each subject had stored only 81 calories of fat. Further testing showed that the men actually lost body fat over the next ten hours because their normal metabolism burned more than the 81 calories of fat that they had gained.

Far from being fattening, carbohydrates from starches, fruits, and vegetables are excellent sources of food for weight reducers. They fill you up, give you something to chew on, can satisfy a sweet craving (at least in the case of fruits), and give you some nutrients, too. Studies have shown that eating bread with meals—long considered a no-no for dieters—makes eaters feel full before they consume their usual quota of calories.

Over the past eighty years, caloric intake by Americans has declined, yet the number of people who are overweight has increased. How is that possible? One place to look for the answer is in carbohydrate and fat consumption. In 1910, almost 60 percent of calories consumed in the United States came from carbohydrates and only 30 percent came from fat. Today, nearly 45 percent of the typical American's calories come from fat. However, switching to a low-fat diet won't help if you still consume a lot of food. Whether a food is low-fat or not, it still contributes to your caloric intake (see The Developing Health Skills box). Where do your calories come from? The *Dietary Guidelines for Americans* recommends that 50 percent of your calories come from carbohydrates and only 30 percent from fat.

Fat as Essential, Fat as Excess

Fat is a general term that can refer to a group of foods or a type of body tissue. In either case, the main components of fat are carbon, hydrogen, and oxygen.

As food, fat is essential to health: without fats in the diet, deficiencies of the fat-soluble vitamins A, D, E, and K would result. Of particular importance to good health are three fatty acids: linoleic, linolenic, and arachidonic acids. Linoleic acid cannot be manufactured by the body but is present in many kinds of foods and is abundant in some oils, including walnut and linseed oil, and some nuts and soybeans.

As tissue, fat is found in all parts of the body. It serves to insulate, cushion, and lubricate the anatomy, but most importantly, it stores energy. The body of the average, healthy young man is 16 percent fat; for the healthy young woman, between 17 and 20 percent body fat is average. Fat from food is stored in the body in the form of **adipose tissue.** The extra fat stored by women (as compared to men) is the equivalent of 144,000 calories, which is enough to provide calories for a pregnancy and about three months of nursing.

One factor related to obesity is the number of fat cells in the body. Theoretically, this number can swell up to three or more times the norm. Once new fat cells are present in the body, they never fully disappear no matter how much a person diets. However, fat cells can change in composition; the amount of fat in them can be reduced.

The number and size of fat cells in the body seem to proliferate naturally in the first year of life. At one year, the fat cells in children begin to decrease in size (but not number). Fat cells increase in both size and number again in early adolescence. Studies show that obese children do not experience the normal drop in fat cell size at age one. Instead, the cells continue to grow and multiply. By the time they are nineteen years old, they have twice as many fat cells as does an average person of the same age. Moreover, these fat cells are 30 to 40 percent larger. Given these findings, a critical factor in controlling obesity is limiting the number of fat cells, particularly in childhood and adolescence. This can be achieved through healthy eating.

Your Body's Energy Needs

Energy needs differ depending on body composition, size, and age. It is obvious that a large person needs more calories to keep the body going than does a small person. Generally, men have higher calorie needs than women, not only because they are larger but also because they have a greater proportion of muscle tissue. The more muscle tissue a person has, the more energy that person uses.

Calorie needs also differ at various stages in life. Calorie requirements are greatest during infancy, adolescence, pregnancy, and lactation (breast feeding). As adults get older, they need fewer calories to keep their bodies functioning. Middle-age spread occurs in part because most people do not alter their intake of food.

There are three major reasons why the body needs less energy with age. To begin with, the demand for food energy is reduced by a drop in the **basal metabolic rate**—the speed with which the body expends calories on basic functions such as breathing. At the same time, the adult body converts more food into fat than it did in earlier years, and fat tissue uses less energy than the same weight

adipose tissue Tissue in which fat from food is stored in the body.

basal metabolic rate The speed with which the body expends calories on basic functions at a resting state.

of muscle tissue would use. On top of this, most people have a tendency to become less active as they grow older.

Taken together, calorie requirements decrease 2 to 8 percent for each decade of life past age twenty. Weight gain should not be a surprise to a fifty-year-old who eats as much as he or she did at age twenty.

Importance of Exercise

Without exercise, it is difficult to lose weight—and keep it off. This is the reason so many diets are not successful: they do not include a program for exercising or for increasing physical activity. The reason a diet without exercise does not work well has to do with the body's metabolism. When you decrease the amount of food you normally eat—that is, when you go on a diet—the body's natural tendency is to conserve energy. This results in a 15 to 30 percent decrease in basal metabolic rate. Exercise is a counteracting force: It speeds up metabolism.

A recent study demonstrates the role of exercise in increasing metabolism. A group of obese people on a low-calorie diet reported a gradual reduction in their metabolism rate over a two-week period. When they started to exercise for twenty to thirty minutes a day, their metabolism rate returned to normal within a few days. Two weeks later, it was even higher than it had been when they began. In contrast, a second group of obese people were put on the same low-calorie diet for four weeks but did not exercise. At the end of the study, their metabolism rate showed a reduction of nearly 20 percent.

Exercise is another way of burning up calories. If you want to cut your calories by 500 a day, you can do this by consuming 200 calories fewer and burning off 300 calories by walking, jogging, biking, playing tennis, or engaging in many other forms of exercise.

The number of calories burned depends on

- the degree of the activity (twenty minutes of running burns more than twenty minutes of walking);
- the length of the activity (the longer the activity continues, the more calories burned);
- air temperature (exercise in colder weather burns up more calories); and

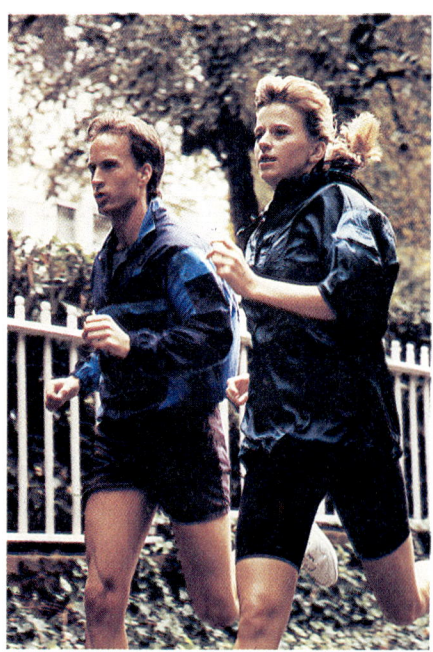

Without doing some form of exercise, it is difficult to lose weight and keep it off. Exercise burns calories and increases metabolism. (Source: © Tony Stone/Gary Nolton)

- your weight (a heavier person uses more energy than a lighter person for the same activity).

Exercise does not have to be strenuous in order to have an impact. There are many ways to burn calories during the day. Stand rather than sit; use the stairs instead of the elevator; walk or bike instead of taking the car. A leisurely walk burns around 300 calories, which is more than twice the number of calories burned when merely standing. In one study, obese women who added a half-hour walk to their daily routines lost twenty pounds in a year's time—even without dieting.

Physical activity also improves a person's sense of well-being and reduces stress. The relationship of this to weight control is that many people eat more when they are under stress. Finally, when people are involved in an exercise program, they are otherwise occupied and cannot be tempted to snack.

Eating Disorders: A Troubled Relationship with Food

A condition of being underweight results from not consuming adequate amounts of foods, participating in excessive exercise, and/or encountering extreme stress. Anyone who is more than 10 percent lighter than average for his or her height and build may be at an increased health risk.

Anorexia nervosa, a condition characterized by starvation behavior, primarily affects adolescent and young women, but it also occurs in men. A person suffering from anorexia usually becomes preoccupied with thinness. She or he diets excessively in an effort to approach a distorted body weight goal that seems progressively out of reach. Anorexic patients seldom see themselves as thin, regardless of their actual appearance. Rather, they are constantly driven to lose more weight.

Anorexia is a relatively rare disease, developing in approximately 1 percent of adolescent girls. A person suffering from anorexia tends to be upper middle class, white, and female. It afflicts ten times as many women as men. The anorexic tends to display perfectionist traits. It is not well understood what causes such a person to acquire this eating disorder. Several factors appear to be related to the disease, including susceptibility to social pressures to be thin, problems in family interaction, and a strong need for control. Unusually severe dieting, particularly in female teens, is considered evidence of risk.

A person who has anorexia can lose up to 30 percent of total body fat. Left untreated, such weight loss can result in starvation and death. Pleas or threats from parents and friends usually do not put a stop to this disease. Treatment usually involves a combination of medical intervention and psychotherapy. Parents and other family members are often involved in psychotherapy along with the anorexic person.

Bulimia is another eating disorder that affects 2 to 3 percent of young women. It is characterized by the extreme behavior of **binge eating** and **purging.** Binge eating refers to eating excessively, consuming greater than the normal amount of food usually taken in one sitting, such as a gallon of ice cream and two large pizzas. A bulimic person can eat 10,000 calories or more at one time. Bingers generally eat alone and usually stop only when they are so full that they cannot continue, when they fall into a stupor, or when they are interrupted. To avoid the weight gain that normally results from such eating behavior, the bulimic follows the binge with an intentional purge of the stomach and bowels. This is accomplished by self-induced vomiting and/or the use of laxatives, ene-

HealthLinks Web
Healthtouch Online
www.healthtouch.com/level1/leaflets/102952/102952.htm
Collection of articles and resources from multiple organizations on all forms of eating disorders.

binge eating Eating excessively; consuming greater than the normal amount of food usually taken in at one sitting.

purging To self-induce vomiting and/or to otherwise rid the body of excessive food; often done after binges by a bulimic person.

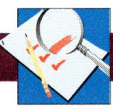

HERE'S LOOKING AT YOU

Are You at Risk for an Eating Disorder?

Losing your appetite on occasion is normal—for example, you may have butterflies in your stomach before a big exam and not want to eat much. But having a serious eating disorder that results in a life-threatening weight loss is totally different: It is not normal, and you should seek out a health care professional who is experienced in working with people who have eating disorders. The student health office should be able to direct you to appropriate care for this problem.

Review the following common symptoms of eating disorders, and ask yourself if you—or someone you know—needs professional help in dealing with eating problems.

Symptom	Anorexia	Bulimia	Binge eating
Excessive weight loss in a relatively short period of time	✔		
Continuation of dieting although bone thin	✔		
Dissatisfaction with appearance; belief that body is fat even though severely underweight	✔		
Loss of monthly menstrual periods	✔	✔	
Unusual interest in food and development of strange eating rituals	✔	✔	
Obsession with exercise	✔	✔	
Eating in secret	✔	✔	✔
Serious depression	✔	✔	✔
Binging—consumption of large amounts of food		✔	✔
Vomiting or use of drugs to stimulate vomiting, bowel movements, and urination		✔	
Binging but no noticeable weight gain		✔	
Disappearance into bathroom for long periods of time to induce vomiting		✔	
Abuse of alcohol or drugs		✔	✔

Source: National Institute of Mental Health

mas, syrup of ipecac, and/or **diuretics.** Although bulimia is typically a disease of young women, young men are at risk as well—particularly wrestlers, runners, dancers, and models.

As with anorexia, the person suffering from bulimia tends to be white, well educated, and perfectionistic. Left untreated, the bulimic is at risk for a variety of complications, including nutritional deficiencies, reproductive problems, and, in extreme cases, death. The treatment for bulimia is similar to that for anorexia—a combination of medical intervention and psychotherapy.

Binge eating disorder, which is found in about 2 percent of the population, resembles bulimia because it involves periods of uncontrolled eating. People with this disorder consume enormous quantities of food and stop eating only when they are uncomfortably full. Unlike bulimics, people who have binge eating disorder do not purge themselves afterwards to get rid of the excess food. And in contrast to both anorexics and bulimics, one fourth to one third of all people who have binge eating disorder are men. One reason for this kind of binge

diuretic A medication that promotes the excretion of excess body fluids and salt in the urine.

binge eating disorder An eating disorder characterized by periods of uncontrolled eating.

eating is related to dieting. Recent research shows that it occurs in about 30 percent of people in medically supervised weight-control programs.

Most people who have eating disorders share certain personality traits. They have

- low self-esteem;
- feelings of helplessness; and
- a fear of becoming fat.

To compensate for these personality traits, they try to gain control through their eating disorders. An anexoric, for example, tries to gain control over her mother who makes disparaging comments about fat people. A bulimic tries to reduce stress and anxiety by eating huge amounts of food and then getting "relief" by purging. Binge eaters and people who have bulimia are also impulsive and are more likely to engage in other risky behaviors, such as alcohol and drug abuse (see the Here's Looking at You box).

Athletes and Dancers at High Risk

Athletes whose performances are judged—gymnasts, divers, and figure skaters—and professional dancers appear to be at high risk for anorexia and bulimia. A recent study of 182 female college athletes representing ten different sports reported that 32 percent of the women interviewed admitted to practicing one of the following pathological behaviors daily for at least a month: self-induced vomiting or use of diet pills, laxatives, and/or diuretics for weight control.

The demand for thinness is highly pronounced in dance. Gelsey Kirkland, a former ballerina, recalled in her autobiography that although she weighed less than 100 pounds, ballet master George Balanchine was still not satisfied. He stopped a class to inspect her body, thumped on the bones of her chest, and said, "Must see the bones. Eat nothing."

According to four studies reported in *Medical Problems of Performing Artists*, teen and adult ballet dancers are between 12 and 18 percent below their ideal weight. In an effort to keep their weight down, dancers often do not eat well. A twenty-four-hour nutritional survey of nineteen dancers from two major ballet companies revealed that more than one half of the dancers consumed less than 85 percent of the recommended daily allowance (RDA) of calories. Four of the dancers fell below 66 percent of the RDA, and two took in less than 50 percent of the RDA. In addition, the young women were putting in three to four hours of dance practice, which is more physically demanding than most other sports.

Teenage dance students have a seven-fold greater chance of developing anorexia than do other high school students. As they advance up the professional ladder, the risk for and incidence of eating disorders increase. Dancers from highly competitive settings have double the incidence of anorexia (7.6 percent) of dancers from less competitive settings (3.5 percent).

Athletes practice pathological eating behaviors to improve their athletic performance and dancers do so to improve their look on stage. In reality, pathological weight loss is likely to cause weakness, hypoglycemia, metabolic acidosis, and other bodily dysfunctions that can result in poor performance for both athletes and dancers.

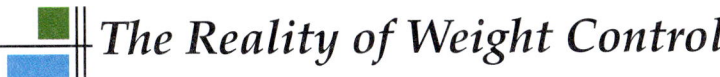
The Reality of Weight Control

The key to long-term weight loss and weight control is to give up the idea of going on a diet. There is simply no magic bullet that can take away unwanted fat. Instead, think of weight control as a combination of two factors: (1) a healthy eating style and (2) appropriate exercise. To enhance your chances for success, you may want to make some changes in your eating environment as well.

Before beginning a weight-control program, however, consult a physician to make sure you do not have a medical condition that would preclude doing exercise or require a special diet. Consulting with a physician can also help you plan a safe weight-control program.

HEALTH SKILLS

Controlling Your Weight

A complete weight-control program begins with a **balanced diet.** This means an emphasis on whole grains, fresh fruits, and vegetables and a de-emphasis on food high in fat, processed foods, red meats, and rich desserts. The best advice from nutritionists calls for consuming about 1,200 calories a day for women and about 1,500 for men trying to lose weight.

Note the word *balanced*. Eating a variety of foods is important. But remember that certain foods can help you lose weight whereas others may hinder weight loss. High-fiber foods are more filling and have fewer calories than do fatty foods. Meanwhile, foods high in fat store in the body more easily than do carbohydrates. High-protein foods reduce blood-sugar level fluctuations that often stimulate hunger. Alcohol lowers blood sugar and stimulates hunger. In addition, alcoholic beverages are a significant source of calories. A regular beer contains about 150 calories. Chapter 5 is a good source of further information about how different foods affect your weight.

You have already read about the importance of exercise in a weight-loss program. For maximum benefits, exercise four or five days a week, starting slowly—perhaps with a five-minute workout—and build up to thirty minutes. Do not forget to do your warm-up and cool-down exercises. Chapter 7 provides a lot more information about exercising to maintain proper weight.

Finally, to help you succeed with a new health style of eating right and exercising, you may need to make some changes in your environment as well as in how you eat. One simple change you can make in your eating environment is to remove the salt shaker from the table. If the salt is out of reach, you will have to think about standing up from the table to get it rather than simply add it to your food out of habit. Extra salt in your diet can derail a successful weight-control program by causing you to retain an abnormal amount of water and thus more weight.

You can also stop buying junk food such as potato chips or cupcakes. If such foods are not around, you will not be tempted to compromise your new weight-control style. As we mentioned in Chapter 5, the way you prepare food can have much to do with its nutritional value. You can learn to prepare foods in order to reduce fat intake. For example, eat baked instead of fried foods, eat uncooked instead of cooked vegetables, and eat grilled fish instead of baked fish in a sauce. You will be surprised how quickly you learn to enjoy the natural taste of vegetables and to find extra sauces and salt to be distasteful. And you will likely lose weight in the process.

Most eating habits were learned a long time ago, and it will take time to unlearn them and to learn new ones. Once you know how to live healthfully with food, you will not have to practice the constant restraint and vigilance that wear down so many dieters. Basically, this involves substituting "thin" strategies for "fat" ones. Consider some of the following ideas:

- Serve yourself on a smaller plate. Smaller portions will fill it up, and you are less likely to feel deprived by a skimpy serving.
- Do not put serving bowls on the table.

- Let your family and friends know that you are changing your eating habits. Ask them not to offer you seconds.
- Get someone else to clear the table and put away the leftovers. Alternatively, clear plates directly into the garbage. Either way, you will be less tempted to nibble after eating.
- Keep a supply of "safe" snacks on hand—raw vegetables, for example.
- If you eat because you are bored or frustrated, think of other activities to get your mind off food—jog, call a friend, walk the dog.
- Drink a glass of water before meals, and sip water while eating. This will help you fill up without overloading on calories.

Dangers of Fad Diets

Dieting is a $50-billion-a-year business in the United States. One reason for this is that most people go on one diet after another in search of the perfect plan, and they are more than willing to spend money on diet doctors, diet foods, diet books, and video cassettes. The fact is that no diet works quickly, and most of them do not work over the long run. Less than 5 percent of people who have lost weight while on a diet have maintained that loss for more than one year. Moreover, people who do **yo-yo dieting**—going on and off diets year after year—may actually be inhibiting future weight loss. In a study of patients enrolled for the second time in a university weight loss clinic, the dieters lost markedly fewer pounds on the second diet (2.1 pounds per week) than on the first (3.1 pounds per week). There is some indication that repetitive dieters tend to gain weight back in fat tissue, which is harder to lose.

From a nutritionist's point of view, it is a good thing that **fad diets** fail and that most people do not stick with them for very long. Virtually every fad diet is nutritionally unbalanced in one way or another because they emphasize eating only a limited number of foods. No combination of only a few foods can provide the essential nutrients. Some fad diets are downright dangerous.

One of the dangers of fad diets is that they may actually work—but too fast. Fast weight loss can be dangerous. It may result from dehydration, or loss of water, a condition that is potentially deadly. Or it may result in an excessive loss of vitamins and electrolytes and a reduction in protein, which can result in malnutrition. Further, if weight loss is due to diet alone, as soon as the diet is ended, the weight will likely be gained back (see the Healthwise Consumer box).

High-protein, low-carbohydrate diets are based on the theory that when, in the absence of carbohydrates, the body burns fat as its major energy source, acidic products called ketones develop, and these are supposed to induce weight loss. However, the accumulation of ketones in the blood **(ketosis)** can cause nausea, vomiting, apathy, fatigue, and low blood pressure.

Low-protein, high-carbohydrate diets consist of a lot of cereal, pasta, fruit, and vegetables. But they are so limited in protein and essential minerals such as calcium and iron that the body is forced to break down its own muscle tissue in order to meet its protein needs. At least one low-protein diet calls for eating so much fruit that it can cause severe diarrhea and result in high fever, muscle weakness, rapid pulse, a severe drop in blood pressure, and shock.

Protein-sparing diets are near-starvation diets. They involve a caloric intake of 300 to 500 calories in a liquid protein formula. Some of these formulas are fortified with minerals and vitamins, but others are not. Weight loss is rapid, averaging three to five pounds a week. These diets were originally designed for use by extremely obese persons and were intended to be carried out under strict medical supervision. Their widespread use among persons with little or no medical supervision has resulted in deaths.

balanced diet An eating pattern that includes a variety of foods in amounts that result in health enhancement.

yo-yo dieting Going on and off diets.

fad diets Diets that are popular for brief periods of time then lose popularity. The loss of popularity usually results when the effectiveness of a fad diet is questioned.

ketosis An accumulation of chemical compounds called ketones in the blood.

HEALTHWISE CONSUMER

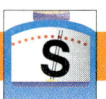

Questions to Ask before Going on a Diet

1. Does the diet provide a reasonable number of calories? This means no fewer than 1,200 calories for the average-sized person.
2. Does it provide enough, but not too much, protein? It should have at least the recommended dietary allowance (RDA) but not more than twice that amount.
3. Does it provide enough, but not too much, fat? No more than 30 percent of the calories in the diet should come from fat.
4. Does it provide enough carbohydrates, particularly complex carbohydrates? No more than 20 percent of the calories should come from concentrated sugar.
5. Does it offer a balanced assortment of vitamins and minerals from whole food sources in all food groups? If a food group is omitted (for example, meat), is a suitable substitute provided?
6. Does it offer variety? Can different foods be selected each day?
7. Does it consist of ordinary foods that are available locally at the prices people normally pay, or does the dieter have to buy special, expensive foods to adhere to the diet?

Note: You may want to refer back to Chapter 5 for a review of nutritional information and what constitutes a healthy diet.

Source: "Questions to Ask before Going on a Diet," from *Understanding Nutrition,* 5th edition, by Eleanor Noss Whieney, Eva May Nunnelley Hamilton, and Sharon Rady Rolfes," © 1990 by West Publishing Company, p. 374. Used by permission of Wadsworth Publishing Company, Belmont, CA

Critical Thinking Question

The goal of fad diets is weight loss—not health enhancement—and they are part of a multimillion-dollar industry. How might they be a symptom of modern lifestyles? Why do they continue to be followed even when proven to be unhealthy?

Total fasting, or not eating anything, as a means of treating obesity is characterized by a progressive reduction in intestinal activity. Among the problems associated with total fasting are dehydration, nausea and dizziness, mineral loss, muscle wasting and kidney impairment. It can also lead to sudden death due to heart rhythm abnormalities. Because about one third of the weight lost during a twenty-four-hour fast is fluid, it is not surprising that this weight is quickly regained.

In addition to weight-loss plans, a variety of drugs are advertised as diet aids. Caution should be used to avoid the problems associated with any drug use: adverse drug interactions and allergic reactions. A new combination of fenfluramine and phentermine, commonly known as fen/phen, was used by some two million dieters before the Food and Drug Administration pulled it off the market in 1997 because of evidence that as many as one third of those using the prescription medications may develop a rare form of heart valve damage that could

total fasting Refraining from eating foods of any type for a period of time.

lead to weakening of the heart. At least three people died from the fen/phen combination.

Water pills or diuretics dehydrate the body, and depending on how much water was in the body, a person may lose three to ten pounds this way. Weight lost due to use of laxatives is also essentially water weight; the way most laxatives work is by increasing the amount of water in the stool. Amphetamines can reduce hunger pangs, but the weight lost is regained as soon as one stops taking the drug. Some people use thyroid hormones to lose weight based on the belief that obese people suffer from a malfunctioning thyroid gland. The fact is that less than 1 percent of overweight people have abnormal thyroid function. The dangers of taking thyroid hormones include heart palpitations and increased heart rate and systolic blood pressure.

Several other gimmicks are advertised as avenues to weight loss. Body wraps, for example, are sold as a method of removing inches from your waistline by means of temporary fluid loss or perspiration. Notice the wording: *inches,* not *fat*. Health spas advertise machines that shake away cellulite, that lumpy fat deposited near the external tissue on hips and thighs. What the ads do not tell you is that cellulite is a fancy word for fat—the same fat that exists anywhere in the body. And shaking fat doesn't make it go away.

Weight-loss organizations such as Weight Watchers and TOPS (Take Off Pounds Sensibly) promote the use of well-balanced meals, and Overeaters Anonymous offers encouragement for dieters. This can be useful for people who can benefit from group support. However, the quality of leadership varies from group to group.

Final Word on Weight Loss

It would be nice if weight loss were simple—if you could take a pill or purchase a product and have the pounds come off. But the fact remains that there is no quick and easy way to lose weight. Anyone who attempts to do so takes risks. It takes time to develop an overweight problem, and it takes time to get yourself back to your desired weight. If you want to lose weight, take the advice of a health professional—a nurse, health educator, nutritionist, physician, or dietitian—not a zealot. Remember: A good weight-control program is one that you want to live with for the rest of your life.

■ *Key Concepts*

1. The inability to maintain proper weight is a serious public health problem in the United States. According to the Centers for Disease Control and Prevention, one in three American adults is overweight.
2. Obesity refers to a surplus of body fat. A person is at increased health risk when body weight is 20 percent above normal. Overweight, on the other hand, refers to an excess of body weight.
3. Anyone who is more than 10 percent lighter than average for his or her height and build is considered underweight and at increased risk of mortality. This is especially true in the case of smokers.
4. The tendency to overweight appears to be related to heredity, eating styles, and exercise patterns.
5. Overweight parents tend to have overweight children, and thin parents tend to have thin children.
6. A calorie is a unit measuring the energy produced by food when oxidized in the body.

7. As food, fat is essential to health. Without fats in the diet, deficiencies of the fat-soluble vitamins A, D, E, and K would result.
8. Weight control results from a lifelong commitment to healthy eating as well as from an appropriate level of exercise, not from going on a diet.
9. Virtually every fad diet is nutritionally unbalanced in one way or another because fad diets emphasize eating only a limited number of foods.
10. Less than 5 percent of people who lose weight while on a diet have maintained that loss for more than one year.

■ Review Questions

1. Explain the difference between overweight and obesity.
2. List five chronic diseases that have been associated with overweight.
3. How are height–weight tables used to assess health risk? How are such tables known to be inaccurate when applied to the general public?
4. Al is six feet two inches tall and weighs 192 pounds. What is his approximate body mass index?
5. Is Al overweight?
6. Overweight parents often have overweight children. Explain why this may occur.
7. Describe how exercise is an important element of a weight-control program.
8. List characteristics of anorexia and bulimia. What is the prognosis if such diseases are left untreated?
9. Define yo-yo dieting and explain the health risks associated with this eating behavior.
10. List several specific actions you can take to help maintain a weight-control program of healthy eating and exercise.

■ Selected Bibliography

Anderson, G.H., and S.H. Kennedy. *The Biology of Feast and Famine: Relevance to Eating Disorders.* San Diego: Academic Press, 1992.
Dietary Guidelines for Americans. Washington, DC: U.S. Department of Agriculture and Department of Health and Human Services, 1995.
Eating Disorders. Bethesda, MD: National Institute of Mental Health, 1994.
Health Implications of Obesity. Bethesda, MD: National Institutes of Health, 1985.
Kucmarski, R.J., et al. "Increasing Prevalence of Overweight among US Adults: The National Health and Nutrition Examination Surveys, 1960–1991." *Journal of the American Medical Association* 272, no. 3 (1994): 205–211.
Methods of Voluntary Weight Loss and Control. Bethesda, MD: National Institutes of Health, 1992.
"Update: Prevalence of Overweight among Children, Adolescents, and Adults—United States, 1988–1994." *Morbidity and Mortality Weekly Report* 46 (March 7, 1997).

■ HealthLinks: Web Sites for Maintaining a Healthy Weight

You can access better health as it relates to this chapter by checking out some of the following sites on the Internet. These and sites identified within the chapter can be accessed directly when you visit the *HealthStyles* Web Site located on the Allyn and Bacon homepage at **http://www.abacon.com.**

Alliance to Fight Eating Disorders (AFED)
www.fsci.umn.edu/~AFED/
A link to an all-volunteer organization comprised of individuals who are fighting or have fought an eating disorder, their family members and friends, and professionals.

Duke University Diet and Fitness Center
dmi-www.mc.duke.edu/dfc/home.html
Visit one of the best programs in the country that focuses on helping people live healthier, fuller lives through weight loss and lifestyle change. This site prides detailed information about weight management and numerous related resources, as well as links to other programs related to weight management.

Health Hotlines: Maintaining Proper Weight

National Association of Anorexia Nervosa and Associated Disorders
(847) 831-3438
Box 7
Highland Park, IL 60035

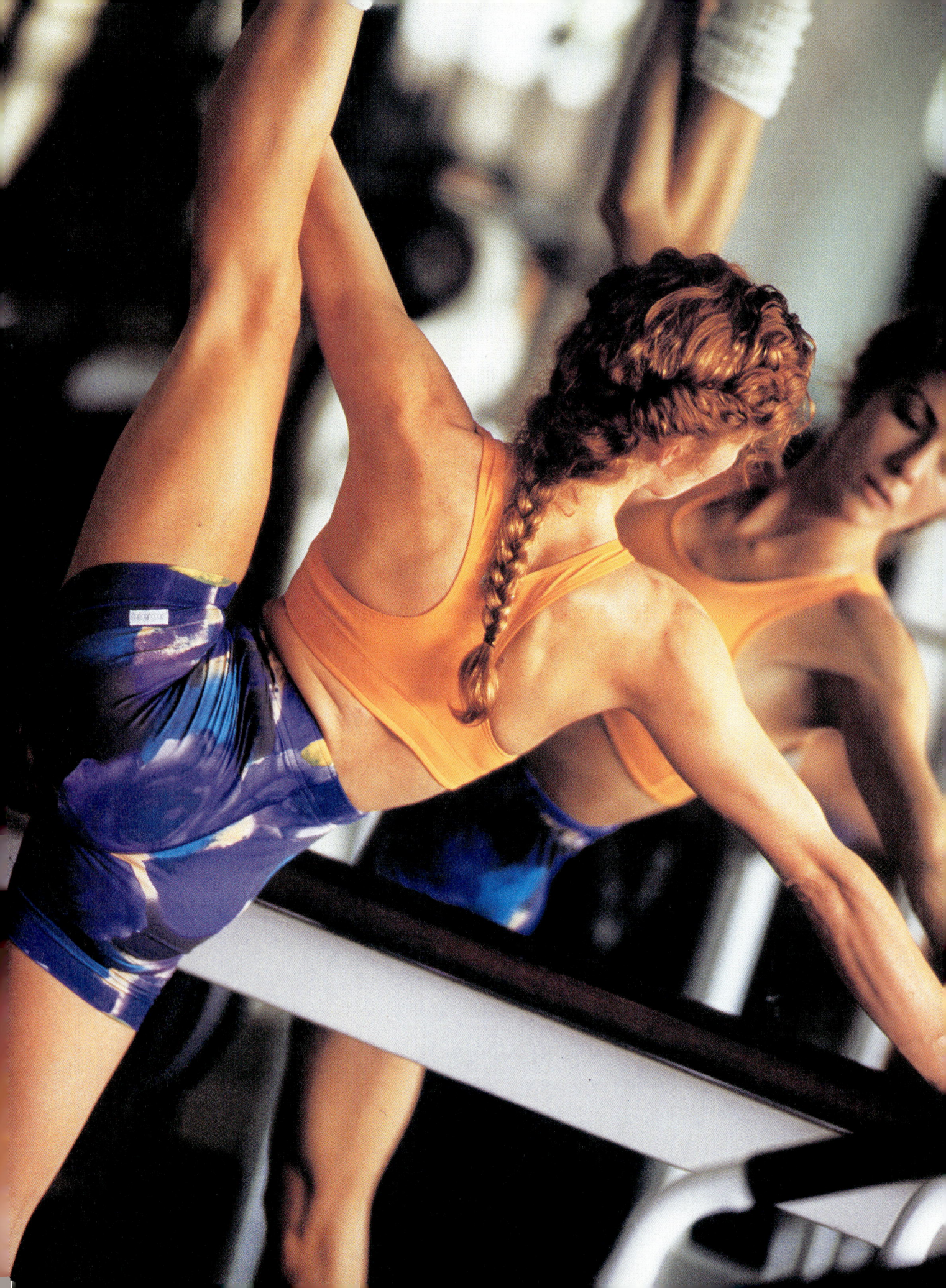

Chapter 7

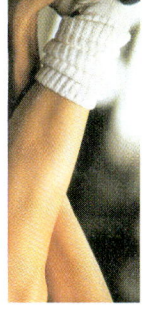
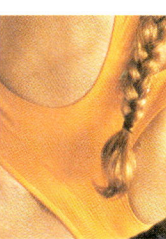
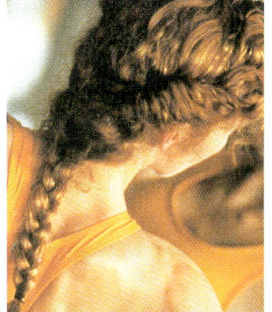

Keeping Fit

Objectives

When you finish reading this chapter, you will be able to:

1. Examine the extent to which people exercise and reasons for the apparent low level of exercise among specific populations.
2. Describe the physical health benefits of exercise.
3. Describe the effect of exercise on psychological well-being.
4. Explain the three major components of fitness: strength, flexibility, and endurance.
5. Differentiate between isokinetic, isotonic, and isometric exercises.
6. Differentiate between aerobic and anaerobic activities.
7. Explain the importance of intensity, duration, and frequency of exercise sessions.
8. Determine your target heart rate for exercise as well as your maximal heart rate.
9. Plan a personal fitness program including warm-up, conditioning, and cool-down periods.
10. List several tactics for maintaining a fitness program.

What Is Your HealthStyle?

Every weekend, Gilda is seen doing one sport activity or another—tennis, swimming, running, rollerblading. It may look like she is serious about her exercise program, but Gilda is a weekend warrior, doing all her exercise in one or two days a week. Because she does not exercise on a regular basis, she is not in shape for the 10K run or half-mile swim that she takes on the weekend. She often ends up with sore joints or blisters and wonders why. She sees herself as a jock. But in reality, Gilda has no true exercise plan for herself, and although she is active, she has no real commitment to fitness.

Toshio has an exercise plan, which he follows carefully. He meets the same group of friends to do brisk walking three mornings a week. No matter how busy he is, Toshio finds time for his walk because he knows that physical fitness results from frequency as much as from intensity. Throughout the day, Toshio builds in additional exercise. He takes the stairs rather than the elevator; he walks to an off-campus building rather than take the free shuttle bus. Toshio has clearly made a choice about his level of fitness. He has established a lifelong commitment to exercise.

In Your Opinion

Gilda and Toshio both look fit, as well they should. Each spends several hours a week in some form of exercise.

- What is wrong with Gilda's fitness program?
- Does it make her physically fit?
- Do you think she will still be fit ten years from now?
- What do you see Toshio doing in ten years?
- How is his current health style related to decisions concerning exercise that he made earlier in his life?

Interest in sports in the United States is at perhaps its highest point in history—but the interest is in spectator sports rather than participation sports. We admire elite athletes but seldom become the athlete ourselves. Advances in technology have contributed to the increasingly sedentary lifestyle of Americans. More and more, work sites are mechanized and automated, making physical fitness no longer a requisite for earning a living. Telecommunications and easy transportation have reduced the need for walking.

At home, television viewing requires little or no physical exertion, especially when a remote control device is used for changing channels. Even people who work out in front of their television sets often do so not to achieve fitness, but rather in pursuit of the promise of "looking good."

Good looks, however, do not always translate into good health and well-being. Evidence suggests that, as a nation, we are not very fit. According to the 1996 Surgeon General's report on physical activity and health, more than 60 percent of American adults are not regularly physically active. And as many as one

Examples of Moderate Amounts of Activity

Washing and waxing a car for 45–60 minutes
Washing windows or floors for 45–60 minutes
Playing volleyball for 45 minutes
Playing touch football for 30–45 minutes
Gardening for 30–45 minutes
Wheeling self in wheelchair for 30–40 minutes
Walking 1¾ miles in 35 minutes (20 min/mile)
Basketball (shooting baskets) for 30 minutes
Bicycling 5 miles in 30 minutes
Dancing fast (social) for 30 minutes
Pushing a stroller 1½ miles in 30 minutes
Raking leaves for 30 minutes
Walking 2 miles in 30 minutes (15 min/mile)
Water aerobics for 30 minutes
Swimming laps for 20 minutes
Wheelchair basketball for 20 minutes
Basketball (playing a game) for 15–20 minutes
Bicycling 4 miles in 15 minutes
Jumping rope for 15 minutes
Running 1½ miles in 15 minutes (10 min/mile)
Shoveling snow for 15 minutes
Stairwalking for 15 minutes

Less vigorous, more time ↑↓ *More vigorous, less time*

Significant health benefits can be obtained with a moderate amount of physical activity, preferably daily. The same moderate amount of activity can be obtained in longer sessions of moderately intense activities (such as 30–40 minutes of wheeling oneself in a wheelchair) or in shorter sessions of more strenuous activities (such as 20 minutes of wheelchair basketball).

Figure 7.1 Examples of Moderate Amounts of Activity. *(Source: Physical Activity and Health: A Report of the Surgeon General, 1996)*

in four are not active at all. Of those who do exercise, few do so at what is considered an appropriate level of activity.

The appropriate level involves physical activity that is both regularly vigorous and regularly sustained. Note the importance of the word *regularly*. On most—if not all—days of the week, you should spend thirty minutes or more on moderate-intensity physical activity, such as brisk walking (see Figure 7.1 for more examples of moderate amounts of activity). Does this sound possible, given your busy student life? The answer is yes, once you make being physically fit a part of your lifestyle.

Who Is Exercising?

In general, males participate in regular exercise more than do females; whites exercise more than do African Americans, Hispanics, and members of other ethnic groups; and college graduates exercise more than do those who have less education. There are also age differences in who is exercising. Young adults are more likely to exercise than are members of any other age group.

But these statistics tell only part of the story. Females do more stretching exercises than do males, while males do more strengthening activities, including weight lifting, than do females (see Table 7.1). Whether it be stretching or strengthening, the key to a good program of physical activity is finding one that you like—and sticking to it.

The key reason people give for why they do not exercise is that they do not have the time or that they lack the good health needed to do so (see Figure 7.2). People who exercise report just the opposite—that they have both the time and the good health needed to maintain an exercise schedule.

The children of the United States are not in much better shape than the adults—and they do not have as many excuses about why they do not exercise. Little is understood about the carry-over effect of physical activity from youth to adulthood, but a reasonable assumption is that active children become active adults and inactive children become inactive adults. The Surgeon General's report found that nearly half of American youth between the ages of twelve and twenty-one are not vigorously active on a regular basis. And about 14 percent of young people report no recent physical activity. The study also found that par-

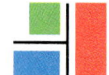

TABLE 7.1 Who Likes to Run…or Walk…or Swim: Exercise Participation by Sex and Age

Percentage of adults aged 18+ years reporting participation in selected common physical activities in the prior 2 weeks.

Activity category	Males 18–29	Males All	Females 18–29	Females All	All ages and sexes
Walking for exercise	32.8	39.4	47.4	48.3	44.1
Gardening or yard work	22.2	34.2	15.4	25.1	29.4
Stretching exercises	32.1	25.0	32.5	26.0	25.5
Weight lifting or other exercise to increase muscle strength	33.6	20.0	14.5	8.8	14.1
Jogging or running	22.6	12.8	11.6	5.7	9.1
Aerobics or aerobic dance	3.4	2.8	19.3	11.1	7.1
Riding a bicycle or exercise bike	18.7	16.2	17.4	14.6	15.4
Stair climbing	10.5	9.9	14.6	11.6	10.8
Swimming for exercise	10.1	6.9	8.0	6.2	6.5
Tennis	5.7	3.5	3.1	2.0	2.7
Bowling	7.0	4.7	4.8	3.6	4.1
Golf	7.9	8.2	1.4	1.8	4.9
Baseball or softball	11.0	5.8	3.2	1.4	3.5
Handball, racquetball, or squash	5.2	2.7	1.0	0.5	1.6
Skiing	1.5	0.9	0.9	0.5	0.7
Cross country skiing	0.1	0.4	0.3	0.4	0.4
Water skiing	1.5	0.7	0.7	0.4	0.5
Basketball	24.2	10.5	3.1	1.5	5.8
Volleyball	6.8	3.1	4.4	1.8	2.5
Soccer	3.3	1.4	0.9	0.4	0.9
Football	7.6	2.7	0.7	0.3	1.5
Other sports	8.6	7.3	4.5	4.1	5.7

Source: *Physical Activity and Health: A Report of the Surgeon General*, 1996

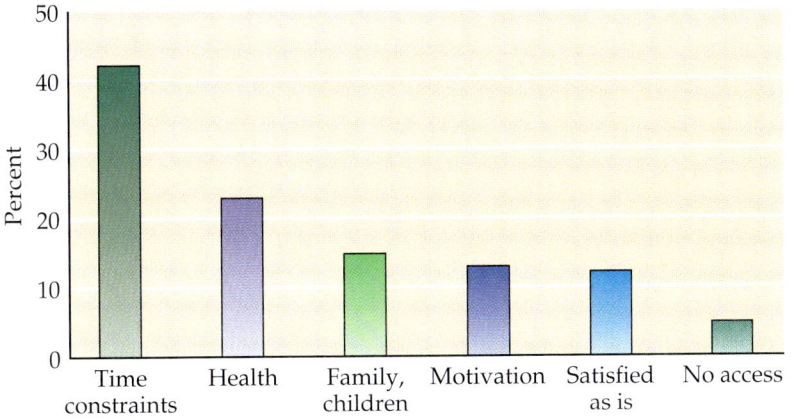

Figure 7.2 Why People Aren't More Active. *Most people who do not exercise say they do not have enough time. This is not the case with people who exercise regularly.* (Source: President's Council on Physical Fitness and Sports, *1993*)

ticipation in all types of physical activity declines strikingly as age or grade in school increases.

Critical Thinking Question

Healthy People 2000 established the following objective: "Increase to at least 50 percent the proportion of school physical education class time that students spend being physically active, preferably engaged in lifetime physical activities." Baseline data show that only 27 percent of students are so engaged. From your experience, do school physical education classes contribute to the fitness of students or to their athletic ability? Why do you think health officials consider active physical education important to our nation's health status?

What will it take to get people—young or old—who are leading sedentary lives to change their habits? For one thing, people need to know that being out of shape can increase health risks, whereas being in shape can reduce those risks. People who exercise regularly already know this. When asked why they exercise, many say they feel and look better when they are physically fit. They have more self-confidence and a better self-image. Others say they are physically active for social reasons—that is, they like to participate in exercise programs such as aerobic dancing because their friends are doing it. Some report that they have simply gotten into the exercise habit and enjoy it. Most physically active individuals, however, say they exercise for the "health" of it.

The Health Benefits of Exercise

It is unfortunate that so few exercise because exercise is a critical component of a healthy lifestyle. In fact, **exercise** may well be the single most important thing you can do if you want to live a long and healthy life. Researchers have persistently found that higher levels of physical activity and physical fitness lead to

exercise Bodily movement undertaken to improve or maintain one or more of the components of physical fitness.

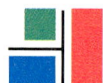

TABLE 7.2 Burning Calories: The Average Caloric Expenditure by Activity (per Hour)

	Body Weight				Body Weight		
	110 lbs.	154 lbs.	198 lbs.		110 lbs.	154 lbs.	198 lbs.
Baseball/softball				Running			
Infield/outfield	220	280	340	5.5 mph	515	655	795
Pitching	305	390	475	7 mph	550	700	850
Basketball				9 mph	720	920	1120
Moderate	435	555	675	Sailing (calm water)	120	155	190
Vigorous	585	750	910	Sawing wood	180	230	280
Bicycling				Shoveling snow	475	610	745
On level 5.5 mph	190	245	295	Skating (ice)			
13 mph	515	655	790	Moderate	275	350	425
Bowling (nonstop)	210	270	325	Vigorous	485	620	755
Bricklaying	160	205	250	Skiing			
Calisthenics	235	300	365	Downhill	465	595	720
Canoeing (4 mph)	490	625	765	Cross-country (5 mph)	550	700	950
Chopping wood	355	450	550	Soccer	470	600	730
Gardening	155	215	280	Swimming			
Gardening and weeding	250	315	380	Backstroke 20 yds/min	165	235	305
Golf				Breaststroke 10 yds/min	210	295	380
Twosome	295	380	460	Butterfly (per hour)	490	630	760
Foursome	210	270	325	Crawl 20 yds/min	235	300	365
Handball/raquetball	610	775	945	Sidestroke (per hour)	230	320	420
Hill climbing	470	600	730	Tennis			
Hoeing, raking, and planting	205	285	370	Moderate	335	425	520
Housework	175	245	320	Vigorous	470	600	730
House painting	165	210	255	Volleyball (moderate)	275	350	425
Motorcycling	165	205	250	Walking			
Mountain climbing	470	600	730	2 mph	145	185	225
Mowing grass				4½ mph	325	450	550
Power, self-propelled	195	250	305	Downstairs	355	450	550
Not self-propelled	210	270	325	Upstairs	720	920	1120
Rowing (20 strokes/min.)	515	655	795	Waterskiing	335	475	610
				Yard work	155	215	275

longer life—and a higher quality of life. Foremost of all the benefits of regular exercise is that it can reduce the risk of coronary artery disease and hypertension.

Regular exercise also helps to control weight. To lose one pound every two weeks from exercise alone, the average person must burn 200 to 250 calories a day in physical activity. Consult Table 7.2 for detailed information about the number of calories burned while performing various activities.

People who have disabilities are less likely to engage in regular physical activity than are people who don't have disabilities, yet they have similar if not greater needs to promote their health and prevent unnecessary disease. Speak with your physician about designing a fitness program that fits your abilities and your interests.

Helping the Heart

Exercise affects your heart in a number of ways. It increases the plasma, thus thinning the blood and allowing it to move smoothly through the vessels. It also

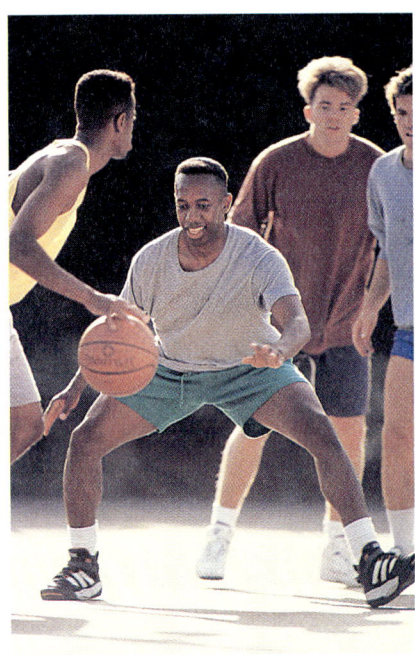

A steady diet of exercise significantly reduces a person's risk of dying from any of the major diseases. (Source: © Tony Stone Images/David Madison)

stimulates the release of a natural enzyme that prevents blood from clotting—**tissue plasminogen activator.** These effects are immediate and provide protection for up to one and a half hours after exercising. Over the long term, exercise can increase the size of the major coronary arteries.

Exercise contributes to lowering blood pressure and reducing the risk for **hypertension** by increasing the number as well as the capacity of capillaries, which carry blood to arteries. In addition, exercise improves the levels of blood cholesterol by raising the "good" cholesterol, the **high density lipoproteins (HDLs),** and lowering the plaque-forming cholesterol, the **low density lipoproteins (LDLs)** (see Chapter 5). It can also help lower blood sugar levels and increase the body's sensitivity to insulin. This is particularly important to diabetics, 70 percent of whom die from heart disease.

FOR MALES ONLY A study of 10,000 male Harvard graduates aged 35 to 74 demonstrated that regular exercise reduced the risk of dying from any of the major diseases. As reported in the *New England Journal of Medicine,* males who had hypertension, particularly, benefited from being fit. Men who had hypertension who exercised reduced their death rate by half. Exercise was also found to reduce the risk of death associated with parental history—specifically, when one or both parents die before age 65. This suggests that inheritance of a weak constitution may be offset by adequate exercise over a long period of time.

FOR FEMALES ONLY A study of female college graduates aged 21 to 80 showed that regular, intensive exercise could help protect against a host of serious diseases. Of the women surveyed by researchers at the Harvard School of Public Health, 2,600 former college athletes (most of whom continued to participate in exercise programs after college) were far less likely than the 2,800 nonathletes to have developed breast cancer, diabetes, or cancers of the reproductive system. For the study, athletes were defined as women who trained at least twice a week in energy-intensive sports such as swimming, tennis, or gymnastics or who ran at least two miles a day five days a week.

The most likely explanation of the lower cancer risk for women athletes, according to the researchers, is related to their lower estrogen levels. **Estrogen** is

tissue plasminogen activator A natural enzyme that prevents blood from clotting.

hypertension High blood pressure.

high density lipoproteins (HDLs) A fatty substance that is the type of cholesterol that is considered good and that prevents atherosclerosis.

low density lipoproteins (LDLs) A fatty substance that is the type of cholesterol that is considered bad and that promotes atherosclerosis.

estrogen The female sex hormone that is produced in the ovaries.

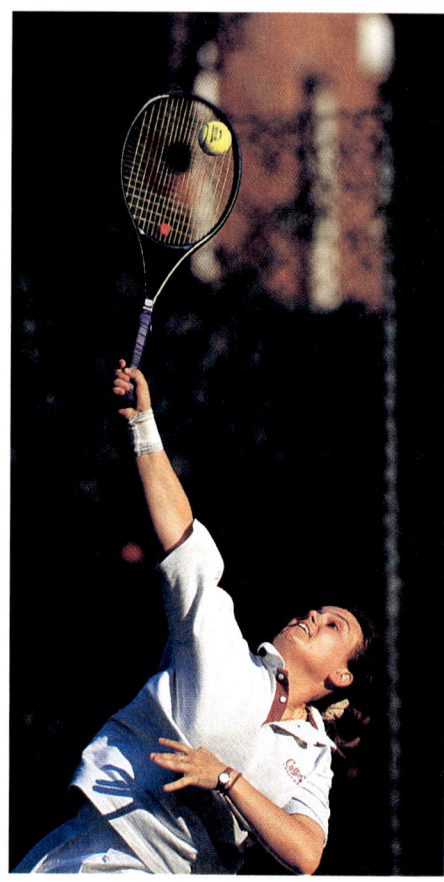

Females who participate in intensive regular exercise—swimming or playing tennis twice a week or running two miles five days a week—are less likely than nonathletes to develop breast cancer, other cancers of the reproductive system, or diabetes. (Source: © Tony Stone Images/Amwell)

a female sex hormone produced in the ovaries. Higher levels of estrogen are associated with some cancers. The greater a woman's body fat, the more estrogen she is likely to produce. Most of the athletes in the study were leaner than the nonathletes. Over the years, the lower estrogen level in leaner women may have reduced the growth of cells that can start tumors. The researchers also found that active exercisers had irregular menstrual cycles and could become infertile when they were in training for a particularly strenuous event such as a marathon or triathlon. It is important to note that exercise does not cause irregular menstruation. Low body fat does. Women who have menstrual problems due to low body fat usually find that when they eat more and exercise less, their menstrual cycles return to normal. The Cultural View box discusses various health considerations of young female athletes.

Preventing Osteoporosis

Another health benefit of exercise is that it helps strengthen bones. Without sufficient weight-bearing exercise, bones become demineralized—that is, they lose their calcium and become brittle. Walking, running, aerobics, and racquet sports are all examples of weight-bearing exercise.

Bones reach their maximum density and strength at around age thirty. After that, bone mass begins to diminish at a rate of about 10 percent per decade. By age seventy, about 45 percent of the total amount of bone mass has been lost. In men, bone mass loss begins approximately twenty years later and proceeds at about half the rate as in women.

Osteoporosis, a crippling condition that is characterized by a thinning of the bones, affects one in four women over age sixty. It develops in men, too, but much less frequently, in part because men have heavier bones to begin with, and,

osteoporosis A disorder in which bone density decreases, making the bones more likely to break.

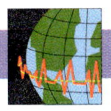

CULTURAL VIEW

Health Problems of Young Women Athletes

When it comes to exercise, too much of a good thing can be harmful. Athletes in training sometimes go overboard, leading to injuries and other health problems. In young women athletes, the start of menstruation may be delayed to beyond 16 years (primary amenorrhea), or young women who have begun menstruating may miss periods for six months or longer (secondary amenorrhea). Both of these conditions are of potential concern because they could signal estrogen deficiency.

The menstrual health and sexual development of young athletes should be monitored. If they stop menstruating, they need to be referred to a doctor for treatment. A decrease in activity level or supplemental estrogen may be recommended.

Eating disorders are common health risks. At the top of the list is anorexia nervosa, a psychological disorder resulting in self-imposed starvation. It may reflect a woman's attempt to conform to an ideal body image, such as the slender or slight shape of a gymnast or dancer. Crash dieting and bulimia (binging and purging) also are harmful and may be practiced to achieve weight limits.

Sometimes young women are horrified by their body's changing shape during puberty and need reassurance from their parents or coaches. Talking with a doctor also will help.

In addition to watching for signs of an eating disorder, parents should monitor the nutrition of their young athlete. She needs about 2,200 calories per day as a baseline during puberty, and about 1,500 additional calories for active participation in sports. She also needs adequate iron intake and about 1,200 to 1,500 milligrams of calcium per day (the equivalent of about five cups of skim milk).

Some athletic injuries are unavoidable. However, some studies of young male athletes suggest that young athletes are at greater risk for soft tissue injuries during growth spurts. Tendons may be unable to stretch fast enough to keep up with the body's changing proportions. When performance suffers, there is a tendency for coaches and trainers to push athletes harder. Instead, a "tapering-off" period may enhance performance.

Coaches of elite or world-class athletes may have differing opinions on how much outside activity is beneficial to top athletes. In general, however, young athletes need influences outside of their sport and time off from training schedules to pursue enjoyable activities. Adolescence is not only a time of physical growth and maturity, but also of emotional and social development. A healthy range of activities will contribute to happiness in the years to come.

Source: Reprinted by permission from American College of Obstetricians and Gynecologists, "Health Problems of Young Women Athletes," *Woman's Health Column* of April 29, 1996

as noted, their bone loss is not as severe as in women. Low estrogen levels come into play again, but in this case, the effect is negative. Bone loss in women sharply accelerates during the years immediately following menopause, when estrogen output is curtailed. Osteoporosis causes 700,000 fractures a year among American women. Of these, 150,000 are hip fractures; more than 15 percent of elderly women who suffer hip fractures die within three months of the injury, usually due to complications of immobility and not to the fracture itself. Osteoporosis can also cause chronic pain and disfiguring spinal deformities.

One of the best defenses against osteoporosis is a lifelong history of weight-bearing exercise. Studies consistently show that people who exercise have a greater bone mineral content than those who do not exercise. Moreover, the greater the load borne during exercise, the greater the bone density. Weight lifters have a greater bone mass than do throwers, throwers greater than do runners, runners greater than do soccer players, and soccer players greater than do swimmers. Recent studies reported by physiologists are finding that exercise can help increase bone mass even among a very elderly and sedentary population.

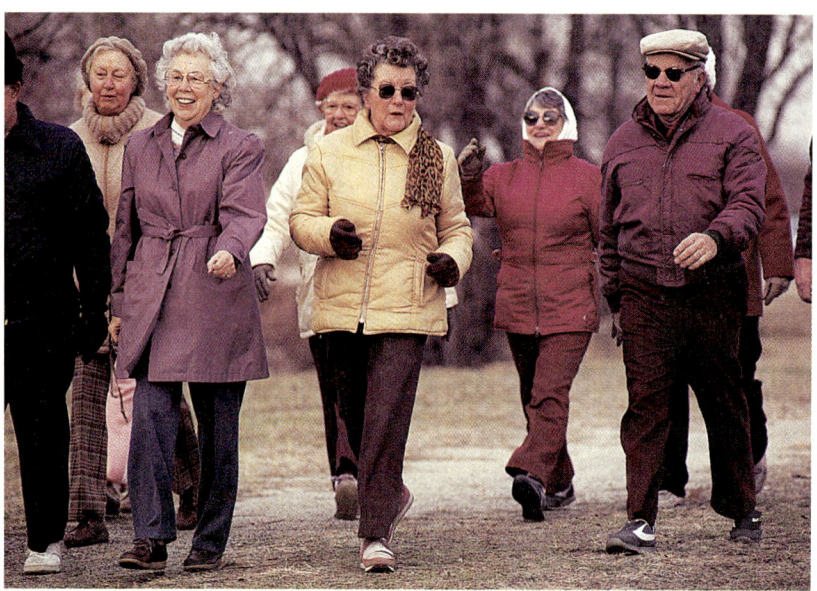

Exercise helps to strengthen bones, thereby reducing the risk of developing osteoporosis, a thinning of bones. It's never too late to benefit: Studies show that bone mass content increases in elderly people who do mild exercise. (Source: The Image Works/© David Wells)

One three-year study of elderly women aged sixty-nine to ninety-six showed that bone mass content increased 4.2 percent among a group doing mild exercise and decreased 2.5 percent among a control group of nonexercisers.

As discussed in Chapter 5, diet also plays a role in preventing osteoporosis. Especially important is the intake of the bone-building mineral calcium.

Warding Off Infection

Few argue about the value of exercise in warding off heart disease and osteoporosis. While more research is needed, there is a growing body of medical findings linking exercise and the immune response. Studies show that runners who exercise regularly have fewer colds and other infectious illnesses than do people who are not regular exercisers.

Moderate exercise often results in a temporary increase in blood levels of various immune cells, which, in turn, may improve resistance to infectious conditions. In one study, men who worked out on an indoor bicycle had an increased number of white blood cells. These cells destroy foreign agents and stimulate production of antibodies and other substances that fight against infections.

Another substance in the body that rises after exercise is a protein that causes fever. After exercise, most people experience a temporary increase in body temperature. It is believed that this rise in temperature—a mimicking of a fever—may help ward off infection.

Psychological Well-Being

Vigorous exercise has psychological benefits as well. People who exercise regularly tend to feel better and to have more energy and less trouble sleeping than do people who do not exercise regularly. Symptoms of anxiety and mild to moderate depression can be reduced through regular exercise. Exercise can reduce stress, and some people claim it gives them a "high." The so-called **runner's high** is due to an increase in the production of the hormone **endorphin,** which is

HealthLinks
Physical Activity and Health Network
www.pitt.edu/~pahnet
PAHNet is a dynamic list of Internet resources that examine the relationship of physical activity and exercise to health.

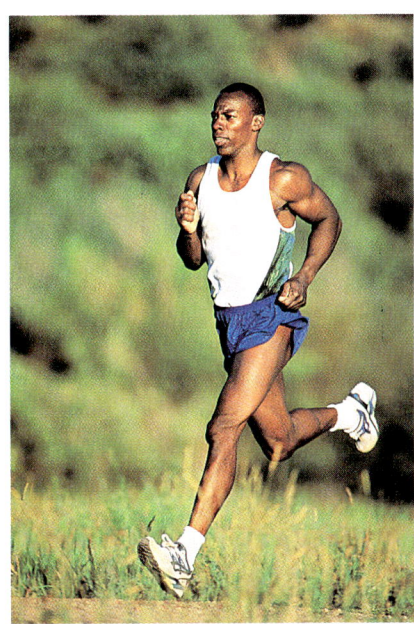

The so-called "runner's high"—a feeling of euphoria—can come after a half hour or so of running. (Source: © Tony Stone Images/Gregg Adams)

thought to cause a feeling of euphoria. This can take place after about thirty minutes of running.

The mental health benefits of exercise are clearly shown in the psychological well-being scores of a group of participants in a twelve-week exercise class that met three times a week. According to researchers from the Department of Sports and Leisure Studies at the University of Connecticut, the participants, who were thirty-six years old on average, reported having less anxiety, greater job satisfaction, and better self-esteem after the twelve weeks. In contrast, a control group of people who did not participate in the exercise class reported having more anxiety, less job satisfaction, or reduced feelings of self-esteem over the same twelve-week period.

Critical Thinking Question

> How can psychological well-being be measured? If you were designing a study of how a person feels after exercise, how might you measure these feelings? How do you know that you can trust your information?

Some evidence suggests that physically fit people learn better and stay mentally alert longer than those who are less fit. Psychologists at Scripps College compared a group of forty-two men and women between the ages of fifty-five and eighty-nine who exercised vigorously for at least seventy-five minutes a week with a group who exercised for less than ten minutes weekly. The more rigorous exercisers scored higher than those in the low-exercise group on a range of mental tests, including reciting a list of numbers backward and solving verbal analogies. Overall, according to the researchers, the high-exercise group showed better memory, quicker reaction, and more accurate reasoning. It is speculated

runner's high The feeling of euphoria due to an increase in the production of the hormone endorphin during or following exercise.

endorphin A hormone produced in the brain that helps give a sense of pleasure and satisfaction.

that regular exercise by older people may forestall some of the degenerative effects of aging on the central nervous system.

In the previously mentioned study of Harvard alumni, the participants who reported higher levels of physical activity also felt younger than their years, enjoyed life more, and felt that they could do more to take care of themselves than did their less physically active cohort.

The Fitness Triangle

The goal of an exercise program is physical fitness. When you think of being physically fit, what do you have in mind? Having muscles? Being able to swim 100 laps or lift 100 pounds? Actually, **physical fitness** is a measure of how efficiently your body works. **Strength, flexibility,** and **endurance** are three major components of fitness that contribute both to the level of exercise performance and to health (see Figure 7.3). These components dynamically interact to ensure that an individual is able to

- Meet the day-to-day demands for movement of the body
- Have a reserve ability for unexpected events requiring movement
- Reduce the risk of certain chronic and degenerative diseases

Strength

Strength is the extent to which you are capable of exerting force as needed. For example, if you are riding a bicycle, you must be able to exert enough force against the pedals to sustain movement. Most of us have enough strength to ride a bicycle but not enough to bench press a heavy weight. You do not have to be a weight lifter to be considered physically fit. You need only enough strength to respond to the day-to-day demands on your body.

Strength is measured in many ways. **Absolute strength** refers to the total force exerted in one effort—for example, lifting a 100-pound weight. This can be an important factor in sports such as football, baseball, and bowling. **Relative strength** takes the effect of body size into account. Larger people generally have larger muscles and therefore tend to have more absolute strength than do smaller people. Relative strength is determined by dividing absolute strength by body weight. Gymnastics is an example of a sport in which relative strength is more important than absolute strength. Generally, women do not have as much strength as men do. In part, this is due to the fact that about 45 percent of men's body weight is muscle whereas women's bodies are about 36 percent muscle.

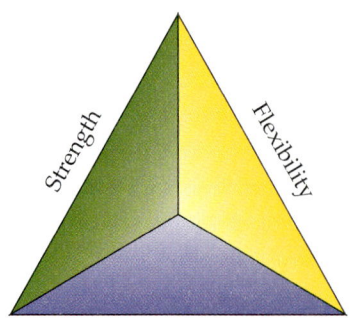

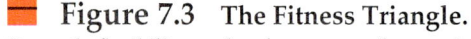 **Figure 7.3** The Fitness Triangle.
Strength, flexibility, and endurance are three major components of fitness.

---

physical fitness How efficiently the body works as measured by strength, flexibility, and endurance.

strength The extent to which an individual is capable of exerting force in one effort, as needed.

flexibility The range of movement an individual can achieve around a joint or group of joints.

endurance The ability to exercise vigorously at a sustained level for a period of time.

absolute strength The total force that an individual can exert when flexing muscles; usually measured in pounds.

relative strength A measure of strength determined by dividing absolute strength by body weight.

isokinetic exercise An exercise in which there are slow-moving contractions throughout a full range of movement against a constant resistance.

isotonic exercise An exercise involving the contraction of muscles against a movable resistance.

isometric exercise An exercise involving the contraction of muscles performed against an immovable object.

aerobic capacity The largest volume of oxygen that your body can consume in one minute; also called maximal oxygen uptake, or VO_2 max.

aerobic To be "with oxygen"; a process of energy production through which carbohydrates, fats, and proteins are used to produce energy and carbon dioxide and water are given off as by-products.

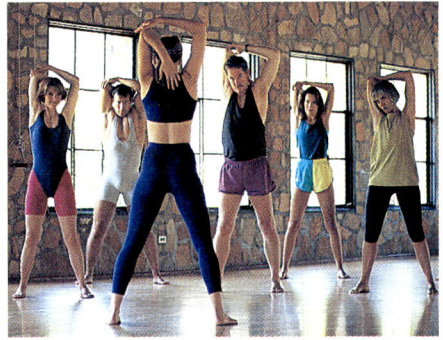 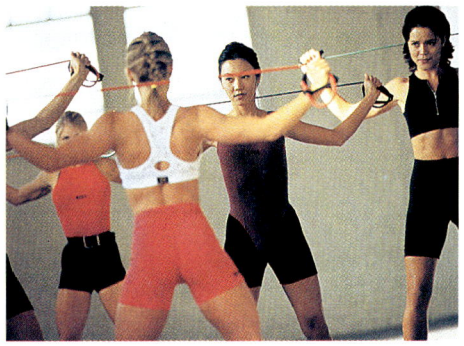

Stretching helps develop flexibility, while exercise bands are a simple way to tone and increase muscular strength. (Sources: LEFT, FPG International/© Stephen Simpson. RIGHT, © Tony Stone Images/Lori Adamski Peek)

Three types of exercise contribute to strength development. **Isokinetic exercise** involves slow-moving contractions throughout a full range of movement against a constant resistance. This form of exercise requires special heavy equipment in a gym. **Isotonic exercise** involves contracting muscles against a movable resistance, as in lifting weights. **Isometric exercise** involves muscle contractions performed against an immovable object, such as a wall. No special equipment is needed for isometric exercise.

Flexibility

Flexibility is the range of movement an individual can achieve around a joint or group of joints. It is usually determined by muscle elasticity. A physically fit person is flexible enough to meet the day-to-day demands for movement of the joints, from reaching for a book on a high shelf to serving a tennis ball.

Good muscular elasticity can increase your agility and your speed, but more importantly, it can reduce your chance of injury to muscles, tendons, and ligaments. Flexibility appears to decrease with age in sedentary people, but there is some consensus among exercise physiologists that flexibility does not decrease significantly in people who do stretching exercises regularly. To test your flexibility, see the Here's Looking at You box.

Endurance and Aerobic Capacity

Endurance is a term for the ability to exercise vigorously at a sustained level for a period of time. A fit person can maintain vigorous activity for at least 20 minutes without taking a break. **Aerobic capacity** is the best way to measure whether you can meet the physiological demands of strenuous exercise. It is usually expressed as maximal oxygen uptake, or VO_2 max. By evaluating how much oxygen you use in a minute, an exercise physiologist can measure your body's respiratory and circulatory ability to support exercise.

Aerobic (meaning "with oxygen") is short for aerobic metabolism, a process of energy production through which carbohydrates, fats, and proteins are used to produce energy, and carbon dioxide and water are given off as byproducts. Because the cells of the body continuously produce energy, aerobic metabolism is under way even when you are sleeping. Aerobic activities include those that can be maintained continuously through rhythmical and repetitive motions. Activities such as running, swimming, cycling, walking, dancing, jumping rope, and aerobic dancing are aerobic exercise. In a fit person, the body's respiratory and circulatory systems can keep up with the muscles' demand for oxygen during aerobic exercise, thus allowing nutrients to metabolize to meet energy needs.

**HealthLinks
ACSM
Online**
www.acsm.org/
A link with the American College of Sports Medicine and all their resources.

HERE'S LOOKING AT YOU

Assessing Your Flexibility

Here are three ways to test your flexibility.

Shoulder Flexibility

Raise your right arm and reach down your back as far as possible. At the same time, place your left arm behind your back and try to reach the fingers of your right hand. If your hands overlap, your arms and shoulders are fairly flexible. Repeat with arms reversed; most people are more flexible on one side than the other.

Sit and Reach Test

This measures the flexibility of the hamstrings and muscles in the lower back. You need a box or step eight to twelve inches high, with a ruler taped to its top so that it extends six inches in front of it. After warming up, sit with your bare soles flat against the box, about four inches apart. Without bending your knees, *gently* reach as far forward as you can toward the box. Have a friend note how far your fingertips reach along the ruler. If you don't stretch regularly, you may not be able to reach the box. Compare your results with the ratings in Figure 7.4.

Hip Flexibility (Hip Flexors)

Lie on your back on a firm surface with your knees bent over the edge. Keeping one leg in place, pull the other knee to your chest and hold it firmly with both hands. Repeat with legs reversed. If you can't keep the lowered leg in place, or if you feel tightness or discomfort in the groin area, you should do hip-stretching exercises regularly.

Rating	How far you reach (inches)
Excellent	over 13
Good	9-13
Fair	4-9
Poor	under 4

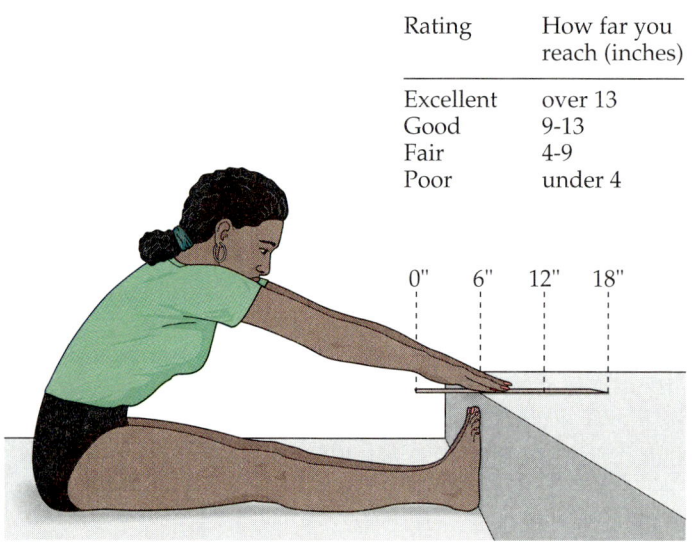

Figure 7.4

Source: "How Flexible Are You?" (not including figure) reprinted with permission from the *University of California at Berkeley Wellness Letter*, December 1987. © Health Letter Associates, 1987. To order a one year subscription, call 800/829-9170.

---

anaerobic To be "without oxygen"; the process of energy production in which surges of energy are needed for a brief amount of time.

exercise intensity The degree of energy that is exerted during exercise.

heart rate The number of heartbeats per minute.

exercise duration The length of time a person exercises.

exercise frequency How often an exercise is done.

The strongest influence on your aerobic capacity is your genetic makeup. Other factors are gender and body size. Men tend to have a higher aerobic capacity than do women for two major reasons. One is that women have lower blood hemoglobin concentrations and therefore less oxygen-carrying capacity. A second is that a woman's heart, compared to total muscle mass, is smaller than a man's.

Aerobic capacity is not a fixed point: It can change for better or worse depending on how much and how often you exercise. If you exercise regularly, you can maintain your aerobic capacity and perhaps even increase it. If you stop exercising regularly, your aerobic capacity decreases. (You can regain it, once you exercise regularly again.) Smoking adversely affects aerobic capacity. It decreases the amount of air that can be taken into the lungs as well as the amount of oxygen the blood can carry.

As one measure of aerobic capacity, college-age men should be able to sustain a pace of about eight minutes a mile while running two to three consecutive miles. College-age women should be able to run the same distance at an eleven-minute-per-mile pace. These are also reasonable goals to try to maintain over a lifetime.

Anaerobic (meaning "without oxygen") refers to the process of energy production in which surges of energy are needed for a brief amount of time. Sprinting and weight lifting are examples of anaerobic exercise. The respiratory and circulatory systems cannot keep up with the demand for oxygen during anaerobic exercise.

Very strenuous anaerobic exercise contributes to muscle strength but does little to enhance cardiovascular health. This is primarily due to the short duration of anaerobic activity. The body simply does not endure anaerobic exercise for periods lasting longer than one or two minutes. Exhaustion is reached, causing an immediate and involuntary reduction in exercise intensity. Both aerobic and anaerobic exercises contribute to the fitness of an individual, but aerobic exercise is clearly the more valuable from an overall health perspective.

Fitness through Exercise

Exercise is bodily movement undertaken to improve or maintain one or more of the components of physical fitness. A planned exercise program has three components: intensity, duration, and frequency. According to the National Health Interview Survey, most Americans do not know how vigorously, how long, and how often they should exercise in order to achieve an appropriate level of activity.

Exercise intensity refers to how hard you exercise. Exercise should be intense enough to be effective but not so intense as to be unsafe for you. For an exercise session to be effective, you need to stimulate your heart, lungs, and muscles to work beyond their normal resting state. You can achieve this state without straining your muscles or forcing your heart to the point of maximum output. The best overall indicator of exercise intensity is **heart rate.** As exercise intensity increases, so does the heart rate, or the number of heartbeats per minute. You can monitor your intensity of exercise by monitoring your heart rate.

Exercise duration refers to how long a person exercises. It is directly related to the intensity of exercise as well. **Exercise frequency** means how often an exercise is done. Because the purpose of exercise is to improve or maintain cardiorespiratory fitness, exercise should be done frequently enough to accomplish this purpose. According to the Surgeon General, the best advice concerning duration and frequency is to work out at your target heart rate at least three times per week for thirty minutes. Not all exercise physiologists believe that such a rigorous exercise plan is necessary to gain health benefits. There is agreement, however, that such a plan is well within the ability of most people and represents a reasonable target for exercise frequency and duration. (See how to calculate your target heart rate on page 167.)

Remember during your busy day to take some time to stop and smell the roses. If you're just beginning an exercise program, you might want to consider walking. Read the Developing Health Skills box to learn about the exercise intensity, duration, and frequency involved in a walking program for becoming fit.

Measuring Your Heart Rate to Monitor Exercise Intensity

HEALTH SKILLS

A very practical health skill, and one that you may use nearly every day, is the skill of measuring your heart rate. The heart is the muscular pump that circulates blood throughout the body. Each contraction, or beat, produces pressure inside

DEVELOPING HEALTH SKILLS

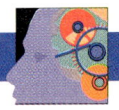

Starting Out: A Walking Program

What is the simplest, safest, least expensive exercise? Walking. Research has shown that walking at speeds of three and a half to four and a half miles an hour—that's brisk walking, not strolling—produces cardiovascular benefits. A woman of average size can walk comfortably at brisk speeds of three and a half to four miles an hour and the average man can walk at four and a half to five miles an hour. Slower walking (two miles an hour) can be advantageous for older people, cardiac patients, or people recuperating from an illness. Walking at a speed of five miles an hour can burn as many calories as moderate jogging, but even slow walking can burn sixty to eighty calories per mile. If weight control is one of your primary goals, a minimum of 30 minutes is required for significant results.

Here are a few tips from the Center for Corporate Health Promotion for a walking program:

1. Find a partner. Walking is an excellent social activity that can be done almost anywhere. Social support will help you adhere to your program and make it more enjoyable.
2. Wear a pair of shoes that provide a comfortable fit, adequate support, and cushioning.
3. Your walking style should be relaxed and efficient. To increase your pace, swing your arms more and maintain a heel-to-toe foot plant.
4. In order to experience an aerobic benefit, your exercise heart rate should be elevated to between 110 and 120 beats per minute for a minimum of twenty to thirty minutes.
5. The use of hand weights (one to five pounds) can increase your workload and provide muscular conditioning to the arms and shoulders. To avoid possible shoulder injury, it is important not to exaggerate your movements by swinging your arms across your body or by using weights that are too heavy.

---

the arteries that causes blood flow and thus the delivery of energy-producing nutrients to the cells.

At rest, a normal person's heart beats anywhere from 60 to 100 times per minute. This number is called the **resting heart rate.** A physically fit individual has a resting heart rate in the lower range, whereas an unfit individual has a higher resting heart rate. People who do aerobic exercises for at least thirty minutes three times per week experience what is called a **training effect.** The exercises actually train the heart to be more efficient—to pump more blood per stroke. The training effect of regular exercise can result in a decline in resting heart rate by as much as twenty beats per minute.

Your heart rate is most easily measured by taking (counting) your pulse. To take your pulse, place your index and middle fingers lightly over an artery at the wrist or neck. The throbs you feel correspond exactly to the beats of the heart. To measure your resting heart rate, the number of beats per minute at a resting state, use a digital watch or a watch with a second hand to count the throbs for ten seconds and multiply by six. The resulting number is the number of beats your heart makes every minute. To be more accurate, take two or three measures of your resting heart rate and calculate an average.

Maximal heart rate denotes the highest number of beats per minute that may safely be achieved during an exercise period. The maximal heart rate for a healthy person is about 220 minus his or her age. This is true for about 70 percent of the U.S. population. Exercise physiologists know that a training effect is accomplished by raising the heart rate during exercise to between 60 percent and 80 percent of the maximal heart rate. This means that for a healthy twenty-

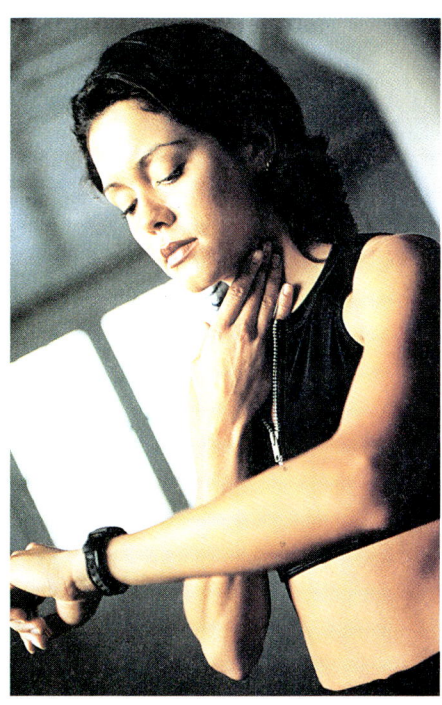

Learning how to take your pulse is a practical skill to learn. You can use it to measure your heart rate before and after exercise to determine your exercise intensity and to monitor one of your vital statistics. (Source: © Tony Stone Images/Lori Adamski Peek)

year-old—a typical college student—the average maximal heart rate is 200 beats per minute, and a training effect is achieved at between 120 and 160 beats per minute.

Achieving a training effect is the goal of an exercise period, thus the term **target heart rate range** is used to denote heart activity high enough to bring about a training effect and low enough to be safe. The target heart rate range of the typical college student is between 120 beats per minute and 200 beats per minute. What is your target heart rate?

To determine your approximate target heart rate range, complete the following formula:

Step 1: 220 – _____ = _____
 (your age)   (maximal heart rate)

Step 2: _____ × 0.60 = _____
 (maximal heart rate)   (lowest heart rate for exercising)

Step 3: _____ × 0.80 = _____
 (maximal heart rate)   (highest heart rate for exercising)

The range between the lowest and highest heart rate for exercising will provide a training effect. If a training program is designed for weight reduction, it should aim to achieve a training effect toward the lower end of the heart rate range.

Planning and Maintaining a Personal Fitness Program

No two people are alike, particularly where fitness is concerned. Therefore, a fitness program has to be personalized. For people who like to exercise with a

resting heart rate The number of heart beats per minute in a resting state.

training effect Health benefits, most notably increased heart efficiency, produced by exercising for a sufficient duration and intensity.

maximal heart rate The maximum number of beats per minute that should be reached during exercise; usually equal to 220 minus the person's age.

target heart rate range Heart activity high enough to bring about a training effect and low enough to be safe.

group, an aerobics or swimming class might make sense. A combination of the two—water aerobics—is another popular alternative. Aerobics and swimming are frequently offered free or at low cost at colleges and other educational facilities. The YMCA or YWCA offers low-cost fitness programs in many communities. Health clubs are another option. Some people prefer to exercise alone—perhaps using a tape or videocassette for guidance or working out on a stationary bicycle while watching the morning news on television. Similarly, some people like running with a group of friends; others prefer solitary running.

One place to start in personalizing your fitness program is with a complete physical examination conducted by a physician. This is essential for anyone over age thirty-five, but can be important regardless of age. Once you get the go-ahead from your physician, you are ready to measure your fitness level.

Critical Thinking Question

> *Healthy People 2000* established the following objective: "Increase the proportion of work sites offering employer-sponsored physical activity and fitness programs." Do you believe that business has found a link between physical fitness of employees and the bottom line—that is, how much profit a company earns? What do you think that link is? How might a company benefit from such a program? How does the employee benefit?

The skill of measuring your fitness level will be valuable not only now but also for the rest of your life because your fitness level will no doubt change. A skill as simple as measuring your heart rate, for example, can provide a means of monitoring such change. As you become more fit, the readings on your heart rate assessment will likely go down. After a period of not exercising, you may discover that your heart rate rises. Whether you apply your own skill in assessing your fitness through simple techniques or seek professional help by employing elaborate clinical assessments, you can monitor change.

There are two important reasons for measuring fitness before beginning a new fitness program:

- Any unknown physical problems can be detected in order to design a modified program that will reduce risk.
- Baseline data can be established so that progress can be measured.

The next step is to decide which exercises best fit your needs and desires and to carry out your personal fitness program in a safe and realistic fashion.

Three Phases of Exercise: Warm-Up, Conditioning, Cool-Down

Regardless of the specific sport or exercise you choose, your complete personal fitness program should include a series of exercise sessions. An exercise session, often referred to as a workout, always involves three segments: the warm-up, the conditioning period, and the cool-down.

During the **warm-up period,** no effort is made to achieve target heart rate. Rather, its purpose is to prepare the body for the exertion that will soon follow.

More importantly, the warm-up period is a means of avoiding unnecessary injury and may be related to a reduction in muscle soreness.

When the body warms up, muscle fibers and tendons become more fluid and can be stretched easily. The warm-up should consist of stretching exercises and low-level exertion. When stretching, take care not to bounce. Bouncing during a stretch can tear muscle fibers. Instead, slowly stretch the muscle and maintain that position for ten to fifteen seconds.

How long should a warm-up last? A good sign that the body is ready for more intense exercise is when body temperature increases by one and a half to two degrees, which is usually the point at which you begin to sweat. About five to ten minutes of warm-up may be sufficient, but it may take as much as fifteen to twenty minutes.

The **conditioning period** varies greatly from individual to individual. For a beginner, the conditioning period may consist of alternating brisk walking and leisurely walking. Someone slightly more fit may alternate periods of jogging and walking. For the fit individual, vigorous exercise sustained for thirty minutes is appropriate. Always remember that a conditioning period is tailored to personal ability and needs. Fitness results from regular exercise, not extreme exertion. Therefore, it is more important to exercise regularly than to exercise vigorously. With regular exercise, the ability for vigorous exercise will increase.

An often overlooked segment of an exercise period is the **cool-down period.** This involves reducing the intensity of exercise to allow the body to recover partially from the conditioning period. During vigorous exercise such as jogging, a lot of blood is pumped to the legs, and there may not be enough to supply the heart and brain. Failure to cool down properly may result in dizziness, fainting, and in rare instances, a heart attack. Walking and stretching are common cool-down activities. In fact, the same procedures used in the warm-up are appropriate for the cool-down. By reducing the level of physical exertion gradually, blood flow is redirected back to the heart and brain.

How long should you cool down? Again, as with the warm-up, about five to ten minutes may be sufficient, but a longer cool-down may be necessary, particularly in warm weather.

Raising Your Safety Consciousness

Despite the benefits of exercise, you need to recognize some risks before embarking on a program. A host of injuries can be attributed to overzealous exercise. When designing your personal exercise program, remember the saying, "Train, don't strain." Initiating a strenuous exercise program too fast can produce injuries such as muscle strains and stress fractures that can bring your exercise program to a standstill. Figure 7.5 points out common athletic and exercise injuries along with the sports with which each is associated.

For some injuries, simple first-aid treatment can help (see the Developing Health Skills box). Resist the urge to return to your usual form of exercise until the injured part of your body can move fully and support the usual weight without pain.

A very important but still unanswered concern is whether regular exercise will lead to degenerative joint disease, or osteoarthritis. Many biomechanical factors may predispose exercisers to joint disease. When a runner leaves the ground momentarily, the leg he or she lands on has to absorb a load two to three times the body weight. When a tennis or basketball player leaps in the air, he or she lands with a force of up to seven times the body weight.

Poor consumer decisions can result in injury. Jogging or walking in improper shoes, for example, can produce injuries to the feet, ankles, and knees. See the Healthwise Consumer box for tips on what to look for when buying a running shoe. Exercising in cold weather in inappropriate attire can result in frostbite and

warm-up period The period of exercise in which the body becomes prepared for exertion.

conditioning period The period of exercise during which a training effect is reached and maintained.

cool-down period The period of exercise in which the intensity of exercise is reduced to allow the body to recover partially from the conditioning period.

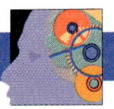

DEVELOPING HEALTH SKILLS

A Timeline for Self-Treatment of Exercise Injuries

For certain soft-tissue injuries, such as muscle, tendon, and ligament injuries, prompt first-aid treatment should promote healing. The correct treatment is called RICE, for *rest, ice, compression,* and *elevation.* Knowing what to do and in what order may accelerate the healing process and may even mean the difference between days and weeks of recuperation.

First Forty-Eight Hours after Injury

- Rest and elevate the injured part of your body (e.g., ankle, knee, arm).
- Begin icing the injury immediately. Apply the ice to the injured area every two waking hours for about ten to twenty minutes. You can make an ice pack by wrapping ice cubes in a towel. A bag of frozen peas works well as an ice pack. Icing constricts the blood vessels and helps reduce inflammation and further tissue damage. It also numbs the nerve endings near the injury and helps to relieve pain.
- Apply a compression to the injured area. For some injuries, an elastic bandage will help. You can make a compression by holding the ice pack in place with a bandage or even a towel.

A Word of Caution

The RICE treatment is not a substitute for calling your doctor in case of a serious injury or if the pain and/or inflammation does not begin to subside.

hypothermia, a loss of body temperature that can result in mental confusion, unconsciousness, and in extreme cases, death.

Perhaps one of the most important safety precautions for joggers and bikers is to wear reflective gear when running or biking at night. Bicycling accidents cause approximately 1,300 deaths and 60,000 injuries a year. Head trauma is the

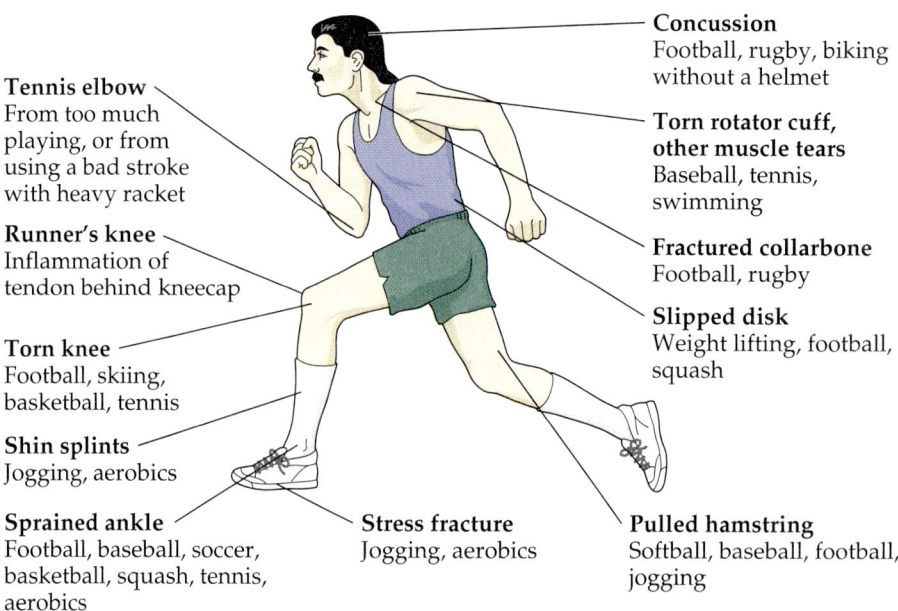

hypothermia A loss of body temperature that can result in mental confusion, unconsciousness, and death.

■ **Figure 7.5 Train, Don't Strain.** *Injuries, such as muscle strains and stress fractures, can bring your exercise program to a standstill.*

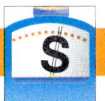

HEALTHWISE CONSUMER

The Right Shoe for You

Buying a running shoe is like buying a computer: There's no accurate answer to the question, Which one is best? The right question is, Which one is best for me? That's because, like computer users, runners have different needs. In running, fitting those needs means finding a shoe that best suits how your body—especially your feet—adapts to the stresses of moving through the gait cycle. (Running geeks call this *biomechanics*.) And as is the case with computers, more isn't always better; unnecessary extras can get in the way after they've drained your wallet.

Running shoes are constructed to address what happens when your feet hit the ground. Ideally, your foot lands on the outside heel, rolls in until your heel is aligned under your lower leg (this is called *pronation*), then becomes rigid as it propels you forward. About half of all runners are blessed with something close to this kind of biomechanics; these people are neutral runners. But many runners' feet roll in too far or continue to roll in as the foot prepares to push off; these people are overpronators. About 10 percent of runners have feet that don't pronate enough; these people are oversupinators. The trick, then, is to determine which type of runner you are and to choose a shoe designed to address your biomechanical needs.

How do you do that? Look at the forefoot of the outsoles (the part that meets the ground) of your old shoes. (Don't bother looking at the heels, because almost all runners land on the outside heel. It's what happens after landing that determines your needs.) Neutral runners usually see wear in the center of the forefoot; overpronators often find wear near the big toe; oversupinators may find wear toward the little toe.

Also, the type of injuries you are prone to can give clues as to your biomechanics. Because of the extra motion required of their muscles, tendons, and ligaments, overpronators tend to get injuries caused by soft-tissue fatigue, such as runner's knee and tendinitis. In contrast, because their feet move through too small a range of motion, oversupinators subject their bodies to great amounts of shock. As a result, they're susceptible to such injuries as ankle sprains, stress fractures, and shinsplints.

Once you have a rough idea of which biomechanical category you fall into, look for these basics of construction.

Neutral Runners

You can run in almost any shoe without risking injury, but you'll enjoy yourself the most in middle-of-the-road models that have a blend of cushioning and stability. These shoes are built on a semi-straight last, meaning that if you look at the outsole, you'll see that the forefoot points slightly in toward the heel. They probably have a small medial post, a chunk of firm material on the inside heel that adds stability. Many are combination lasted. This means that if you remove the insole, you'll see a firm board last that extends from the back of the shoe to the arch area. The front of the shoe, meanwhile, is slip lasted, that is, the upper of the shoe has been stitched directly to the midsole, much like a moccasin.

Overpronators

You need stability features. This usually means a shoe that looks straight when examined from underneath, that has a large medial post, and that is combination or board lasted (in which the board runs the length of the shoe). More severe overpronators should look for a midsole that's at least part polyurethane; this material is heavier and denser than EVA, which most midsoles are made from, and provides greater stability. If you can't distinguish between materials yourself, ask a salesperson for help. Some models also have a small anti-roll bar made of thermoplastic or similar material in the inner heel.

Oversupinators

You need flexibility features that will encourage your feet to work through a greater range of motion. This usually means a curved shape to the shoe and a soft midsole without a medial post. The shoe is also likely to be slip lasted from heel to toe.

Virtually all manufacturers make shoes geared toward each of these needs. Since each company uses a different shape of last, chances are you'll find certain manufacturers' shoes, fit your foot better than others. Once you determine whether you are an overpronator, an oversupinator, or a neutral runner, try on shoes from the different manufacturers that suit the type of runner you are. That's how you'll find the best shoe—for you.

Source: Reprinted by permission from Scott Douglas, "The Right Shoe for You," *Women's Sports & Fitness,* September 1997, pp. 47–48.

most frequent cause of death in these cases. Wearing a helmet, using hand signals, and abiding by traffic laws can result in safer exercise programs on bicycles. As with most health-promoting behavior, the watchwords for a safe exercise program are moderation and common sense.

Patience and Adherence

Few quick results can be expected from an exercise program. Over time, however, you will notice clear evidence of improved fitness. Therefore, be patient. How long do you have to wait to see results? This varies from individual to individual, but younger exercisers will see evidence of improved fitness levels more quickly than will older exercisers. Establishing baseline data on your strength, flexibility, and aerobic capacity before exercising can help you monitor subtle and otherwise not visible improvements in your fitness level. This will help reinforce your adherence to a fitness program.

Critical Thinking Question

> Before reading further, formulate a list of tactics you can use to help you adhere to an exercise program. Begin by listing the barriers to adherence. Then identify a concrete way to overcome each barrier.

For a variety of reasons—including a mismatch between the person and the activity—more than 50 percent of exercisers do not adhere to an exercise program for more than twelve months. The key to success is finding the right match with an exercise activity that you will enjoy and continue to do. Sometimes, this involves a period of experimentation. Care also needs to be taken to design an exercise program that fits the time you have available—or want to make available—and that will meet your expectations for short-term and long-term effects.

Tactics for Maintaining a Fitness Program

Here are some tips on how to get a fitness program that works for you going.

- Choose an activity that you like and that you feel competent and safe doing.
- Set a regular time and place for your exercise. Make sure it is easily accessible to you on a regular basis.
- Establish realistic goals that you can achieve.
- Don't be pressured to do an exercise program that you cannot afford either financially or in time needed to do it correctly.
- Alternate the physical activities you do—brisk walking one day, swimming another.
- Be aware of physical activities you can do as part of your day-to-day living, such as cleaning the house, shoveling the walk, or gardening.
- Avoid injuries by not overdoing your exercise program. Gradually work up to fitness.

- Feel good about what you are doing. Give yourself something you want when you reach significant goals.
- Guard against giving yourself excuses for not exercising, such as, "I'm too busy."

Key Concepts

1. Most Americans do not exercise on a regular basis, and of those who do, few exercise at the appropriate level of activity.
2. The benefits of regular exercise include reduced risk for coronary artery disease, hypertension, and osteoporosis and increased psychological well-being.
3. Exercisers report feeling better and having more energy and less trouble sleeping. Some evidence suggests that physically fit people learn better and stay mentally alert longer than those who are less fit.
4. Fitness involves the efficient use of muscles and bones to bring about movement, maintain posture, and/or sustain a healthy appearance.
5. Strength, flexibility, and endurance are three major components of fitness.
6. A planned exercise program has three components: desired intensity of exercise (how much); desired duration of exercise (how long); and frequency of exercise (how often).
7. A good measure of fitness is the resting heart rate. Physically fit individuals tend to have a lower resting heart rate than those who are less fit.
8. The best fitness programs are personalized and begin with a complete physical examination conducted by a physician.
9. An exercise session consists of the warm-up, the conditioning period, and the cool-down, three relatively distinct and important stages.
10. Few dramatic changes result from an exercise program. The health benefits of fitness develop over time.

Review Questions

1. Describe the exercise pattern of most Americans adults and that of most American children.
2. Identify three chronic diseases associated with a sedentary lifestyle and explain the impact of exercise on each disease.
3. Support the statement, People who exercise regularly tend to feel better.
4. What are the three major components of fitness? Describe the types of exercise that develop each component.
5. Differentiate between isokinetic, isotonic, and isometric exercises.
6. Give examples of both aerobic and anaerobic activities.
7. How do exercise intensity, exercise duration, and exercise frequency affect the quality of an exercise session?
8. What is the difference between a resting heart rate, a maximal heart rate, and a target heart rate?
9. Why is a warm-up period important to an exercise plan? What about a cool-down period?
10. List several tactics for maintaining a fitness program.

Selected Bibliography

Biddle, S.J.H. *Foundations of Health-Related Fitness in Physical Education.* London: Ling, 1987.

Fletcher, G.F., et al. "American Heart Association Medical/Scientific Statement: Position Statement on Exercise: Benefits and Recommendations for Physical Activity Programs for All Americans." *Circulation* 86 (1992):340–344.

Journal of Physical Education, Recreation and Dance. Reston, VA: American Alliance for Health, Physical Education, Recreation and Dance (published monthly).

Paffenbarger, R.S., Jr., et al. "The Association of Changes in Physical Activity Level and Other Lifestyle Characteristics with Mortality among Men." *New England Journal of Medicine* 328 (1993):538–545.

Pate, R.R., et al. "Physical Activity and Public Health: A Recommendation from the Centers for Disease Control and Prevention and the American College of Sports Medicine." *Journal of the American Medical Association* 273, no. 5 (1995):402–407.

Physical Activity and Cardiovascular Health (Consensus Development Conference Statement). Bethesda, MD: National Institutes of Health, 1995.

Physical Activity and Health: A Report of the Surgeon General. Atlanta, GA: Centers for Disease Control and Prevention, 1996.

Research Quarterly for Exercise and Sport. Reston, VA: American Alliance for Health, Physical Education, Recreation and Dance (published quarterly).

HealthLinks: Web Sites for Keeping Fit

You can access better health as it relates to this chapter by checking out some of the following sites on the Internet. These and sites identified within the chapter can be accessed directly when you visit the *HealthStyles* Web site located on the Allyn and Bacon homepage at **http//:www.abacon.com.**

American Alliance for Health, Physical Education, Recreation, and Dance
www.aahperd.org
Home page for the national organization dedicated to the advancement of Health, Physical Education, Recreation, and Dance education standards.

FitnessLink
www.fitnesslink.com/feature/assoc2.htm
FitnessLink provides the resources you need to get fit and stay fit. This link provides the latest fitness news and contains a comprehensive list of health and fitness associations and organizations.

Health Hotlines: Keeping Fit

American Running and Fitness Association
(800) 776-2732
4405 East-West Highway, Suite 405
Bethesda, MD 20814

Women's Sports Foundation
Information and Referral Service
(800) 227-3988
Eisenhower Park
East Meadow, NY 11554

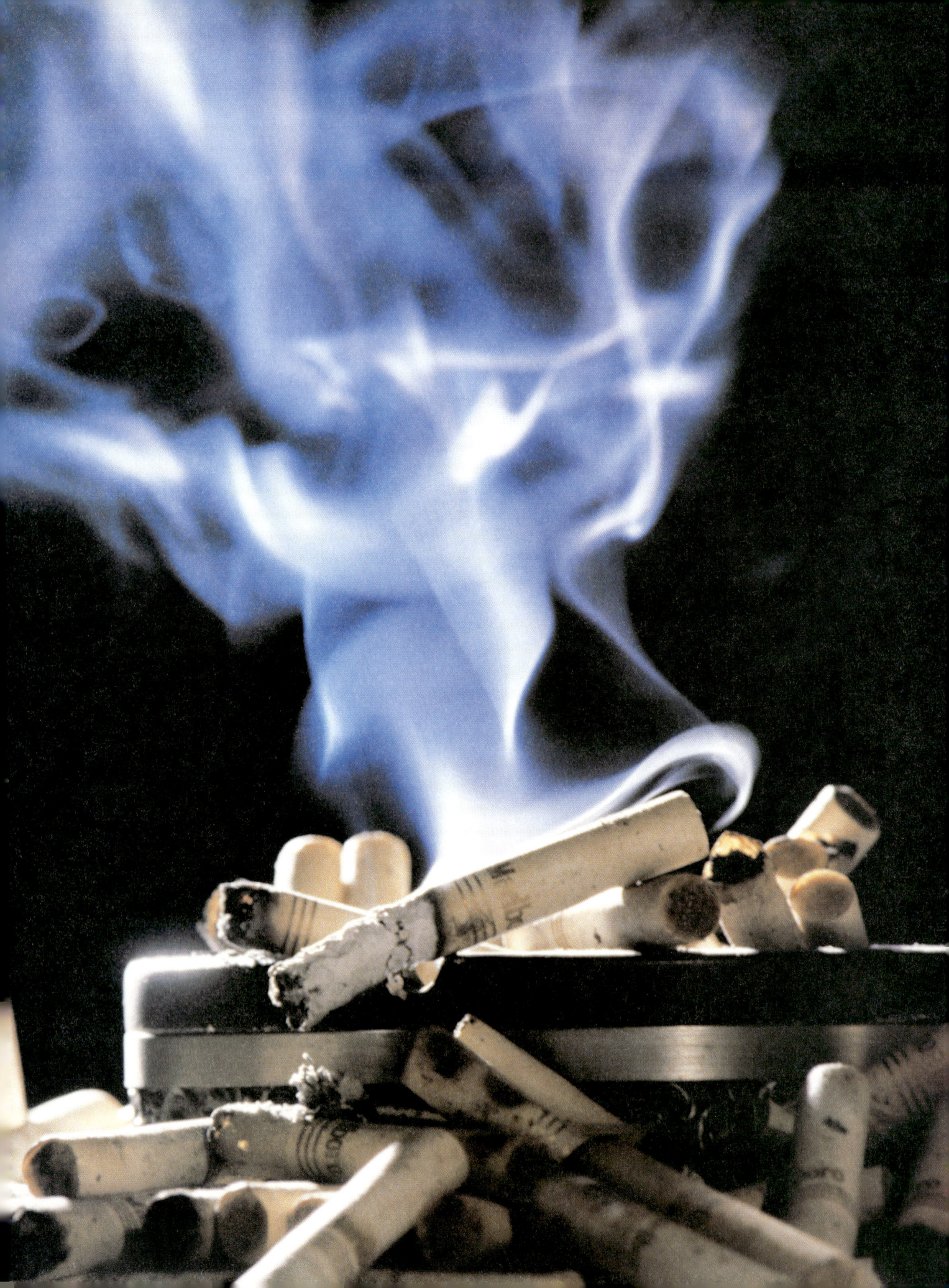

Chapter 8

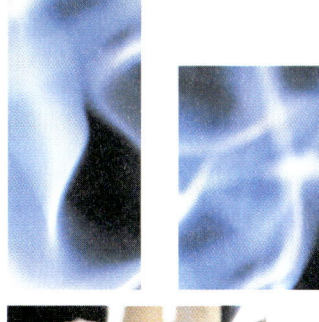

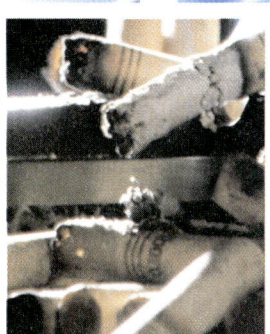

Smoking Out Tobacco

Objectives

When you finish reading this chapter, you will be able to:

1. Describe typical smokers and give reasons for their choice to use tobacco.
2. Identify the similarities between dependence on tobacco products and drug addiction.
3. Describe how advertising has influenced the rate of tobacco use.
4. Describe assertive ways to avoid tobacco use.
5. List three major components of cigarette smoke and identify the health risks of each.
6. Describe how tobacco use contributes to cancer, heart disease, and lung disease.
7. Identify the effect of smoking on the developing fetus of a pregnant woman.
8. Define passive smoke and identify the risk associated with this involuntary exposure to tobacco.
9. Differentiate and compare the effects of smoking and the use of smokeless tobacco.
10. List three means of smoking cessation and compare the advantages of each.

What Is Your HealthStyle?

Manuel tried to quit smoking several times, but each time, he went back to smoking. This time, he had not had a cigarette in three weeks, and here he was—stuck in his car in a traffic jam while driving to school. He was frustrated and he was alone. He reached into the pocket where he used to keep his cigarettes, but none were there. He reviewed some of the techniques he had learned in a smoking-cessation clinic: Think of something enjoyable—sailing, listening to music, a world without traffic jams. Pull off the road and take a five-minute stretch break. Remind yourself that smoking won't change the situation.

Manuel tried these techniques, but he got too frustrated and pulled into a gas station to buy a pack of cigarettes. Once he had them in his hand, his resolution to stop smoking left him immediately. He smoked. "Maybe next time," he said, "I'll really quit."

Donetta was also taking a smoking-cessation class, and she, too, had tried to quit before without much success. But this time, she was really determined to do it after nine smoke-free days. Her will was tested one night after studying when she and three friends were at a popular coffee bar. They were having a good time when suddenly, Donetta started feeling jumpy and on edge; she wanted to smoke. What worried her was that she knew she could bum a cigarette from one of her friends.

Just as Manuel did, Donetta reviewed some of the tricks she had learned in smoking-cessation class. She told her friends that she was no longer a smoker and asked them not to offer her a cigarette. She got up twice from the table when she felt the urge to smoke and went to the ladies room, where she washed her face, combed her hair, and put on perfume. She played with her spoon to keep her hands busy and even chewed gum at the table. But she didn't smoke.

That evening was a turning point for Donetta. After that, she knew she would not go back to smoking. And she was right.

In Your Opinion

Manuel and Donetta both wanted to quit smoking, but only one of them succeeded—at least for the time being.

- Why do you think Donetta succeeded in quitting while Manuel did not?
- What skills did Donetta possess that helped her resist the temptation to smoke?
- What should Manuel do the next time he wants to quit?
- If you smoke, what would you do in the situations in which Manuel and Donetta found themselves?
- Is there a way you can help a friend who is trying to quit?

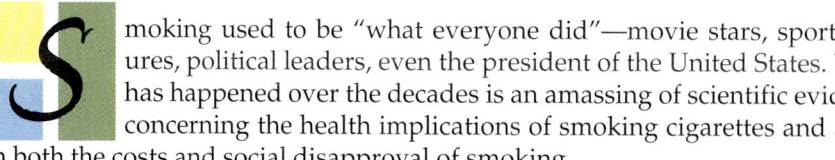

Smoking used to be "what everyone did"—movie stars, sports figures, political leaders, even the president of the United States. What has happened over the decades is an amassing of scientific evidence concerning the health implications of smoking cigarettes and a rise in both the costs and social disapproval of smoking.

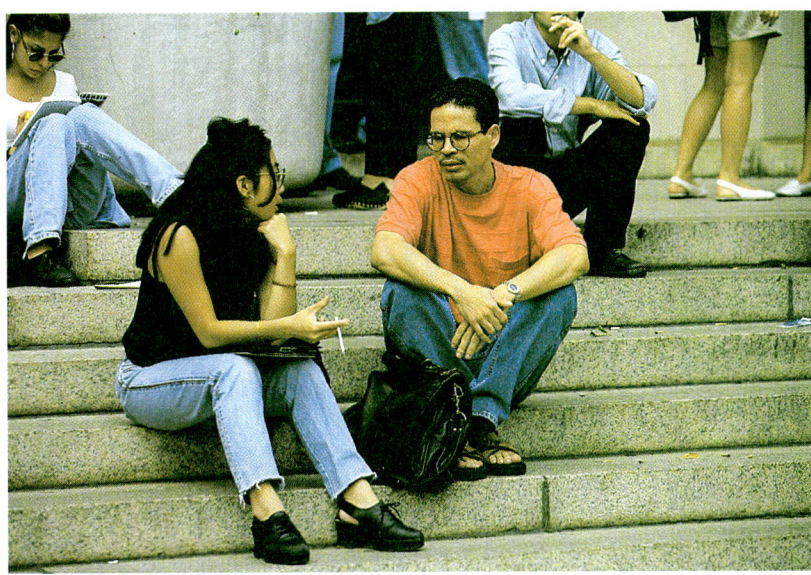

Despite the negative health effects, smoking among young people continues to pose a serious problem. By the time they are ready for college, more than 60 percent of high school seniors have smoked at least once. (Source: Stock, Boston/© Peter Vandermark)

Much of this is documented in the U.S. Surgeon General's reports on smoking and disease. Smoking causes cancer and lung and heart disease. So, too, does **sidestream smoke,** which comes from the burning end of the cigarette between puffs and can affect nonsmokers standing nearby. Smokeless tobacco in the form of snuff and chewing tobacco also causes serious health problems. Tobacco use is the single most preventable cause of death in the United States. The morbidity and mortality associated with tobacco are at an epidemic level, but unlike disease-caused epidemics, this one is manufactured.

Fortunately, millions of Americans have stopped smoking, and most never even start. But many who still smoke say they wish they could stop but cannot because nicotine is addictive—as addictive as other drugs such as alcohol and cocaine.

Who Smokes?

About 25 percent of adult Americans, or 48 million people, smoke—down from 42 percent in 1965, the first year the Public Health Service assessed cigarette smoking and a year after the Surgeon General first reported that smoking increased the risk of lung cancer. The typical smoker is a blue-collar man who does not have a high school diploma. But that tells only part of the story. Women smoke almost as much as men today, whereas three decades ago, women smoked far less than men (in 1965, 32 percent of women and 50 percent of men smoked).

One fifth of all youth between twelve and seventeen years old have smoked at least once, and by the time they are seniors in high school, more than three fifths have smoked at least once, according to national surveys. Each day, more than three thousand American teenagers start smoking. Young smokers also tend to be heavy smokers. These statistics on teenage smoking behavior could have a profound effect on the future of smoking and public health because 90 percent of smokers pick up the habit in adolescence.

sidestream smoke The smoke originating from the burning end of the cigarette between puffs, that adversely affects the health of individuals nearby.

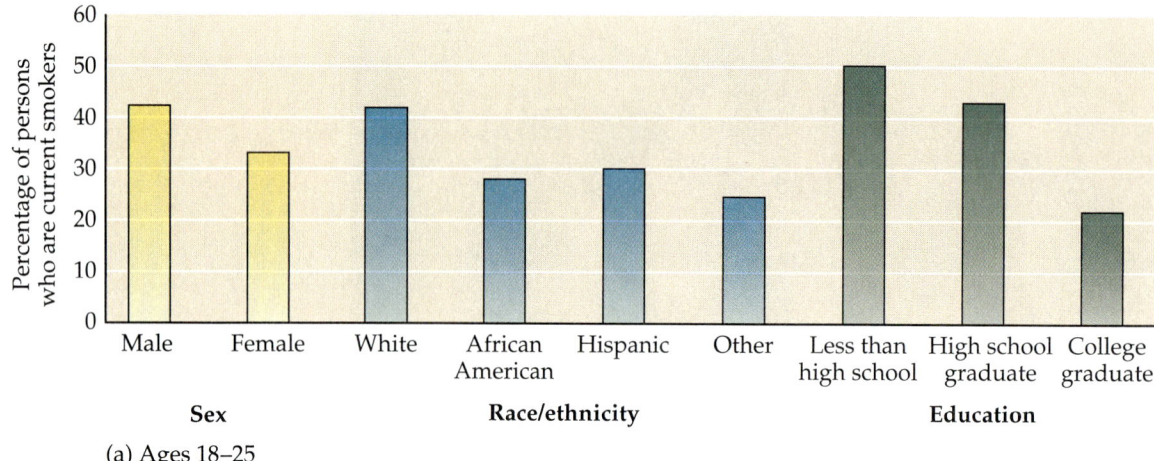

(a) Ages 18–25

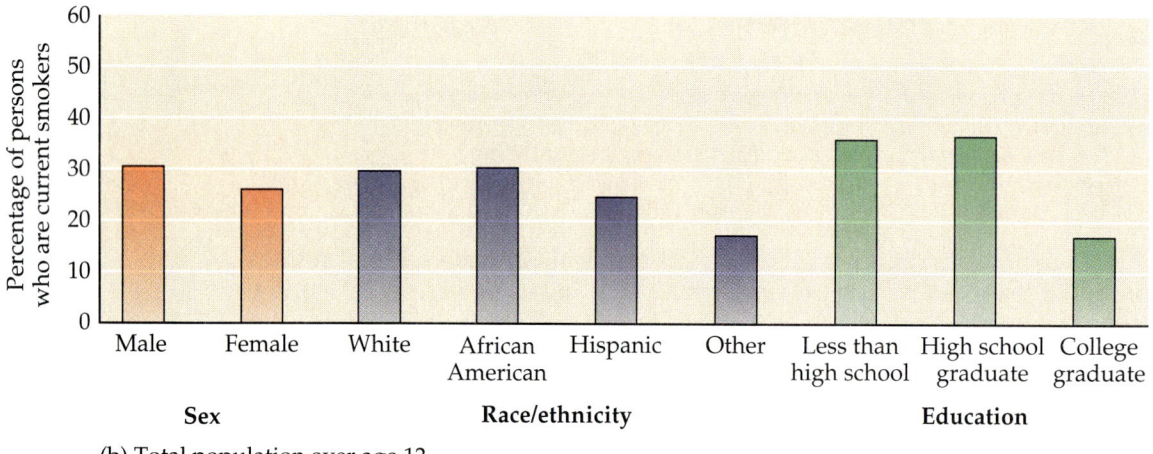

(b) Total population over age 12

Figure 8.1 Look Who's Smoking. *Americans are smoking less, but African Americans are more likely to smoke than whites and males are more likely to smoke than females. Education level also is a factor in who smokes. (Source:* Substance Abuse and Mental Health Administration, *National Household Survey on Drug Abuse, 1996)*

Smoking is increasingly becoming a habit of minority groups. A gap exists between the health status of minority groups and the health status of the general population. This gap, according to public health researchers, is partly a result of the use of tobacco products by minorities. Studies have long documented that African Americans are more likely to smoke—and to die from smoking—than are whites, and the African–American–white gap is expected to widen in coming years. Recent data from the Centers for Disease Control and Prevention (CDC) show that Native Americans and Alaska Natives are more likely to smoke than is the population at large (see Figure 8.1).

No matter what their race or gender, people who have less education have higher smoking rates than do those who have more education. Nearly 40 percent of people who have not graduated from high school smoke, in contrast to about 12 percent of college graduates. Similarly, people who have lower incomes smoke more than do those who have higher incomes.

Another recent finding of the National Center for Health Statistics is that smokers tend to have other bad health habits. A nationwide survey of adults showed that heavy smokers were more likely to skip breakfast, snack more during the day, drink more alcohol, and remain physically less active than nonsmokers. According to a health statistician analyzing the survey data, there are two possible factors at work here. One is that this cluster of bad health habits is associated with a lifestyle oriented toward consumption—smoking, drinking, and eating. Another is that smokers demonstrate more risk-taking behavior and pay less attention to the healthier practices of life.

Why People Smoke

With so much publicity about the health consequences of smoking, what makes a person smoke that first cigarette and continue to smoke? The key reasons are: influences from family and friends; the allure produced by advertising; a quest for relaxation; and the addictive nature of tobacco.

Influence from Family and Peers

Typically, children first become exposed to smoking at home or through friends. Children of smoking parents are more likely to smoke than are children of nonsmoking parents, and smoking teenagers are more likely to have friends who smoke than are nonsmoking teenagers.

Parents' influence is strongest on younger adolescents. For example, teenagers are more likely to smoke when they live in a home where cigarettes are available and family members show indifference toward smoking. Interestingly, parental restrictiveness and harsh criticism are also associated with a greater likelihood of a teenager smoking. Conversely, affection, emotional support, and participation in meaningful conversations at home more often result in the teenager not smoking.

Studies consistently support the notion that peers also play an important role in the questions of whether to smoke and whether to use smokeless or chewing tobacco. Teens tend to seek out groups with which they identify, and these group affiliations may be related to tobacco use. For example, in a study of high school students, a predominantly male group called "the dirts" was characterized by smoking, problem drinking, poor academic performance, and cutting classes. Another group, called "the hot shots," was made up mostly of popular female leaders in academic and extracurricular activities, among whom there was rela-

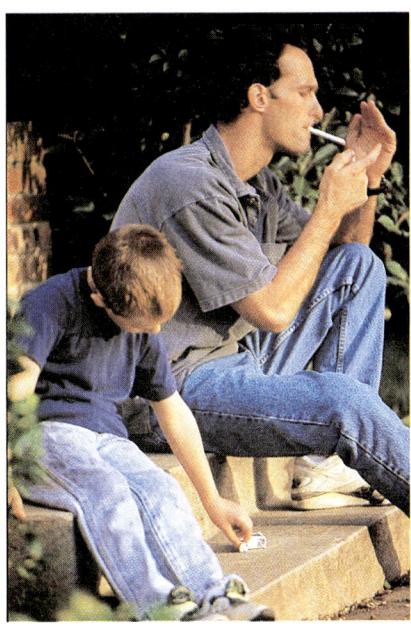

Many children first become exposed to smoking at home. Teenagers are more likely to smoke if their parents do. (Source: © Tony Stone Images/Peter Poulides)

tively little smoking. A third group, "the jocks," exhibited many of the macho attributes of the dirts, but as athletes, they tended not to drink or smoke.

Critical Thinking Question

In *Healthy People 2000,* the following objective is listed: "Reduce the initiation of cigarette smoking by children and youth so that no more than 15 percent have become regular cigarette smokers by age 20." In 1994, 30 percent had become regular smokers by that age. What could be done to accomplish this objective: Implement strict laws concerning accessibility? Fund tobacco education programs? What can be done to promote nonsmoking role models for children and youth?

Advertising Hype

An even greater influence on teenagers is cigarette advertising. A study published in the *Journal of the National Cancer Institute* found that teens are twice as likely to be influenced to smoke by cigarette ads as by peer pressure. Illustrating the power of advertising, the *Journal of Marketing* reported that 86 percent of youth who smoke prefer Marlboro, Camel, and Newport—the three most heavily advertised brands.

Youth have been especially targeted by advertisers as a way to attract new smokers and brand loyalty early on. Research shows that the cartoon figure Joe Camel, designed to promote Camels, was recognized by children as young as three years old, and that among twelve- to fifteen-year-olds, the Joe Camel ads were the favorite. In 1997, as part of the backlash against smoking and the tobacco industry, R.J. Reynolds Tobacco Co., the manufacturer of Camels, ended the Joe Camel ad campaign (see Figure 8.6 on p. 201).

Although banned from television and radio since 1970, cigarette advertising has continued indirectly. If you watch an automobile race on television, you will see cigarette ads in the form of decals and billboards placed in front of the TV camera. This is true of many athletic events. Tobacco companies purchase advertising space next to a scoreboard, with the primary purpose of having its brand name carried on national television each time the score is shown. One study found that the viewers of tobacco-sponsored car races broadcast on network television in 1993 included 2.6 million children and 2.2 million teenagers. The way tobacco products are advertised and promoted will probably change due to proposed federal regulations that would control cigarette advertising aimed at youth.

The tobacco manufacturers have long stated that their advertising is intended to promote brand switching and capture market share, not to promote smoking by youth. Health educators and others, however, question whether the industry would spend more than $6 billion a year on advertising and promotional activities, such as the sale of T-shirts sporting cigarette brand logos and the sponsoring of sports and musical events at which the name of the company or brand of cigarettes is displayed, if these efforts did not increase overall tobacco use. Since smoking has declined significantly among adults, many health educators believe that tobacco companies need to look to younger people who will become heavy smokers as adults. Research shows that those who begin smoking in their early teens are more likely to be heavy smokers than are those who begin smoking as adults.

Pleasure and Relaxation

Many people say that they smoke for pleasure and relaxation. "A cigarette after breakfast gives me a lot of pleasure," says a college junior. "It relaxes me and gets me ready for the day."

She isn't alone in her thinking. Most smokers believe that smoking relaxes them, whereas in fact cigarettes—just like coffee—can increase a state of tension and cause the jitters. Research indicates that smoking a cigarette causes a rise in blood pressure by five to ten points and an increase in heart rate by ten to twenty beats—the opposite of relaxation.

Ask a friend who smokes to lie down on a bed, sofa, or floor and relax as much as possible. Then, have your friend smoke a cigarette while he or she remains relaxed. Monitor your friend's heart rate before, during, and after the cigarette. Did it rise? Remain the same? Now, how would you answer the question, Does cigarette smoking cause the body to relax?

Addiction to Nicotine

Once they start to smoke, people continue because they are addicted to cigarettes—specifically, to the **nicotine** in them. Within seconds after a smoker inhales a cigarette, nicotine reaches the brain. Over time, a chemical change takes place that causes the smoker to feel the need for additional nicotine. As with **addiction** to other drugs, such as crack cocaine and heroin, people who have a **nicotine addiction** smoke in spite of the clear harm. They talk about the desire to quit, but the addiction makes it difficult for them to do so. Those who do quit go through **withdrawal symptoms.**

In a classic study showing that, once addicted to cigarettes, smokers need to maintain a certain level of nicotine in their blood, research subjects received an intravenous drip that sometimes contained and sometimes did not contain nicotine. This was continued for six hours a day over a fifteen-day period. During the time when there was no nicotine in the intravenous solution, the subjects smoked more cigarettes (10.1 over the six-hour session) and smoked each cigarette longer. When nicotine was in the solution, they smoked fewer cigarettes (7.3 over the six-hour session) and left longer butts. The consistent difference, according to the researchers, demonstrated that the subjects smoked only the amount they needed to maintain a nicotine level in the blood.

Many smokers say, "It's just tobacco—not a drug." But the nicotine in tobacco *is* a drug, and it has the same characteristics concerning drug addiction as do heroin and cocaine:

Primary Characteristics of Tobacco and Drug Addiction

- Highly controlled or compulsive pattern of drug use
- Psychoactive or mood-altering effects involved in the pattern of drug taking
- Drug functioning as reinforcer to strengthen behavior and lead to further drug use

Additional Characteristics of Tobacco and Drug Addiction

- Tolerance (increased doses either tolerated without discomfort or needed to achieve desired effects)
- Physical dependence (withdrawal syndrome upon termination of drug taking)
- Use despite harmful effects
- Relapse following drug abstinence
- Recurrent drug cravings
  Source: U.S. Public Health Service

nicotine The ingredient in tobacco smoke that causes addiction.

addiction A strong desire or need to continue using tobacco, alcohol, or another drug.

nicotine addiction The state of being physically and emotionally dependent on nicotine.

withdrawal symptoms Symptoms ranging from mild discomfort to very traumatic events when a drug is not present in the body.

HEALTH SKILLS

Avoiding Tobacco Use

There is no evidence that tobacco can be used wisely: Any level of tobacco use carries risks. Therefore, the only health-promoting approach to tobacco is to avoid its use. Basically, this means say, "No." Social assertiveness is a skill that can be applied not only to avoiding tobacco product, but also to avoiding other drugs or behaviors that might present a health threat.

The decision to say no to tobacco is best made before trying any tobacco products. The best way to be able to stick by the decision is to be equipped with solid reasons. And the best reasons are derived from unbiased, reliable information, such as that contained in this chapter. It is always wise to consider the source when acquiring information about tobacco. Tobacco companies may attempt to mislead the public, but scientific studies are clear, consistent, and absolute in their indictment of tobacco as a threat to health.

Once you are committed to the decision not to smoke, here are three assertive comments you can make when pressured to smoke:

- "No. I am not willing to take the risk."
- "No. Smoking causes cancer."
- "No. Smoking will make everything I own smell bad."

If the person pressuring you to use tobacco insists that you participate in an activity that causes cancer and will make you smell bad, you should seriously question how much to value that person's opinion.

To avoid sidestream smoke, or even being in a room with smokers, another aspect of social assertiveness can come into play—one that deals with environmental restructuring. For example, you may want to place a sticker or a sign on your door that reads, "No smoking, please!" This will alert all visitors that your room, home, or office is a smoke-free zone. By adding the word *please,* the sign can be assertive but polite. You may be surprised how cooperative others are in complying with your wishes. To reinforce this, you may also want to remove all ash trays.

You can also show social assertiveness on a community level by working with a coalition for a total ban on smoking in your dorm, apartment building, or workplace. It is likely that the majority of your friends will support the idea—including many current smokers.

The Components of Cigarette Smoke

Each time a smoker inhales a cigarette, he or she gets a dose of nicotine, tar, carbon monoxide, hydrogen cyanide, and other dangerous particles and gases. All in all, tobacco smoke contains more than four thousand separate substances, many of which have some biological activity. At least forty-three are known to be **carcinogens**—that is, agents capable of causing cancer. Some of the chemicals in cigarette smoke are better known for their use in cleaning solvents, including benzene, acetone, and formaldehyde. The following are the primary harmful ingredients in tobacco smoke.

Nicotine

The major reason nicotine is harmful is that it is the ingredient in tobacco smoke that causes addiction. Nicotine is a poison that is deadly if concentrations are high enough. For smokers who inhale, 90 percent of the nicotine is absorbed in the bloodstream. Only 20 to 50 percent of the nicotine goes into the bloodstream

carcinogen An agent capable of causing cancer.

tar The most carcinogenic substance in cigarettes; the gummy mixture left over from burning.

carbon monoxide A dangerous, poisonous, odorless gas produced in the burning process.

if the cigarette is just puffed—smoke is taken into the mouth and then exhaled. Even if you never puff on a cigarette, nicotine can get into your bloodstream if you are exposed to sidestream smoke.

Once in the body, nicotine causes release of adrenaline—the hormones that cause the fight or flight reactions. Nicotine also causes the heart to beat faster and coronary blood flow and blood pressure to increase. These effects create additional oxygen requirements by the heart muscle and are associated with increased risk of a heart attack.

Tar

Tar is the gummy mixture left over from burning tobacco. It consists of more than two hundred chemicals and is the most carcinogenic substance in cigarettes. Smoking damages the cilia, which are hair-like structures in the respiratory system that sweep debris, such as tar, out of the lungs. With the cilia damaged, tar and other debris can easily enter the lungs and remain there. One chemical in tar, benzopyrene, is one of the most toxic of all carcinogens. Tar also affects the respiratory system by blocking the normal action of mucus. As a result, foreign materials are not screened from the lungs and irritants attack lung tissue. A nonlethal example of what happens as a result of this is the hacking smoker's cough. To learn if low-tar, low-nicotine cigarettes are safe, see the Healthwise Consumer box on page 192.

Carbon Monoxide

Most of the compounds in cigarette smoke are gaseous, and many of them are toxic. By far the most hazardous of these gases is **carbon monoxide,** the same gas that is emitted from the exhaust pipe of a car. The difference is that there are community or statewide standards to keep carbon monoxide auto emissions within a safe level, whereas no standards exist for cigarette smoke. The amount of carbon monoxide that stays in a smoker's blood is related to activity levels. During the day, carbon monoxide remains in the blood for two to four hours; during sleep, however, it remains for up to eight hours. This is why smokers awake in the morning with substantial amounts of carbon monoxide in their blood despite not smoking overnight.

Carbon monoxide also affects the hemoglobin's ability to carry oxygen. This causes smokers to get out of breath when doing exercise—running, playing tennis, or even walking. It also causes problems for people already suffering from or at risk for cardiovascular diseases. Chain smokers are particularly vulnerable to the effects of a buildup of carbon monoxide in the body. The highest concentrations of carbon monoxide leave the body within five minutes after smoking, but chain smokers do not allow their bodies to experience this decrease.

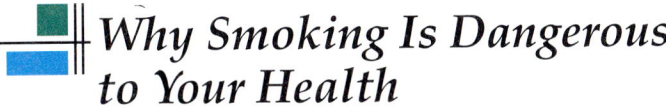

Why Smoking Is Dangerous to Your Health

It is printed on every package of cigarettes sold in the United States—smoking is dangerous to your health. But the warning label cannot document just how dangerous it is. Cigarette smoking is responsible for approximately one out of every five deaths in the United States. Each year, some four hundred thousand people die from cigarette-related diseases. These deaths often result from a variety of cancers, including lung cancer, and from heart and lung disease. Another smoking-related cause of death is fire due to a burning cigarette left unattended. It is estimated that one half of all regular smokers will die due to this addictive behavior. It is estimated by the CDC that smoking-related illnesses cost the nation $50

Figure 8.2 Smoking: An Expensive Habit. *Smoking-related illnesses carry a $50 billion-a-year price tag for health care costs for conditions that are largely preventable. (Source: Centers for Disease Control and Prevention)*

Total health care costs related to smoking	$50.0 million
Hospital expenses	26.9
Physician payments	15.5
Nursing home care costs	4.9
Prescription drug charges	1.8
Home health care bills	.9

billion per year in health care costs for conditions that are largely preventable (see Figure 8.2).

Critical Thinking Question

Who should foot the bill for tobacco-related illnesses? This is an important question given the financial implications of tobacco use. What are some possible ways to pass the expense of smoking along to the tobacco user and away from the nonuser?

In terms of morbidity, smokers are less healthy than nonsmokers. Workers who smoke are 50 percent more likely to be hospitalized than nonsmokers. They are also 50 percent more likely to be absent from their jobs. The best news about smoking and health is that quitting smoking carries major and immediate benefits for people of all ages (see Figure 8.3). To test your knowledge of the physical effects of smoking, see the Here's Looking at You box.

Links to Cancer

Cigarette smoking is the leading cause of cancer deaths in the United States. Lung cancer has long been the most common form of cancer in men, and starting in 1986, lung cancer caught up with and has now surpassed breast cancer as the leading cause of cancer deaths in women. Most lung cancer deaths—87 percent—are attributable to cigarette smoking.

Lung cancer mortality depends in part on how many cigarettes are smoked, how deeply the smoker inhales, and the age at which the smoker started. Figure 8.4 reveals, as one would expect, that the likelihood of dying from lung cancer increases with the number of cigarettes a person smokes, the deeper the smoke is inhaled, and the younger the initiation age. Figure 8.5 shows that the mortality rates for lung cancer dramatically reverse with the number of years a person has stopped smoking. After twenty years of not smoking, a former smoker's risk of dying of lung cancer is nearly equal to that of someone who has never smoked.

A number of components of cigarette smoke have been implicated as carcinogens, including ethylene oxide, benzene, styrene, and benzopyrene. Each of these is found in high concentrations in the homes of smokers because of all the carcinogens they exhale.

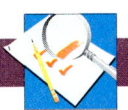

HERE'S LOOKING AT YOU

The Physical Effects of Smoking

This test consists of twenty statements about the effects of smoking. Put a check to show whether you think each statement is true or false. If you don't know whether a statement is true or false, put a check under "Don't know."

	True	False	Don't know
1. Smoking low-tar and low-nicotine cigarettes reduces the risk of all smoking-related diseases.	( )	( )	( )
2. Carbon monoxide is inhaled when a person smokes.	( )	( )	( )
3. How deeply a smoker inhales is not related to that smoker's chance of developing lung cancer.	( )	( )	( )
4. Most experts agree that the harmful effects of smoking on health are not as great for women as for men.	( )	( )	( )
5. Cigarette smoking increases the risk of developing breathing problems.	( )	( )	( )
6. Cigarette smoke can increase the air pollution of homes and offices.	( )	( )	( )
7. Cigarette smoking increases the health dangers associated with taking birth control pills.	( )	( )	( )
8. Frequent pipe and cigar smokers are more likely than nonsmokers to develop lung cancer.	( )	( )	( )
9. The average life expectancy of a smoker is the same as that of a nonsmoker.	( )	( )	( )
10. People who smoke filter cigarettes inhale less carbon monoxide than do people who smoke nonfilter cigarettes.	( )	( )	( )
11. Almost all people gain weight when they quit smoking.	( )	( )	( )
12. Smokers have an increased risk of developing a lung infection after an operation.	( )	( )	( )
13. Smoking during pregnancy does not increase baby's risk of death.	( )	( )	( )
14. Pipe smokers have a greater risk of developing cancer of the mouth than do cigarette smokers.	( )	( )	( )
15. Smoking causes the heart to beat more slowly.	( )	( )	( )
16. The health risks due to smoking do not change even after a person stops smoking.	( )	( )	( )
17. The more a person smokes, the greater the chance of developing heart disease.	( )	( )	( )
18. Cigarette smoke in the air can cause eye soreness in nonsmokers.	( )	( )	( )
19. On average, babies born to mothers who smoke during pregnancy are smaller than babies born to nonsmokers.	( )	( )	( )
20. Nicotine does not cause dependence similar to other addictive drugs.	( )	( )	( )

Answers
1 F; 2 T; 3 F; 4 F; 5 T; 6 T; 7 T; 8 T; 9 F; 10 F; 11 F; 12 T; 13 F; 14 T; 15 F; 16 F; 17 T; 18 T; 19 T; 20 F

Source: U.S. Department of Health and Human Services, Office of Disease Prevention and Health Promotion

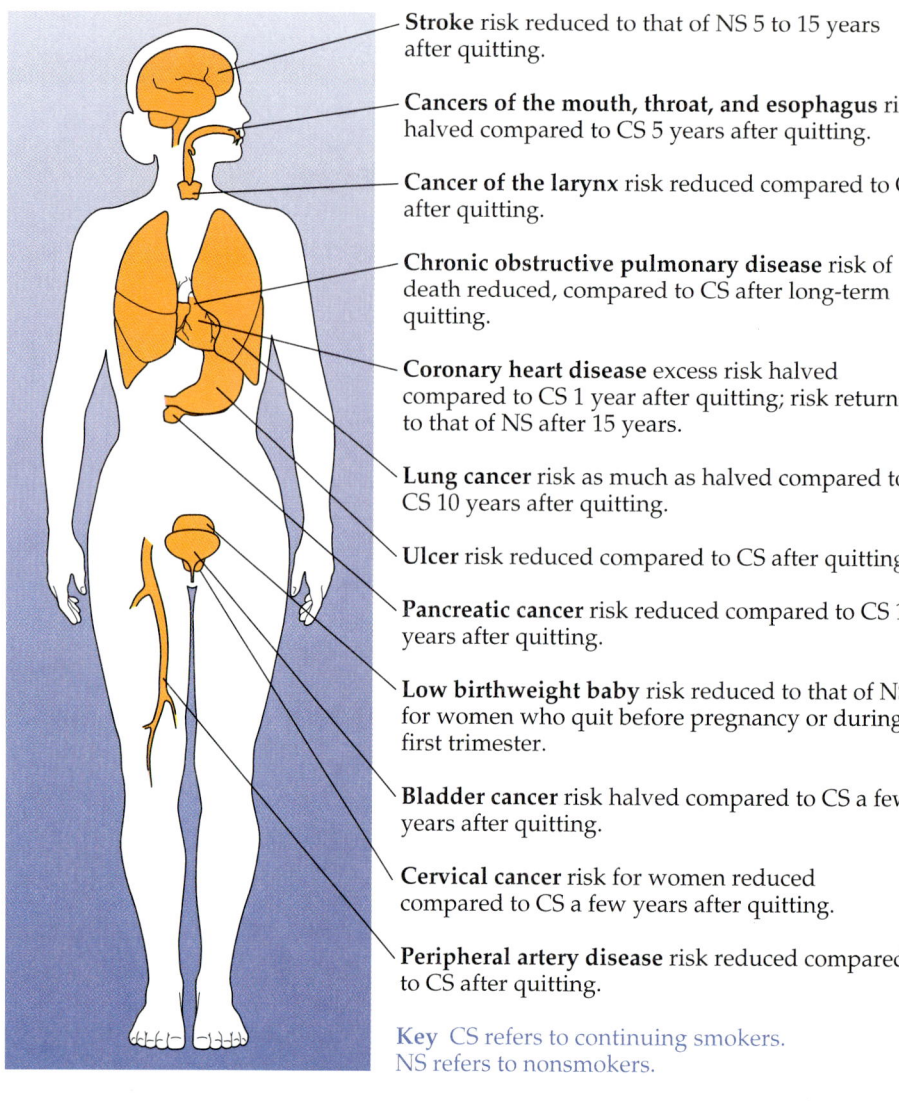

Figure 8.3 Good News about Smoking: Health Benefits from Stopping. *You can substantially reduce your risk of cancer and other diseases by quitting smoking. (Source: Centers for Disease Control and Prevention, Office on Smoking and Health)*

Smokers exposed to toxic agents in the environment are particularly vulnerable to cancer, especially lung cancer. For example, the lung cancer risk associated with radon is estimated to be six to eleven times higher in smokers than in nonsmokers. Asbestos workers who smoke are also at a significantly increased risk of developing lung cancer. In addition to lung cancer, smokers are at increased risk for cancer of the mouth, larynx, esophagus, kidney, bladder, pancreas, stomach, and cervix.

Heart Disease and Stroke

Heart disease is a term that refers to a broad range of conditions from **atherosclerosis** (hardening of the arteries) to **myocardial infarction** (major heart attack). It results from many factors, one of which is cigarette smoking. Cigarette smoking accounts for approximately 21 percent of all coronary heart disease deaths.

Although smoking does not actually cause heart disease, it contributes to nearly every physiological factor associated with it. For example, smoking dou-

atherosclerosis Damage to the circulatory system brought about by a buildup of plaque on the inner walls of arteries. Sometimes called hardening of the arteries.

myocardial infarction Damage of heart tissue caused by an interruption of blood supply to the heart that can result in death.

angina Chest pain that occurs when the heart muscle does not get enough blood supply.

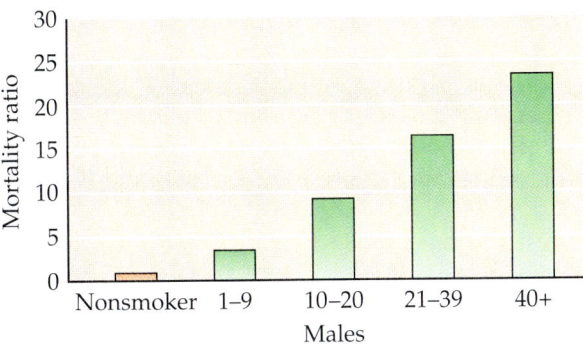

(a) Risk according to cigarettes smoked per day

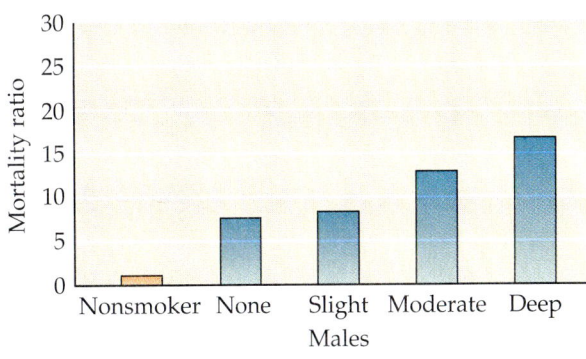

(b) Risk according to the degree of inhalation

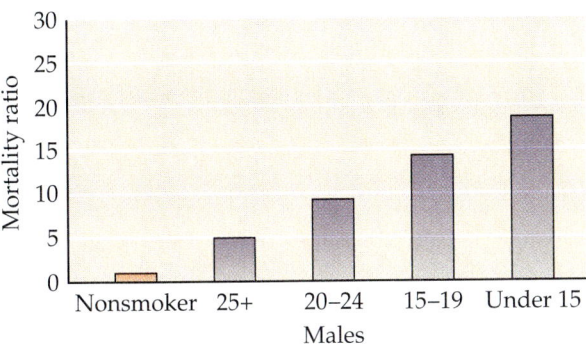

(c) Risk according to the age smoking began

■ **Figure 8.4** **The Risks for Lung Cancer from Smoking.** *These three bar graphs describe risk in terms of mortality ratio. Mortality ratio is the ratio of deaths among those who fall into a certain group (in this case, smokers) compared to those not in the group (nonsmokers). (Source: U.S. Public Health Service)*

bles the risk for having **angina** (chest pains that occur when the heart muscle does not get enough blood supply). Smoking also increases the risk for dying of a heart attack. And smokers experience heart attacks at an earlier age than do nonsmokers. Smoking also increases the risk for a second heart attack among people who have already had one. The risk for heart disease for people who smoke more than one pack of cigarettes a day is three times higher than for nonsmokers. Although, in general, women die of heart disease less often than men,

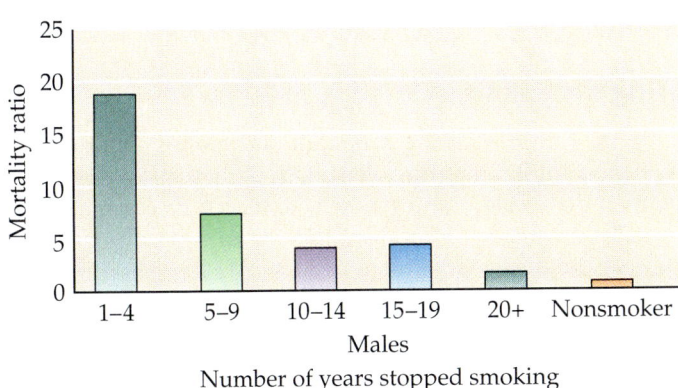

■ **Figure 8.5** **The Effect of Smoking Cessation on Lung Cancer.** *With each year of not smoking, a former smoker's risk of dying of lung cancer decreases. (Source: U.S. Public Health Service)*

women who smoke have a higher incidence of heart disease than do women who do not smoke.

The two major components in smoke that contribute to heart disease are nicotine and carbon monoxide. Nicotine increases blood pressure, heart rate, the amount of blood pumped by the heart and the blood flow in the arteries; carbon monoxide reduces the amount of oxygen available to the heart, and other parts of the body.

The third leading cause of death in the United States (after heart disease and cancer) is stroke. It is also a major cause of morbidity, with more than four hundred thousand Americans suffering nonfatal strokes a year. Much of this is avoidable because smoking is the major cause of stroke. The mechanism at work here is a decrease in cerebral blood flow, which is associated with smoking. In addition, smoking increases the risk for heart disease and congestive heart failure, both of which increase the risk for stroke.

Women who smoke and take birth control pills are three times more likely to die of heart attack or stroke than are nonsmoking women on the pill. This risk is considered so great that the U.S. Food and Drug Administration (FDA) requires that all birth control pill products have the following label: "Women who use oral contraceptives should not smoke."

Smoking cessation can dramatically reduce the risks for both heart disease and stroke. Some studies show a benefit within two years of quitting, but others suggest that the former smoker's risk gradually decreases over a period of several years.

Lung Damage

Smoking is a major cause of emphysema, chronic bronchitis, and other lung diseases. **Emphysema** is a disease of the lungs, particularly the small air sacs. Smoke damages the lungs' natural self-cleaning mechanism—the hairlike cells along the lining of the bronchial tubes. Over time, the lungs lose their ability to expand. **Chronic bronchitis** is a condition in which the bronchial tubes become inflamed as a result of irritation. One cause of bronchial irritation is smoke.

A smoker's risk for death from these two diseases is six and a half to fifteen times that of a nonsmoker. The lungs of smokers with respiratory disease generally show a thickening and a narrowing of airways. Both of these changes produce airflow obstruction and make it difficult to breathe.

The influence of smoking on these diseases is so great that it is believed that emphysema, chronic bronchitis, and other obstructive lung diseases would be uncommon without cigarette smoking. About as many people die each year from these lung diseases as from lung cancer. In addition, thousands more who have chronic bronchitis and emphysema live for many years, suffering from breathing difficulties and other discomforts that often compromise the quality of their lives. Smokers are also prone to a hacking cough and lowered resistance to colds and other minor upper respiratory infections. When smokers have pneumonia or other serious respiratory conditions, it takes them longer than nonsmokers to recover.

Complications during Pregnancy

Two of the most basic things in life—getting pregnant and having a baby—are compromised for women who smoke cigarettes. To begin with, those who smoke take longer to conceive than do nonsmoking women. Researchers calculate that the fertility of smokers is 72 percent that of nonsmokers. (Fertility is not affected by the husband's smoking, but the sperm of male smokers are decreased in density and motility and have more abnormalities than those of nonsmokers.)

Once pregnant, a smoker seriously harms her growing fetus in many ways. Even so, 20 percent of American women smoke at some point during their preg-

---

HealthLinks
American Cancer Society
www.cancer.org

The home page for the largest private organization dedicated to fighting cancer. The site includes antismoking games, news, and other information.

nancies. The carbon monoxide in cigarette smoke crosses the placenta and is transported into the fetal blood. Carbon monoxide deprives the fetus of oxygen, which slows down the fetal growth process. At the same time, nicotine in the mother's blood constricts blood flow to the placenta and reduces oxygen and nutrients until the effects of the nicotine have worn off. With the baby's growth compromised, the risk for having a spontaneous abortion (miscarriage), stillbirth, neonatal death, and/or premature birth are greater. As many as 7.5 percent of miscarriages and 14 percent of premature deliveries in the United States may be caused by maternal smoking.

Risks continue after the baby is born. Nicotine is found in the breast milk of smoking mothers and is passed on by nursing mothers to their infants. These babies are likely to be restless and irritable and to vomit and have diarrhea more often than breast-fed babies of nonsmoking mothers. Also during infancy, the risk of sudden infant death syndrome (SIDS) is increased among babies of mothers who smoked during pregnancy. Children whose parents smoke have more respiratory infections and hospitalizations in the first year of life.

Babies born of smoking mothers have lower birth weights, and they lag measurably in physical growth during childhood. Smoking may also have effects on their behavior and cognitive development throughout childhood and perhaps longer.

The good news for babies of smoking mothers is that if a mother gives up smoking early during pregnancy, her baby will probably develop normally.

Other Health Effects of Smoking

Smokers are at risk for increased illness and death from a range of other health conditions, including digestive diseases (cigarette smoke stimulates more digestive acid secretions from the stomach) and circulatory diseases (the carbon monoxide in smoke constricts the already damaged blood vessels).

Smoking contributes to many problems that, although not life threatening, reduce the quality of life. For example:

- Smoking is associated with increased upper respiratory infections such as colds and influenza.
- Smoking contributes to allergy symptoms such as coughing and sneezing.
- Smoking reduces the effects of medications, especially antianxiety drugs and painkillers.
- Smoking more than a pack a day doubles the likelihood that a person will develop cataracts, a clouding of the lenses of the eye.
- Smoking contributes to macular degeneration, which is an important cause of loss of vision in older Americans (defined as 20/200 or worse in the better eye).
- Smoking damages cells and tissues in many ways, which can result in delayed wound healing, poor circulation in the lower legs, and psoriasis (an unsightly and discomforting skin condition).

For some people, the threat of wrinkles may be a powerful motivator to stop smoking. Smoking causes a thickening and fragmentation of elastin, elastic fibers that are long and smooth in healthy skin. It also decreases the formation of collagen, the skin's main structural component, and it may reduce the skin's water content. All of this can increase wrinkling and cause what is called smoker's face. According to a report in *Dermatology,* distinctive characteristics of smoker's face—shriveled, gray-colored skin with purplish blotches—were found in 46 percent of current smokers studied but in only 8 percent of former smokers or nonsmokers.

emphysema A disease of the lungs, particularly the small air sacs, in which the lungs lose their ability to expand as a result of an accumulation of fluid in the tissue.

chronic bronchitis A condition in which the bronchial tubes become inflamed as a result of irritation.

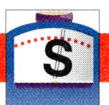# HEALTHWISE CONSUMER

Are Low-Tar, Low-Nicotine Cigarettes Safe?

There is no such thing as a safe cigarette, but people who smoke low-tar and low-nicotine cigarettes can reduce some of the health risks associated with smoking. According to an American Cancer Society study, the average lung cancer mortality of low-tar, low-nicotine cigarette smokers is 26 percent lower than that of people who smoke regular cigarettes. Overall, mortality of low-yield cigarette smokers is 16 percent lower than that of high-yield cigarette smokers.

Although low-yield cigarettes might sound attractive if you have not been able to quit smoking, consider the following facts:

- Low-tar, low-nicotine cigarettes do not reduce the risk for nonfatal heart attacks among either male or female smokers under age sixty-five.
- Low-tar, low-nicotine cigarettes do not reduce the amount of carbon monoxide and other poisonous gases. These gases are critical factors in coronary heart disease and fetal growth retardation. Cigarette filters do not provide much safety on this front, either. Certain filtered brands have actually been found to deliver more carbon monoxide than those without filters.
- People who smoke low-tar, low-nicotine cigarettes tend to compensate for the lower yield by taking more frequent puffs, inhaling more deeply, smoking more cigarettes, and smoking them closer to the end. In effect, they smoke to get the same level of nicotine in their blood as before.

An editorial in the *New England Journal of Medicine* concludes that while the movement toward low-yield cigarettes makes sense from a public health perspective, "the only reliable way to reduce the adverse health consequences of smoking is to stop."

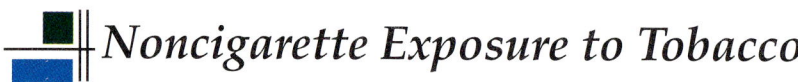## Noncigarette Exposure to Tobacco

So far, this chapter has discussed the act of smoking cigarettes and the health effects of that on the smoker. There are other ways to be exposed to tobacco, including inhaling the cigarette smoke around you, smoking cigars, and chewing tobacco.

Passive Smoke: Who Asked for It?

Inhaling environmental tobacco smoke, also called **passive smoking,** is an acknowledged health hazard. After many years of debating the issue, the Surgeon General concluded in a 1986 report that sidestream smoke can cause lung cancer in healthy nonsmokers. Sidestream smoke is the smoke that comes from the burning end of the cigarette between puffs; **mainstream smoke** is the smoke inhaled and exhaled by the smoker.

Because both sidestream and mainstream smoke are generated from the same source—the burning tip of the cigarette—it is not surprising that their compositions are similar. The quantities of chemicals in the smoke, however, differ. Curiously, sidestream smoke has higher concentrations of dangerous and irritating substances than does mainstream smoke. The concentrations of tar and nicotine in sidestream smoke are as much as two times higher than in mainstream smoke. Sidestream smoke also contains three times as much carbon monoxide and benzopyrene, a cancer-causing agent. In addition, the particles in sidestream smoke have a smaller diameter than those in mainstream smoke and are therefore more likely to infiltrate the lung. Sidestream smoke also irritates the eyes, noses, and throats of others in the room.

Young children are especially affected by sidestream smoke. One reason for this is that they breathe faster and inhale more air for their body size than do adults. Another is that they have not yet fully developed their natural immunities to fight disease. The children of parents who smoke have an increased frequency of hospitalization for bronchitis and pneumonia during the first year of life compared with children of nonsmokers. They also have more acute respiratory illnesses and infections, including middle ear infections.

Another vulnerable group are people who have angina and other heart conditions. Angina patients are more prone to attacks when they are in smoke-filled rooms. Similarly, the risk of a nonsmoker for dying from heart disease increases if that person's spouse is a smoker. These findings from the Surgeon General are based on studies of both men and women.

Cigar and Pipe Smoking

Cigar and pipe smoking dramatically dropped in popularity in the United States between the 1960s and the 1990s—from 9.1 billion cigars a year in 1964 to a low of 2.1 billion in 1993. Since then, cigar smoking has been slowly rising and has become increasingly popular among women as well as men. There are private cigar clubs, cigar cruises, and cigar nights for sampling brands. Sales are brisk for premium cigars—the kind that sell for $2.50 a piece or more. The cigar industry estimated in 1996 that more than 10 million Americans regularly smoke cigars, an increase of 2 million since 1993.

Cigar and pipe smokers have higher lung cancer rates than do nonsmokers but lower rates than do those who smoke cigarettes. Cigar and pipe smokers are more at risk than cigarette smokers for cancer of the mouth, lips, and tongue. This is due to the way people smoke pipes and cigars. Most do not inhale; rather, they hold the smoke in their mouths and release it. As with users of other tobacco products, cigar smokers are more likely than nonsmokers to develop chronic obstructive lung disease and heart attacks.

Another problem with cigars and pipes is that they are more polluting than cigarettes. One cigar, for example, produces more carbon monoxide than do three cigarettes. This sidestream smoke is worse for the smoker as well as others in the room.

The Risks of Smokeless Tobacco

Smokeless tobacco became popular among men in their teens and twenties as an alternative to smoking. It was seen as a macho thing to do, and, at the same time, it was thought to be safe.

As it turns out, this is not the case. Smokeless tobacco contains carcinogens that cause oral cancer. It also causes **leukoplakia** (white patches on the oral mucosa that may transform into a malignancy) and periodontal diseases, including gingivitis and receding gums. In addition, smokeless tobacco is highly addictive. Although it takes longer for the nicotine to reach the brain from smokeless tobacco than from cigarettes, users are exposed to blood levels of nicotine equal to those of cigarette smokers.

There are two forms of smokeless tobacco: chewing tobacco and snuff. In chewing tobacco, the leaf is usually shredded, combined with a sweetener or flavoring, and pressed into bricks (called plugs) or dried and twisted into rope-like strands (called twists). A portion is either chewed or held in place in the cheek or between the lower lip and the gum.

Snuff is a coarse powder. In its dry form, it is sniffed through the nose. In the United States, it is more popularly sold as a moist powder, and a pinch is held in

passive smoking Inhaling tobacco smoke from the environment, as a result of someone else smoking.

mainstream smoke The smoke inhaled and exhaled by the smoker.

smokeless tobacco Tobacco products that are chewed, placed in the mouth, and/or sniffed through the nose.

leukoplakia White patches on the oral mucosa that may transform into a malignancy.

DEVELOPING HEALTH SKILLS

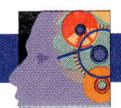

Smokeless Tobacco Users: Check Monthly for Early Signs of Disease

The early signs of cancer of the mouth and tongue may be detected by self-examination. Dr. Elbert Glover, director of the Tobacco Research Center at West Virginia University, and the American Cancer Society recommend that the following self-check procedures be conducted every month:

- Check your face and neck for lumps on either side. Both sides of your face and neck should be the same shape.
- Look at your lips, cheeks, and gums. Look for sores, white or red patches, or changes in your gums by pulling down your lower lip. Check your inner cheeks, especially where you hold your tobacco. Gently squeeze your lip and cheeks to check for lumps or soreness.
- Put the tip of your tongue on the roof of your mouth. Place one finger on the floor of your mouth and press up under your chin with a finger from your other hand. Feel for bumps, soreness, or swelling. Check around the inside of your teeth from one side of your jaw to the other.
- Tilt your head back and open your mouth wide. Check for color changes or bumps or sores in the roof of your mouth.
- Stick out your tongue and look at the top. Gently grasp your tongue with a piece of cloth and pull it to each side. Look for color changes. Feel both sides of your tongue with your finger for bumps.

If you use smokeless tobacco and find anything that looks or feels unusual, see your dentist or physician as soon as possible.

---

place between the lip or cheek and the gum. Another popular variety of snuff is bagged in cheesecloth, like a tea bag, to give a "neat" way to hold the snuff in the mouth. This bag is popularly called a "bandit." The carcinogens in the tobacco, along with the nicotine, are absorbed through the oral tissue.

The use of smokeless tobacco is increasing among young people—particularly teenage males. Of the estimated 10 million smokeless tobacco users, 3 million are younger than twenty-one years old. Two thirds of men who have ever used smokeless tobacco began before age twenty-one, and more than one third began before age sixteen. Young women also use smokeless tobacco, but much less than men. Among high school students, 20 percent of males use smokeless tobacco, while only 2.5 percent of females do. If you ever used smokeless tobacco, be sure to see the Developing Health Skills box.

Critical Thinking Question

Healthy People 2000 establishes the following objective: "Increase the average (state and federal combined) tobacco excise tax to at least 50 percent of the average retail price of all cigarettes and smokeless tobacco." This would represent an increase from 31 percent in 1994. Do you believe that "sin taxes" are an effective means of public health promotion? Support your answer with evidence from states (e.g., California and Massachusetts) where such taxes have been used extensively.

Kicking the Habit: How to Stop

Most smokers want to quit, but the task is so difficult that surprisingly few try and fewer succeed. Surveys conducted by the CDC show that 70 percent of current cigarette smokers have tried to stop at least once. These statistics clearly illustrate the addictive nature of nicotine. For an unusual approach to smoking cessation, see the Cultural View box.

Physical Problems of Quitting

The initial problems that smokers have to face when they stop smoking are symptoms related to withdrawal from nicotine. As with any drug withdrawal, these symptoms can cause great discomfort. Withdrawal symptoms—which are experienced in varying degrees from mild to severe—include craving for tobacco, irritability, anxiety, restlessness, dry mouth, difficulty sleeping, and impaired concentration, judgment, and motor coordination. These symptoms usually last one to two weeks. In some cases, however, they can last several months.

In addition to the problem of nicotine addiction, many people also have a psychological dependence on smoking. Cigarettes are used automatically along with simple everyday activities such as starting the car, waiting for the bus, or reading the newspaper. For many people, lighting a cigarette is perceived as a way to reduce stress in a social or business situation—on a first date or when making a presentation in front of a group of people. These events are called triggers because they trigger the urge to smoke.

Look at the following list of triggers. If you smoke or someone close to you smokes, which ones do you think trigger an urge to light up?

- Drinking coffee
- Talking on the phone
- Reading a newspaper
- Writing a paper
- Waiting for a bus
- Having a beer
- Playing cards
- Watching someone smoke
- Taking a study break
- Studying under pressure
- Watching television
- Having a family argument
- Meeting with your professor
- Driving in a car
- Waiting for food in a restaurant
- Feeling lonely
- Finishing a meal

Another reason some people have a problem quitting is that they think they will gain a lot of weight. This is particularly true for female smokers (some women smoke to control weight). The fact is that most people will gain some weight when they stop smoking—on average fewer than 10 pounds—but health researchers note that this weight gain is a negligible health threat compared with the risks of continued smoking. Moreover, there is evidence that people who stop smoking can see favorable changes in the distribution of their body fat.

The best advice from clinicians to people worried about weight gain: Put your concerns about weight on the back burner. Tackle one problem at a time. *After* you have quit smoking successfully, start talking about how to reduce your

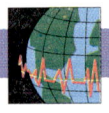

CULTURAL VIEW

How One Village Kicked the Habit

Talk about life imitating art. In the 1970 movie *Cold Turkey*, an entire California town tries to quit smoking in order to collect a $25 million prize. Now a small village in Fiji has attempted the same feat. But unlike their celluloid counterparts, the residents of Nabila were successful.

How'd they do it? For years, an international team of public health experts tried to get the villagers to quit via Western strategies like counseling—and failed spectacularly. The turning point came when the Nabila elders made tobacco taboo. In a special ceremony, the villagers drank a sacred potion and called for supernatural retribution against anyone who violated the cigarette ban. Twenty-one months later, Nabila was smoke-free, except for the four octogenarians given official permission to inhale.

Several factors contributed to the community's success, reports Australian psychologist Gary Groth-Marnat, Ph.D. Media attention on the "village that quit smoking" added incentive, as did Fiji's cultural emphasis on social cohesion. But perhaps the best motivation came courtesy of the three smokers whose resolve faltered. Within days of giving in to their urge for cigarettes, one lacerated his scalp, another suffered swollen testicles, and a third was attacked by a dog. In a society where mystical beliefs hold sway, the other villagers got the message.

Source: "Life: How One Village Kicked the Habit," reprinted with permission from *Psychology Today Magazine*, January–February, 1997. Copyright © 1997 Sussex Publishers, Inc.

---

weight. For now, think about eating plenty of fruit and vegetables, getting regular exercise, getting enough sleep, and not eating a lot of fats.

Getting Motivated

As with any addicting drug, smoking is possible to give up if the motivation is strong enough. The thought of having a heart attack, lung cancer, or advanced emphysema should be a powerful enough incentive. A substantial number of smokers, however, still do not believe that smoking increases the risk for developing these diseases.

What, then, motivates people to quit? Generally, people quit because of something personal (see the Here's Looking at You box). Perhaps they want to make an impression on a new (and nonsmoking) boyfriend or girlfriend. The following are some of the reasons people give for quitting:

- I don't want to be a slave to a habit. I want to be more in control of my life.
- I want to get rid of my smoker's cough.
- Smoking around nonsmokers makes me feel uncomfortable, and I'm tired of going outside by myself to smoke when I'm at a party.
- Smoking is costing me a lot of money. I am going to save my cigarette money and buy something special for myself.
- Smoking makes my clothes and breath smell.
- My office will be smoke-free in six months, and the company will pay for smoking cessation classes.
- Even though I deny anything bad will actually happen to me, I know that smoking is bad for my health.

Cessation Approaches

As difficult as it is to stop smoking, nearly half of all people who have ever smoked have quit. Most—90 percent—did it on their own, but plenty of **smoking-cessation** help is available for those who want it.

smoking cessation The process of breaking a smoking habit. Stopping the use of tobacco.

behavior modification Therapy designed to change the learned behavior of an individual.

nicotine replacement Therapy in which a person who smokes gets nicotine by means other than tobacco.

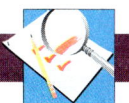

HERE'S LOOKING AT YOU

How Did You Avoid Smoking This Week?

Listed below are ways that some people avoid smoking. Put a check to show how frequently in the *past week* you successfully used each of these activities to avoid smoking.

	Often	Sometimes	Never
1. Exercising	( )	( )	( )
2. Eating or drinking something	( )	( )	( )
3. Thinking about the effort you've put into quitting	( )	( )	( )
4. Chewing gum	( )	( )	( )
5. Using relaxation/deep breathing	( )	( )	( )
6. Calling a friend	( )	( )	( )
7. Giving yourself a "pep talk" not to smoke	( )	( )	( )
8. Promising yourself a reward for not smoking	( )	( )	( )
9. Leaving a situation that makes you want to smoke	( )	( )	( )
10. Thinking about the negative effects of smoking (e.g., poor health, bad breath)	( )	( )	( )
11. Talking to a supportive ex-smoker	( )	( )	( )
12. Keeping busy (e.g., getting involved in a craft or hobby)	( )	( )	( )
13. Reminding yourself of the benefits of not smoking (e.g., better health, money saved)	( )	( )	( )
14. Reading a book or magazine, or watching television	( )	( )	( )
15. Thinking about something besides smoking	( )	( )	( )
16. Putting off having a cigarette until the urge passes	( )	( )	( )
17. Avoiding places that make you want to smoke	( )	( )	( )
18. Doodling	( )	( )	( )
19. Avoiding frequent contact with people who smoke	( )	( )	( )
20. Giving yourself a reward for not smoking	( )	( )	( )

Source: U.S. Department of Health and Human Services, Office of Disease Prevention and Health Promotion

One approach is **behavior modification,** in which smokers learn to change their behavior pattern of smoking. Taking a short walk after dinner, for example, is one way to break the pattern of having a cigarette at the end of the meal. Other tactics include calling a buddy when you are tempted to smoke, switching to brands lower in nicotine, and forcing yourself to break patterns by smoking only on the odd hour—7, 9, 11. About 40 percent of smokers completing behavior modification classes sponsored by the American Cancer Society, the American Lung Association, and private groups such as Smokenders are free from cigarettes a year later.

Hypnosis helps about 20 percent of the people who try it to stop smoking. When the smoker is in a trance state, the hypnotist coaches him or her how to stop. Motivation is the key to making hypnotism work, and researchers say that the more a smoker wants to quit, the better hypnosis works. There is no solid evidence that acupuncture lessens the physical symptoms of withdrawal, yet many people who try it are able to stay off cigarettes.

Nicotine replacement is also proving successful in getting smokers to quit, according to clinical practice guidelines developed by the federal Agency for

HealthLinks
American Lung Association
www.lungusa.org

The home page for the largest private organization dedicated to the prevention of lung disease and respiratory disorders, as well as tobacco control and environmental health.

Health Care Policy and Research. Through this technique, the smoker gets nicotine by means other than tobacco, and the urge to smoke is lessened.

The nicotine in a special gum is absorbed by the body as the person chews and intermittently "parks" it between the cheek and gum for about 30 minutes. The recommended course of treatment for nicotine gum is up to three months. By itself, the gum helps 11 percent of smokers to quit for at least a year. Using the gum in conjunction with counseling, 29 percent remain smoke-free. Between 5 and 10 percent actually become addicted to the gum. Other problems are compliance, ease of use, social acceptability, and an unpleasant taste.

Another form of nicotine replacement is a **transdermal nicotine patch**. When applied to the skin (usually on the upper torso or the upper arm), the patch releases the drug at a constant rate. It is absorbed by the skin and enters the bloodstream. Studies show a success rate of about 25 percent when the patch is used for six to eight weeks. The patch does not have the problems noted above for nicotine gum, and researchers believe it is a more acceptable way for most smokers to quit. The patch presents a risk, however, to those who use it and continue to smoke. When the patch and smoking are combined, the level of nicotine in the system is actually increased and can reach dangerously high levels in some people.

Nicotine is also available as a nasal spray. The nicotine is absorbed into the bloodstream through the lining of the nose. Researchers have not yet compared the spray with nicotine gum or the patch, but studies show that 25 percent of those who used the nasal spray stopped smoking for at least a year, compared with 13 percent of smokers who tried to quit without help.

Critical Thinking Question

> Several legal cases have centered on the financial responsibility of tobacco companies to pay for medical costs of smoking borne by taxpayers. Should the tobacco companies be held responsible for the costs of providing tobacco-related health care services to low-income people who receive health care through Medicaid, a federal-state program? If not, who should bear the cost?

The Changing Climate of Public Acceptance of Tobacco Use

The social and political climate concerning smoking has changed substantially over the years. Nonsmokers are less willing to accept smoke in their environment, and increasingly, smoking is banned in public places where people congregate. Almost every state requires smoke-free indoor air to some degree or in some public places. There are smoke-free offices, hospitals, rental cars, planes, fast-food restaurants, hotels—every room is guaranteed to be "clean"—and even smoke-free jails. There are also financial dividends for nonsmokers, including discounts on life, health, disability, home, and automobile insurance policies.

transdermal nicotine patch A form of nicotine replacement that, when applied to the skin, releases nicotine into the system at a constant rate.

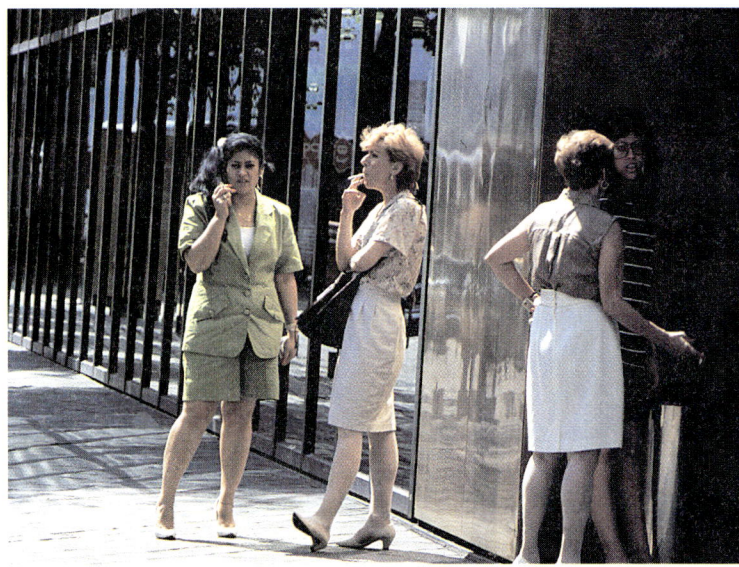

In an effort to protect employees from sidestream smoke, many businesses ban smoking inside their buildings, forcing smokers to the exits. (Source: The Image Works/© Lee Snider)

And a growing number of pharmacists who fill patients' prescriptions are refusing to sell them tobacco products.

The legal and regulatory environment has also changed. Law suits have been filed against tobacco companies by smokers who had lung cancer and/or by their families for false advertising and negligence. The Supreme Court ruled in one case that the federal labeling law, which requires that all cigarette packages and advertisements carry a warning that smoking is dangerous to your health, does not shield tobacco firms from liability. States have sued tobacco companies for reimbursement for Medicaid costs of treating indigent smokers with tobacco-caused diseases. And widely publicized congressional hearings in 1994 focused on whether and when the tobacco companies knew that smoking is a health hazard and that nicotine is addictive.

The National Cancer Institute and several states are working to change the social environment in which people decide to smoke—for example, by getting local coalitions to change laws affecting tobacco taxes. In California, activists helped get a state referendum passed that raised cigarette taxes and directed the funds to be used in antismoking campaigns. In seven years, tobacco use in California dropped 26 percent.

It is against the law in every state to sell and distribute tobacco products to anyone under age eighteen, but most teenagers—an estimated two thirds—report having no problem buying cigarettes. To help enforce these laws, the Food and Drug Administration issued regulations in 1997 that require retailers to get identification showing proof of age before selling tobacco products to young people.

Public health interests also won a major victory in 1997 with the public acknowledgment by some tobacco manufacturers that smoking can be a health hazard. In addition, the tobacco companies began to settle with the forty state attorneys general that had sued them to recover money the state spent treating tobacco-related diseases for people on Medicaid. The settlement will cover annual payments to the states as well as set goals to reduce smoking by youth and put significant curbs on advertising. Figure 8.6 documents key events that link tobacco to health hazards, regulatory and legislative measures, and changes in the percentage of adults who smoke.

Chapter 8 Smoking Out Tobacco

Percentage of adults who smoke:	Year	Event
	1964	The U.S. Surgeon General reports that smoking causes lung cancer and other diseases.
42.4	1965	
	1966	Warning labels are required on cigarette packages and, eventually, on cigarette advertisements.
37.4	1970	
	1971	Cigarette advertising is banned from radio and television.
37.1	1975	Soldiers in the U.S. military no longer receive cigarettes as part of their daily rations.
	1977	Berkeley, California, passes the first comprehensive smoking law, requiring restaurants to establish nonsmoking areas. Since then, similar laws have been passed throughout the nation. Some restaurants quickly move to a smoke-free policy.
	1978	
	1979	
33.2	1980	
	1982	The U.S. Congress doubles the cigarette sales tax.
	1983	
30.1	1985	
	1987	
	1988	The U.S. Surgeon General issues a report saying that nicotine is an addictive drug that acts in much the same fashion as cocaine and heroin. Smoking is banned on two-hour or shorter domestic flights. The ban is extended to six-hour or shorter flights two years later. Eventually, airlines worldwide adopt a smoke-free policy.
25.5	1990	
	1991	
	1993	The Environmental Protection Agency declares second-hand smoke a health hazard.
	1994	
24.7	1995	*Journal of American Medical Association* publishes a series of articles documenting that the tobacco industry has long known that nicotine is an addictive drug and that smoking causes cancer and other diseases. Mississippi sues tobacco companies to recover Medicaid costs for treating smoking-related illnesses. Other states follow.
	1996	President Clinton announces that the FDA has authority to treat nicotine as a drug, giving it control over tobacco products for the first time.
	1997	Tobacco manufacturers begin to settle with the 40 states that have sued them for tobacco-related Medicaid costs. R.J. Reynolds Tobacco Co. eliminates its Joe Camel ad campaign.

Figure 8.6 Tobacco Timeline. *(Source: Centers for Disease Control and Prevention)*

Given these events, what might be the worst present on record was the one given by the natives of San Salvador to Christopher Columbus on his birthday in 1492: tobacco leaves. Some of the New World tribes restricted use of tobacco to ceremonies or medicines, but others dried the leaves, set them afire, and inhaled the smoke for pleasure. The explorers and their crew picked up the smoking habit and took it back to Europe with them.

People around the world have been smoking tobacco for pleasure ever since—and suffering as a result. It is estimated by the World Health Organization

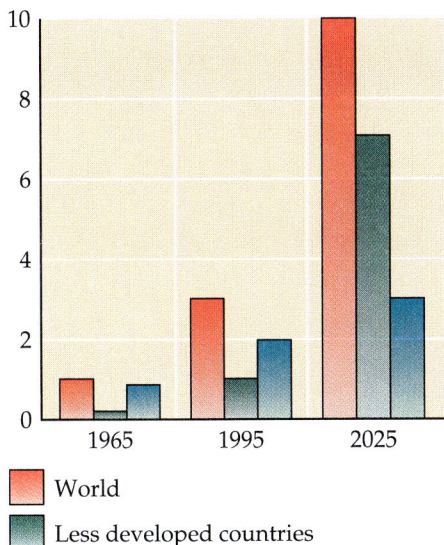

Figure 8.7 Annual Deaths Attributed to Tobacco Worldwide.
Ten million people will die of tobacco-induced illnesses by 2025. Most of those deaths will occur in less developed countries. (Source: Data are World Health Organization estimates)

that if current smoking rates continue, about 10 million people worldwide will die in 2025 of tobacco-induced illnesses. Seventy percent of these deaths will occur in less developed countries, where tobacco use will account for 15 percent of all deaths (see Figure 8.7).

WHO's predictions for 2025 need not come to pass. Whether through education or legislation, the reduction of tobacco use is clearly in the best interest of the world's health.

Of more immediate importance, avoidance of tobacco is in the best interest of your health when you are confronted with the question of whether to smoke or not to smoke. As legal and public opinion accepts the irrefutable scientific evidence that smoking is dangerous to your health and to the health of people around you, perhaps tobacco use will become a dying habit.

Key Concepts

1. Tobacco use is the single most preventable cause of death in the United States.
2. Currently, about 48 million Americans smoke.
3. The main reasons people smoke are family and peer influence, advertising hype, pleasure and perceived relaxation, and the addictive nature of nicotine.
4. Tobacco smoke contains more than four thousand separate substances, many of which produce some biological activity.
5. Cigarette smoking is the leading cause of cancer deaths and is related to nearly every risk factor associated with heart disease.
6. A pregnant woman who smokes harms herself and her baby because the chemicals in cigarette smoke cross the placenta.
7. Passive smoking presents many of the same hazards as direct smoking. Young children are especially vulnerable to passive smoke.
8. Smokeless tobacco contains carcinogens that cause oral cancer.
9. Nearly half of all people who have ever smoked have quit.

10. Smoking-cessation approaches include behavior modification, hypnosis, and nicotine replacement.

Review Questions

1. Describe how smoking behavior has changed over the last century.
2. Explain four reasons why people smoke and explain each reason.
3. Compare dependence on tobacco products and drug addiction.
4. Define passive smoke and identify the risks associated with this involuntary exposure to tobacco.
5. Explain the health risks of nicotine, tar, and carbon monoxide.
6. Describe how tobacco use contributes to cancer, heart disease, and lung disease.
7. Pregnant women are encouraged not to smoke. Explain this advice by describing the influence of tobacco smoke on pregnancy.
8. Explain the risks of smokeless tobacco use. How do they compare to the risks of smoking?
9. Make a list of assertive statements that can be used to avoid tobacco use.
10. Identify three approaches to smoking cessation and compare the advantages of each.

Selected Bibliography

Brunton, S., and J. Henningfield. *Nicotine Addiction and Smoking Cessation.* New York: Medical Information Services, 1991.

Glantz, S.A., et al. "Tobacco Litigation: Issues for Public Health and Public Policy." *Journal of the American Medical Association* 277, no. 9 (1997): 751–753.

Gostin, L.O., et al. "FDA Regulation of Tobacco Advertising and Youth Smoking." *Journal of the American Medical Association* 277, no. 5 (1997): 410–418.

Health Implications of Smokeless Tobacco Use Bethesda, MD: National Institutes of Health, 1986.

Healthy People 2000 Review 1995–96. Hyattsville, MD: National Center for Health Statistics, 1996.

Journal of the American Medical Association 275, no. 16 (1996), (entire issue devoted to smoking).

Paul, C.L., and R.W. Sanson-Fisher. "Experts' Agreement on the Relative Effectiveness of 29 Smoking Reduction Strategies." *Preventive Medicine* 25 (1996): 517–526.

Reducing the Health Consequences of Smoking: 25 Years of Progress, A Report of the Surgeon General. Washington, DC: U.S. Department of Health and Human Services. 1989. See also other reports of the Surgeon General.

Smoking Cessation (Clinical Practice Guideline Number 18). Rockville, MD: U.S. Department of Health and Human Services, Agency for Health Care Policy and Research. 1996.

HealthLinks: Web Sites for Preventing Tobacco Use

You can access better health as it relates to this chapter by checking out some of the following sites on the Internet. These and sites identified within the chapter can be accessed directly when you visit the *HealthStyles* Web Site located on the Allyn and Bacon home page at **http://www.abacon.com.**

Office on Smoking and Health: Tobacco Information & Prevention Sourcepage (TIPS)

www.cdc.gov/nccdphp/osh/tobacco.htm

Federal agency dedicated to eliminating tobacco use, primarily among young people. This site provides numerous links to educational materials and resources, as well as providing tips for cessation.

Robert Wood Johnson Foundation

www.rwjf.org/

Home page for the nation's largest philanthropy devoted to assuring that all Americans have access to basic health care at reasonable a cost; to improving the way services are organized and provided to people with chronic health conditions; and to reduce the personal, social, and economic harm caused by tobacco, alcohol, and illicit drugs.

Health Hotlines: Smoking Out Tobacco

Campaign for Tobacco-Free Kids
(202) 296-5469
1701 L Street NW, Suite 800
Washington, DC 20036

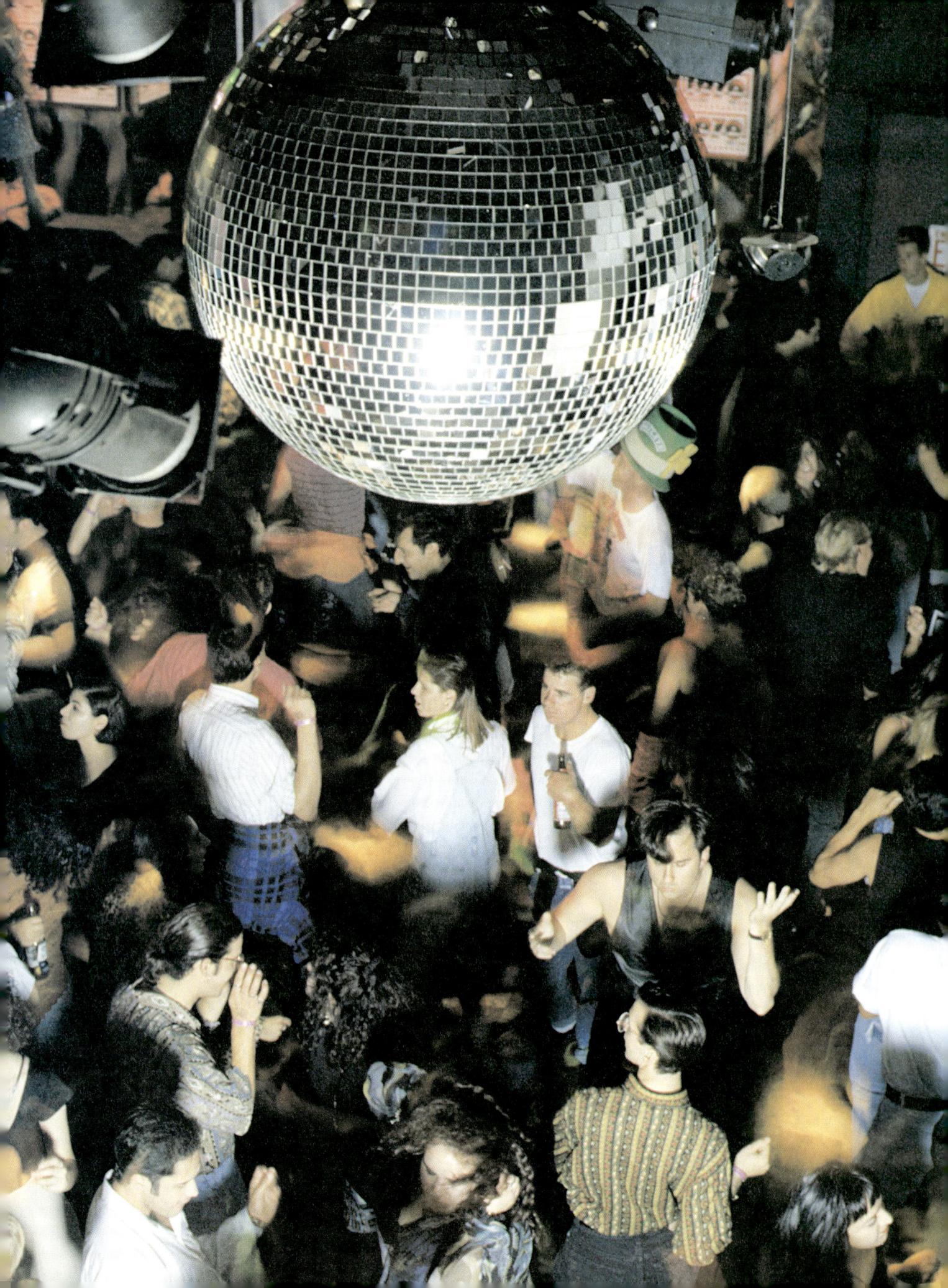

Chapter 9

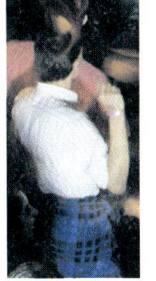
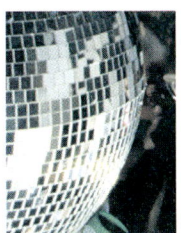
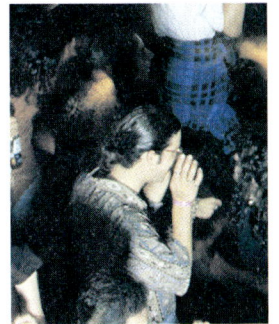

Dealing with Drinking

Objectives

When you finish reading this chapter, you will be able to:

1. Differentiate between the drinking patterns of the adult population, college students, and adolescents.
2. Explain why people drink alcohol.
3. Describe the dangers of binge drinking.
4. List the health hazards of alcohol use and abuse.
5. Relate alcohol use to the incidence of suicide, homicide, and unintentional injuries.
6. Define alcoholism as a disease.
7. Differentiate between the occasional drinker, the social drinker, and the problem drinker.
8. Identify treatment options for alcoholism.
9. Explain how to avoid problem drinking. Include in your explanation the importance of social assertiveness skills.
10. Explain why prevention is the ultimate answer to the problems associated with alcohol use.

What Is Your HealthStyle?

Fiona and William were up for celebrating. They had just finished their exams and had a few days before the next semester began. They invited classmates to a bring-your-own party and planned for dancing, drinking games, and a lot of junk food. Aware of the dangers of drinking and driving, they asked people to bring sleeping bags and stay over.

What they didn't count on was people getting sick, throwing up, and leaving the mess for them to clean up. They also didn't count on the police busting up the party and arresting five students who were under age twenty-one—the legal drinking age. When the weekend came to an end, Fiona and William were physically exhausted and psychologically stressed out from the experience. They were not fully fit when they started second-semester classes on Monday.

Lois and Eduardo were busy working on a school play, but they still wanted to do something special to celebrate the end of exams. Because they had just completed a history course, they decided to invite their friends to come to a party dressed up as a historical person and to bring food and drink that was representative of the times. Marie Antoinette brought cake, George Washington a cherry pie, Charlemagne mead, and Dionysius wine. Johnny Appleseed brought apple juice.

There was plenty to eat and drink, but no one got drunk. The objective was to relax, let loose, and have fun for the evening, not to get sick. Lois and Eduardo spent the rest of the weekend working backstage on sets and lighting, and they were ready for the new semester.

In Your Opinion

Both couples had planned a celebration party, but only one was successful.

- What was the problem with Fiona and William's party from the very beginning?
- Why did Lois and Eduardo's party turn out better?
- Did Lois and Eduardo possess health skills that Fiona and William lacked?
- How would you describe the different role of alcohol at the two parties?
- How would you plan a postexam celebration?

Excessive use of alcohol, which can lead to problem drinking and alcoholism, is a major public health problem. Alcohol-related motor vehicle accidents caused by drinking are a major cause of death, especially for adolescents and young adults (those aged fifteen to twenty-four). Alcohol is associated with an increased incidence of certain forms of cancer and liver disease, and it contributes to the breakup of normal family life. Alcohol is also a source of some blatantly mixed messages in our society concerning health values. For example, consider the mixed message given when a convenience store sells both gasoline and beer when anyone who drives knows that it is not safe to drink and drive.

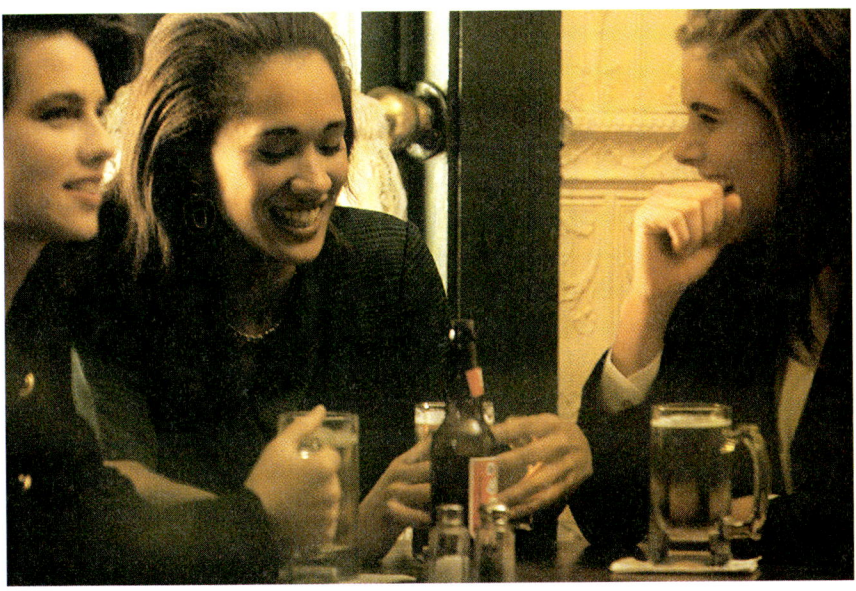

Drinking habits are changing among women. Many young women are consuming alcohol about as frequently as young men. (Source: FPG International/© Ed Taylor Studio)

Most American adults consume and report having had at least one drink in the past month. Many who consume alcohol never experience the negative health and social effects that problem drinking can cause. Others, however, experience serious health threats, both physical and social. Why such a different response to the use of the same chemical substance—alcohol? Perhaps the answer begins with the question, Who drinks?

Who Drinks: A Picture of Alcohol Consumption

Drinking alcoholic beverages is common behavior in this culture as well as in most cultures around the world. There is reason to believe, however, that the nature of alcohol consumption is changing in the United States and that people are drinking less. One reason for this is a changing public perception about alcohol use. According to a Harvard School of Public Health researcher, the public message used to be, "It's cool to get smashed." Now, the message is, "It's dumb to get drunk." This change in perception may be due to extensive—and effective—alcohol education efforts that stress the message "If you do drink, drink in moderation." This recognizes the fact that adults, college students, and adolescents drink, even though it is illegal for people under age twenty-one to drink. Most college students fall into this category.

Adult Drinkers

According to the National Institute of Alcohol and Alcohol Abuse, about 60 percent of the adult population drinks. Differences in drinking patterns exist between men and women. The NIAAA reports that women drink less often, drink heavily less often, and suffer fewer problems associated with drinking than do men. Women tend to abstain from drinking at nearly twice the rate of men. And men tend to report themselves as heavy drinkers three times as often as women.

Women's new lifestyles, however, may be affecting their drinking habits. Women have tended to be more secretive than men about their drinking, but in recent years, there has been an increase in the number of reported female **alcoholics,** and differences between working women and full-time homemakers are showing up. One study of female alcoholics showed that the professional woman is the least secretive about her drinking and the suburban housewife is the most secretive. Married women who have paying jobs outside the home are somewhat less likely than full-time homemakers to be heavy drinkers. However, moderate drinking is more common among married women who work.

As people age, they generally cut back on drinking. Accordingly, alcohol use is lower among the elderly than in the general population. But the elderly, too, have problems with alcohol. About 10 percent of elderly men have a drinking problem. Because older people reflect drinking patterns rooted in a past way of life, only 2 percent of elderly women have a drinking problem.

College Student Drinkers

There are important differences between the drinking behaviors of college students and of the general adult population. Studies of college students show that 85 to 95 percent choose to drink alcohol. Alcohol is twice as popular among college students as the next leading drug, marijuana, and more than five times as popular as cocaine.

College students also tend to drink more often—and more often to excess—than the general adult population. A study conducted at 140 campuses by researchers at the Alcohol Studies Program at the Harvard School of Public Health found that 44 percent of college students are binge drinkers. **Binge drinking** is defined as having five drinks in a row for men or four in a row for women on at least one occasion in the two weeks before the survey. (Because women generally have more fat in their bodies than do men, it takes women longer to metabolize alcohol; they are therefore affected equally by lesser amounts.)

Binge drinking can cause significant health and social problems. According to the study, binge drinkers were seven times as likely to have unprotected sex as nonbinge drinkers, ten times as likely to drive after drinking, and eleven times as likely to fall behind in school.

It is not fully understood why college students drink alcohol more than the general public does, but factors such as newly found independence and social pressure likely contribute. For example, the Harvard study found that 41 percent of entering freshmen who reported no binge drinking in high school said they began to binge shortly after arriving at college, and almost half said they were drinking more since arriving at college than they did in high school. As for social pressure, 86 percent of fraternity residents and 80 percent of sorority residents reported binge drinking. This compares to 45 percent of men not affiliated with fraternities and 36 percent of women not affiliated with sororities.

There are also differences by region of the country and by type of school. Colleges in the northeastern and north-central states had higher rates of binge drinking than did those in the West or the South. Women's colleges and historically African American colleges had lower rates than others.

At the same time that binge drinking is taking place, other research shows that more and more college students are abstaining. A study conducted by the University of California at Los Angeles of more than three hundred thousand students nationwide found that nearly half of the students said that they do not drink—even an occasional beer—up from one in four students in 1971 who abstained. There are several possible reasons for this:

- There is a perceptible change in attitude, and college students do not automatically turn to drinking on the weekend.

alcoholic Someone who suffers from alcoholism and who has lost control over his or her drinking.

binge drinking Having five drinks in a row for men or four in a row for women on at least one occasion in the past two weeks.

- College students have grown up with tough drunk driving laws and are aware of the consequences of drinking and driving.
- For African American and other students following Muslim tenets, drinking is forbidden, and many do not want to be around people who are drinking.
- The average age of college students has risen. Priorities change, and for many older students, spending time and money drinking is not at the top of their list—or even on it.

To curb college drinking, and to respond to the needs of non- and moderate drinkers, many schools have developed strict policies about alcohol use on campus—for example, banning kegs at football games and at fraternity house parties. At a growing number of schools, student–administration coalitions are working together to develop—and enforce—these policies. Check with your school's administration to see if your campus has an alcohol-use policy.

Critical Thinking Question

Healthy People 2000 contains the following objective: "Reduce the proportion of college students engaging in recent occasions of heavy drinking of alcoholic beverages to no more than 32 percent." In 1994, 40 percent of college students reported doing heavy drinking in the past two weeks. Who should bear responsibility for reaching this goal? The college? The local police? The educational efforts of the state or federal government? What would you propose to assure that this objective is met?

Adolescent Drinkers

The use of alcohol among high school students slowly but steadily declined from the early 1980s to 1994, but it began to rise in 1996, according to the annual University of Michigan "Monitoring the Future Study." The study, which surveys eighth, tenth, and twelfth graders, found an increase in lifetime alcohol use by eighth and tenth graders and a continued decline by twelfth graders. While fewer high school seniors are drinking, many of those that do drink are heavy drinkers. More than 30 percent said that they had had more than five drinks in the last two weeks and 31 percent said that they had been drunk in the past month.

These teens are at high risk for becoming alcoholics. The earlier a person starts drinking, the greater the chance of addiction. A teenager who drinks has two to three times the risk for becoming addicted to alcohol as does a teenager who does not drink but who later drinks as an adult.

Why Do People Drink?

People choose to drink alcohol for a variety of reasons. Some people drink because of social circumstances ("All my friends do it") or as a way to release inhibitions ("I just want to let loose after a rough day"). Others drink to celebrate special occasions such as the end of the school year, a promotion, or a birthday.

DEVELOPING HEALTH SKILLS

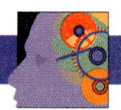

Why College Students Choose to Drink

College students consume alcohol for a variety of reasons. The following list includes some reasons often mentioned by college students. What reasons have you heard for drinking? Check them off on the following list and add any additional reasons you've heard people use. After the list is complete, examine each reason. Is it based on good information? What values influenced the reason the most? Is the reason well thought out, or do you think it is just an excuse for drinking? Do any of the reasons suggest alcohol dependence?

- Drinking makes me accepted by my peers.
- Drinking gives me winning qualities.
- Drinking increases my popularity.
- Drinking reduces tension.
- Drinking makes me sexier.
- Drinking gives me a feeling of power.
- Drinking makes me feel independent.
-
-
-

---

occasional drinker A person who drinks an alcoholic beverage every now and then but seldom consumes enough alcohol to become intoxicated.

intoxicated Consuming enough alcohol to experience its effect. Usually indicated by a high blood alcohol concentration, delayed muscle coordination, and impaired judgment.

social drinker A person who drinks regularly in social settings but seldom consumes enough alcohol to become intoxicated.

Some people, however, do not make a conscious decision to drink. Rather, they drink because of a compulsion to do so because they are addicted to alcohol.

The manner in which a person chooses to drink or the setting in which alcohol is consumed can vary widely and can have many different results. It is not the product—an alcoholic beverage—but rather how and where the product is consumed that determine whether it acts as a relatively harmless beverage or as a drug that may produce serious metabolic changes in the body. Having an occasional drink for social reasons presents quite a different result than binge drinking on an empty stomach for the purpose of getting drunk.

Social Reasons

The risks associated with the consumption of alcohol are determined in part by how much an individual drinks. An **occasional drinker** is a person who drinks an alcoholic beverage once in a while. The occasional drinker seldom becomes **intoxicated.** Such drinking presents little or no threat to the health of the individual. A **social drinker** is someone who drinks regularly in social settings but seldom consumes enough alcohol to become intoxicated. Social drinking, like occasional drinking, does not necessarily increase health risks.

One reason people choose to drink is the peer pressure to do so from friends and acquaintances. Self-reports of the drinking behavior of college students illustrate the strong desire for peer acceptance. According to one study of 120 male students, as reported in the *Journal of Studies on Alcoholism,* the heavier drinkers rated themselves more positively on a range of so-called winning qualities: masculine, successful, sophisticated, strong, mature, sociable, excitable, adventurous, and aggressive. Heavier drinkers rated their nondrinking male classmates more negatively on these social qualities than did lighter drinkers. The men who preferred beer or mixed drinks rated themselves as more drunk—viewed by them as a positive, masculine quality—than did males who preferred wine or nonalcoholic beverages.

Many college students are motivated to drink because they believe that drinking will increase their interpersonal skills, allow them to be more socially assertive, produce feelings of power, and reduce tension. Such logic is erroneous. Drinking does not lead to social assertiveness—in fact, social assertiveness is one of the best means of controlling drinking as you will read later in this chapter. College students may also believe that drinking alcohol will increase sexual feelings. Again, this is erroneous. Studies show that alcohol can result in less sexual arousal. It can cause testosterone levels in men to fall as much as five times below normal and can hinder women's ability to have satisfying interactions with men. If you drink, explore the possible reasons why by completing the Developing Health Skills box on page 210.

Role models who drink—particularly sports heroes and movie stars—are known to influence drinking behavior. Drinking is portrayed as the thing to do by the media, where it is promoted as an important aspect of work and social life.

Advertisements for alcohol are associated with increased consumption among adults and serve as an informal source of information about alcohol for teenagers. However, research is inconclusive on the association between exposure to alcohol ads and consumption of alcohol by younger drinkers.

Culture and Tradition

Drinking is nothing new. Historians trace the use of intoxicating beverages to 6400 B.C. Egyptian physicians included beer and wine in about 15 percent of their prescriptions, according to medical documents dating back to 1500 B.C. Alcohol consumption is evident throughout history, so it should not be surprising to find that many people consume alcohol today because such consumption is culturally ingrained, traditional, or simply taken for granted.

In some cultures, drinking is forbidden, but most ethnic groups and nationalities include alcohol as part of their social and religious lives. Even within ethnic groups, there are wide variances in drinking patterns. For example, the proportion of Native Americans who drink alcohol varies according to the tribe. Some Native American religions forbid the use of alcohol under any circumstance; others use alcohol as a part of their formal religious ceremony.

One tradition found in many cultures is that alcohol is consumed outside the home among peer groups and not in the company of family members. The motivation, at least in part, is social. It is more fun to drink with friends than with parents. But the pattern also suggests a recognition of the potential harm of alcohol consumption and that it is something you do not want to do in front of your parents.

Alcohol Dependence

Perhaps the most health-threatening reason for the consumption of alcohol is dependence on it, despite the user's knowledge of the adverse social and medical

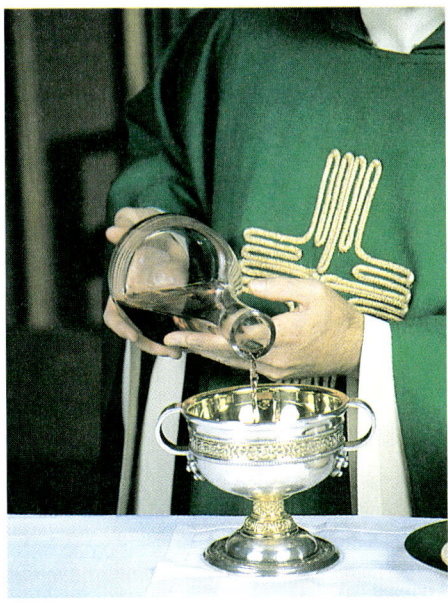

Alcohol is part of many cultural traditions, including religious ceremonies. Some religions, however, forbid the use of any alcohol—even for ceremonial purposes. (Source: © Tony Stone/Myrleen Cate)

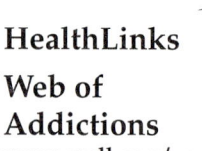

**HealthLinks
Web of
Addictions**
www.well.com/user/woa
Links with various organizations providing information on addictive behaviors, including addiction to the web.

consequences associated with drinking too much. **Alcohol dependence** occurs when a person is so physically attached to alcohol that he or she cannot live comfortably without it. Dependence usually develops over a long period of time and after a pattern of excessive alcohol consumption. In some individuals, however, it may develop in an extremely short time frame and after limited alcohol consumption. The need for alcohol may vary from a mild craving to a compulsion to use the drug.

The term **alcohol addiction** refers to a severe degree of alcohol dependence. The person addicted to alcohol is so dependent on the drug that the acquisition and use of alcohol become the focus of his or her entire life. Virtually all of the negative health effects of alcohol use are found, often to an exaggerated degree, among those who are considered either alcohol dependent or addicted to alcohol.

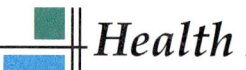

Health Hazards of Alcohol

Alcohol can affect nearly every part of the body. It can alter memory and reflexes, lower sex drive, lead to birth defects, cause heart muscle deterioration, and produce fatal liver damage. Cancers of the tongue, mouth, esophagus, larynx, and liver occur in higher numbers among alcohol users than among nonusers. At the same time, there is evidence that moderate drinking has health benefits. According to the 1995 *Dietary Guidelines for Americans,* moderate drinking—defined as no more than one drink a day for women and no more than two drinks a day for

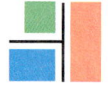

TABLE 9.1   Alcohol and Calories: The Price You Pay

Alcoholic beverages are high in calories but low in nutrients. People who want to lose weight or maintain weight at a desirable level should limit their intake of alcoholic beverages to make room for foods with needed nutrients. The table below gives you an idea of how different alcoholic beverages compare in calories. Pay close attention to serving size when comparing items. A serving of beer is 12 fluid ounces—the size of the average bottle or can—while a serving of wine is only 5 fluid ounces—a little more than one-half cup. How big is *your* wine glass?

Drinks	Approximate calories	Carbonated drinks	Approximate calories
Beer		If you're making a mixed drink, you have to count the calories in the mixer too:	
Regular beer	12 fl. oz. = 150		
Light beer	12 fl. oz. = 95	Fruit-flavored	6 fl. oz. = 90
		Root beer	6 fl. oz. = 80
Liquor	(jigger = 1½ fl. oz.)	Cola	6 fl. oz. = 80
Gin, rum, vodka, and		Ginger ale	6 fl. oz. = 55
whiskey (86-proof)	jigger = 105	Quinine soda	6 fl. oz. = 60
Vermouth, sweet	jigger = 70	Low-calorie soda (contains artificial	
Vermouth, dry	jigger = 55	sweeteners)	6 fl. oz. = 0–1
Wine		Club soda	6 fl. oz. = 0
Sweet	5 fl. oz = 200	**Fruit and vegetable juices**	
Dry table, red	5 fl. oz. = 110	**(unsweetened)**	
Dry table, white	5 fl. oz. = 115	Pineapple	6 fl. oz. = 105
Cordials and liqueurs	jigger = 145	Orange	6 fl. oz. = 90
		Grapefruit	6 fl. oz. = 75
		Tomato	6 fl. oz. = 35

Source: U.S. Department of Agriculture, Human Nutrition Information Service

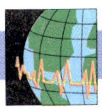

CULTURAL VIEW

The French Experience: Does Red Wine Reduce the Risk for Heart Disease?

Reports on television and elsewhere have said that the French can get away with eating more fat than Americans can because the wine they drink flushes away fat platelets, clearing the arteries and reducing their risk for heart attacks. But experts say this is only part of the story and thus is misleading.

There is a relationship between moderate wine intake (one to three glasses a day) and a reduced risk of heart ailments. But the strikingly lower incidence of heart disease in France suggests something special about the country's wine consumption. One possible explanation is that the French generally consume red wine with meals, slowing its absorption and perhaps prolonging its positive effects.

However, the downside is that the French are prone to other diseases linked to alcohol consumption, such as cancer of the esophagus, stomach cancer, cirrhosis of the liver, and chronic liver disease. The French are also more likely to die in alcohol-related accidents and suicides. Interestingly, the French diet is not all that fatty either. The French tend to eat smaller portions of red meat and other flesh foods; also, their diet is relatively high in fiber and vitamin-rich fruits and vegetables as well as grains.

Apparently, the influence of alcohol on health is far more complicated. In fact, we should be wary of any statement suggesting that the dietary and drinking pattern of another culture is responsible for the reduction of a single disease—without looking at disease and mortality rates overall.

Source: "The French Experience: Does Red Wine Reduce the Risk of Heart Disease?" *Work and Family Life,* October 1992. Reprinted by permission.

---

men—may lower the risk of heart attacks. However, there are many other factors that need to be considered. For example, read the Cultural View box.

Some people think of alcohol as a food because it is consumed in the same manner and often at the same time as food. If it were a food, alcohol would rate poorly. As a food, alcohol provides empty calories in that it is high in calories but low in nutrients (see Table 9.1). Unlike food, it requires no digestion. As noted earlier, it may be absorbed through the stomach and begin circulating in the blood in a matter of minutes.

Central Nervous System Effects

Alcohol has its most significant impact on the central nervous system. It depresses, or slows down, the activities of the central nervous system. Within minutes after consumption, the brain's normal functioning changes. Alcohol alters judgment, increases the time it takes to react to something, reduces muscle control, and affects reasoning.

Alcohol acts primarily on four parts of the brain: the cerebrum, the cerebellum, the thalamus, and the medulla. The **cerebrum** is the part of the brain that is responsible for reasoning and inhibitions. When alcohol sedates this area, thought processes can become disorganized and memory and concentration are dulled. The **cerebellum,** a portion of the brain that contributes to the control of movement, also becomes restricted, often resulting in the impairment of motor processes and quick changes in moods.

The **thalamus** plays a part in controlling the senses. Accordingly, alcohol levels in the blood can affect vision, hearing, smell, taste, and touch. Specifically, it becomes more difficult to hear and see. The **medulla** controls breathing. In extreme cases, drinking can cause impaired respiration and can result in death.

alcohol dependence When a person is so physically attached to alcohol that he or she cannot live comfortably without it.

alcohol addiction Extensive dependence on alcohol; this dependence is so acute that the acquisition and use of alcohol becomes the focus of everyday life.

cerebrum The part of the brain responsible for reasoning and inhibitions.

cerebellum The portion of the brain that contributes to the control of movement.

thalamus The part of the brain that plays a part in controlling the senses.

medulla The part of the brain that controls breathing.

Alcohol may produce a feeling of relaxation and may reduce **inhibitions.** Inhibitions are controls placed on emotions and behaviors. Once inhibitions are reduced, people may say and do things they would normally never consider. For example, a person under the influence of alcohol may express anger in a violent or destructive manner or may practice unsafe sex.

Some people believe that alcohol is an aphrodisiac, but this is a myth. In small amounts, it may decrease inhibitions and make a person more relaxed about sex. As alcohol intake increases, however, it reduces sexual interest.

A **hangover** is characterized by nausea, upset stomach, anxiety, and a headache. The symptoms normally appear a few hours after heavy drinking and disappear over time. Hangovers have no permanent damaging effect. Contrary to some beliefs, there are no quick cures for a hangover. Coffee is a stimulant, and drinking a cup or two is just the opposite of what your body needs, which is rest. Taking two aspirin will not help, either. Aspirin does not speed up the rate at which the alcohol in your body is metabolized. Only after the alcohol is completely out of your body will you lose your headache. So only time will cure a hangover.

Blackouts may occur with almost any level of alcohol in the body, although they usually are experienced by people who have consumed high levels of alcohol and/or are intoxicated. A blackout is a temporary form of **amnesia.** The individual appears to be conscious of what he or she is doing but the next day cannot remember much or any of what happened. Blackouts are a clear warning sign of problem drinking.

One of the most serious central nervous system impairments is the Wernicke-Korsakoff syndrome, a form of alcohol amnesia and personality disorder. It usually is not reversible. Other mental disorders associated with alcohol use are alcohol psychosis, delirium tremens (DTs), and acute alcoholic hallucinosis.

Liver Problems

Alcohol is processed by the liver. It eventually handles virtually all the alcohol in the bloodstream, but it does so at a constant pace—usually about 0.5 to 1 ounce per hour. This is why the amount of alcohol consumed is directly related to how long it takes a person to become intoxicated.

Cirrhosis of the liver is a condition that is seven times more common in heavy drinkers than in nondrinkers and results at least in part from the strain placed on the liver by excessive amounts of alcohol. What happens is that blood is diverted to those areas of the liver that are processing the alcohol. Cells in other parts of the liver are deprived of blood and eventually die. The process of filling in these regions with scar tissue leads to cirrhosis. Although the incidence of cirrhosis has been declining in recent years, it began to rise in 1994 and is among the top ten leading causes of death of adults in the United States.

Fetal Alcohol Syndrome

Most substances that circulate in the blood of a pregnant woman can pass through the placenta and enter the fetus. Alcohol is one such substance. It diffuses readily through the placental membranes and into the fetus's circulation system. Because alcohol is present in fetal blood in about the same concentration as in maternal blood, the amount of alcohol that a pregnant woman drinks is an important indicator of the risk for birth defects.

A pregnant woman who drinks moderately (four or five drinks per week) has a much higher chance of having a spontaneous abortion or a low-birth-weight infant than a pregnant woman who does not drink. Moderate amounts of drinking during pregnancy may affect the fetus—a malady referred to as **fetal alcohol effect (FAE).**

---

inhibitions Self-imposed controls on emotions and behavior intended to assure socially acceptable interactions with others.

hangover A condition caused by excess alcohol consumption and characterized by nausea, upset stomach, anxiety, and a headache.

blackout A temporary form of amnesia in which the individual appears to be conscious of what he or she is doing but later cannot remember much if any of what happened.

amnesia Partial or total loss of memory.

cirrhosis of the liver A disease in which scar tissue replaces normal liver tissue and interferes with the liver's ability to function.

fetal alcohol effect (FAE) Impairment of fetal development linked to the mother's use of alcohol during pregnancy; may include some of the attributes of fetal alcohol syndrome.

fetal alcohol syndrome (FAS) A birth defect caused by alcohol consumption during pregnancy that is characterized by mental retardation, poor motor coordination, hyperactivity in childhood, facial deformities, and other abnormalities.

Large amounts of alcohol consumption by a pregnant woman significantly increase the risk for having a baby who has **fetal alcohol syndrome (FAS).** This syndrome includes irreversible mental retardation, poor motor coordination, hyperactivity in childhood, facial deformities, and other abnormalities. It is the third leading cause of birth defects accompanied by mental retardation, and it is the only one of the top three causes of birth defects that is preventable.

Critical Thinking Question

Fetal alcohol effect and fetal alcohol syndrome have an impact that reaches far beyond the individual and his or her family. These tragic but preventable birth defects affect the schools, the medical care system, and, in some cases, law enforcement. Should the use of alcohol during pregnancy be criminalized? If not, how can the best interests of the individual, as well as the public, be protected against alcohol-related birth defects?

Not all women who drink abusively during pregnancy have babies who suffer fetal alcohol syndrome. Little is known about this, but it is thought that some fetuses may be genetically more susceptible to alcohol damage than others; conversely, some maternal factors may produce a protective effect. Susceptibility to fetal alcohol syndrome might be related to a mother's previous history of drinking problems and the beverage consumed. Studies indicate that although all alcoholic beverages pose a risk to developing fetuses, heavy beer consumption during pregnancy seems to be associated with an even greater risk. Binge drinking, even for relatively brief periods of time, has been clearly associated with the development of fetal alcohol syndrome.

More than 16 percent of American women drink at some point when they are pregnant. Because a safe level of alcohol consumption during pregnancy is not known, the office of the Surgeon General, the National Council on Alcoholism and Drug Dependence, and other health-related groups recommend complete abstinence during this time.

Drinking and Death

In contrast to the chronic health conditions discussed above, which develop over time, sometimes drinking too much can result in immediate death. A single dose of alcohol, if large enough, can be lethal. During freshman hazing season in the fall, usually several students die each year from alcohol poisoning. For example, one freshman died of alcohol poisoning after drinking a gallon of wine in forty-five minutes during a hazing session. As with most depressant drugs, death due to alcohol poisoning usually results from respiratory failure. Generally a blood alcohol concentration of 0.40 percent is considered lethal, but some persons may be at risk for alcohol poisoning at a lower level.

Alcohol use is also linked to suicide, homicide, and other violent deaths. Alcoholics are about thirty times more likely to commit suicide than is the general population. According to the National Council on Alcoholism and Drug Dependence, thirty-five thousand deaths occur annually from alcohol-related homicides, suicides, and non–motor vehicle accidents, such as drownings and fires. Nearly half of those who die in fires are legally drunk at the time of death, and alcohol is probably an important risk factor for fire and burn injuries associated with cigarette smoking. In general, drinking does not mix well with recreational or work activities. More than two-thirds of drownings and fatal falls and two-fifths of work accidents are alcohol related.

Critical Thinking Question

Healthy People 2000 contains the following objective: "Extend to 50 states legal blood alcohol concentration tolerance levels of 0.08 percent for motor vehicle drivers aged 21 and older and zero tolerance (0.02 percent and lower) for those younger than age 21." Currently, only eleven states use tolerance levels of 0.08 for adult drivers, and twenty-one states use a zero tolerance policy concerning under-age drivers. Is this goal realistic? Is it an effective means of reducing deaths and injury due to automobile crashes? Does it represent an excessive infringement on personal freedom?

Perhaps the most life-threatening use of alcohol occurs when an individual chooses to drink and then to drive (see Figure 9.1). Alcohol is closely linked with about 40 percent of all traffic fatalities, or an estimated 13,000 motor vehicle deaths each year; in addition, millions more are injured. Generally, the risk of motor vehicle accidents increases in proportion to the **blood alcohol concentration (BAC)** of the driver. All of these statistics are based on the tragedies of real people who have hurt or been hurt because of alcohol-related injuries and deaths. One such person is the founder of Mothers Against Drunk Driving (MADD), whose daughter died because of a drunk driver. Read about the citizen

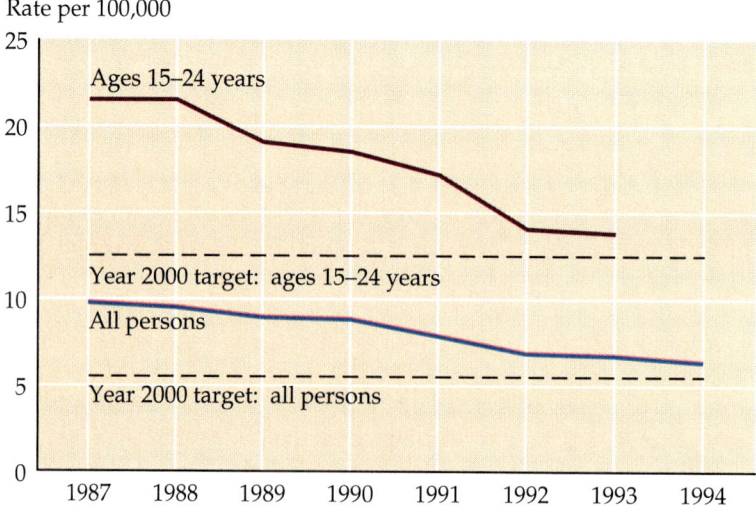

Figure 9.1 Alcohol-Related Motor Vehicle Crash Deaths: United States, 1987–94, and Year 2000 Targets. *(Source: U.S. Department of Transportation, Fatal Accident Reporting System)*

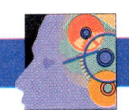

DEVELOPING HEALTH SKILLS

Speaking Out Against Drinking and Driving

A growing number of citizen groups are concerned about drunk driving. The goals of these groups are to make people aware of the problem and to make it socially unacceptable for anyone to drink and then drive.

Mothers Against Drunk Driving (MADD) was started by Candy Lightner, whose daughter Cari was killed by a drunk driver near her home in Fair Oaks, California. The driver was not only drunk but also had a prior arrest for hit-and-run driving and drunk driving and had been released from custody on bail only two days before killing Cari. MADD was formed to protest a judicial system that allows someone with an extensive history of drunk driving to continue to drive. As a national organization, MADD has been successful in reducing the legal blood alcohol concentration in various states.

Students Against Driving Drunk (SADD) started as part of a health education program at Wayland High School near Boston, Massachusetts, after two high school students were killed by a drunk driver. Now called Students Against Destructive Decisions, SADD educates students about the problem of drinking and driving and develops peer counseling programs for students about alcohol use. Perhaps its most important contribution to opening communication about drinking between parents and teenagers is its "Contract for Life," in which both parties agree to a lifestyle of safe, sober driving. SADD has adapted this for college students, expanding it beyond sober driving to include other safe lifestyle decisions.

COLLEGE CONTRACT FOR LIFE

Between Friends

STUDENTS AGAINST DESTRUCTIVE DECISIONS

As students at _____, we recognize that we will be faced with many decisions. Throughout our college experience we might have to deal with issues such as alcohol and drug use, AIDS, sexuality, date rape, drunk driving, relationships, and many more confusing subjects.

Therefore we have entered into a contract in which we agree that we will always attempt to choose the best option considering our own well-being, health, and safety. In addition, we will confront any of our friends that we see making destructive decisions and help them find any assistance they need.

If I find myself in a situation that makes me uncomfortable or that I feel unequipped to handle, I will discuss this with someone I trust.

_____   _____
signature of 1st party   signature of 2nd party

_____   _____
date   date

Students Against Destructive Decisions • Inc.

SADD and all SADD logos are registered with th. United States Patent and Trademark Office and other jurisdictions. All rights reserved by SADD Inc. a Massachusetts non-profit corporation. Copying of this material is prohibited unless written permission received. SADD, Inc. sponsors Students Against Driving Drunk, Students Against Destructive Decisions and other health and safety programs.

SADD, Inc., P.O. Box 800 Marlborough, MA 01752, Tel. 508-481-3568 • 508-945-5122

Source: The "College Contract for Life" is reprinted by permission of Students Against Destructive Decisions (SADD)

---

action groups called MADD and SADD (Students Against Destructive Decisions) in the Developing Health Skills box.

Teenagers are particularly at risk for drinking and driving, in part because they often do not recognize the consequences of their actions. Unfortunately, statistics clearly link teenage drinking and driving with morbidity and mortality. For example, 62 percent of motor vehicle accidents involve sixteen- to nineteen-year-olds having measurable blood alcohol levels, and alcohol-related motor vehicle accidents are the leading cause of death among Americans aged fifteen to twenty-four. Fortunately, though, young people are getting the message, and the number of alcohol-related deaths of fifteen- to twenty-four-year-olds is dropping.

blood alcohol concentration (BAC)
A measure of the amount of alcohol in the blood.

Alcoholism as a Disease

Controversy exists among researchers concerning **alcoholism.** Is it an addictive behavior like cocaine addiction? Is there a hereditary or environmental link? For whatever reason, of adults who drink today, 7 to 10 percent will become chronic alcoholics within fifteen to twenty years from the time they began to drink. It is possible to become an alcoholic in a shorter period of time, and many college-age students are already addicted. Further, there has been considerable controversy in the past over the actual definition of alcoholism. Much of this controversy, however, was laid to rest with a definition of alcoholism developed in 1992 by the National Council on Alcoholism and Drug Dependence and the American Society of Addiction Medicine.

Defining Terms

Although alcoholism is referred to as a single disease, it is in fact a syndrome—a constellation of symptoms that can lead to death. In the same way that the term *cardiovascular disease* refers not to a specific disease but to a variety of diseases, *alcoholism* refers to a number of health problems related to the uncontrolled use of alcohol. Because drinking gets more and more out of control, alcoholism is a progressive disease. Each of these factors was taken into consideration when a new definition of alcoholism was developed. The 1992 definition acknowledges genetic, psychosocial, and environmental factors in alcoholism and at the same time emphasizes behavioral aspects, including denial.

In 1976, the official council and society definition of alcoholism read:

Alcoholism is a chronic, progressive, and potentially fatal disease. It is characterized by tolerance and physical dependency or pathologic organ changes or both.

In contrast, the 1992 definition read:

Alcoholism is a primary, chronic disease with genetic, psychosocial, and environmental factors influencing its development and manifestations. The disease is often progressive and fatal. It is characterized by impaired control over drinking, preoccupation with the drug alcohol, use of alcohol despite adverse consequences, and distortions in thinking, most notably denial.

Additional terms are associated with alcoholism. The American Psychiatric Association, in its *Diagnostic and Statistical Manual of Mental Disorders IV—Revised,* defines **alcohol abuse** as a pattern of pathological use of alcohol that results in impaired social or occupational functioning. Alcohol dependence, according to the psychiatric manual, is manifested by an individual's **tolerance** for alcohol and **withdrawal symptoms** that are relieved by drinking after a period of cessation of or reduction in drinking.

Tolerance is the progressive change in the body's reaction to alcohol causing an individual to need more and more alcohol in order to achieve the same mood-modifying effects. A high tolerance for alcohol does not necessarily mean that an individual is alcohol dependent, but it is a common precursor to addiction. A person who develops a physical need for alcohol usually experiences withdrawal symptoms when alcohol is not present in the body. These symptoms range from mild discomfort at first to very traumatic events, including DTs, seizures, and hallucinations.

Alcoholism begins gradually, when the casual or social drinker becomes a **problem drinker.** Using alcohol in a manner that causes physical, psychological, or social harm to the drinker or others is considered problem drinking. A problem drinker is in need of help but has not totally lost control over his or her drinking behavior. The problem drinker retains the ability to choose to drink or not to

---

alcoholism A progressive disease related to the uncontrolled use of alcohol that interferes with the drinker's health and social functioning.

alcohol abuse A pattern of pathological use of alcohol that results in impaired social or occupational functioning.

tolerance The progressive change in the body's reaction to a drug, causing an individual to need more and more of the drug to achieve the same effect.

withdrawal symptoms The symptoms ranging from mild discomfort to very traumatic events when a drug is not present in the body.

problem drinker A person who uses alcohol in a manner that causes physical, psychological, or social harm to the drinker and/or others.

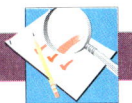

HERE'S LOOKING AT YOU

A Self-Assessment of Your Drinking

	Yes	No
1. Are you unable to stop drinking after a certain number of drinks?	___	___
2. Do you need a drink to get motivated?	___	___
3. Do you often forget what happened while you were "partying" (have blackouts)?	___	___
4. Do you drink or "party" alone?	___	___
5. Have others annoyed you by criticizing your alcohol use?	___	___
6. Have you been involved in fights with your friends or family while you were drunk?	___	___
7. Have you done or said anything while drinking that you later regretted?	___	___
8. Have you destroyed or damaged property while drinking?	___	___
9. Do you drive while drunk?	___	___
10. Have you been physically hurt while drinking?	___	___
11. Have you been in trouble with the school authorities or the campus police because of your drinking?	___	___
12. Have you dropped or chosen friends based on their drinking habits?	___	___
13. Do you think you are a normal drinker despite friends' comments that you drink too much?	___	___
14. Have you ever missed classes because you were too hung over to get up on time?	___	___
15. Have you ever done poorly on an exam or assignment because of drinking?	___	___
16. Do you think about drinking a lot?	___	___
17. Do you feel guilty or self-conscious about your drinking?	___	___

If you answered yes to three or more of these questions, or if your answer to any of the questions concerns you, you may be using alcohol in ways that are harmful. Do not waste your time blaming yourself for past binges or any other alcohol-related behavior. If you think you have or might be developing problems in which drinking plays a part, act now. You can get help.

For more information and counseling, contact your campus health or counseling center community mental health facility, or Alcoholics Anonymous (AA). Information about local AA meetings may be available from your local library or telephone directory as well as from the national AA office at P.O. Box 459, Grand Central Station, New York, NY 10163; telephone: (212) 686-1100.

Source: Reprinted from *Alcohol: Decisions on Tap* with permission from the American College Health Association, P.O. Box 28937, Baltimore, MD 21240–8937

---

drink, how much to drink, and in what situations to drink. Such an individual is completely capable of stopping drinking prior to becoming intoxicated but often chooses not to. An alcoholic is someone who has lost at least some, and often total, control over his or her drinking behavior. You can assess your drinking behavior by responding to the questions posed in the Here's Looking at You box.

The Role of Genetics and the Environment

Researchers looking for a genetic link to alcoholism have found a lot of evidence, but no one gene. Rather, it is likely that alcoholism can be controlled by a major genetic effect involving a number of genes located at two or more chromosome locations.

Particularly compelling data supporting a genetic linkage come from studies of sons of alcoholic mothers or fathers who had been adopted by other families at an early age. These sons have about a threefold greater chance of becoming alcohol abusers or alcoholics than do adopted sons of nonalcoholics. Because most of the alcoholic adoptees studied had been separated from their biological parents within the first few months of life, they presumably were removed from any of the predisposing environmental influences of an alcoholic home. Other studies show abnormal brain patterns among both young sons of alcoholics and their fathers. These abnormalities are present in the sons long before they begin to drink.

Studies on twins also suggest a strong genetic link. Researchers believe that if vulnerability to alcoholism has a genetic basis, identical twins—who are genetically alike—should tend to develop more similar drinking patterns and problems than would fraternal twins—who are no more genetically alike than nontwin siblings.

In a review of current research, the National Institute of Alcohol Abuse and Alcoholism reports that the **concordance rate** (which indicates the extent to which a trait is found in both membesr of a twin pair) for alcohol abuse, alcohol dependence, or both is 0.76 for identical twin males and 0.61 for fraternal twin males. The concordance rate is 0.36 for identical twin females and 0.25 for fraternal twin females. (A concordance rate of 0.5 indicates that when one member of a pair expresses a trait, the other member also expresses the trait in 50 percent of the cases.) The differences between identical and fraternal twins is even more dramatic when looking at alcohol dependence only. In this case, concordance rates are 0.59 for identical twin males and 0.36 for fraternal twin males and 0.25 for identical twin females and 0.05 for fraternal twin females.

Does this settle the case for a genetic component? Not entirely. Environment alone can cause it too. More than 35 percent of alcoholics have no family history of alcohol abuse. Alcohol abuse among the homeless in the United States—clearly an extreme environmental factor—ranges between 20 and 45 percent.

A significant relationship has been found between a person's self-esteem and alcoholism. Researchers have found that alcoholics often have dependent personalities and lack a good self-image. However, many people who have low self-esteem never become alcoholics. It is not clear how, if at all, self-esteem relates to genetic factors. It is now widely accepted by researchers in the field that alcoholism can result from the interaction of heredity and environment.

Treatment Options

A variety of treatment programs and approaches are designed to help the alcoholic control his or her disease. More than half a million people are in treatment on any one day in the year. Hospitals and private facilities offer services for alcoholics and their families, including detoxification, drug treatment, and social support. These services are available on an inpatient and outpatient basis.

For many alcoholics, the first step in the treatment process is **detoxification.** This process of removing all alcohol from the person's body is usually an inpatient treatment conducted in a hospital or similar medical facility. The complete process can take days, or even weeks, depending on the amount of alcohol the individual has consumed. During detoxification, the alcoholic experiences withdrawal symptoms. These can be extremely dangerous; medical attention therefore is important. Once alcohol has been removed from the body, other treatments are possible.

Drug treatment for alcoholism has been attempted for many years and with a variety of drugs, including tranquilizers and antidepressants. To date, no one drug appears to be the answer. Disulfiram (Antabuse) is a widely prescribed drug and has been required by courts for some cases involving alcohol abuse. It

concordance rate   The extent to which a trait is found in both members of a twin pair.

detoxification   The process of removing all alcohol from an individual's body.

Alcoholics Anonymous   A member organization of recovering alcoholics who provide social support for avoiding the use of alcohol.

abstinence   The choice of not consuming alcoholic beverages in any form.

codependency   A relationship in which one person contributes to another person's dysfunctional behavior by accepting it or masking it from others.

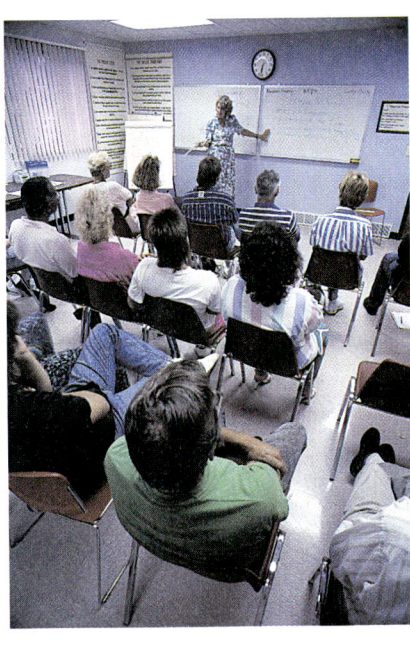
Members of Alcoholics Anonymous (AA) meet regularly with the goal of attaining sobriety one day at a time. (Source: FPG International/© Terry Quing)

causes severe reactions to the ingestion of alcohol, including nausea, vomiting, accelerated heart rate, and severe dizziness. Disulfiram has demonstrated some effectiveness with alcoholics who voluntarily enter a drug therapy program. Similar results, however, have not been produced when the alcoholic involuntarily enters a program.

Perhaps the most widely known and successful treatment program is **Alcoholics Anonymous.** AA, as it is commonly called, is a self-help approach for the problem drinker. Members are required to admit that they are alcoholics and that they desire to stay sober while helping other alcoholics do the same. The goal of AA is sobriety—not for a lifetime but for one day at a time.

The focal point for the more than 750,000 members of AA in the United States is its meetings. In the Washington, D.C., area alone, AA sponsors about 1,100 meetings a week. Evidence exists that attendance at AA meetings is positively correlated with maintaining **abstinence.** A review of the literature on outcomes in AA suggests that between 26 and 50 percent of its members are fully abstinent after one year of sobriety.

Al-Anon and Alateen are social support programs for the family members of alcoholics. There are also social support groups specifically for adult children of alcoholics. There are 28 million children of alcoholics in the United States. These youngsters grow up in drastically different home environments than do children of nonalcoholics. Many are haunted by a sense of failure because they could not save mommy or daddy. Children of alcoholics are more likely than the general population either to become alcoholics or to marry alcoholics or other troubled people. This may be because they are familiar with the life associated with having an alcoholic family member and may be willing to accept an alcoholic's behavior. This is called **codependency.** A codependent person contributes to another person's dysfunctional behavior by accepting it or masking it from others. Children of alcoholics and family members need help coping with the alcoholic's behavior. They also need support in better understanding their own problems, which often include low self-esteem, excessive feelings of responsibility, difficulties reaching out, and depression.

No matter what the form of treatment, abstinence from alcohol has long been regarded as a major goal. One of the most controversial topics in alcoholism treatment is whether alcoholics can go back to social drinking once they are cured. Moderation Management (MM) is a treatment program and support

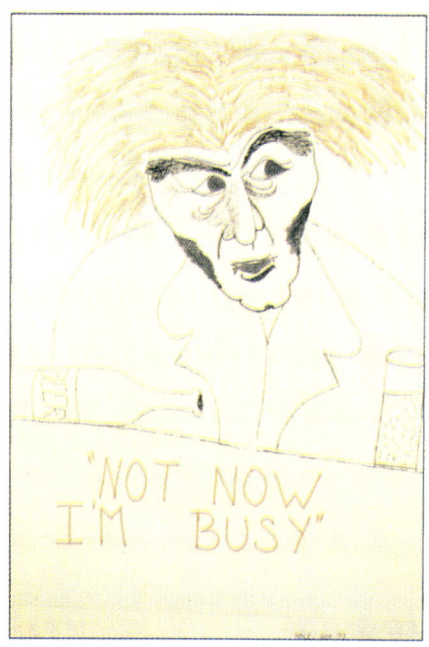
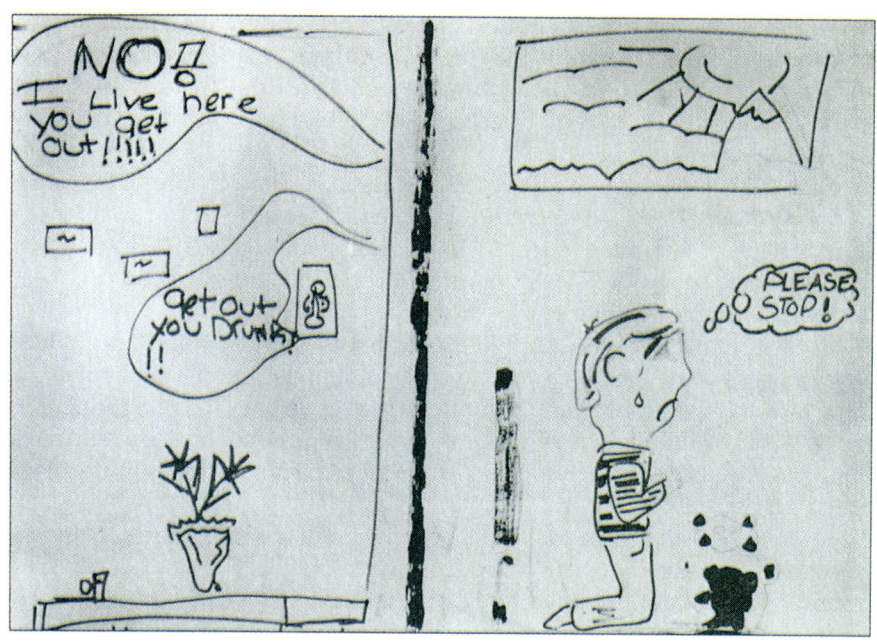

Children of alcoholics are familiar with the problems associated with drinking and want to help their parents. As can be seen in these sketches by children of alcoholics, there can be emotional effects. Children of alcoholics are at greater risk of becoming alcoholics or marrying alcoholics than is the general population. (Source: Courtesy of Children of Alcoholics. Used with permission)

group for problem drinkers that is based on the belief that some—but not all—people who abuse alcohol can learn to moderate their drinking. MM begins with thirty days of abstinence followed by limits on how much alcohol can be consumed in any one week. The number of problem drinkers who can learn to drink in moderation is believed to be very small—between 4 percent and 14 percent of those who try it. Critics of MM point out that most of the people who try it will not succeed and may be tempted to resume drinking; if they had gone to AA instead, they might have achieved sobriety.

The bulk of clinical evidence appears to support the interpretation that once significant physical dependence has occurred, the alcoholic no longer has the option of returning to social drinking. Relapse occurs in most cases when an alcoholic begins drinking socially, and given the high mortality rates for alcoholics who continue to misuse alcohol, relapse can be serious. Given this, abstinence remains the most appropriate goal for alcoholics.

Controlling Access to Alcohol

The effects of alcohol use and alcoholism have been known for generations, and many approaches have been undertaken to control access to alcohol. At one time, it was thought that limiting access to alcohol would adequately control its consumption. The Eighteenth Amendment to the Constitution, passed in 1919 and effective one year later, prohibited the manufacture, sale, or transport of intoxicating liquors in the United States. Until the amendment was repealed in 1933, it caused more harm than good. During the period popularly called **Prohibition,** the use of alcohol did not cease. In fact, the amendment produced social problems far beyond expectations. Because people were unable to buy alcoholic products whose quality was controlled by responsible manufacturers, they drank impure liquids sometimes containing methyl alcohol, which resulted in blindness and death. In addition, contempt for the law developed, and bootlegging, organized crime, and other illegal activities flourished. It also set back scientific research on alcoholism by decades.

Critical Thinking Question

> Why do you think Prohibition was such a failure? Can you think of similar laws that have not met with such resistance and that have been successful in controlling the use of substances by the general public? Are there drugs for which another Prohibition should be considered? Is alcohol one of those drugs?

Legal age restrictions are one remnant of the prohibition concept. As stated earlier, every state requires that a person be twenty-one years old in order to purchase alcohol. In reality, alcohol products are widely available to young people. Although it is illegal to do so, many college students obtain fake IDs proving that they are of age. Another age-related restriction relates to the level of alcohol in the blood of minors. Six states (Arizona, Illinois, Oklahoma, Oregon, Utah, and Wisconsin) have legislation making it illegal for minors who drive to have any amount of alcohol in their blood. This is called a blood alcohol concentration (BAC) of 0.00 percent.

Another remnant of the prohibition concept is a dry county ordinance. In counties that have passed such a law, alcoholic beverages cannot be sold to the general public. Easily acquired club memberships, however, can make alcohol available in these counties.

A higher tax on alcohol products has been cited as another way to restrict accessibility, but because alcohol remains so inexpensive relative to other consumer items, an increased tax is not likely to deter anyone from buying it. In fact, the relative cost of alcohol has declined substantially over the last twenty years. The cost of nonalcoholic beverages has increased four times over, and the cost of all consumer goods has almost tripled since 1967. Over the same period, the cost of alcohol has not even doubled.

Despite public health policies and laws limiting access to alcohol or making it prohibitively expensive, drinks continue to be served in most restaurants, and alcohol continues to be available in convenience stores seven days a week. Most

Prohibition A period of time in U.S. history when the manufacture, sale, or transport of intoxicating liquors was prohibited by law.

homes have at least some alcoholic beverage on hand. The prevention of problem drinking, therefore, has not been successfully accomplished by limiting access to alcohol. Perhaps it can be accomplished through individual choice. The choice not to drink—or to drink wisely—may boil down to the skill with which each person interacts with the drinking culture.

HEALTH SKILLS

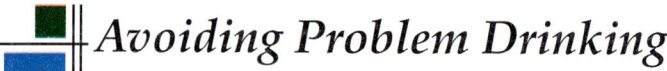
Avoiding Problem Drinking

Avoiding the problems associated with the consumption of alcohol is not complicated. It does, however, require basic knowledge of the effects of alcohol on the body, knowledge of how those effects can be minimized, and the skills needed to handle the social settings in which alcohol consumption takes place.

Practice Not Drinking

You have probably heard, and even made fun of, the saying "Just say no to drugs." Actually, this saying has its origin in reality. The most obvious and effective means of avoiding problem drinking is simply not to drink. Not drinking, often referred to as abstinence, is practiced by a large percentage of the population as a means of avoiding problem drinking. Two options are widely practiced: **total abstinence,** to abstain from alcohol use at all times, and **situational abstinence,** to abstain from alcohol use in situations in which use would present a risk.

People who totally abstain from alcohol use do so for a variety of reasons, including the following:

- Their religion forbids it.
- They have an allergic reaction to some of the components in alcohol products.
- They have a genetic predisposition to problem drinking.
- They are aware of the health and social effects of drinking and do not want to have anything to do with it.
- They simply do not like the taste or smell of alcohol.

Situational abstinence is far more prevalent. One common situation in which it is not appropriate to drink alcohol is just before driving. The reasons for this are obvious: to avoid a potential automobile crash and to obey the law. Another situation in which abstinence is appropriate is when entering a risky social situation, such as a party where there is a lot of drinking. As you have read, alcohol is a contributing factor in unwanted sexual practices, including unprotected sex and date rape. Abstinence can help reduce the risks associated with such situations.

Pace Your Drinking

If you choose to drink, there are some practices that can help you drink wisely and reduce the risks of drinking. One important practice is to pace the amount of alcohol you consume. By doing so, you can avoid intoxication and the problems that result.

When alcohol is consumed at the pace of one drink per hour, the body is generally able to process the alcohol. One drink is measured as one and a half ounces of eighty-proof liquor, five ounces of 12 percent wine, or twelve ounces of five percent beer (this usually means one jigger of liquor, one glass of wine, or one bottle of beer). **Proof** refers to the percentage of pure alcohol in a beverage. The percentage of alcohol is half the proof: 40 percent alcohol is 80 proof.

total abstinence The choice never to consume alcoholic beverages.

situational abstinence The choice not to consume alcoholic beverages in situations in which the consumption of alcohol would present a health risk.

proof The percentage of pure alcohol in a beverage; the percentage of alcohol is half the proof.

Having one drink results in a 0.01 percent alcohol concentration in the blood of a 150-pound man (see Table 9.2). In one hour, nearly all the alcohol from one drink is eliminated from the blood through sweating, respiration, urination, and metabolism in the liver. Four drinks consumed within a one-hour period could raise the BAC to 0.07, and six drinks could bring it up to 0.11. It takes a person more than six hours to eliminate six ounces of alcohol from the blood.

Alcohol begins to influence the brain, vision, and decision making at BAC levels of 0.02, and from this point on, driving is impaired. Between 0.10 and 0.20, an individual may have difficulty walking a straight line or touching his or her fingers together, two common tests used during highway sobriety checks. Blood concentration levels of 0.40 can be lethal.

Be Aware of the Full Stomach Factor

Before you drink, make sure you have had something to eat. Drinking on a full stomach has a different effect than drinking on an empty stomach. Alcohol is diluted by the stomach juices and is very quickly distributed throughout the body. The rate of absorption depends on the type of beverage, how much is consumed, and how full the stomach is. Alcohol consumed on an empty stomach may be absorbed directly through the stomach wall into the bloodstream. The fuller the stomach, the longer it takes alcohol to be absorbed. When alcohol mixes

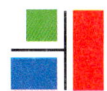

TABLE 9.2 Blood Alcohol Concentration (BAC): A Measure of Drunk Driving

Within minutes after having a drink, the brain's normal functioning is changed. One measure of how your brain, vision, and decision making might be impaired is how much alcohol is in your blood. This is called the blood alcohol concentration.

Your Weight	Number of drinks (over a two-hour period) 1.5 oz. 80 proof liquor or 12 oz. can of beer
100	1 2 3 4 5 6 7 8 9 10 11 12
120	1 2 3 4 5 6 7 8 9 10 11 12
140	1 2 3 4 5 6 7 8 9 10 11 12
160	1 2 3 4 5 6 7 8 9 10 11 12
180	1 2 3 4 5 6 7 8 9 10 11 12
200	1 2 3 4 5 6 7 8 9 10 11 12
220	1 2 3 4 5 6 7 8 9 10 11 12
240	1 2 3 4 5 6 7 8 9 10 11 12

Social	Warning	Intoxicated
Drive with caution BAC to 0.05%	Driving impaired 0.05–0.09%	Do not drive 0.10% and up

This table is only a guide. Information presented is based on averages and may vary according to particular circumstances or from individual to individual.

Source: U.S. Department of Transportation, National Highway Traffic Safety Administration

with food, it passes more slowly into the small intestine and from it into the blood. Foods high in protein and carbohydrates—cheese and meats—are especially good snacks to serve with drinks. Drinking after a complete meal slows the absorption of alcohol into the blood by as much as 50 percent. On the other hand, alcohol taken together with carbonated beverages—gin and tonic, rum and coke, scotch and soda—is usually absorbed more rapidly.

Don't Mix Alcohol and Drugs

Perhaps the most important concept to understand about the consumption of alcohol is that it is a drug. And when two drugs are mixed, dangerous results can occur.

The **synergistic effects** of alcohol plus another drug—even if the other drug is prescribed or obtained over-the-counter at the pharmacy—can be disastrous. Synergism means that the whole is greater than the sum of its parts. When this concept is applied to drug use, it means that when the effects of one drug, for example, alcohol, are added to the effects of another drug, such as a barbiturate, the combined impact of the two drugs is greater than would be expected if each drug's effects were simply added together. You might say that synergism means that 2 + 2 = 7. The hazard of synergistic effect is especially important to the elderly because many of them take prescription drugs.

Antihistamines and other cold medications induce drowsiness to begin with. When combined with another depressant such as alcohol, side effects are increased and driving becomes even more dangerous. Sedatives, antidepressants, or antianxiety drugs plus alcohol can depress the central nervous system to the point of coma, respiratory arrest, and death.

Be Socially Assertive

Because drinking is most often a social activity, the primary skill necessary for reducing the health risk of alcohol is social assertiveness. The most effective way to be socially assertive is to know exactly how much alcohol you will consume before entering into a social situation where drinking takes place. By doing so, you are assured that your limits are based on clear thinking, not social pressure. You need to decide how you will answer the following questions:

- How much are you going to drink (e.g., no more than two)?
- How fast will you have those drinks (e.g., no more than one an hour)?
- Under what conditions are you going to drink?
- What type of alcohol will you drink? Different alcoholic beverages contain different quantities of alcohol. Four ounces of wine produce less effect on you than four ounces of hard liquor.
- With whom are you going to drink?
- With whom are you *not* willing to drink?
- How will you get home after attending a function where you have been drinking?

Once you have made your decisions and set limits on your drinking, stick to them. If you don't set limits for yourself, make sure someone else in your group sets limits for him- or herself. Identify a designated driver—someone who agrees not to consume alcohol during the evening and who will drive you and the others who do drink home. Some bars provide nonalcoholic beverages free to designated drivers—a positive incentive to avoid the risk of driving under the influence of alcohol. One national beer company pays for a taxi service that takes people home from a party if they are unable to drive. In a growing number of states, courts have held that if a person leaves a party drunk, gets in a car, and is

---

HealthLinks

Mothers Against Drunk Driving
www.gran-net.com/madd/madd.htm

Link to the national organization dedicated to eliminating drinking and driving.

---

synergistic effect Occurs when two or more substances present at the same time result in a total effect much greater than the sum of the effects of each substance.

involved in a crash, the host or hostess can be held liable. Restaurants and bars in many states are also legally responsible for drunk patrons.

Assertively maintain the conditions under which you are willing to drink. If someone attempts to force you to drink at a faster pace than you have decided is safe for you, say, "Not tonight. I am not willing to take the risk." If someone attempts to get you to drive after drinking, say, "Not tonight. I am not willing to take the risk." While you may feel socially uncomfortable, in the long run you will avoid the health risks associated with alcohol use. The paraplegic college student injured by a drunk driver would suggest that it is far better to feel a little socially uncomfortable than not to feel at all.

Prevention: The Ultimate Answer

Preventing health and social problems associated with alcohol use is a major personal and public health task. Prevention programs for college students are designed to raise awareness of the dangers of alcohol abuse and encourage the social skills needed to avoid alcohol abuse. Many colleges have an office for alcohol abuse prevention where students can get this information. In addition, National Collegiate Alcohol Awareness Week is held on many campuses across the country every fall. Some schools hold meetings on campus about university regulations concerning alcohol and work with bars in the community to enforce drinking-age laws and to require servers to have alcohol abuse awareness training.

The risk factors of alcohol use change somewhat with age and, accordingly, so do the prevention messages. Many prevention efforts for children take into account risk factors related to taking the first drink because alcohol use is not widespread in this age group. Risk factors related to children include a family history of alcoholism and/or antisocial behavior or other indicators of family dysfunction. It is interesting to note the importance of family in these risk factors. Adolescents tend to be influenced much more by peers than by family members, and effective prevention programs for teenagers often involve teaching skills to prepare them for situations that involve peer pressure to use alcohol.

If alcohol abuse were prevented in the first place, the difficult and costly road to recovery for alcoholics could be avoided. The number of alcohol-related auto crashes could be reduced. The number of alcohol-related traumas, including date rape, could be reduced. The best hope is that prevention strategies will collectively create a climate, for children and college students alike, in which alcohol consumption in the years to come does not lead to the extensive and costly public health problems seen in today's society.

Key Concepts

1. Approximately 60 percent of the adult population drinks. Studies of college populations show that 85 to 95 percent of college students drink.
2. It is not the product—an alcoholic beverage—but rather how and where the product is consumed that determine whether it acts as a relatively harmless beverage or as a drug that may produce serious metabolic changes in the body.
3. Pressure from family, peers, and the media is important in the choice to drink or not to drink.
4. Drinking does not lead to social assertiveness.
5. Alcohol has its most significant impact on the central nervous system. It depresses, or slows down, the activities of the central nervous system.

6. Cirrhosis of the liver is a condition that is seven times more common in heavy drinkers than in nondrinkers.
7. Alcohol consumption has been associated with a variety of problems and tragedies, including liver disease, fetal alcohol syndrome, suicide, homicide, and accidents.
8. Alcoholism is thought to result from the interaction of heredity and environment.
9. A problem drinker is a person who uses alcohol in a manner that causes physical, psychological, or social harm to the drinker or to others.
10. The primary skill necessary for reducing the health risks of alcohol is social assertiveness. Prior to beginning to drink, a socially assertive person decides how much and under what conditions he or she is going to drink and with whom he or she is *not* willing to drink.

Review Questions

1. How do the drinking patterns of college students differ from those of adult drinkers? From those of adolescent drinkers?
2. Describe how alcohol acts on the central nervous system.
3. Differentiate between a hangover, a blackout, and delirium tremens.
4. Define fetal alcohol syndrome and how to prevent it.
5. Differentiate between the 1976 definition of alcoholism and the 1992 definition of alcoholism.
6. Identify three different treatment options for alcoholism and explain the advantages of each.
7. List examples of legal efforts to control access to alcohol. How successful have these efforts been?
8. Explain the importance of the pace of consumption and the full-stomach factor in avoiding the problems associated with alcohol use.
9. Explain how being socially assertive can help prevent the problems associated with alcohol use.
10. How would you propose changing health promotion and education efforts relating to alcohol use in order to improve their success rate?

Selected Bibliography

Alcohol and Health, 8th Special Report to the U.S. Congress from the Secretary of Health and Human Services. Rockville, MD: Alcohol, Drug Abuse, and Mental Health Administration, 1993.

Alcohol, Tobacco, and Other Drugs May Harm the Unborn. Rockville, MD: Alcohol, Drug Abuse, and Mental Health Administration, 1990.

Cychosz, C.M. "Alcohol and Interpersonal Violence: Implications for Educators" *Journal of Health Education* 27, no. 2 (1996): 73–77.

Holder, H.D. "Can Individually Directed Interventions Reduce Population-Level Alcohol-Involved Problems?" *Addiction* 92, no. 1 (1997): 5–7.

Holloway, F.A. "Low-Dose Alcohol Effects on Human Behavior and Performance" *Alcohol, Drugs and Driving* 11, no. 1 (1995): 39–56.

Monitoring the Future Study. Rockville, MD: National Institute on Drug Abuse, 1996. (published annually.)

Morse, R.M., et al. "The Definition of Alcoholism." *Journal of the American Medical Association* 268, (1992): 1012–1014.

Roman, P.M., and T.C. Blum. "Alcohol: A Review of the Impact of Worksite Interventions on Health and Behavioral Outcomes." *American Journal of Health Promotion* 11, no. 2 (1996): 136–149.

Schlaadt, R.G. Wellness: *Alcohol Use and Abuse*. Guilford, CT: Dushkin, 1992.

Wechsler, H., et al. "Health and Behavioral Consequences of Binge Drinking in College." *Journal of the American Medical Association* 272, no. 21 (1994): 1672–1677.

HealthLinks: Web Sites for Dealing with Alcohol

You can access better health as it relates to this chapter by checking out some of the following sites on the Internet. These and sites identified within the chapter can be accessed directly when you visit the *HealthStyles* Web Site located on the Allyn and Bacon home page at **http://www.abacon.com.**

National Institute on Alcohol Abuse and Alcoholism
www.niaaa.nih.gov/
National goverment agency provides information on the latest findings in alcohol research, including direct links to statistical information, abstracts, and surveillance reports.

Prevention Online
www.health.org
A special site from the National Clearinghouse for Alcohol and Drug Abuse. PREVLINE offers electronic access to searchable databases and substance abuse prevention materials that pertain to alcohol, tobacco, and drugs.

Health Hotlines: Dealing with Drinking

Al-Anon, Alateen Family Group Hotline
(800) 344-2666
(800) 245-4656 (within New York)

Children of Alcoholics Foundation
(800) 359-COAF (359-2623)

National Clearinghouse for Alcohol and Drug Information
(800) SAY-NOTO (729-6686)

National Drug and Alcohol Treatment Routing Service
(800) 662-HELP (662-4357)

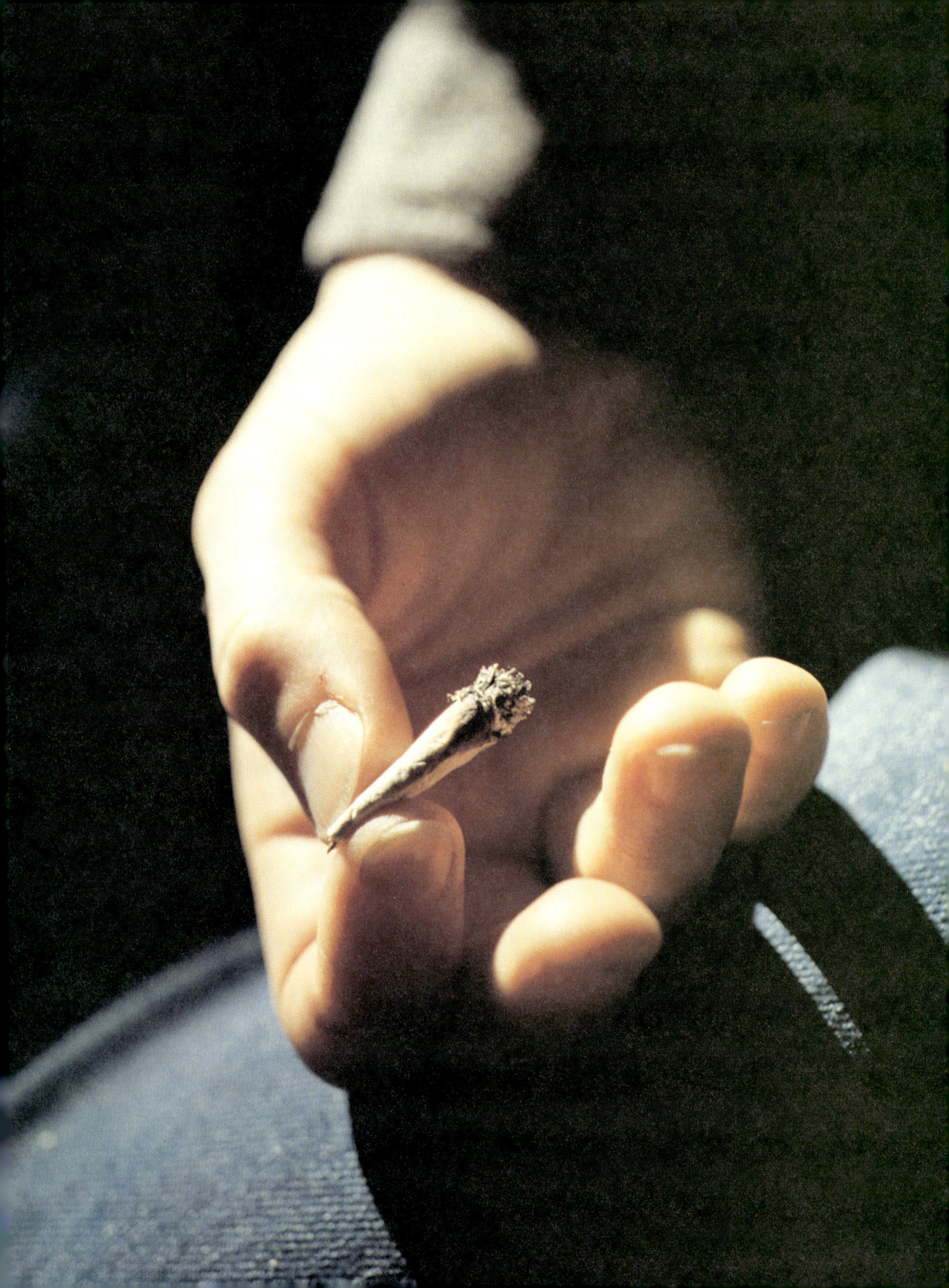

Chapter 10

Understanding the Dangers of Drug Use

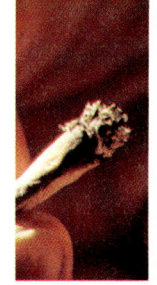
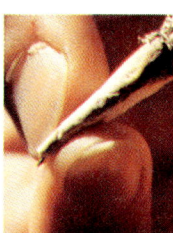
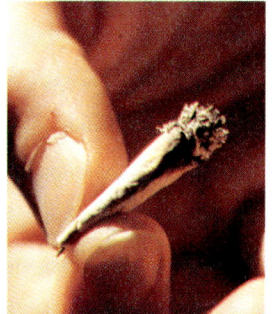

Objectives

When you finish reading this chapter, you will be able to:

1. Differentiate between over-the-counter drugs, prescription drugs, and dangerous or illegal substances.
2. Describe who uses drugs and cite the most often used drugs among college students.
3. Explain the concept of staging as it relates to drug use.
4. Differentiate between main effects and side effects of drugs.
5. Explain the dangers of mixing drugs and describe additive, inhibitory, and synergistic effects.
6. Group drugs according to the way they are taken, their effects, and the motive of the user.
7. Describe the cost to society of drug abuse.
8. Describe the health risks associated with drug abuse.
9. Describe three treatment alternatives for individuals experiencing a drug problem.
10. Suggest specific actions you can take to avoid drug abuse.

What Is Your HealthStyle?

Suzy studies hard, and her grades show it. But she is also a very tense person and enjoys relaxing by smoking marijuana. Suzy started smoking cigarettes when she was in high school, so smoking marijuana was an easy move for her.

After studying the night before an exam, she smoked a couple of joints with some friends. The next day, Suzy remembered very little of what she had reviewed. She didn't know that marijuana can affect short-term memory; instead, she rationalized that she hadn't studied enough—after all, she did take some time off to be with friends. She didn't associate the lower grade with her marijuana smoking.

Even though he studies a lot, James is not a top student. He has to work hard to get B's and C's. So James takes all of his exams seriously. He reviews his class notes ahead of time—not just the night before an exam. And he goes over review questions with classmates to help him feel more confident when answering the real test questions.

James knows that all work and no play isn't a healthy balance, so, like Suzy, he took some time the night before the exam to be with friends. But he didn't want to cloud his judgment and be fuzzy about facts and concepts during the exam, so he steered clear of friends who smoke pot and hung out with friends who relax in a drug-free way.

In Your Opinion

Suzy never questioned whether marijuana was responsible for her lower grade and James never took the risk of smoking it before an exam.

- Given that Suzy is an intense person, do you think smoking cigarettes and marijuana really helps her relax?
- Which health skills would have helped Suzy make a different decision, and why?
- James chose not to smoke marijuana. Do you think he felt left out because of this decision? Would you feel left out?
- Which health skills did James exhibit by choosing to hang out with friends who do not smoke marijuana?

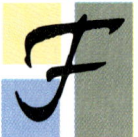

From morning through night, some form of drug seems to be used—or abused. Coffee helps people wake up in the morning, and sleeping pills help them sleep at night. Aspirin helps them get rid of headaches that occur during the day, and beer and other alcoholic drinks help them relax in the evening. In addition, crack, heroin, uppers and downers, poppers and snappers, and hundreds more illicit or street drugs are available.

Drug use and drug abuse are national problems that have enormous consequences for your personal health and safety and for that of the American public. Among these health consequences are sterility, stroke, severe mental disorders, irreparable brain damage, the spread of AIDS, and death. Drugs are associated with violence in many cities, and increasingly, in suburbs and rural communities as well.

Drugs are used by people from virtually all economic, racial, and ethnic backgrounds. College students, even some top academic performers, use drugs.

Some have experimented with drugs in high school—particularly marijuana—and the increased availability of drugs on the college campus plus the absence of parental guidance make further experimentation tempting.

What the Term Drug Means

The word **drug** refers to a chemical substance that causes a change in the body's functioning, including physiological and psychological activity. This definition encompasses over-the-counter and prescription drugs; legal substances such as beer, wine, and coffee; and illegal substances such as marijuana, cocaine, and heroin (see the Healthwise Consumer box). A drug is considered dangerous when it is believed to be a threat to the health of the user.

Over-the-counter drugs (OTCs) are chemical compounds that can be bought in pharmacies and supermarkets without restriction. They include analgesics (pain relievers) such as ibuprofen and aspirin and any number of aspirin compounds. Other examples of OTCs include cold capsules used to reduce the symptoms of colds and the flu; cough syrups used to reduce the symptoms of sore throat; laxatives used to treat irregular bowel activity; vitamin and mineral supplements used to enhance nutrition; and ointments used for the treatment of minor abrasions or fungal infections. There are thousands of over-the-counter drugs, but they all have one thing in common—they are available without restriction. This lack of restriction presents the possibility of health risks if the drugs are overused or used in certain combinations with other drugs.

Prescriptions drugs are chemical compounds that can be acquired legally only under a physician's direction. When a prescription is written, the physician gives the pharmacist specific information about which drug and how much of it to provide and gives the patient directions on how and when the drug is to be taken. When taken in a manner other than prescribed or when taken by someone other than the person receiving the prescription, they may be considered dangerous drugs. It is illegal to sell prescription drugs for other than the primary intended purpose. In many states, prescriptions for certain drugs must be written in triplicate, with one copy sent to the state drug enforcement agency. Such a step can help prevent the overprescription of dangerous drugs. Penalties for selling con-

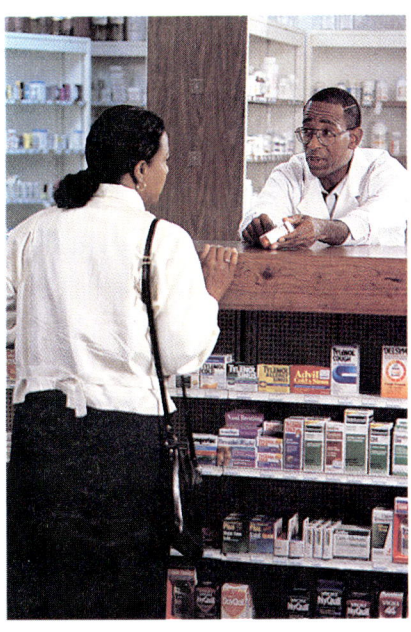

Your pharmacist can explain the safe use of a prescription drug. Prescription drugs can be considered dangerous if they are used for purposes other than the one intended by a physician. (Source: FPG International/© Ron Chapple)

drug A chemical substance that causes a change in the body's functioning, including physiological and psychological activity.

HEALTHWISE CONSUMER

The Caffeine High

Caffeine is the most popular and widely consumed drug in the world. It is in coffee, tea, soft drinks, chocolate, and medications, including cold pills (see Table 10.1). Caffeine is the only drug in the food supply, and like all drugs, it causes an array of physiological changes.

As a stimulant, caffeine has a direct effect on the brain and the central nervous system. It can ward off drowsiness, improve alertness, and speed reaction times in people who are tired and increase the muscles' capacity for work. It can also lead to nervousness, anxiety, jitteriness, and loss of sleep.

Like other stimulants, caffeine is addictive. People develop a tolerance for it and need more to get through the day. According to researchers at the Center for Science in the Public Interest, coffee drinkers tend to become dependent on caffeine at daily doses of about 3½ cups of coffee. As with other drug-related dependencies, caffeine produces withdrawal symptoms when regular users stop drinking coffee. These symptoms include lethargy, irritability, nervousness, and severe headaches.

Some people can consume large amounts of caffeine without noticing any effect. Others become jittery after one cup of coffee or a can of cola. Similarly, people differ in the duration of caffeine's effect. Caffeine has a half-life of three to seven hours for the typical nonsmoking adult. This means that half its effects wear off in that time. For reasons not fully understood, the half-life is shorter for smokers and longer for pregnant women.

Most experts agree that two cups of coffee a day pose little or no health hazard to adults. But the scientific evidence about high use is unclear. Some animal studies have implicated caffeine in birth defects, heart disease, and cancer. Even without conclusive evidence, the Food and Drug Administration recommends that women avoid or significantly reduce their intake of caffeine during pregnancy.

Alternatives to caffeine include decaffeinated coffee (which is not without health hazards itself because it contains additives that may cause liver cancer in mice), herbal tea, and grain-based drinks. For those who need their daily fix of junk food, there are caffeine-free sodas and chocolates.

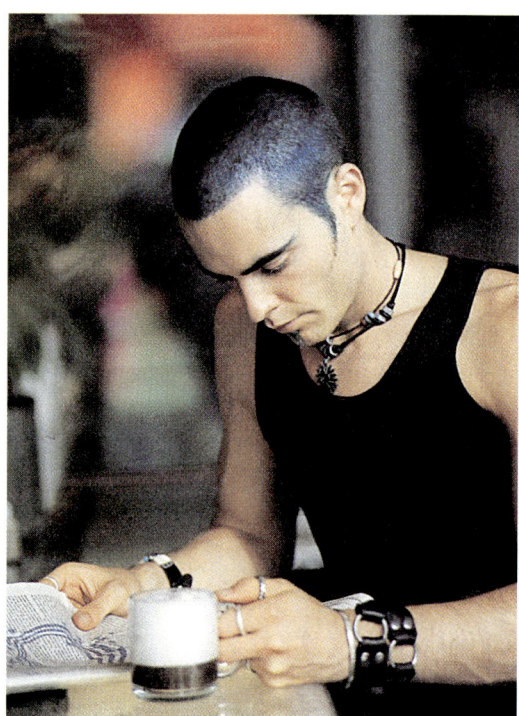

Coffee is a legal, socially accepted substance, but you can still become addicted to it. (Source: FPG International/© Ron Chapple)

trolled substances or for illegal use of dangerous drugs range from fines to stiff jail sentences. For more on medicinal drugs, see Chapter 21.

Some substances are not thought of as drugs, yet they are abused substances and are often included when identifying drugs of abuse. For example, freon, glue, gasoline, and correctional fluids are abused substances when they are

TABLE 10.1 Common Sources of Caffeine

Item	Milligrams caffeine	Item	Milligrams caffeine
Coffee (5-oz. cup)		Instant	25–50
Brewed, drip method	60–180	Iced (12 oz.)	67–76
Brewed, percolator	40–170	Cocoa beverage (5-oz.) cup	2–20
Instant	30–120	Chocolate milk beverage (8 oz.)	2–7
Decaffeinated, brewed	2–5	Milk chocolate (1 oz.)	1–15
Decaffeinated, instant	1–5	Dark chocolate, semi-sweet (1 oz.)	5–35
Tea (5-oz. cup)		Baker's chocolate (1 oz.)	26
Brewed, major U.S. brands	20–90	Chocolate-flavored syrup (1 oz.)	4
Brewed, imported brands	25–110		
Soft drinks (12-oz. serving)			
Sugar-Free Mr. Pibb	58.8	Big Red	38.4
Mountain Dew	54.0	Pepsi-Cola	38.4
Mello Yello	52.8	Diet Pepsi	36.0
Tab	46.8	Pepsi Light	36.0
Coca-Cola	45.6	RC Cola	36.0
Diet Cola	45.6	Diet Rite	36.0
Shasta Cola	44.4	Canada Dry Jamaica Cola	30.0
Mr. Pibb	40.8	Dry Diet Cola	12
Dr. Pepper	39.6		
Prescription drugs			
Cafergot (for migraine headache)	100	Fiorinal (for tension headache)	40
Nonprescription drugs			
Weight control aids		Vanquish	33
Dex-A-Diet II	200	Soma Compound (pain relief, muscle	
Dexatrim, Dexatrim Extra Strength	200	relaxant)	32
Maximum Strength Appedrine	100	Darvon Compound (pain relief)	32.4
Prolamine	140	Diuretics	
Alertness tablets		Aqua-Ban	100
Nodoz	100	Permathene	200
Vivarin	200	Cold/allergy remedies	
Analgesic/pain relief		Triaminicin tablets	30
Anacin, Maximum Strength Anacin	32	Dristan Decongestant tablets and	
Excedrin	65	Dristan A-F Decongestant tablets	16.2
Midol	32.4	Duradyne-Forte	30

Source: U.S. Food and Drug Administration

inhaled. Because such substances are easily available and legal to buy, they are often thought of as harmless. However, when abused they can result in respiratory failure and death.

Problems caused by the use of illegal substances such as marijuana, cocaine, and heroin have become so widespread and serious that the word *drug* is often used to refer specifically to *dangerous or illegal substances.* Newspapers report drug-related crimes and details about drug rings. The use of the term *drug* to mean dangerous and illegal is evident in phrases such as "Just say no to drugs" and "the war on drugs."

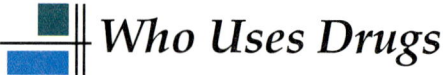

Who Uses Drugs

The first drug young people usually experiment with is tobacco. Studies show that a substantial number of children smoke or at least puff cigarettes by age nine. Boys start to test drinking around age twelve, girls a bit later. Marijuana becomes more popular in high school, and in 1995, more than 16 percent of youths aged twelve to seventeen reported having smoked it at some time. By the time they are college age (eighteen to twenty-five years old), as much as 41 percent of the population has smoked marijuana at least once, and many students have tried a wide range of other drugs.

According to the 1996 National Household Survey on Drug Abuse, the college-age population continues to use illicit drugs extensively. Nine percent of youths ages twelve to seventeen, nearly 16 percent of young adults aged eighteen to twenty-five, 9 percent of people aged twenty-six to thirty-four, and about 3 percent of people aged thirty-six and over reported using an illicit drug in the past month (see Table 10.2). As the table shows, drug use dropped between 1985 and 1995 but began to rise again in 1996. These statistics may underestimate drug use because the household survey does not interview homeless people—a vulnerable group at high risk for using drugs.

Progression from Cigarettes to Marijuana

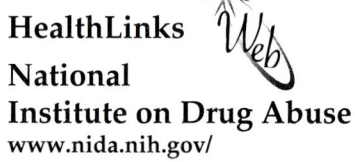

**HealthLinks
National
Institute on Drug Abuse**
www.nida.nih.gov/
Home page of this national government agency with information on the latest statistics and findings in drug research.

What does early involvement with drugs predict for future use? According to drug abuse researchers, past behavior can be the best predictor of future behavior. For example, a person is not likely to smoke marijuana without having smoked cigarettes first. In the typical progression of drug use, a person starts with cigarettes, beer, or wine (also referred to as the **gateway drugs**). He or she then moves on to marijuana and hard liquor and subsequently to other illicit drugs such as amphetamines, heroin, and cocaine. This concept is called **staging.** According to the National Institute of Drug Abuse, for someone who has ever smoked or drunk, the risk for moving on to marijuana is 5 times higher than for a person who has never smoked or drunk; the risk for moving on to cocaine is 104 times higher for someone who has smoked marijuana at least once in his or her

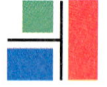

TABLE 10.2 Drugs of Choice for College Students
(Percentage of young adults aged 18 to 25 who used in the past month)

Drug	1985	1990	1995	1996
Any illicit drug	25.3	15.0	14.2	15.6
Alcohol	70.1	62.8	61.3	60.0
Alcohol binge use	34.4	29.5	29.9	32.0
Cigarettes	47.4	40.9	35.3	38.3
Cocaine	8.1	2.3	1.3	2.0
Marijuana	21.7	12.7	12.0	13.2

Source: Substance Abuse and Mental Health Services Administration, 1996 National Household Survey on Drug Abuse

lifetime than for a person who has never done so. This progression, however, is not inevitable. That is, it cannot be said that smoking and drinking at young ages are the cause of later drug use.

Critical Thinking Question

> The concept of staging drug use has been understood for generations, yet much of the effort to address the drug problem focuses on the user of hard drugs, not the user of gateway drugs. Would our efforts to curb drug abuse be better spent addressing gateway drugs? Can you suggest a strategy for reducing the jump from a gateway drug to a more immediately dangerous substance?

Why College Students Take Drugs

Even though more people aged eighteen to twenty-four use illicit drugs than people in any other age group, the fact is that most college students do not take drugs. Why do some students experiment with drugs while others do not? Perhaps this is because the drug problem is essentially a people problem, and not all people are at risk for taking drugs.

Researchers have identified several risk factors for drug abuse among older teenagers and young adults, including college students. Peer pressure is the strongest and most consistent of all factors. In fact, two questions reveal much about the risk of drug use among teenagers and young adults: "Do your friends use drugs?" and "Do your close friends disapprove of your using drugs?" A positive answer to the first question coupled with a negative answer to the second question suggests a very high probability of drug use. Opposite answers suggest a low probability of drug use.

Families can influence drug use behavior. Children are more at risk for using drugs if their parents use drugs and alcohol. Being involved in their parents' habits—as in getting mom or dad a beer from the refrigerator or lighting a cigarette for them—also increases their likelihood of using alcohol, cigarettes, and marijuana. Young adults appear to continue habits begun in late childhood. Parental influence may be positive as well as negative. Living at home with parents, in contrast to living in the dorm or other student housing arrangements, results in statistically lower rates of marijuana use by college students.

Additional risk factors include rebelliousness, low grades, and little commitment to school, psychological variables such as low self-esteem and emotional variables such as stress, depression, and the need for excitement. As the number of risk factors increases, the chances of drug use also increase.

Many college students take drugs to get through periods of intensive studying—cramming for final exams or staying up all night to finish a term paper. Taking drugs for this reason, however, is not likely to lead to the desired result. Although some stimulant drugs might keep you awake, they can also play tricks with your mind. Tranquilizers can calm you down before taking a test. But they can also remove the competitive edge you need to do well. A more predictable way to improve test performance is to study properly and experience a little test anxiety.

There is also a relationship between low grades and marijuana use. Researchers at the University of Maryland, College Park, found that students who

gateway drugs Drugs such as tobacco, alcohol, and marijuana that most users of illicit drugs have tried before their first use of cocaine, heroin, or other illicit drugs.

staging The use of drugs in a predictable progression beginning with gateway drugs, such as tobacco and alcohol, and progressing to hard drugs, such as crack cocaine and heroin.

had the lowest grade point averages (below 2.5) were four times more likely to have used marijuana in the past month than those students who had the highest grade point averages (3.6 and above). It could be that low grades are a risk factor for smoking marijuana, that marijuana use can result in low grades, or both.

There is no simple answer to the question of why college students—or anyone else for that matter—take drugs. Among the reasons may be to escape, to reduce pain, to be less inhibited, to feel pleasure, to reduce stress, or to gain energy. The fact remains that some college students do choose to use drugs, often with harmful consequences. However, researchers at the University of Michigan recently reported that maturity—specifically the responsibilities of marriage and family—diminishes drug use. In what they called the "marriage effect," the researchers found that marijuana use dropped on average by more than one third when young adults got married.

Availability and Legality of Drugs

A person who wants illicit drugs can get them in almost any community in the United States. To a great extent, the small-time pusher assures the availability of illicit drugs to college students. At its simplest level, this is the person who buys beer for friends under the drinking age at the local convenience store. Other pushers buy marijuana, LSD, crack, and other drugs from dealers and then sell them in the dorms and other student hangouts. Availability and accessibility of drugs are more a matter of demand than of law.

The drug Rohypnol (Roofies), for example, is not approved for medical use in the United States, yet is available on the streets, where it is referred to as the date-rape drug because it impairs mental judgment, results in amnesia, and is used to incapacitate innocent people who are then exposed to violent assaults such as rape. As long as a demand exists for a certain drug, there will be a way to get it.

Perhaps the best indicator of the availability of drugs is the price, because the drug business—like any other business—is subject to the economics of supply and demand. As the availability of drugs increases, the price drops. Currently, the price of drugs, particularly crack, has reached a level at which only a few dollars buys a "hit."

Even though drugs are widely available, it is illegal in all states to possess, deliver, or manufacture controlled substances or dangerous drugs. A **controlled substance** is a drug or chemical that has been identified through legal review as a threat to an individual or to society. Controlled substances include marijuana, LSD, cocaine, heroin, morphine, secobarbital, and methamphetamine. Some states have added steroids to their list of controlled substances.

Critical Thinking Question

The *Healthy People 2000* objectives include the following: "Reduce drug-related deaths to no more than 3 per 100,000 people." In 1993, the last year for which there are available data, drug-related deaths stood at 4.8 per 100,000 people. How accurate are these data? They were collected by the CDC and are available through the National Vital Statistics System, but are they the best indicator of the nation's drug problem? Can you suggest a better way to measure it?

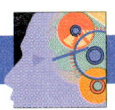

DEVELOPING HEALTH SKILLS

At Issue: Should Americans Be Allowed to Smoke Marijuana as Medicine?

Yes Patients all over the world use marijuana. Cannabis reduces vomiting and nausea in cancer patients and has helped people with AIDS gain weight. It lowers internal eye pressure, helping preserve the vision of glaucoma patients, and people with multiple sclerosis have used it successfully to treat muscle spasms. Some patients with migraines say they get instant relief from smoking marijuana. Yet because marijuana was dropped from the U.S. pharmacopoeia list in 1941, it was not grandfathered into the federal comprehensive drug act of 1970 in a category that would allow doctors to prescribe it as they can morphine and cocaine.

The government says marijuana must gain the Food and Drug Administration's approval to be used as medicine yet until recently has not allowed any small trials to go forward. And what drug company would invest in the huge trials needed to earn FDA approval when it can't patent the product?

I do worry about lung damage from smoking marijuana. Marijuana smoke may be dirtier than tobacco smoke. But I can't imagine patients smoking as much as tobacco users do. Ultimately the medically useful ingredients in marijuana will be extracted and inhaled as vapors by patients.

Doctors' prescribing morphine as medicine hasn't increased its abuse. The same will hold true for marijuana. In the new millennium people will look back and say, "Did we really behave that way?"

Lester Grinspoon is a psychiatrist and professor at Harvard Medical School and the coauthor of *Marijuana: The Forbidden Medicine.*

No There isn't enough known at this point for doctors to safely recommend marijuana to patients for anything other than a life-threatening illness. Marijuana probably has some value as an appetite stimulant. And it does seem to decrease nausea and vomiting for patients undergoing chemotherapy and radiation. For patients with AIDS or cancer, it may help their quality of life without great risk.

But it's different for people who have glaucoma or migraines and might need treatment all their lives. If you ask ophthalmologists how marijuana compares to other drugs as a treatment for glaucoma, they say they wouldn't recommend it. If you ask neurologists if they would suggest the drug for migraines, they say no.

Smoking anything is a worry to doctors. Tobacco smoke clearly has profoundly negative effects on health. It's logical that marijuana would have a similar toxic effect on the lungs. We also know that marijuana is very addictive psychologically. There are people who can't get through the day without it. Opposing the use of marijuana is not a moral judgment; it's a commonsense health issue.

It's true that marijuana is so politicized we've almost been afraid to find out if it has therapeutic benefits. That's wrong. Most doctors favor limiting use of medical marijuana to controlled studies for patients with life-threatening conditions. That's the scientific way to move ahead.

Jack Lewin is a family practitioner and the chief executive officer of the California Medical Association.

Source: "Should Americans Be Allowed to Smoke Marijuana as Medicine?" *Health,* March 1997, p. 29. Reprinted by permission of Time Inc. Health

---

The penalties associated with drug possession or the sale of drugs raise important societal and ethical questions. To date, there is little evidence to indicate that criminal law has stemmed the illegal use of drugs. Should drugs be legalized? In 1996 as a first step, California voters made it legal for doctors to prescribe marijuana for medical use (for example, to relieve the pain of critically ill patients and to increase the appetites of patients wasting from cancer or AIDS), and Arizona voters made it legal for doctors to prescribe heroin and LSD as well as marijuana. Read the Developing Health Skills box to gain insight about the complexity of this controversy.

controlled substance A chemical that has been identified through legal review as a threat to an individual and/or to society.

From Drug Use to Drug Abuse

Drug use is the use of a chemical substance for the purpose intended. **Drug misuse** is taking prescribed medication without consulting a physician—for example, using someone else's prescription for cramps. **Drug abuse** is the intentional misuse of a chemical. The person who misuses tranquilizers by taking them to feel at ease socially becomes a drug abuser when he or she can't get through the day without several doses of tranquilizers. People who abuse tranquilizers usually obtain them illegally. Drug abuse is more often associated with illicit drugs such as cocaine and heroin.

A person who is **drug dependent** (a drug addict) is a drug user who, in most cases, has a tolerance for and dependence on the drug. **Tolerance** is a physical adaptation to a substance that causes it to become less effective with repeated use. As a result, a person has to take more of the drug to get the intended effect. For example, a heroin user may go from a 3-mg dose to a 1,000-mg dose in a few months.

Dependence occurs when a person is so physically attached to the drug that he or she cannot live comfortably without it. Physical dependence occurs when the body becomes accustomed to the presence of the drug and requires the drug to function normally. Another term for physical dependence is **addiction.** A person who has a physical dependence on a drug goes through **withdrawal** symptoms when he or she stops taking the drug. Withdrawal symptoms are usually unpleasant and sometimes dangerous. For example, withdrawal from heroin can include nausea, vomiting, joint and muscle pains, heightened blood pressure, racing pulse, tremors, and fever. Psychological dependence occurs when the person believes that he or she needs a drug to function normally. The drug is usually associated with specific feelings or moods. A person who is psychologically dependent may not experience physical withdrawal symptoms when the drug is not taken, but the process of stopping use is still very difficult.

Drug Action and Drug Interaction

Drug actions are usually spoken of in terms of effect—the impact of the chemical substance on the body. The **main effect** of a drug is the effect for which the drug is taken. In the case of diet pills, the main effect might be reduced hunger. Diet pills, however, are introduced through the stomach into the bloodstream, and thus throughout the system. They therefore cause other effects, some of which are not intended. A **side effect** is an effect that a drug has on the body that is not the primary effect, or the effect intended. A side effect of diet pills might be anxiety, nervousness, or sometimes hallucinations.

Drugs don't act just anywhere in the body. They act on specific organs or tissues. A **receptor site** receives natural chemicals made and used by the body to carry out its day-to-day functions. A drug can attach itself to a receptor site if its molecules have the right size, shape, and chemical and electrical characteristics. The brain, for example, makes its own natural opiates that produce pleasure and mask pain. Heroin and other drugs in the opiate family are taken up by those same cells, or receptors (see Figure 10.1).

Receptor sites may also hold some clues as to why users develop a tolerance to a drug and need increasing doses of it to get a high. According to one theory, chronic heroin use causes the brain to stop producing its own natural opiates, so highs have to come from outside the body. Another theory is that heroin users are more likely to have naturally underactive opiate systems.

---

drug use The use of a chemical substance for the purpose intended to bring about a change in the way the body functions.

drug misuse The use of a prescribed medication without consulting a physician.

drug abuse The intentional and chronic misuse of a chemical substance.

drug dependent A drug user who relies on the use of a drug to carry out normal day-to-day activities; dependence may be physical or psychological.

tolerance The progressive change in the body's reaction to a drug causing an individual to need more and more of the same drug to achieve the same effect.

dependence A condition in which a person is so physically and/or psychologically attached to a drug that he or she cannot live without it.

addiction Physical or psychological dependence on a drug, often involving tolerance and withdrawal.

withdrawal A group of symptoms that occur when a person stops taking a drug.

main effect The desired (intended) physical or mental response of the body to a drug; sometimes called the primary effect.

side effect An unwanted or even dangerous physical or mental effect caused by a drug or medicine.

receptor site The location in the body at which a drug triggers a response.

drug interaction The simultaneous presence of two or more drugs in the body that causes a detrimental effect.

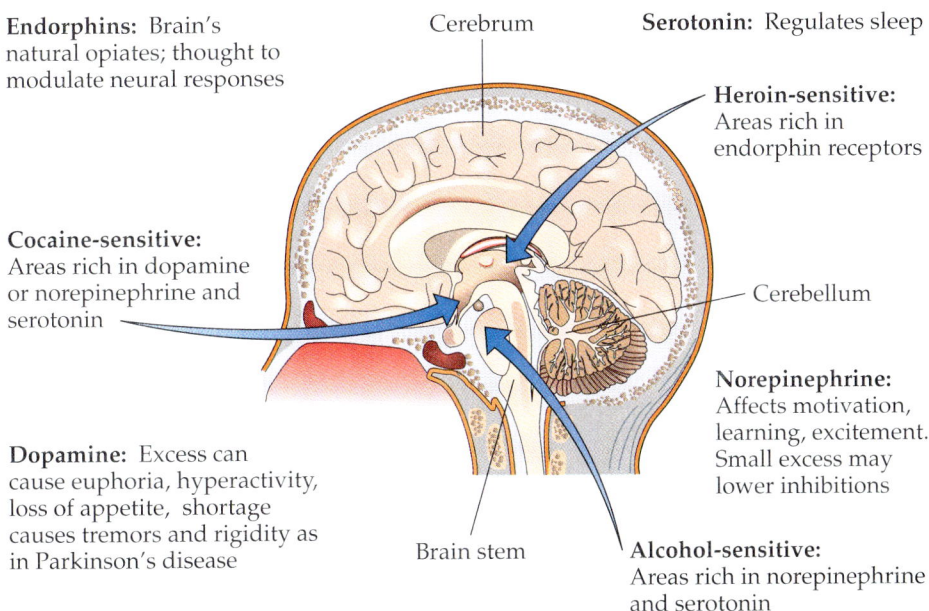

Figure 10.1 The Effect of Drugs on the Brain. *Alcohol, cocaine, and heroin affect different parts of the brain. There are many theories about what happens in the brain and why.*

Factors other than the drug itself or the receptor site can have a significant effect on the results of drug use. For example, the physical characteristics of the person taking a drug are critical to the actions of that drug. The same dosage of a drug taken by a 210-pound person may be far more potent if taken by a 120-pound person.

What are sometimes called the "set" and "setting" may also play a role in the effectiveness of a drug. *Set* refers to a person's psychological state, including mood or motive. A person who expects a positive reaction to a drug may experience that positive reaction more often than someone who expects a different result. *Setting* refers to the environment in which a drug is consumed. A drug consumed at a party with friends may have a different effect than a drug consumed alone or on the street.

Without thinking much about the consequences, many people take more than one kind of drug a day—from a cold pill to a cigarette to marijuana. Taking more than one drug at a time is a very tricky business. The presence of two or more drugs in the body may result in an adverse **drug interaction.**

Drugs may interact in three ways:

- *Additive effects.* The total effect of two drugs taken at the same time is equal to the simple sum of the two drugs' effects.
- *Inhibitory effects.* Two drugs are present at the same time, and the effect of one reduces or blocks the effect of the other.
- *Synergistic effects.* Two drugs present at the same time result in a total effect much greater than the simple sum of the two drugs' effects.

The additive effect of drugs can be seen when a cold remedy, which can be as much as 25 percent alcohol, is taken at the same time as an alcoholic beverage. This can lead to a blood alcohol content much higher than expected. An example of the inhibitory effects of two drugs takes place when antibiotics are taken with birth control pills—the effectiveness of both is reduced. (The effects of drug interactions from prescription and over-the-counter drugs are discussed in Chapter 21.)

The synergistic effects are particularly potent when two psychoactive drugs are used. As an example of how dangerous synergistic drug interactions can be, barbiturates and alcohol taken together have up to four times the depressant effect that either a barbiturate or alcohol would have alone. Mixing barbiturates and alcohol can result in death. Basically, the two drugs together depress the central nervous system to the point that vital functions such as breathing cease.

A term often used to describe the undesired effects of taking a large amount of a single drug is **overdose.** An overdose can occur under two conditions: (1) when enough drug is consumed to produce exaggerated effects, or (2) when the person taking the drug is *hypersensitive* to the substance and thus physiologically or psychologically responds to even a small amount of the drug in an exaggerated manner. Most deaths attributed to cocaine use result from overdose. The fact that the drug is prepared without regulation means that concentrations of the drug vary from dose to dose because the purity of the product varies from purchase to purchase.

How Drugs Differ

Drugs come in many shapes, sizes, and forms. One way to gain a better understanding of drugs is to group them. This is done primarily in two ways: by the way they are taken and by their effects. Some drugs, however, do not fit easily into either grouping. Rather, they must be understood in terms of the motive of their users. Designer drugs, for example, came into existence as a way to circumvent the law. Some drugs fit into more than one group, making any effort to create categories difficult. Consider the following groups as an effort to understand the similarities and differences of drugs, not as a definitive categorization of drugs.

By the Way They Are Taken

Drugs may be inhaled, smoked, swallowed, injected, or absorbed through the skin. Drugs travel around the body differently, depending on how they are taken.

Some drugs are inhaled through the nostrils. In the case of legal drugs such as medication for asthma, the drug may be packaged in an inhaler to facilitate easy transmission. In the case of inhaled products such as airplane glue, which

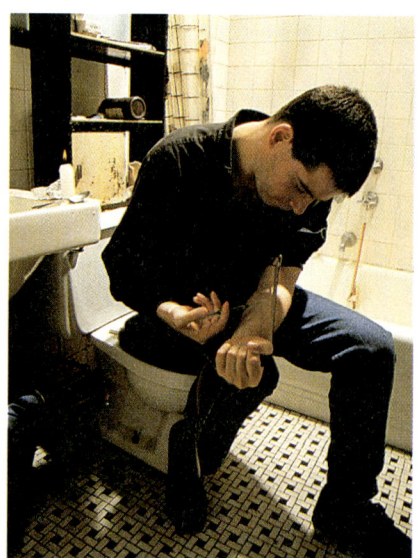

Illicit drugs are inhaled, smoked, swallowed, injected, or absorbed through the skin. Injecting drug use carries the additional danger of contracting and spreading HIV. (Source: Photo Researchers, Inc./ © James Prince)

are taken to produce a high, the substance is put in a plastic or paper bag or on a rag and inhaled or sniffed. The results of inhaling a drug are almost immediate because the entry into the blood and in turn access to the brain is quick and easy through the lungs. Marijuana and crack are two drugs that are usually *smoked.* The drug passes into the bloodstream and is carried to the brain in seconds.

Inhalants are drugs that cause a quick rush to the brain. Popular abused inhalants are airplane glue, paint thinner, and dry cleaning solution. These substances are easily obtained at hardware stores. Restaurant and ice cream supply stores are the source of another abused inhalant—nitrous oxide capsules, which are used for making whipped cream. Some other inhalants have no commercial value other than to get the user high. An example of this type of inhalant is butyl nitrite. Because of their easy means of transmission, and in some cases easy access, inhalants are often abused by children.

When a drug is *swallowed,* as with most pills or in a marijuana brownie, the chemical reaches the brain more slowly because digestive processes are needed to release the psychoactive ingredients of the substance.

A more effective means of administering a drug is through *injection.* This occurs when a syringe is used to inject the drug directly into a vein. This is called an *intravenous injection.* Injections may also be *intramuscular* (into the muscle) or *subcutaneous* (under the skin). When a drug, such as heroin, is injected, it affects the brain within seconds. Injection, however, carries many health risks that are unrelated to the actual drug itself. HIV transmission, for example, can occur when unclean needles are used for administering illicit drugs.

Another means of transmission is *dermal* or *subdermal absorption*—often called topical application. Absorption, whether through use of a suppository, a transdermal patch, or a stamp, is a very effective means of transmitting drugs. LSD *(lysergic acid diethylamide),* for example, is often sold on stamp-like sections of paper to be placed on the tongue. The LSD on the stamp is absorbed through the tissue of the tongue. A transdermal patch impregnated with nicotine is used to transmit the drug to people who are trying to quit smoking yet still crave nicotine.

By Their Effects

Drugs are often classified by their psychoactive effects, or how they affect the mind. This provides a good way to compare and contrast drugs. There are five groups of substances: *stimulants, depressants, hallucinogens, narcotics,* and *cannabis.*

Stimulants speed up the body's functions and movements through actions on the central nervous system. A group of powerful stimulants is *amphetamines.* These stimulants are available by prescription only and are considered safe when taken under a physician's supervision. But they may also be abused. The effects of stimulants wear off quickly, so the abuser of these drugs may be left feeling depressed. Once depressed, the abuser may take more stimulants to counter the depression. Stimulants are habit forming and may be life threatening.

Cocaine is a powerful but short-acting stimulant. Cocaine abusers sniff the drug into their noses, inject it into their bloodstreams, or smoke it. When smoked, crack—cocaine in its rock form, which vaporizes when heated—goes straight to the lungs and is released into the bloodstream, where it is pumped to every organ in the body within eight to ten seconds. In addition, crack is transported from the lungs to the brain directly. It bypasses the liver, which would normally detoxify the cocaine. Cocaine is highly addictive, and tolerance develops rapidly.

Depressants slow down the body's functions and movements through actions on the central nervous system. Depressants relax a person and cause sleep. *Tranquilizers* are a form of depressant that slow nerve activity and relax muscle tension. They are safe when used as directed by a physician. They are used to treat anxiety, but can be habit forming. *Barbiturates,* another depressant, are also considered safe when taken under a physician's supervision. But both drugs are often abused. A tolerance for barbiturates or tranquilizers is developed

overdose A serious reaction to an excessive amount of a drug that can result in coma or death.

inhalant A chemical that is inhaled through the nostrils to cause a quick rush to the brain; abused inhalants include airplane glue, paint thinner, and butyl nitrite.

stimulant A drug that speeds up the body's functions and movements.

depressant A drug that slows down the body's functions and movements.

quickly, causing the abuser to need more and more of the drug in order to feel the desired effects.

Narcotics are any depressant drug made from or chemically similar to opium. Narcotics reduce pain and induce sleep. *Opium* is a drug obtained from the seed pod of a poppy plant. *Morphine* and *codeine* are natural narcotic compounds that are contained in opium.

Heroin, a popularly used narcotic, is usually injected. Heroin addiction produces harsh withdrawal symptoms, including sweating, shaking, chills, nausea, and cramps. The user of heroin is always at risk for overdose because dealers often "cut," or dilute, the drug by adding other substances. This means that one purchase of heroin may be diluted while another may be pure.

Hallucinogens cause a change in perception, including causing people to see, hear, and feel things that are not really there. Hallucinogens are unpredictable—they may stimulate or depress the central nervous system. The strongest known hallucinogen is LSD. Users (all might be considered abusers) experience hallucinations in which they may see colorful visions and mistakenly feel that they have superhuman powers. Side effects are sometimes harsh, including unpleasant visions sometimes called "bad trips." The user of LSD may experience flashbacks, an unexpected return to the hallucinogenic state long after recovery from drug use. Other hallucinogens are *mescaline,* the psychoactive component of peyote cactus; *psilocybin,* which is obtained from a mushroom; and *phencyclidine* (PCP), an anesthetic used in veterinary medicine.

Cannabis, better known as marijuana, does not fit into any of these classes because it can act like all of them. Under different circumstances, cannabis can be a stimulant, depressant, narcotic, or hallucinogen. This is because marijuana is not a single drug. It contains nearly 400 chemicals, at least 60 of which are unique to the *Cannabis sativa* plant. When marijuana is smoked, tetrahydrocannabinol (THC) enters the lungs, passes into the bloodstream, and is carried to the brain in seconds. Marijuana may act as a depressant because one or more chemicals having a depressing effect are present at a higher concentration at any given time in the body following marijuana use. It may act as a stimulant for similar reasons. Or it may cause a variety of reactions depending on the user's rate of metabolism of the various chemicals.

Table 10.3 describes the major dangerous and illegal drugs, classified by psychoactive effects. The street names used are examples of what people popularly call them. These names change from one city to another and from time to time. New names—and new drugs—come into use quickly.

By the Motive of the Abuser

Some drugs are best understood in terms of the motivation of the abuser. An example is designer drugs. **Designer drugs** are made in clandestine laboratories and are designed specifically to circumvent the law. They look like drugs already on the market (both legal and illegal) but have something altered in their molecular structure so that they are "new" drugs. By being new drugs, they circumvent the law that defines controlled substances. For example, one designer drug is a heroin substitute but is much more powerful and longer lasting. It has been linked to overdoses. Another designer drug, popularly called ecstasy, is similar to amphetamines but produces hallucinations and feelings of euphoria.

Many naturally occurring substances become abused drugs. An example of such a substance is anabolic steroids. **Anabolic steroids** promote tissue growth and lead to increased muscle mass and improved strength and power. These substances occur naturally in the body. But when extra amounts of anabolic steroids are taken, the effects can be dramatic. Steroids are taken either by mouth in pill form or by injection. Sharing needles has resulted in a new health hazard associated with steroid use: HIV infection and AIDS. (Text continues on p. 251.)

narcotic A drug that reduces pain and induces sleep.

hallucinogen A drug that causes a great change in perception.

cannabis Marijuana, hashish, ganga; the dried flowering tops of the hemp plant, *Cannabis sativa.*

designer drug A drug that looks like a drug already on the market but has something altered in its molecular structure so that it is a "new" drug and not explicitly banned.

anabolic steroid A drug that promotes tissue growth and leads to increased muscle mass and improved strength and power.

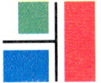

TABLE 10.3 A Primer on Drugs and Their Effects on Health

Stimulants

Amphetamines

What are they called?
Speed	Pep pills	Benzedrine
Uppers	Copilots	Dexedrine
Ups	Bumblebees	Footballs
Black beauties	Hearts	Biphetamine

What do they look like?
Capsules   Tablets   Pills

How are they used?
Taken orally   Inhaled through nasal passages   Injected

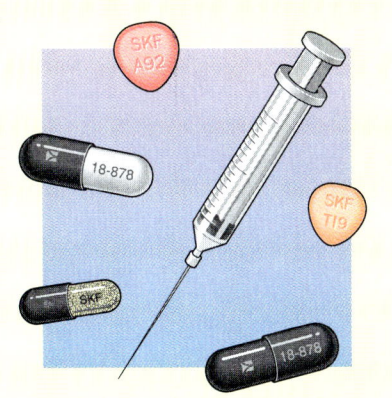

Methamphetamines

What are they called?
| Crank | Crystal | Speed |
| Crystal meth | Methedrine | Meth |

What do they look like?
White powder   Pills   A rock that resembles a block of paraffin

How are they used?
Taken orally   Injected

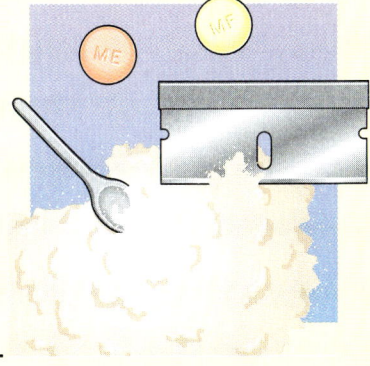

Other stimulants

What are they called?
Ritalin	Didrex	Tenuate	Sandrex
Cylert	Pre-State	Tepanil	Plegine
Preludin	Voranil	Pondimin	Ionamin

What do they look like?
Pills   Capsules   Tablets

How are they used?
Taken orally   Injected

Short-term health hazards for all stimulants
| Excitation | Rapid speech | Convulsions |
| Restlessness | Irritability | Death |

Long-term health hazards for stimulants
| Insomnia | Hallucinations | Malnutrition |
| Excitability | Severe mental disorders | Death |

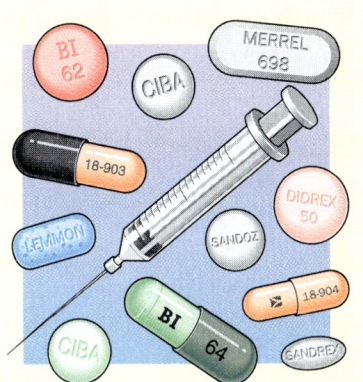

Cocaine

What is it called?
Coke	White	Big C
Snow	Blow	Snowbirds
Flake	Nose candy	Lady

What does it look like?
White crystalline powder, often diluted with other ingredients

How is it used?
Inhaled through nasal passages   Smoked   Injected

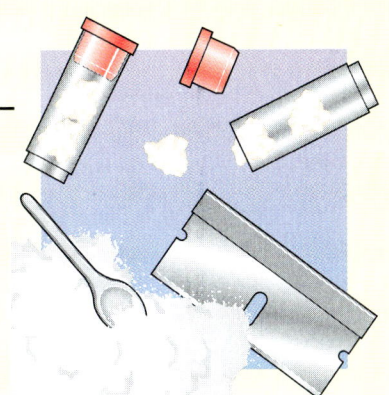

TABLE 10.3 A Primer on Drugs and Their Effects on Health (continued)

Crack

What is it called?
Crack   Freebase rocks   Rock

What does it look like?
Light brown or beige pellets or crystalline rocks

How is it used?
Smoked

Short-term health hazards for crack and cocaine
Irritability   Mental disorders   Death   Depression

Long-term health hazards for crack and cocaine
Damage to lining of nose and blood vessels when sniffed
Severe mental disorders
Death

Depressants

Barbiturates

What are they called?
Downers   Yellow jackets   Seconal
Barbs   Yellows   Amytal
Blue devils   Nembutal   Tuinals
Red devils

What do they look like?
Red, yellow, blue, or red and blue capsules

How are they used?
Taken orally

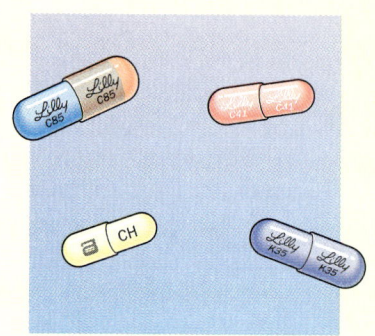

Methaqualone

What is it called?
Quaaludes   Ludes   Sopors

What does it look like?
Tablets

How is it used?
Taken orally

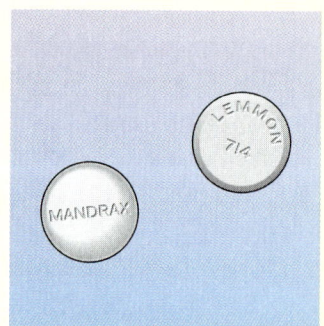

Tranquilizers

What are they called?
Valium   Miltown   Tranxene
Librium   Serax   Xanax
Equanil

What do they look like?
Tablets   Capsules

How are they used?
Taken orally

Short-term health hazards for all depressants
Decreased alertness   Drowsiness
Confusion   Irritability
Poor coordination and judgment   Death

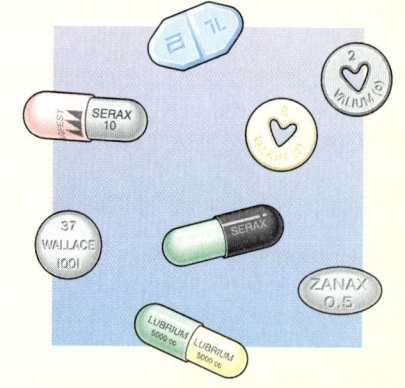

TABLE 10.3 A Primer on Drugs and Their Effects on Health (continued)

Long-term health hazards for all depressants
- Loss of appetite
- Sleeplessness
- Nausea
- Addiction
- Death

Hallucinogens

Phencycidine

What is it called?
- PCP
- Angel dust
- Loveboat
- Lovely
- Hog
- Killer weed

What does it look like?
- Liquid
- Capsules
- White crystalline powder
- Pills

How is it used?
- Taken orally
- Injected
- Smoked—can be sprayed on cigarettes, parsley, and marijuana

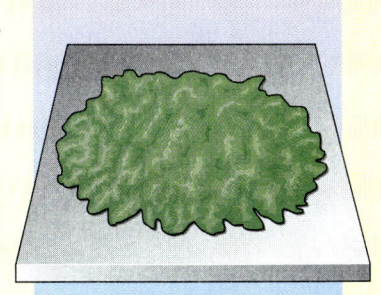

Lysergic acid diethylamide

What is it called?
- LSD
- Acid
- Green or red dragon
- White lightning
- Blue heaven
- Sugar cubes
- Microdot

What does it look like?
- Brightly colored tablets
- Thin squares of gelatin
- Impregnated blotter paper
- Clear liquid

How is it used?
- Taken orally
- Licked off paper
- Gelatin and liquid can be put in eyes

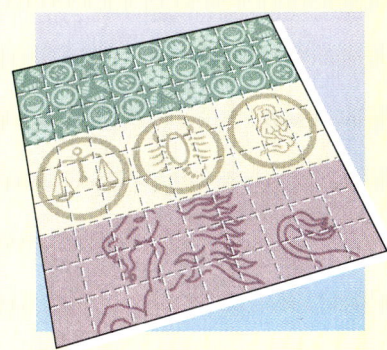

Mescaline and peyote

What are they called?
- Mesc
- Buttons
- Cactus

What do they look like
- Hard brown discs
- Tablets
- Capsules

How are they used?
- Discs—chewed, swallowed, smoked
- Tablets and capsules—taken orally

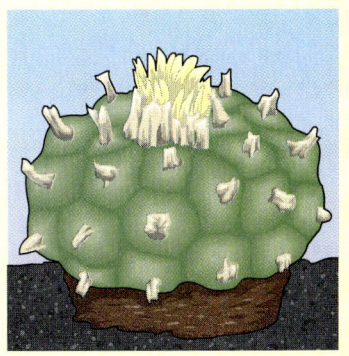

Psilocybin

What is it called?
- Magic mushrooms
- Shrooms
- Mushrooms

What does it look like?
- Fresh or dried mushrooms

How is it used?
- Chewed and swallowed
- Mixed with beverage such as tea or juice and swallowed

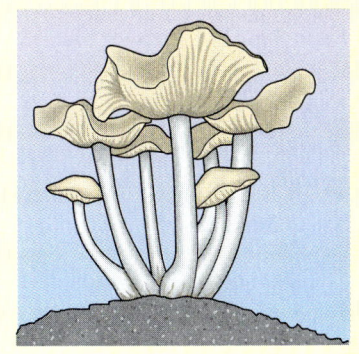

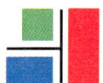

TABLE 10.3 A Primer on Drugs and Their Effects on Health (continued)

Short-term health hazards for all hallucinogens
- Confusion
- Agitation
- Changes in perception
- Impaired memory
- Anxiety
- Hallucinations
- Loss of coordination
- Vomiting
- Panic
- Mental disorders
- Death

Long-term health hazards for all hallucinogens
- Delusions
- Severe mental disorders
- Increased panic
- Death

Narcotics

Heroin (natural)

What is it called?
- Junk
- Horse
- Brown sugar
- Smack
- Mud
- Big H
- Black tar

What does it look like?
- Powder, white to dark brown
- Tar-like substance

How is it used?
- Injected
- Smoked
- Inhaled

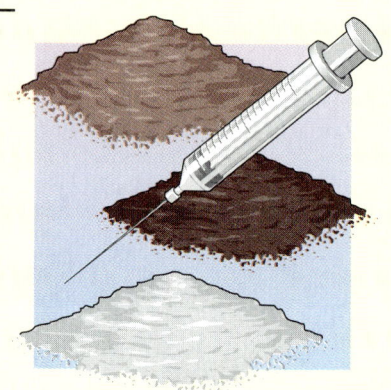

Methadone (synthetic)

What is it called?
- Colophine
- Amidone
- Methadose

What does it look like?
- Solution
- Tablets
- Caplets

How is it used?
- Taken orally
- Injected

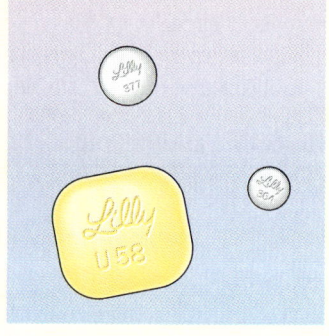

Codeine

What is it called?
- Empirin compound with codeine
- Tylenol with codeine
- Codeine
- Codeine in cough medicine

What does it look like?
- Dark liquid varying in thickness
- Capsules
- Tablets

How is it used?
- Taken orally
- Injected

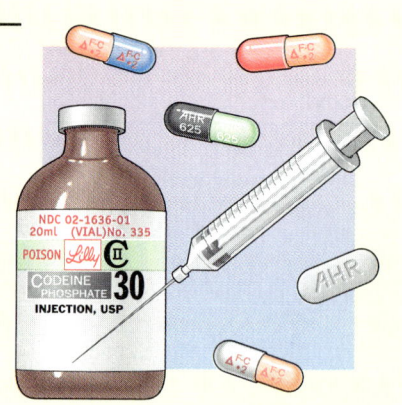

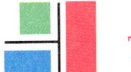

TABLE 10.3 A Primer on Drugs and Their Effects on Health (continued)

Morphine

What is it called?
   Pectoral syrup

What does it look like?
   White crystals   Injecting solutions   Hypodermic tablets

How is it used?
   Injected   Taken orally   Smoked

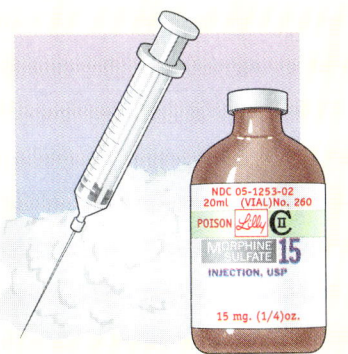

Meperidine

What is it called?
   Pethidine   Demerol   Mepergan

What does it look like?
   White powder   Tablets   Solution

How is it used?
   Taken orally   Injected

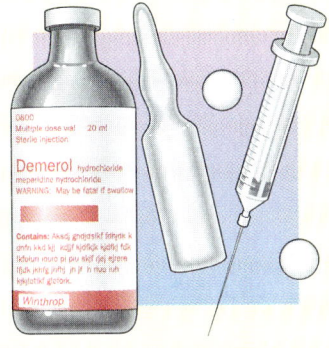

Opium

What is it called?
   Paregoric   Parapectolin   Dover's powder

What does it look like?
   Dark brown chunks   Powder

How is it used?
   Smoked   Eaten

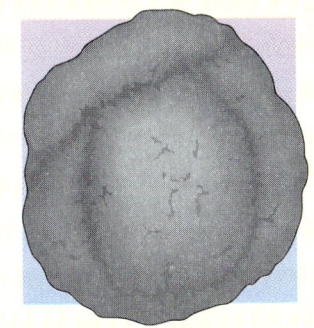

Other narcotics

What are they called?
   Percocet   Fentanyl   Talwin
   Percodan   Darvon   Lomotil
   Tussionex

What do they look like?
   Tablets   Liquid   Capsules

How are they used?
   Taken orally   Injected

Short-term health hazards for all narcotics
   Decreased alertness   Stupor   Vomiting
   Confusion   Slurred speech   Unconsciousness
   Hallucinations   Nausea   Death

Long-term health hazards for all narcotics
   Constipation   Convulsions   Coma
   Temporary sterility and impotence   Addiction   Death
   Hepatitis and HIV from dirty needles

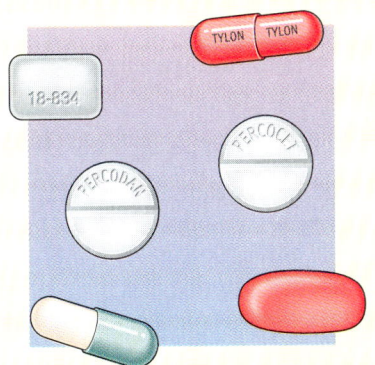

TABLE 10.3 A Primer on Drugs and Their Effects on Health (continued)

Cannabis

Marijuana

What is it called?
- Pot
- Grass
- Weed
- Dope
- Mary Jane
- Sinsemilla
- Acapulco gold
- Thai sticks
- Tea
- Reefer

What does it look like?
Dried parsley mixed with stems that may include seeds

How is it used?
Eaten   Smoked

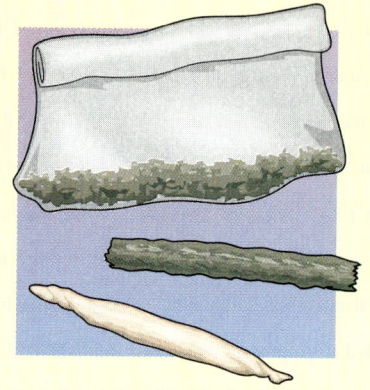

Hashish

What is it called?
Hash

What does it look like?
Brown or black cakes or balls

How is it used?
Eaten   Smoked

Hashish Oil

What is it called?
Hash oil

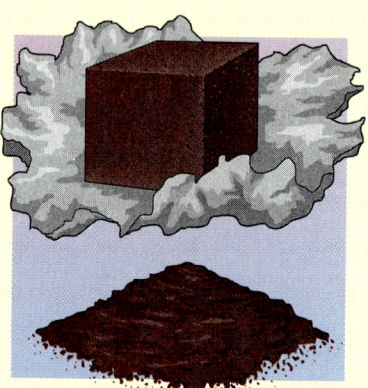

What does it look like?
Concentrated syrupy liquid varying in color from clear to black

How is it used?
Smoked, mixed with tobacco

Tetrahydrocannabinol

What is it called?
THC

What does it look like?
Soft gelatin capsules

How is it used?
Taken orally   Smoked

Short-term health hazards for all cannabis
- Reduction of inhibitions
- Impaired memory
- Loss of interest and motivation
- Changes in perception
- Panic
- Paranoia
- Loss of coordination

Long-term health hazards for all cannabis
- Interference with psychological motivation
- Miscarriage or stillborn baby
- May impair heart function and immune systems
- Psychological dependence
- Possible sterility

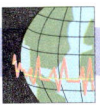

CULTURAL VIEW

Adolescent Girls Abuse Steroids, Too

What do anabolic steroids have in common with amphetamines, tobacco, diet pills, laxatives, and anorectics? They all are also drugs used by adolescent girls seeking to stay thin, says Dr. Linn Goldberg of Oregon Health Sciences University. The use of these drugs, which often goes hand in hand with eating disorders, is particularly prominent among adolescent girls engaged in athletic activities ranging from track and field, soccer, basketball, and volleyball to school dance and drill teams, Dr. Goldberg says.

Dr. Goldberg and his colleague Dr. Dianne Elliot have been conducting preliminary research, funded by the National Institute on Drug Abuse (NIDA), to identify risk factors that influence adolescent girls' use of harmful drugs. Among other things, the researchers have found that many adolescent girls use drugs to maintain thinness, Dr. Goldberg says. National surveys indicate that girls account for about one third of the high school students who abuse steroids, Dr. Goldberg says. "The primary reason that these girls use steroids is to lose fat and gain lean muscle," he says.

Dr. Elliot and Dr. Goldberg have already developed an effective steroid prevention program for male high school athletes. (By educating student athletes about the harmful effects of anabolic steroids and providing nutrition and weight training alternatives to steroid use, the program has increased football players' healthy behaviors and reduced their intentions to use steroids.) Now, they are developing a similar drug abuse prevention program for adolescent girls. In their future research, the researchers hope to test the effectiveness of the intervention in reducing drug use and eating disorders among females athletes in Oregon's public middle and high schools.

Source: National Institutes of Health, National Institute on Drug Abuse, "Adolescent Girls Abuse Steroids, Too," *NIDA Notes*, July–August 1997.

Critical Thinking Question

The *Healthy People 2000* objectives include the following: "Reduce to no more that 3 percent the proportion of male high school seniors who use anabolic steroids." In 1994, 4.8 percent of high school males reported that they had taken anabolic steroids. Taking anabolic steroids could be dangerous. Some experts feel it can even lead to death. With the risks so high, why do many male high school students continue to use this substance?

Along with getting bigger, males who take steroids can experience numerous adverse side effects, including developing breasts; hair loss; impotence and shrunken testicles; painful, prolonged erections; increased acne on the back, chest, and face; abnormally aggressive behavior, moodiness, and "bodybuilders' psychosis"; liver, kidney, and heart damage; stunted bone growth; cancer; and coma and death.

Steroid use isn't restricted to males, however. Recent indications suggest that more and more females are using steroids as well, as noted in the Cultural View box. Women, too, can have adverse reactions to steroids, including deepening of the voice, scalp hair loss, body hair growth, and clitoral enlargement that is often irreversible.

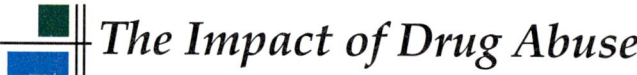

The Impact of Drug Abuse

The cost of drug abuse is staggering: $66.9 billion per year in drug-related illness, death, and crime. It ruins individuals, families, and neighborhoods. Drug abusers drop out of school and work, and the loss of their potential and self-esteem is immeasurable. The National Institute on Drug Abuse estimates that typical drug users spend $100 a day—$36,500 a year on their habits. The only way for most people to get this kind of money is to do something illegal—stealing, pimping, prostitution, or selling drugs. It is estimated that an addict has to steal three to five times the actual cost of the drugs he or she abuses to maintain his or her habit. This means stealing about $110,000 to $180,000 worth of goods a year. There are no accurate figures on drug-related prostitution, but about one of every three or four prostitutes in major cities is thought to be a heroin addict.

The Threat to Public Health

Drug abuse is a national problem that has enormous consequences for your personal health and safety and for that of the U.S. public. Among the health consequences are sterility, stroke, severe mental disorders, irreparable brain damage, and death.

Drug-related hospital emergency room episodes provide a useful snapshot of the health consequences of drugs (see Figure 10.2). Cocaine-related emergencies are at a historic high. Overall rates are higher for men than for women and for African Americans than for whites. In fact, deaths caused by cocaine use have increased for all people since 1990 but rates have increased by almost 50 percent for Hispanics and African Americans.

The Toll from AIDS

Of all the drug-related health problems, AIDS exacts the greatest toll because of its impact on the individual involved as well as on society at large. AIDS is the fastest growing cause of all illegal-drug-related deaths, and more than one third

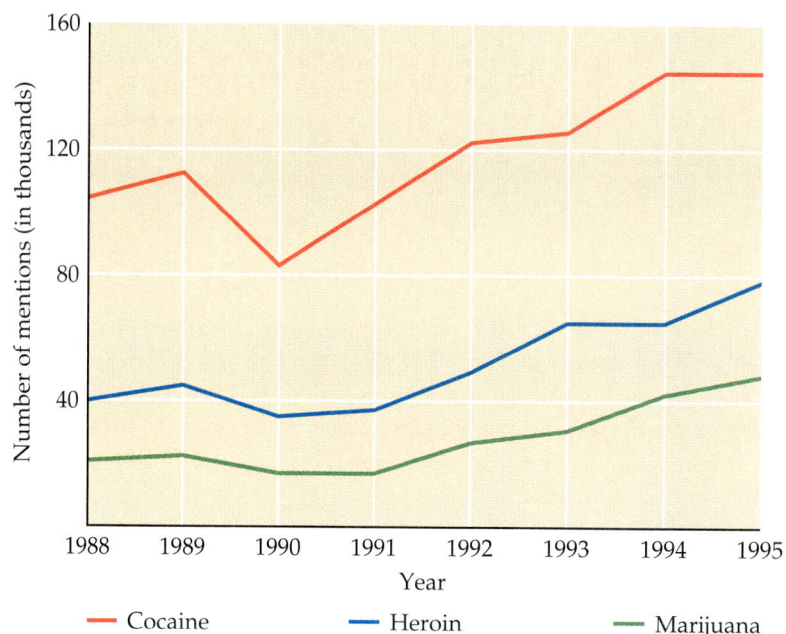

Figure 10.2 Trends in Drug-Related Emergency Room Mentions of Cocaine, Heroin and Marijuana. *Emergency room episodes related to drugs reflect the serious health hazards associated with cocaine, heroin, and marijuana. (Source: Drug Abuse Warning Network, National Institute on Drug Abuse (1988–91) and Substance Abuse and Mental Health Services Administration (1992–95))*

of all new AIDS cases affect injecting drug users and their sexual partners. There has also been a considerable increase in the number of babies born to women who are injecting drug users.

According to epidemiologists, injecting drug users who also smoke crack are seven times more likely to become infected than are injecting drug users not on crack. This is attributed to addicts swapping sex with their suppliers for crack or selling sex for money to buy the drug. This makes crack a significant contributing risk factor for AIDS.

People who inject drugs get the virus by sharing their needles, syringes, and other drug paraphernalia with users who already have HIV in their blood. AIDS is caused by a virus that destroys the body's immune system. It is passed from one person to another in bodily fluids, including blood, semen, and vaginal secretions. It can also be transmitted from an infected mother to her newborn baby (see Chapter 15).

In an effort to stop the increase in AIDS among injecting drug users, cities from New York City to Portland, Oregon, have experimented with programs in which clean needles are distributed free to addicts. Researchers studying needle exchange programs are reporting positive results—that is, fewer cases of HIV infection. In addition, many communities are providing street information, bleach to clean needles, and condoms to drug users. These programs are controversial because they aid the continuation of an illegal activity—possession of heroin, cocaine, and other drugs that are injected.

Even noninjecting drugs have a connection to AIDS. Drugs and sexual promiscuity often go together. Because drugs alter judgment, drug users are prone to engage in indiscriminate and unsafe sex, thus putting themselves and their partners at higher risk for getting HIV. Recent research indicates that HIV may require the presence of an already damaged immune system before it can cause disease. Some drugs, including amphetamines, marijuana, and inhalants, may first damage the immune system, leaving the user open to the further risk of AIDS. In addition, inhalants (particularly poppers and amyl nitrites) may be a cofactor in the development of Kaposi's sarcoma, a cancer associated with AIDS.

Special Concern for the Fetus

Concern about drug use during pregnancy has increased greatly in recent years, particularly as medical evidence mounts to show the adverse effect that drugs can have on the mother who takes them and on her unborn child. Overall, more than 10 percent of American babies are at risk for medical complications because their mothers abused drugs during pregnancy.

The effect of a drug on a fetus depends on many factors, including the drug, the amount taken by the mother, and the stage of pregnancy at which it is taken. The fetus is in greatest danger during the first three months of pregnancy, when its major organs are developing.

Studies show that cocaine use at any time during pregnancy—even once—can cause lasting fetal damage. When cocaine crosses the placenta, a large proportion of it is converted into norcocaine, a water-soluble substance that does not leave the womb. It is thought that norcocaine is more potent than cocaine itself. At the very least, the fetus is continually exposed to it. Norcocaine is excreted into the amniotic fluid and the fetus swallows it and thus is reexposed to the drug. Not only are many of these children born addicted to cocaine, but also they tend to suffer strokes and to have retarded growth, including smaller-than-normal-size heads and brains, and delayed motor development.

In general, pregnant women who are injecting drug users or sexual partners of injecting drug users greatly increase the risk of infecting their fetuses with HIV. However, it is not known why, but about 70 percent of all babies born to mothers with HIV do not themselves become infected.

Who should protect an unborn child from drugs? Lawsuits have been brought against women who have given birth to drug-addicted babies or have otherwise compromised their babies' lives by taking drugs during pregnancy. This has created much discussion within the legal community. Some of the issues involved in this controversy are an individual's right to privacy, the problem of proving intent to harm, and the conflict between fetal rights and women's rights.

Drugs in the Workplace

According to a study of drug-positive urine samples taken from the U.S. workers, marijuana is the most frequently detected drug. Nearly 60 percent of positive workplace drug tests conducted in the first six months of 1997 were positive for marijuana, followed by cocaine (18 percent), opiates (8 percent), and tranquilizers (5 percent).

Employers are increasingly testing workers for drugs on the job—and before they are hired. Ninety-eight percent of Fortune 200 companies—the nation's largest—used drug tests to screen potential employees, and an increasing number of midsize and small businesses are also screening. In a recruiting program, one large bus company found that 30 percent of applicants—all experienced bus drivers—tested positive for marijuana. Some drug testing programs have been successfully challenged in court on the basis of individual workers' right to privacy. Others have withstood this challenge and remain in force.

Another aspect of drug testing concerns employee morale and loyalty. As an executive in an engineering company in Pennsylvania said, "When you say to an employee, 'You're doing a great job; just the same I want you to pee into this jar and I'm sending someone to watch you,' you've undermined that trust." On the other hand, nearly 40 percent of white- and blue-collar workers surveyed by Gallup and the Institute for a Drug Free Workplace said they believe drug testing is necessary. Said an air conditioning and furnace installer, who applauds the fact that he and his coworkers are tested periodically, "If you have someone working on an electrical panel who has been using drugs and he turns on the power when he's not supposed to, and you're on the other end of the line, you're the one who's going to get hurt."

Harm Reduction: Preventing Drug Trafficking

One way to reduce the harm caused by illicit drugs is to reduce their entry into the United States. The number-one point of entry of drugs is the United States–Mexico border, where cocaine, heroin, methamphetamine, and marijuana come in hidden among the millions of cars, people, and drugs that cross thirty-eight ports of entry spanning nearly 2,000 miles. The second largest drug trafficking route into the country is through the Caribbean, specifically via Puerto Rico and the U.S. Virgin Islands. Drugs, especially heroin, also come in from southeast Asia.

Each year, thousands of pounds of drugs worth millions of dollars are seized by U.S. government officials. Despite national and international efforts to disrupt trafficking—including reducing coca cultivation abroad and increasing arrests at home—drugs still come into the United States illegally. To consider different points of view on the drug issue, see the Developing Health Skills box.

maintenance program A treatment program that involves providing a less dangerous drug to prevent withdrawal symptoms.

detoxification program A treatment program that involves a gradual but complete withdrawal from an abused drug.

therapeutic community A residential treatment center where people who abuse drugs can live and learn to adjust to drug-free lives.

Treatment Alternatives: The Long Road Back

A wide range of treatment alternatives are available for drug users, including maintenance and detoxification programs, therapeutic communities, hotlines, rap centers, and self-help groups.

Maintenance Programs

Maintenance programs involve substituting a more socially acceptable and less dangerous drug for the drug of choice. The substitute is provided free or at low cost. Maintenance programs are mainly used for heroin addiction. Methadone, a synthetic drug, is used to alleviate an addict's craving for the natural drug heroin and to prevent withdrawal symptoms. There are many benefits of methadone:

- It is easy to administer (a pill).
- Its effects last twenty-four to thirty-six hours, compared with heroin's action of four to eight hours.
- It does not produce a feeling of euphoria.
- It is safe at maintenance levels.
- It frees users from a physical dependence on heroin so they can spend their energy putting their life back together—being part of a family, working.
- It is legal.

Methadone's primary purpose is to prevent withdrawal symptoms. It can help heroin addicts seeking another "hit" to avoid criminal behavior. The main disadvantage of methadone is that it substitutes one addiction for another. It does not change the underlying addictive behavior.

Detoxification Programs

The goal of a **detoxification program** is to reduce drug intake to zero and to give the addict medical and psychological assistance during withdrawal. This approach can work well, especially for alcoholics. The majority of heroin addicts who enter a detoxification program drop out after a few days because, even though the discomfort of withdrawal is minimized, the craving for heroin still remains. Some detoxification centers are housed in hospitals or clinics; others are in outpatient settings with the addicts attending programs and therapeutic sessions all day.

Therapeutic Communities

The goal of **therapeutic communities** is to deal with the psychological cause of drug dependence and to bring about a complete lifestyle change. This includes

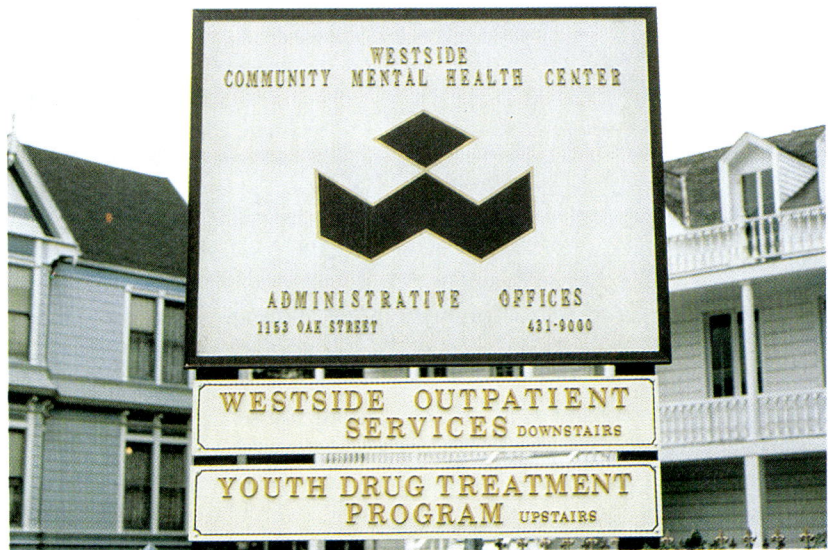

There are a range of drug treatment programs available in every community—from inpatient and outpatient counseling to acupuncture. The first step in treatment is seeking help. (Source: Stock, Boston/© Stephen Frisch)

moving toward abstinence from drugs, development of employable skills or return to school, self-reliance, and honesty.

The first therapeutic community for drug addicts was Synanon, which started in 1958. Others include Daytop Village and Phoenix House. Part of the treatment includes encounter group therapy and group pressure. All members of the community are assigned jobs in the community and eventually on the "outside." Staff members are mostly former drug addicts who have been rehabilitated in the same or a similar therapeutic community.

One of the drawbacks of this approach is that it takes about fifteen months before a resident is ready to leave the community, and there is a high dropout rate. Some people get bored or frustrated with the program or aren't ready for such a complete change in their lifestyles. Among those who remain, there is a relatively high success rate.

Other Treatment Modalities

Although these results are not clinically documented, some people report successful treatment for drug addiction with acupuncture, biofeedback, and hypnosis. In addition, there are groups including Narcotics Anonymous, rap centers, free clinics, and hot lines, which are used for self-help and crisis intervention and to direct people to appropriate resources in the community. The growth of drug abuse treatment facilities in recent years reflects an increase in the demand for such services.

Caution should be exercised when deciding to seek professional help for a substance abuse problem. A reliable way to check a treatment center's credentials is through your physician, college health clinic, a local medical school, or a psychiatric society.

Critical Thinking Question

One of the most recognized health promotion campaigns is "Say no to drugs." There is some evidence that it was successful with some segments of the U.S. public and not so successful with others. With what groups might such a campaign be most effective? What groups do you think would be less likely to respond positively? Why?

HEALTH SKILLS

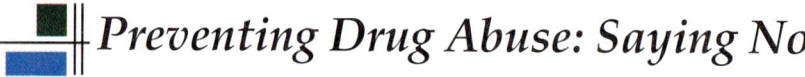
Preventing Drug Abuse: Saying No

Is it possible to learn how to say no? Here are some strategies that health education specialists recommend. Think about how you can incorporate them as a part of your lifestyle.

Build self-esteem and self-confidence. Drug abuse is a symptom of low self-esteem. For the person who values social acceptance above his or her own health, drug abuse is an option. For the person who values him- or herself above the all-too-brief social acceptance of a night out, drug abuse is not an option.

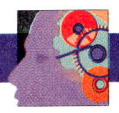

DEVELOPING HEALTH SKILLS

Perspectives on Solving the Drug Problem: What Will Work

Public opinion polls consistently show that Americans are greatly concerned about the extent of drug use in their country. There is no consistent response, however, on how to solve the drug problem. Attitudes toward drug use are diverse and conflicting and proposed solutions range from jailing all first-time offenders to legalizing drugs to making treatment and rehabilitation available to drug users.

Consider the following personal perspectives on the drug problem:

An Advocate of Stronger Law Enforcement

"What we need in this country are stronger laws, more laws, and more law enforcement officers. Test everybody for the presence of controlled substances within their system, and whoever fails should go to jail or pay a stiff fine. If we can simply get the pusher off the street and stop the flow of drugs across our borders, then our problems will be solved. The way to do this is to build more prisons and require that drug users and pushers serve time. In fact, we should take a hint from some of our foreign friends and cut off the hands of drug pushers. They would have a difficult time pushing so hard if they had no hands."

- Would the money spent on building jails and hiring law enforcement officers be better spent on drug rehabilitation and prevention?
- If everyone is tested for drug use, won't civil rights be abused?

An Advocate of Legalizing Drugs

"Make drugs legal, and the corruption and violence associated with them will disappear. Our cities will be safe again. The Prohibition Era proved that making a substance illegal simply doesn't work. That's why the eighteenth amendment was repealed. It was done with alcohol, and now it's time to legalize drugs."

- Won't this lead to more people taking drugs?
- Isn't there a big difference between legalizing marijuana and legalizing cocaine?

An Advocate of Education and Prevention

"The only answer lies in prevention. We must get to the children before they take their first drug. Let's tell them how to say no in social situations. Let's give them the facts about the dangers of drugs. If we are ever going to have a drug-free society, we must begin with a drug-free population—our children."

- Children recognize split messages such as, "Do as I say and not as I do." How can we ask them to say no to drugs when so many adults say yes?

A Former Addict

"Nobody knows what I know. When you take drugs you lose control. You forget about society, you forget about honesty, you forget your values and your moral upbringing. You'd kill your mother for a $5 hit. Nobody knows who has never been there. The answer is to rehabilitate the drug users—bring them back from the dead through intensive intervention and support. If we do that for everyone, then we'll be on the road to solving the drug problem."

- What does rehabilitation cost, and who will pay for it—employers? The federal government?
- Can former addicts really be effective proponents of "say no" when they have said yes for so long?

Make decisions about drugs rationally, not emotionally. Be proactive, not reactive. The decision to use or not to use a drug should not be a spur-of-the-moment choice. It should be done well ahead of the real-life confrontation with drugs. Good decision-making skills include (1) honestly assessing a situation and identifying the problems that might result, (2) examining solutions to the problems and the possible consequences of each solution, (3) taking action that is in the best interest of yourself and those around you, and (4) evaluating the choices.

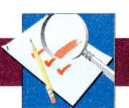

HERE'S LOOKING AT YOU

Reacting to Situations: Are You Able to Say No?

Below are ten situations involving drugs. Read each situation, then circle the letter next to the action that you would be most likely to take.

1. During lunch, a friend claims that "everyone" should smoke marijuana, just to find out what it is like. This friend offers to get you high. What would you be most likely to do in this situation?
   A. Tell your friend that you don't care what getting high is like.
   B. Avoid the subject by asking if anyone would like to go to a movie later.
   C. Point out to your friend that you know enough about marijuana to know that it's no good.
   D. Accept your friend's offer to try marijuana.

2. You are at a large party. You meet some people who are snorting cocaine. They invite you to sit down and "do some coke." What would you be most likely to do in this situation?
   A. Sit down and snort the cocaine.
   B. Turn and leave without speaking.
   C. Sit down, but say, "Not right now," to the offer of cocaine.
   D. Explain that you don't use cocaine.

3. The actions of a close relative have made you extremely upset. When you discuss this with a friend, he offers you some tranquilizers to calm you down. What would you be most likely to do in this situation?
   A. Accept the pills from your friend, but throw them away once your friend leaves.
   B. Accept the tranquilizers and take them.
   C. Refuse the pills and ask your friend to leave.
   D. Thank your friend for the offer, but refuse the pills.

4. You go out for the evening with a new friend whom you like very much. On your way to dinner, your friend asks if you would like to smoke some very good hashish. You can tell that your friend is trying to do something special for you. What would you be most likely to do in this situation?
   A. End the evening right then and go home.
   B. Tell your friend that you're not ready to try smoking hashish yet.
   C. Smoke the hashish and make your friend happy.
   D. Decline the hashish and hope that you don't hurt your friend's feelings.

5. You must work many hours without rest to finish a project. A person working with you offers you some "speed" (amphetamines) to help you stay awake. What would you be most likely to do in this situation?
   A. Say that you are concerned that taking speed would make you less able to do your work.
   B. Accept the pills, but throw them away when you go to get a glass of water.
   C. Say that you would rather keep drinking coffee to try to stay awake.
   D. Accept the speed, and take it.

6. A long-time friend asks you to try LSD. Your friend has never taken LSD and wants to find out what it is like. Your friend wants the two of you to take it together. What would you be most likely to do in this situation?
   A. Tell your friend to take the LSD alone or with someone else.
   B. Take LSD with your friend, as long as you can find a safe time and place to do it.

Assertively resist peer pressure. If you make a decision that protects your health, stick to it. Peer pressure exists at all levels of society and at all ages. Just because you have survived adolescence, it doesn't mean you are free from peer pressure. Being assertive is important in dealing with many health-related behaviors. Whether the pressure is to drink or to become involved with harder drugs like crack cocaine, resistance is a matter of assertively standing up to people—and for yourself.

Reduce stress. Stress is one of the primary reasons people turn to drugs. By developing coping skills and learning breathing exercises and other tech-

C. Suggest that the two of you find something safer to do than take LSD.
D. Tell your friend that you might take LSD, but then hope that your offer is forgotten.

7. You are having dinner with several friends who are cigarette smokers. When the coffee is served, most of them light up. One offers you a cigarette. What would you be most likely to do in this situation?
   A. Say that you don't smoke.
   B. Decline the offer, saying that you want to wait awhile.
   C. Have a cigarette.
   D. Tell the person that you can't smoke because you have a chest cold.

8. Your new neighbors invite you over for dinner. After dinner, one of them says that they sometimes smoke marijuana in the evening. They invite you to smoke with them. What would you be most likely to do in this situation?
   A. Decline the offer and go home.
   B. Decline the marijuana, but stay and talk.
   C. Smoke the marijuana.
   D. Tell them that you would rather smoke it some other time.

9. You are under great pressure at work. You feel nervous all the time and have begun to lose sleep. A good friend suggests that you take some Valium (tranquilizers) until the pressure eases off. Your friend has a prescription for the drug and can easily give you the pills. What would you be most likely to do in this situation?
   A. Try the pills to see if they help.
   B. Accept the pills, but throw them away.
   C. Refuse your friend's offer.
   D. Tell your friend that you would like to think about it.

10. You attend a party of people from work. To your surprise, several of your coworkers are snorting cocaine ("coke") together. It is apparent that they have done this before, and they encourage you to join them. These are people you work with every day, and you like them. What would you be most likely to do in this situation?
    A. Tell the group that your ride is leaving, so you don't have time to use the cocaine.
    B. Snort the cocaine.
    C. Tell the group that you don't use drugs.
    D. Refuse the offer by saying that you're not in the mood to snort cocaine.

Below is a key to the answer choices that entail using drugs. For each of these selected, assign no points. For any other response selected, assign one point. Sum your scores.

Item no.	Drug use response
1	D
2	A
3	B
4	C
5	D
6	B
7	C
8	C
9	A
10	B

A maximum score of ten indicates that you believe strongly that you will not take drugs if offered. A minimum score of zero indicates that you believe strongly that you will take drugs if offered.

Source: U.S. Department of Health and Human Services, Office of Disease Prevention and Health Promotion

niques, you can reduce stress and, in turn, reduce the potential for succumbing to drug abuse.

Get involved in hobbies and recreational activities. Hobbies and recreational activities can provide excitement and challenge. The healthy nature of such activities leaves little room for the unhealthy activity of drug abuse.

Remain informed. Get accurate and up-to-date information about drugs, including the short- and long-term risks. By knowing the facts, you are equipped to resist the temptation to engage in health-compromising behaviors.

Develop your own strategies for saying no. By having lots of reasons not to use drugs, you reduce your potential for drug use. Check your ability to say no with the Here's Looking at You box.

Key Concepts

1. The term *drug* refers to a chemical substance that causes a change in the body's functioning, including physiological and psychological activity.
2. Drug abuse normally occurs in stages, with a typical progression starting with cigarettes, beer, or wine; moving on to marijuana and hard liquor; and subsequently moving on to illicit drugs such as heroin and cocaine.
3. Drug use among college-age men and women dropped between 1985 and 1995 and began to rise again in 1996.
4. When used properly, many drugs, such as antibiotics, offer great benefit. Others, however, offer no benefit and present a clear danger to individuals and to society as a whole.
5. Dependence occurs when a person is so physically and/or psychologically attached to a drug that he or she cannot live comfortably without it.
6. A drug may affect only a limited portion of the body, or it may affect the entire body. Drugs also can be transmitted across the placenta and compromise the normal development of a fetus.
7. Marijuana is not a single drug. It contains nearly 400 chemicals, several of which are unique to the substance.
8. Designer drugs are a variation on illegal drugs. They are made in clandestine laboratories and are designed specifically to circumvent the law.
9. The National Institute on Drug Abuse estimates that typical drug users spend $100 a day—$36,500 a year—on their habits.
10. Treatments for drug addiction include maintenance and detoxification programs, therapeutic communities, hot lines, and self-help groups such as Narcotics Anonymous.

Review Questions

1. Define the term *drug*, and explain how over-the-counter drugs, prescription drugs, and dangerous or illegal substances all fit the definition.
2. List the drugs most often used by college students.
3. What is a gateway drug and how is it related to the concept of staging?
4. Differentiate between main effects and side effects of drugs.
5. Illustrate, using mathematics, additive, inhibitory, and synergistic effects that result when two or more drugs are taken at the same time.
6. Explain the differences between grouping drugs according to how they are taken, by their effects, and by the motive of the user.
7. List ways that injecting drug use harms health.
8. Of all the health risks associated with drug abuse, why is the fetus in a most vulnerable position?
9. Describe three treatment alternatives for individuals experiencing a drug problem.
10. List specific actions you can take in order to avoid drug abuse.

Selected Bibliography

Cahalan, D. *An Ounce of Prevention: Strategies for Solving Tobacco, Alcohol, and Drug Problems.* San Francisco: Jossey-Bass, 1991.

Monitoring the Future Study. Rockville, MD: National Institute on Drug Abuse, (published annually).

National Household Survey on Drug Abuse. Rockville, MD: Substance Abuse and Mental Health Services Administration, (published annually).

Strain, E.C., et al. "Caffeine Dependence Syndrome." *Journal of the American Medical Association.* 272, no. 13 (1994): 1043–1048.

Understanding Drug Treatment. Washington, DC: National Institute of Medicine, National Academy Press, 1990.

HealthLinks: Web Sites for Preventing the Illegal Use of Substances

You can access better health as it relates to this chapter by checking out some of the following sites on the Internet. These and sites identified within the chapter can be accessed directly when you visit the *HealthStyles* Web Site located on the Allyn and Bacon home page at **http://www.abacon.com.**

Center for Substance Abuse Research (CESAR)
sss.bsos.umd.edu/cesar/cesar.html
Based at the University of Maryland, the Center for Substance Abuse Research collects, analyzes, and disseminates information on the nature and extent of substance abuse and related problems. The Center also heads up initiatives on prevention and abuse programs and provides training and technical assistance on prevention programs.

Partnership for a Drug-Free America
www.drugfreeamerica.org
The most complete and accurate compilation of information about drugs on the Web. The site includes information on the slang names of drugs, identification of different drugs, and tips on how to talk to your kids about drugs.

Health Hotlines: Understanding the Dangers of Drug Use

Cocaine Anonymous
3740 Overland Avenue, Suite H
Los Angeles, CA 90034
(800) 347-8998

Families Anonymous
(Families coping with drug abuse and alcohol)
P.O. Box 3475
Culver City, CA 90231–3475
(800) 736-9805

National Clearinghouse for Alcohol and Drug Information
P.O. Box 2345
Rockvillw, MD 20852
(800) SAY-NOTO (729-6686)

National Drug and Alcohol Treatment Routing Service
107 Lincoln Street
Worcester, MA 01605
(800) 662-HELP (662-4357)

MUNI Line 19

If you are beaten
If you are hurt
If you are scared
If you need help

GET OUT

Call
(415) 864-4555

San Francisco Domestic Violence Consortium

Liz Claiborne

Chapter 11

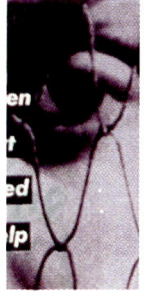
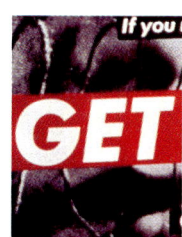
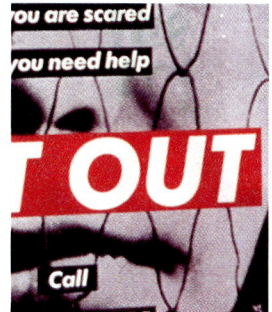

Recognizing Violent Behavior

Objectives

When you finish reading this chapter, you will be able to:

1. Recognize violent behavior as a threat to personal health as well as a threat to the health of the general public.
2. List several characteristics of the typical criminal, the person who commits acts of violence.
3. List several characteristics of the typical victim, the person who experiences violent crime.
4. Explain when and where violent crime usually takes place.
5. Describe how television, drugs, and the availability of handguns are factors in violent crime.
6. Conduct a mediation session between two individuals experiencing a conflict.
7. Cite several examples of violent behavior found in the home or on the job.
8. Describe the prevalence of abuse carried out against women in the United States.
9. Recognize an abusive relationship.
10. Differentiate between different types of rape and describe the attacker in each case.

What Is Your HealthStyle?

After graduating from college in her small hometown, Faye moved to the city for better job opportunities and more excitement. She knew that big cities offer dangers along with the excitement. But she felt that the trade-off was worth it.

When actually confronted with big-city living, Faye found herself too frightened to enjoy it. Instead of taking advantage of the numerous cultural and educational activities, she went home after work to her apartment. Although it was boring, she felt safe there. When she ventured out, even in the daytime, she looked at everyone as a possible mugger, rapist, or robber. After several months of living in fear and anxiety and seeing her quality of life diminish, Faye returned to her hometown.

When LaVerne moved to the city after graduating from college in a rural community, she was ready for some excitement, but she also wanted safety. She had taken karate in college, and she practiced it regularly. Now she took a course at the Y in women's assertiveness training so that she would be less intimidated if someone confronted her on the street.

LaVerne evaluated her environment and figured out what was safe, and unsafe, to do. For example, at school she had jogged in the evenings after studying. In the city, she switched to a lunchtime run, in daylight and with lots of other people on the streets. She also went out a lot at night—to listen to live jazz and to go to the latest movies—but she always went with friends, stayed on well-lit blocks, and took other safety precautions.

In Your Opinion

To protect herself from crime on the streets, Faye stayed at home. In contrast, LaVerne took positive steps to protect herself against some of the dangers of living in a big city.

- What steps could Faye have taken to make her life more manageable yet at the same time safe?
- What would you do to protect yourself if you moved to a high-crime city?
- What health skills does LaVerne have that Faye seems to be missing?
- How would living in a big city enhance or compromise the quality of your life?

Hardly a day goes by that a harsh, violent act is not a front-page story. If you tune into the news on television, you are likely to see a report of a man firing a handgun at a room full of people in a public building; of an angry, abused teenager killing her father; or of a suicide pact carried to completion. Violence in the United States is a public health emergency. Some possible reasons for violence are drugs, availability of firearms, urban poverty, and a variety of sociological factors.

Violence is not something that happens only to someone else. You have a good chance of being a victim of some act of violence in your lifetime. Moreover, you are likely to be victimized more than once. Being a victim can be traumatizing, even though not all crimes are life threatening or even require medical attention—for example, having your car vandalized or stolen.

Violence is often viewed as a law enforcement problem and, in this context, is associated with questions about gun control, policing, sentencing, and parole policy. In this textbook, however, we discuss violence as a personal and public health problem. It is a major cause of death for adolescents and young adults and a source of mental anguish, stress, and anxiety among the population as a whole. From the health perspective, crime and the fear of crime are eroding the quality of life.

By definition, **violence** is the use of force with the intent to harm oneself or another person. Each year, according to a recent report from the National Institute of Justice, 49 million people are victims of violence in the United States. This includes homicide, child abuse, rape, arson, and other assaults. The price tag is high: $105 billion annually in medical expenses and property and productivity losses. This amounts to what the researchers call a "crime tax" of roughly $425 per man, woman, and child in the United States. And when the values of pain, long-term emotional trauma, and disability are put into dollar terms, the costs rise to $450 billion annually, or $1,800 per person.

The intangible, quality-of-life losses—the emotional scars—are often larger than tangible costs such as medical care. For example, the tangible costs for a rape victim are calculated to be $5,100, but the intangible costs are $81,400. One woman who was raped in her apartment said, "My whole life has been invaded, violated, and not just by the act itself. There have been times when I wish the rapist had killed me. It would have been kinder."

For many other victims as well, life after a violent crime is never the same as before the event. Some victims are afraid to go out in public; others change their jobs or schools or move from one community to another to escape bad memories. Children who are victims of violent crimes may suffer delays in physical, social, and emotional development, and battered women are at a greatly elevated risk for alcoholism, drug abuse, and suicide attempts.

Even if you are not a victim, violence can affect the overall quality of your life. If one household in your neighborhood is affected by a crime, the entire neighborhood may feel more vulnerable. An increasing number of Americans, particularly the elderly, report in surveys that they are afraid to go out alone at night. They are afraid of the possibility of being a victim of violence.

The Criminal: Who Commits Acts of Violence?

There is no one type of person who commits violent crimes. Neither is there a gene that predisposes someone to such behavior. Nevertheless, it is possible to make some generalizations about who commits a crime, based on the Federal Bureau of Investigation's (FBI) *Uniform Crime Report* and Bureau of Justice Statistics surveys of inmates in local jails and state correctional facilities:

- Violent crimes tend to be committed by young men. In more than half of arrests for violent crime, the offender is under twenty-five years old.
- Most violent offenders are white, but African American arrest rates are significantly higher than for whites. Although African Americans make up about 12 percent of the population, they account for at least 50 percent of the arrests for homicide, rape, aggravated assault, and robbery. These figures may misrepresent the extent of the involvement of African Americans in violent acts. For example, it is possible that police prejudice results in greater surveillance of African Americans and a greater willingness to arrest them.
- A relationship exists between family background and delinquency. Many offenders have been abused as children. Some studies suggest that adoles-

violence The use of force with the intent to harm oneself or another person.

cents subjected to extreme abuse and violence at home may develop violent behavior because they never learn how to relate to others effectively and continue to model the aggressive behavior of their parents. About 40 percent of prison inmates have immediate family members (father, mother, brother, sister, spouse, or child) who have been in prison.

- Alcohol and drugs often play a role in the life of offenders. To begin with, drug use is usually illegal. As many as 80 percent of jail and prison inmates report having used drugs, and about one third of state felony convictions are for drug offenses.
- The average level of education attained by offenders is far below the national average. About 28 percent of prison inmates have completed high school, compared with 85 percent of all men aged twenty to twenty-nine.
- Employment bears some relationship to violent behavior. About 45 percent of all men in jail were unemployed at the time they were incarcerated. Adult felons are more likely than the general population never to have worked at all or to have held a wide variety of short-term jobs. Given this, it is not surprising that the average inmate was living at the poverty level before entering jail.

The Victim: Who Is at Risk for Being Assaulted?

Victims share many similar demographic characteristics with people who commit crimes, such as gender, race, income, and age (see Figure 11.1).

- Overall, crime is a male experience: Far more men than women commit and/or are victimized by violent crimes. Women are victims more often than men in only two categories: rape and personal larceny. (Purse snatching is an example of personal larceny.)

Characteristic of victims	Rate of personal crime per 1,000
Sex	
Male	64.4
Female	38.5
Age	
12–15	110.9
16–19	110.3
20–24	79.8
25–34	55.9
35–49	35.8
50–64	15.6
65 or older	6.9
Race	
White	44.6
Black	58.4
Other	43.8
Hispanic origin	
Hispanic	56.1
Non-Hispanic	45.0
Household income	
Less than $7,500	74.6
$7,500–14,999	49.7
$15,000–24,999	49.2
$25,000–34,999	48.1
$35,000–49,999	45.8
$50,000–74,999	44.1
$75,000 or more	37.9
Region	
Northeast	41.1
Midwest	46.7
South	39.6
West	61.5
Residence	
Urban	59.9
Suburban	43.5
Rural	35.5

Figure 11.1 Who Are Victims of Crime? *Men, African Americans, and young adults are at higher risk for being a victim of crime than women, whites, and middle-aged people. (Source: Bureau of Justice Statistics, 1995)*

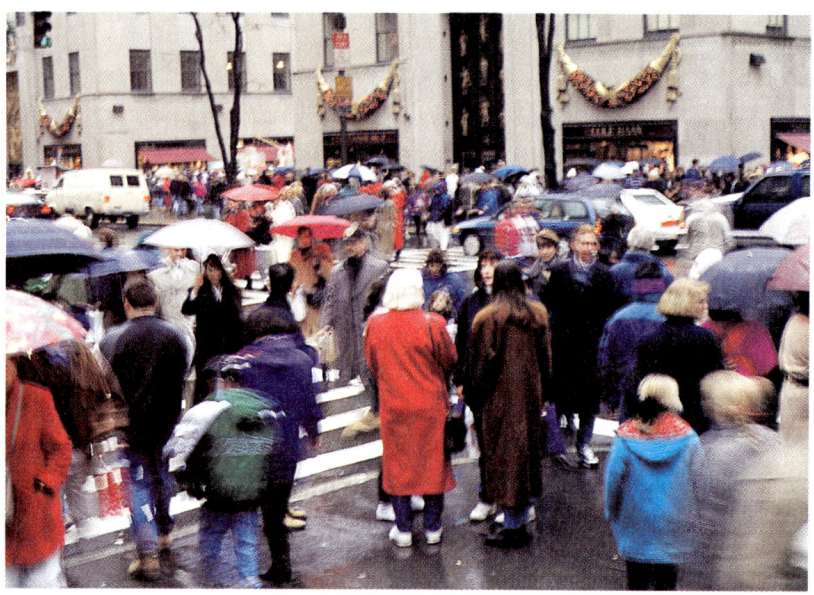

More crimes take place in cities, but the suburbs and rural communities are not without their problems. Violence knows no boundaries. (Source: © Tony Stone/Cosmo Condina)

- African Americans are victims of crimes at a higher rate than whites, particularly for robbery and burglary. For instance, an African American's risk for being robbed is three times higher than a white person's. In part, this is because African Americans live in high-crime neighborhoods to a greater extent than do whites.
- The lower his or her income, the greater a person is at risk for being a victim of crime. Poorer people are more likely to be raped, robbed, or assaulted seriously. As annual family income increases, the incidence of violent crime generally decreases. There is one exception to this: Higher-income households are more likely to be robbed than are lower-income households.
- Teenagers and young adults are more likely to be victims of crime than are older people. However, the elderly are a particularly vulnerable crime target. They tend to live alone, often in high-crime, urban neighborhoods; eyesight and hearing losses reduce their alertness to danger signs; physical weakness and chronic conditions such as osteoporosis or arthritis reduce the chance that they will fight back aggressively; and they are lonely and more likely to trust someone, thus making them more susceptible to fraud.
- Violence against gay people has increased significantly, according to a study by the National Gay and Lesbian Task Force. Incidents of victimization include verbal harassment and threats, physical assault, and police abuse.
- Nearly half of all victims know, or have seen, the person who has committed the crime against them. According to the Bureau of Justice Statistics, 38 percent of violent crimes were committed by acquaintances and friends and 9 percent by relatives.

HealthLinks Web
Department of Justice Information Center
www.ncjrs.org
A collection of clearinghouses providing extensive information, documents, and links about criminal and juvenile justice.

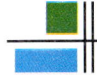 When and Where Crimes Take Place

Crime does not take place in a random fashion. Just as it is possible to make general characterizations about people who commit crimes and about victims, it is also possible to characterize where and when crimes take place.

More crimes take place in cities than in suburbs, and more crimes take place in suburbs than in rural areas. In recent years, the difference in crime rate between cities and suburbs has been decreasing. In part, this is because the suburbs have become more city-like in population mix, commercial development, and feeling of anonymity. Rural areas, too, are no longer as isolated and homogeneous as they once were and are not without their problems.

Crime rates also differ within cities, depending on neighborhoods. Low-income neighborhoods, usually in the deteriorating and older parts of a city, are more likely to have higher proportions both of people who commit crimes and victims than more affluent sections.

Crimes tend to concentrate during certain time periods. The weekend, particularly Saturday night between 8 P.M. and 2 A.M., is highly associated with homicide and rape. Saturday night is the traditional time for fun, carousing, and letting loose. Money, alcohol, and drugs flow more freely on the weekend, thus setting a conducive environment for crime.

Robbery is more evenly distributed throughout the day and the week. Robberies in homes tend to take place during the day when people are at work, at school, shopping, or otherwise away. Robberies in stores and other commercial properties are more prevalent in the evening, when customers and employees are not likely to be there.

The statistics on crime are intimidating, particularly those that suggest that there is a good chance that you may experience a crime yourself. As with all health threats, however, prevention is the key to avoiding becoming a victim of crime. Examine the Developing Health Skills box for pointers on prevention.

DEVELOPING HEALTH SKILLS

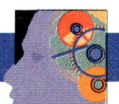

How to Avoid Being a Victim of Crime

It is not possible to know in advance how you will respond to an act of violence–being robbed, raped, beaten, threatened, or abused. Trying to reason with the attacker or putting up resistance might make sense in one situation but not another. An act of "bravery" in the face of an armed assailant could be foolish and might result in injury or death.

Overall, most people do not behave passively when they are violently attacked. Eight of ten victims of forcible rape and more than 50 percent of robbery victims attempt some kind of self-protective measure, ranging from trying to get help to using physical force.

Many preventive measures can be taken so that you can avoid being a victim of crime. The following tips come from various police departments.

At Home or in a College Residence

- Lock the windows and doors—including sliding glass doors—when you go out.
- Make your home appear occupied when you go out by using a timer to turn on lights and a radio.
- Do not keep large sums of money at home or leave valuables such as jewelry in open view.
- Never let a stranger into your home without checking his or her identification. Install a peephole in your door and use it.
- Do not give the impression that you are at home alone if strangers telephone or come to the door.
- If you live in an apartment, avoid being in the laundry room or garage by yourself, especially at night.
- If you come home and find a door or window open or other signs of forced entry, do not go in. Go to the nearest phone and call the police.
- Get to know your neighbors and keep their phone numbers handy for emergencies.
- Take care of your keys. Do not give anyone the chance to duplicate them. Do not hide extra house keys under a doormat or in other obvious spots.

On the Street

- Walk purposefully and look confident. Walk close to the curb. Avoid doorways, bushes, and alleys. Be alert to your surroundings.
- Use well-lighted, well-traveled routes and try to walk with friends.
- Avoid shortcuts through isolated areas, including parking lots and underground garages.
- Be careful when people stop to ask you for directions. Always reply from a distance and never get too close to the car.
- If you believe you are being followed, walk into a store or knock on a house door.
- If you are in trouble, attract help any way you can. Scream, yell for help, or yell, "Fire!"
- Have your house key in your hand as you approach your home.
- Carry change for emergency telephone and transportation use.

In Your Car

- Lock all doors and close all windows when leaving your car.
- Park in well-lighted areas and try not to walk alone in parking areas at night.
- Have your keys ready when you approach your car. Check the inside for intruders before entering and lock the door immediately after getting in your car.
- Always keep your gas tank at least half full.
- If you have a flat tire, drive on it until you reach a safe, well-lighted, and well-traveled area.
- If your car breaks down in an isolated area, raise the hood. Stay in the locked car. If someone stops to help, ask them to call the police. Sound your horn if you are threatened.
- Never pick up strangers.

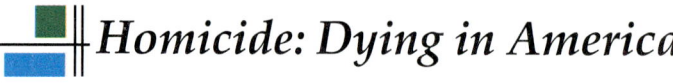

Homicide: Dying in America

"It's a jungle out there," said a political leader of one of the largest cities in the United States. What he was referring to is the **homicide** rate in U.S. cities. Homicide rates rose from the mid-1980s to 1993—up from 8.2 per 100,000 population in

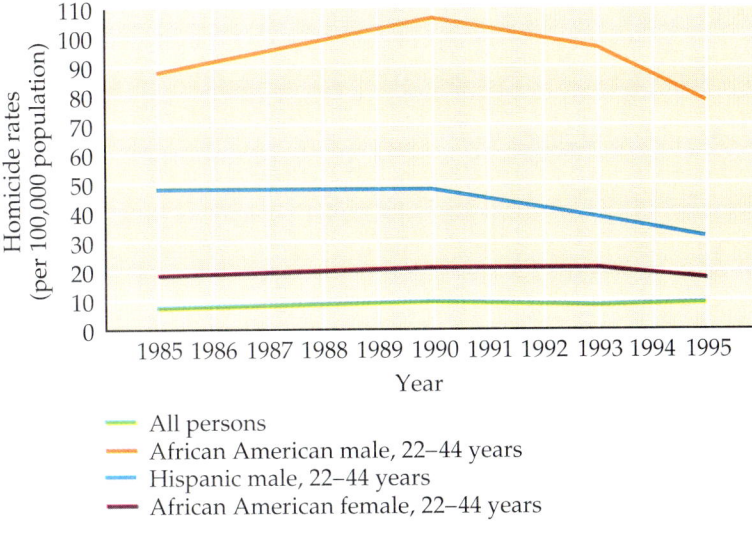

Figure 11.2 Homicide Rates for Minorities (per 100,000 population). *African-American and Hispanic males have a significantly higher risk of dying as a result of a homicide than do other Americans. (Source: National Center for Health Statistics, 1997)*

1985 to 8.9 per 100,000 in 1995. For African Americans, the rate was much higher: 77.9 per 100,000 males aged 22 to 44 (see Figure 11.2). The overall homicide rate began to drop, and by 1996, it was about 7.3 per 100,000. Criminologists do not have an adequate theory to explain why the homicide rate has fallen, but many experts point to more aggressive police tactics and tougher gun control laws.

Another change in homicide trends is less positive. Most homicides used to be committed by family members or acquaintances, but that is no longer the case. In 1965, nearly one third of all murders in the United States were family-related; today, only about one tenth are. Increasingly, murders are committed by persons of "unknown relationship" to the victim.

Offenders give a wide range of responses as to the single reason they killed someone. A recent study of homicides in Ohio conducted by the Ohio Department of Health reported that 40 percent of the respondents said that they killed someone because of some type of threatened or actual physical abuse that had occurred just before the incident; 10 percent suggested alcohol and/or drugs were the immediate reason; 10 percent blamed jealousy, money, or the general stresses of living together; 12 percent said their crimes were accidental; and the rest of the motives for killing were listed as "other" or "unknown."

Several factors prevalent in U.S. society are linked with violence. Three of the most widely discussed and debated factors are: the availability of handguns, drug and alcohol consumption, and viewing violence on TV.

Gun Killings

Guns were the cause of more than 39,000 deaths nationwide in 1993. Forty-eight percent of them were suicides, 46 percent were homicides, and the rest were unintentional. Guns are widely available in the United States, where more than one of every three households has a gun, according to a recent Justice Department survey. Roughly 44 million Americans own 192 million guns in total. No other country comes near this record. In Canada, for example, only 6 million guns are legally owned (see Cultural View box).

Gun ownership is highly correlated as a risk factor for homicide in the home. In the Ohio homicide study, handguns accounted for 76 percent of the homicides. Most of the guns were kept loaded and in an unlocked location in the household in which the homicide took place.

Researchers have calculated just how risky having a gun at home can be:

- If you have a gun at home, you are eight times more likely to be killed by or to kill a family member or close acquaintance.

homicide The killing of one human being by another.

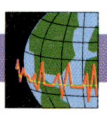

CULTURAL VIEW

How Other Countries Get a Grip on Gun Control

The United States has more guns per household—and a higher gun homicide rate—than does any other country. Do more handguns lead to more killings no matter where you live? Or is there something in the culture of a country that drives the mortality rate from guns up—or down? By studying Figure 11.3, you will see that Northern Ireland has a very high gun homicide rate but a low rate of gun ownership. Conversely, Canada and Switzerland have relatively high rates of gun ownership but low gun homicide rates.

The high rate of gun homicides in Northern Ireland can be explained by the decades of deadly fighting between Catholics and Protestants. The following provide insights about guns and homicide in three countries.

Taking Action in Canada

After a 1989 massacre of fourteen college women in Quebec by a gunman with a semiautomatic rifle, the Canadian government began tightening its gun control measures. To start with, big-rifle magazines and semiautomatic versions of automatic weapons were banned in 1991. After two more highly publicized gun shootings, even stricter laws were passed. Canada now requires gun owners to pass a test, get a license, and register every gun by the year 2003.

Handgun registration has long been in effect in Canada, so the new law is aimed mostly at unregistered rifles and shotguns in more rural areas. Polls consistently show that more than 70 percent of Canadians are in favor of tougher gun laws.

The Swiss Tradition

The Swiss have a high level of gun ownership, but that is because they have a militia rather than a standing army. Under the compulsory military service laws in Switzerland, most men remain active soldiers until their early 40s, and they keep their assault rifles and an allotment of ammunition at home. Nevertheless, there are relatively few gun homicides in Switzerland—there were 113 in 1995. In part, this is because there are a lot of regulations, including requiring police authorization to purchase a gun. Another reason is that the Swiss revere their guns, and they respect the confidence that the state puts in each citizen to protect the country.

A Cultural Change in Japan

Thirty-four people were murdered with guns in Japan in 1995 out of a population of 125 million. While this is a very low rate of gun homicide, gun control officials in Japan are concerned because the

- If you get involved in a fight with a family member or close acquaintance and one of you has a gun in the home, you are twelve times more likely to kill or to be killed.

Critical Thinking Question

Following a mass killing in Tasmania in 1996, Australia banned all handgun ownership and banned the possession of most guns altogether. Given the staggering amount of handgun violence in the United States, what are the chances that such a ban will become law in the next five years? What might prompt quicker action in the United States? Has the "right to bear arms" clause in the U.S. Constitution become outmoded?

number of Japanese being threatened or murdered by guns is increasing.

Japan's gun laws are already very strict. For example, it is against the law for virtually anyone except law enforcement officials to own a handgun. And while rifles and shotguns are permitted for hunting and target shooting, licensing requires a background check and training in proper use of the firearm.

Laws, however, cannot stop cultural products that are promoting the gun-and-violence trend. According to one gun salesman: "A violent hit movie can boost sales."

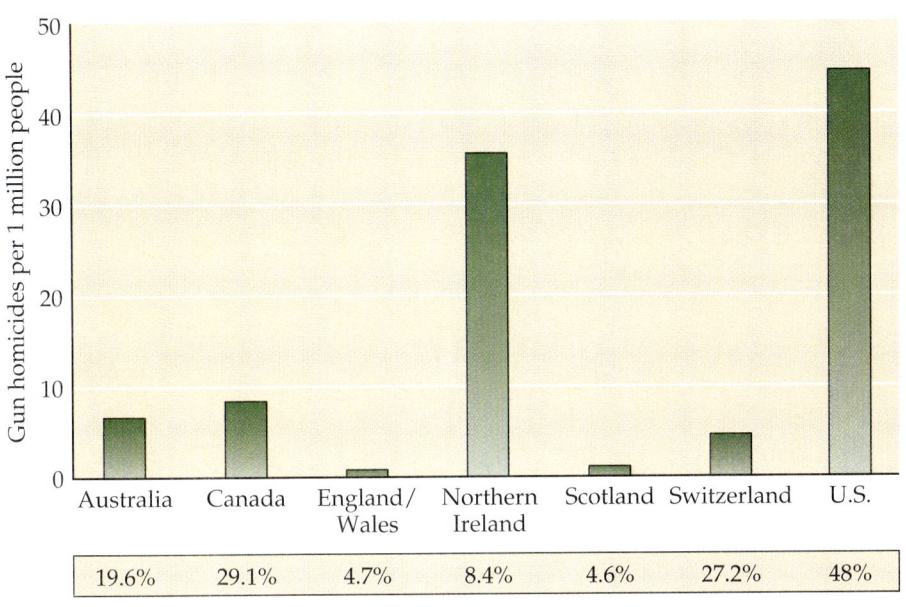

Figure 11.3 Homicide Rate and Gun Ownership. *(Source: Data from Coalition for Gun Control, Canada)*

The Influence of Drugs

A factor contributing to the overall homicide rate is the increase in drug-related killings. For example, of 465 homicides in Houston, Texas, evidence confirmed that 106 killings were directly linked to drugs. The homicides were associated mostly with drug dealing or attempts to get money to purchase drugs.

The consumption (in contrast to the sale) of drugs and alcohol also has a link to violent behavior. Classic studies of homicides show that the killer, the victim, or both were drunk in more than half the cases studied. According to the Ohio homicide study, 62 percent of the offenders were reported to have consumed alcohol before homicide incidents, and 88 percent of the offenders or victims were reported to have consumed alcohol and possibly other drugs.

Drug and alcohol consumption is a predictor of serious "career criminality," according to a National Institute of Justice study, which showed that the majority of the most serious offenders among prison inmates had histories of heroin use, frequently in combination with alcohol and other drugs.

Although a close relationship between substance abuse and homicide does exist, these and other studies do not prove conclusively that drugs and alcohol

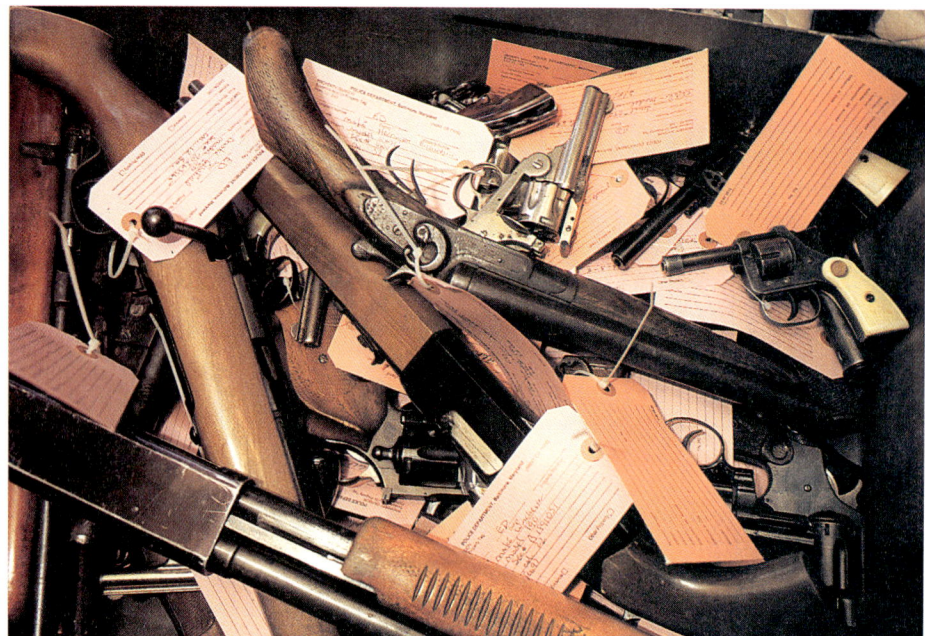

One of three American households has a gun. If you have a gun at home, you are eight times more likely to be involved in a homicide—as victim or murderer—than if you didn't have a gun. (Source: The Image Works/© Stephen Rubin)

cause crime. In a report on drinking and crime prepared for the National Institute of Justice, researchers note that people may first decide to commit their crimes and then get drunk to muster courage or allay fears.

The Role of Television

The average child in the United States watches 8,000 murders and 100,000 other acts of violence on television by the time he or she leaves elementary school. This, according to the American Psychological Association, influences the behavior of children, particularly as it relates to racial and sexual prejudices and inciting violence. Television has long been accused of causing a host of social ills in the United States, including low levels of literacy. A recent Gallup poll found that nearly two-thirds of the adult population think that there is a relationship between violence on television and crime.

Numerous studies do show a possible link between viewing television violence and engaging in violent behavior. Children most likely to be aggressive are the ones who watch violent programs most of the time they are on, who believe that the shows portray life just as it is, and who identify strongly with the aggressive characters in the shows. In addition, these children tend to have aggressive fantasies and are unpopular with the other children in their grade.

For youngsters such as these, exposure to violence on television could increase the probability of their behaving violently. This argument has been used in criminal cases in which the defense claims a television show or video may have inspired a youth predisposed to violence to "see what it was like to kill someone."

For most television watchers, the evidence is less clear and to date does not fully support the view that watching violence on television causes an increase in violence in the real world. On the other hand, the relationship between watching violent shows and committing violent acts cannot be entirely dismissed. Several studies suggest that repeated exposure to violent acts in films and on television "desensitizes" people to violence, making an experience that would at first be repulsive seem commonplace or even acceptable.

Fortunately, there are nonviolent ways of dealing with violence. See the Developing Health Skills box to learn about conflict resolution techniques.

domestic violence A range of abusive behaviors perpetrated by one person against another within the domestic sphere.

spouse abuse Any intentional physical, sexual, or psychological assault by a spouse.

Violence at Home and on the Job

Many people do not find refuge from violence even in their own homes. Spouse and child abuse are so widespread that it is a statistical probability that some form of family violence is going on across the street or down the block from where you live. Violence that takes place at home has for many years been regarded as a very private matter, perhaps a source of embarrassment, and at times, even a source of pride. However, in recent years, this attitude has changed; studies indicate an increased awareness of domestic violence as a threat to both personal health and the health of a community.

Violence at home knows no boundaries. It takes place in the finest sections of town as well as in the inner city. It occurs among people of all races and religions and among the wealthy as well as among low-income people. According to the American Medical Association, between 2 and 4 million women and nearly 2 million children are battered every year in the United States. Researchers estimate that some form of violence occurs in 25 percent of all marriages. It is also possible that some of the couples you see around the college campus are "battling it out," because the rate of violence among nonmarried couples may approach that found within marriage.

As high as these figures are, experts believe that many cases of family abuse are not reported, so the actual incidence of abuse is even higher. This is because, despite changing attitudes, many victims of violence in the home remain too ashamed or fearful to tell anyone about their experiences. Some victims continue to believe that their experiences do not represent a reportable crime.

Domestic Violence

Domestic violence is defined as a range of abusive behaviors perpetrated by one person against another within the domestic sphere. This can be interpreted to mean one member of the family against another or one partner against another. Although men suffer from domestic violence, the incidence and severity of victimization of men are lower than for women. In fact, physical abuse against women rose sharply in the early 1990s (see Figure 11.4), and much of this is the direct result of domestic violence.

"To have and to hold, to love and to cherish." An abused spouse might well wonder what happened to those traditional wedding vows. **Spouse abuse** is defined as any intentional physical, sexual, or psychological assault by a spouse. Domestic abuse cases involve an assault by a nonmarital partner—a boyfriend, girlfriend, lover, or date. Both are forms of domestic violence under the law.

Critical Thinking Question

One objective listed in *Healthy People 2000* states: "Reduce physical abuse directed at women by male partners to no more than 27 per 1,000 couples." Not only is this objective not being met but also the data suggest that the incidence rate of physical abuse against women is actually rising. Can you explain this rise? Are there more incidents of abuse of women? Or are more events of abuse being reported?

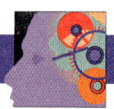

DEVELOPING HEALTH SKILLS

Conflict Resolution

Many forms of violence begin as simple conflicts between two individuals but escalate into violent encounters. This is the case with fights that begin with an indirect insult, such as, "You took my chair; I was here first," or a more direct one, such as an obscene gesture made by one driver to another who passed improperly. Road rage—a new term to describe this anger—can escalate to a car chase and result in serious injury to the drivers and people in nearby cars. Insults may also arise from racial or religious prejudices, feelings of unfair treatment, learned hatred, and simple miscommunication. Regardless of the source of insult, the outcome does not have to become violent.

One method of assuring that conflicts do not escalate into violent encounters is a process known as conflict resolution. **Conflict resolution** is a process of negotiation between two individuals. It is facilitated by a third party. The goal of conflict resolution is, as the term suggests, to resolve the conflict.

You might want to use conflict resolution to handle a difficult encounter in your dorm or your community. Here are some guidelines for conducting a mediation session, the actual meeting between the two individuals in conflict:

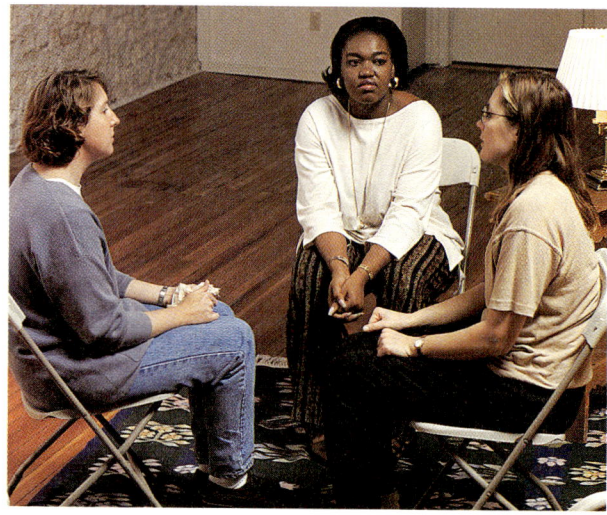

Conflict resolution is a process of negotiation between two people. It is facilitated by a third, neutral party. What situations have you been in that could have been resolved through conflict resolution? (Source: Stock, Boston/ © Bob Daemmrich)

---

conflict resolution A process of negotiation between two individuals, facilitated by a third party, with the goal of resolving differences.

physical abuse The infliction of physical injury that causes substantial harm over a period of time.

psychological abuse Acts that lead to mental anguish, such as threats insults, and unreasonable demands and that damage the victim's self-esteem over time.

battery Any illegal beating or touching of another person.

Kicks, punches, and chokings are typical examples of the **physical abuse** to which men and women are subjected in cases of domestic violence. These abuses often result in black eyes, split lips, broken noses, fractured jaws, damaged vocal cords, permanent eye damage, broken ribs, internal bleeding, ruptured spleens, lacerated livers, sexual organ damage, and numerous other injuries.

Another form of battering is **psychological abuse.** A spouse or partner can verbally batter the abused person with insults and threats, which can severely damage the victim's self-esteem. Victims are often required to perform demanding, demeaning, and unreasonable tasks. One abused woman reported that her husband was the only one permitted to wear shoes in the house. If she or their children forgot to take off their shoes, she risked being beaten.

Although each case is different, there are some identifying characteristics of both the abused and the abusers. Women who were abused as children, or who saw their mothers being abused by their fathers, are at risk for marrying someone who will abuse them. Abused women tend to be submissive, lacking in self-confidence, and in need of security and a strong male figure. As one formerly battered woman said, "My husband had always put me down and told me I was incapable of making decisions."

Similarly, men who grew up in abusive households are at risk for abusing their own families. According to studies reported in the *Journal of Family Violence,*

1. *Emphasize your neutrality.*
   Introduce the mediation session by establishing your neutrality. Make it clear to each party that you do not have a personal interest in the outcome. Say, "I am neutral. I will not take sides or decide who is right or wrong. My role is to help you find a solution that is acceptable to both of you."
2. *Establish guidelines.*
   It is important to agree upon some rules that must be followed throughout the mediation session. Both parties must agree to

- keep everything that is said confidential;
- be as honest as possible;
- avoid name calling and swearing;
- refrain from interrupting the other person;
- participate in proposing solutions that they can agree to; and
- follow through on any agreed-upon solution.

3. *Allow each person to state his or her views.*
   Give each person a chance to state his or her view of the situation. Listen carefully and ask questions to clarify anything that is unclear. To make sure you understood what was said, restate something and ask, "Is that what you mean?"

   Do not go on to the next person until you really understand the first person's viewpoint. While you are listening and asking questions, try to get at the principle behind each person's position. That is, you should try to gain a deeper understanding of what each person truly cares about, not just what the person is saying.
4. *Explore possible solutions.*
   If participants seem relaxed, ask them to brainstorm a list of possible solutions together. Remind them that, during brainstorming, they should not judge the other person's proposed solution. Encourage the participants to invent new and different solutions and to use the other's suggestions to spark ideas in their minds.
5. *Do not give up.*
   It is not always easy to find a win–win solution, but it can be done. It is important to keep the focus on the common principle or goal that is behind the two different positions. Also, try to keep the participants actively involved in the process of proposing solutions. The more involved they are, the greater interest they will have in resolving the problem.

   If, however, you are unable to find an agreeable solution, it may be necessary to ask for help. You may want to encourage the two individuals to seek counseling from a trained mediator.

---

wife beaters developed a need to dominate their wives (and often their children) based on their childhood experiences, in which their mothers as well as they were dominated by their fathers. They, too, often feel insecure, but rather than being submissive about it, they may use violence to vent the bad feelings they have about themselves. One wife abuser describes why he physically forced his wife to stay with him at a social gathering: "I felt that she didn't have the right to make the decision to leave. Her decision to leave was not as important as mine to have her stay…. When all else fails, violence is the way to keep control and maintain your identity. It is a way to lay down the law."

There is a big difference between laying down the law and taking the law into your own hands. Beating up someone, or **battery,** is a crime. Although laws exist to protect an abused person, the courts have often ruled in favor of the sanctity of the family. Even without a court ruling, most people stay in the abusive household year after year. One of the main reasons they stay is fear. Typically, women are afraid of angering their husbands and of the consequences of that anger being directed against them or their children. They are also afraid because most abused women are financially dependent on their husbands and have lost the job skills they had in their independent years. If a battered woman has her husband arrested, he may not be able to support her. Many male abusers also blame their female partners, creating a cycle of guilt and shame that traps them

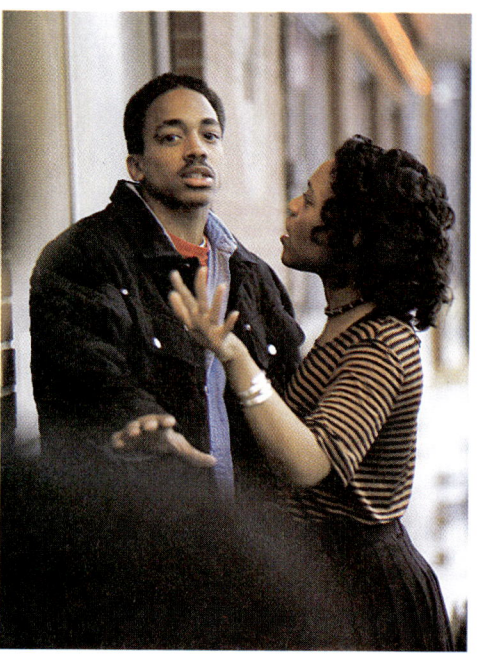

Left unchecked, a heated argument can escalate to domestic violence. Statistics from recent years indicate a rise in the incidence of domestic violence. This rise includes couples dating at college as well as married couples. (Source: FPG International/© Ron Chapple)

in the marriage so that no one uncovers their secret. Reasoning such as this likely increases abused women's feelings of apprehension and helplessness about the future, even if they do finally leave.

In recent years, attention has been given to the plight of battered women. All large cities and an increasing number of smaller ones have places where an abused woman (and her children) can go, such as an emergency shelter. Recognizing the problem of abuse among young people in dating situations, colleges have begun to operate shelters for battered women students. Also, more than half the states have mandatory laws requiring police officers to arrest abusive men when called to a home (see the Here's Looking at You box).

When Children Get Hurt

Children usually look to their parents for the kind of love and nurturing that will help them develop into healthy adults. The tragedy for many children is that what they get instead is abuse that could physically and emotionally harm them for the rest of their lives.

More than 3 million children were victims of **child abuse** in 1996, according to data collected by the National Committee to Prevent Child Abuse, and at least 1,000 of these cases resulted in death. In most cases, the children were killed at home with a blunt instrument by a parent.

In general, child abuse falls into four categories: emotional abuse, physical neglect, physical abuse, and sexual abuse.

Emotional abuse is the most subtle form of child abuse. Although there are no visible scars, there are tell-tale signs in terms of learning problems, extremes in behavior (being withdrawn or aggressive), and a depressed and apathetic demeanor. Parents can inflict emotional abuse on a child by depriving him or her of the self-esteem needed to thrive. Ways in which this happens include continually degrading or belittling the child, telling the child he or she is bad or evil, threatening severe punishment or abandonment, and ignoring the child.

A child exposed to **physical neglect** is often deprived of the basic necessities of life, including food, clothing, sanitary living conditions, and medical care. Another form of physical neglect involves leaving a child in a situation in which

HealthLinks
National Committee to Prevent Child Abuse (NCPCA)
www.childabuse.org

Excellent reference for essential information and statistics related to child abuse, as well as violence prevention tips, parenting tips, and a calendar of upcoming NCPCA events.

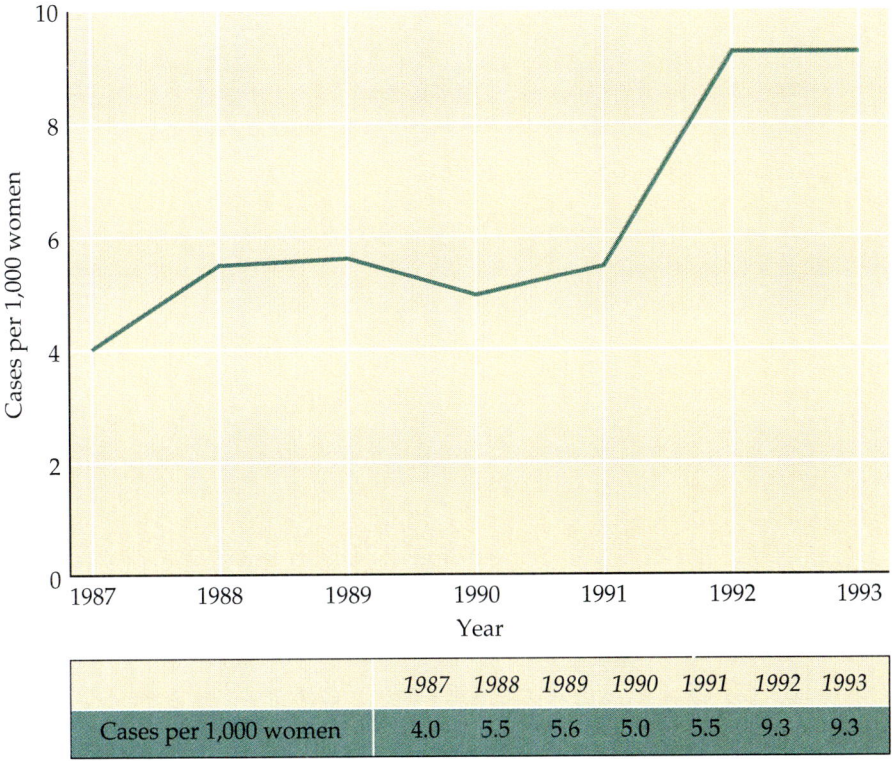

Figure 11.4 Physical Abuse Directed at Women by Male Partners.
Mostly as a result of domestic violence, physical abuse against women has been rising.
(Source: Bureau of Justice Statistics)

he or she would be exposed to danger. For example, 20 percent of all child fatalities caused by fire occur when children are unattended or unsupervised.

Physical abuse of a child is defined as a physical injury that causes substantial harm over a period of time. A continuum of physical abuse starts with mild spanking on the buttocks, which many people consider to be an acceptable disciplinary action. Even mild spanking may be abusive when delivered in anger.

At some point, discipline becomes overdiscipline, and it is no longer acceptable behavior. The battered child may be hit anywhere on the body, including the head. Belts, paddles, and switches are often used. Signs of physical abuse include burns, welts, lacerations, scars, and fractures. Children who are physically abused tend to be easily frightened and fearful. They have a short attention span and do not do well in school. They crave affection from adults yet relate poorly to children their own age.

Sexual abuse covers a wide range of activities. Some of these involve physical acts, such as fondling, oral sex, and intercourse. Other kinds of sexual abuse do not involve physical contact. A child may be forced to look at the genitals of an older child or adult or to undress or otherwise expose himself or herself. Having intercourse intentionally in front of a child and staging or watching obscene photographs or films with a child are also forms of sexual abuse.

Children who are abused sexually develop poor self-concepts, which can lead to depression, withdrawal, and suicide. In some cases, so much anger is pent up after years of abuse that the child finally fights back with a vengeance. One teenager, who was an incest victim for six years, had a friend kill her father.

Several myths exist about sexual abuse. For example, many people think it is done by a stranger or that it is an isolated incident in the life of a child. In 90 percent of the cases, however, the offender is a person the child knows. The child

child abuse Any intentional physical, sexual, or psychological assault on a child.

emotional abuse Depriving a child or close relative of love and affection; belittling or degrading another person.

physical neglect A deprivation of the basic necessities of life, including food, clothing, sanitary living conditions, and medical care.

sexual abuse A criminal offense in which a person is used for sexual purposes.

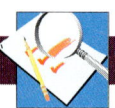

HERE'S LOOKING AT YOU

Detecting an Abusive Relationship

You probably know someone who has experienced an abusive relationship. Perhaps a friend's boyfriend behaved in a manner that made you suspect a problem. Or perhaps a friend shared anxiety or fear with you about a relationship. Getting out of an abusive relationship begins with recognizing that abuse exists. This is sometimes more evident to those on the "outside" than to the person on the "inside."

How can you detect an abusive relationship? Consider the following questions:

- Does one person often yell and scream at the other?
- Is one person occasionally frightened of the other?
- Does one person stop the other from seeing family or friends?
- Does one person force the other to have sex?
- Does one person occasionally hurt or threaten the other?

An answer of yes to any one of these questions is an indication that the relationship is not fair, that is, that one person expresses more power within the relationship than the other. An abusive relationship may exist.

An answer of yes to more than one of these questions is an indication that an abusive relationship does exist and outside help, in the form of counseling or legal aid, may be needed to end the abuse.

An answer of yes to all five questions is an indication that this may be a dangerous relationship and that the well-being of one of the partners may be at risk.

If you suspect that abuse is part of a friend's relationship, the most important action you can take is to talk to him or her about it and to suggest that he or she seeks professional help, such as from a mental health counselor or physician.

---

abuser is most often a relative or a friend of the family, but that person could be almost anyone in the community—a baby-sitter, teacher, youth leader, or shopkeeper. The child is likely to be abused by that person over and over again.

HEALTH SKILLS

Reporting Child Abuse

As with abuse within an adult relationship, child abuse may be more easily recognized from a point of view outside the family than from inside. If you suspect child abuse, would you know what to do?

When child abuse is suspected, it must be reported. This is not only a good idea, in most states it is the law. Law enforcement officials advise that if you have reason to believe a child is being abused, do not try to investigate it or confront the abuser. Report your reasonable suspicions. It is the responsibility of law enforcement authorities to investigate the case. Even if your report does not bring immediate action, it will help establish an official record that could be useful in helping the child at a later date.

For help in reporting a suspected case of child abuse, contact your local physician. Review Figure 11.5 to find out when to suspect child abuse.

Sexual Harassment: An Abuse of Power

Although seldom a violent crime, sexual harassment is a criminal offense involving the abuse of power. It is found on the job, in the classroom, and, in some cases, at home. It may be obvious, as in the case of a boss or professor imposing unwanted sexual attention or requests for sexual favors. It may also be less direct, such as the creation of a hostile, intimidating, or offensive work or class

Suspect child abuse when you see:

- Frequent injuries such as bruises, cuts, black eyes, or burns, especially when the child cannot adequately explain their causes
- Frequent complaints of pain without obvious injury
- Burns or bruises in an unusual pattern that may indicate the use of an instrument or a human bite; cigarette burns on any part of the body
- Aggressive, disruptive, and destructive behavior
- Lack of reaction to pain
- Passive, withdrawn, and emotionless behavior
- Fear of going home or of seeing parents
- Injuries that appear after the child has not been seen for several days
- Unseasonable clothes that may hide injuries to arms or legs

Suspect child neglect when you see:

- Obvious malnourishment
- Lack of personal cleanliness
- Torn and/or dirty clothes
- Obvious fatigue and listlessness
- A child unattended for long periods of time
- Need for glasses, dental care, or other medical attention
- Stealing or begging for food
- Frequent absence from or tardiness to school

Suspect child sexual abuse when you see:

- Physical signs of sexually transmitted diseases
- Evidence of injury to the genital area
- Pregnancy in a young girl
- Difficulty in sitting or walking
- Frequent expressions of sexual activity between adults and children
- Extreme fear of being alone with adults of a particular sex
- Sexually suggestive, inappropriate, or promiscuous behavior
- Knowledge about sexual relations beyond what is appropriate for the child's age
- Sexual victimization of other children

Figure 11.5 When to Suspect Child Abuse. *(Source: Office of the Attorney General, Texas)*

environment by actions or speech of a sexual nature based on gender. On the college campus, sexual harassment might take the form of offers of a good grade in a course or special treatment in exchange for sexual favors, repeated staring in a suggestive way, or unwanted touching. Even sexual comments, jokes, or personal questions that are offensive or distracting to the person who feels harassed may constitute sexual harassment.

Most commonly, it is women who are harassed, usually by men in a position of power or authority over them. However, men may be harassed by women, and either men or women may be harassed by persons of the same sex. If harassers are left unchallenged, others may become victims because harassers are usually repeat offenders. A new form of sexual harassment is taking place over the Internet (see the Healthwise Consumer box).

The following are recommended actions developed by a university panel addressing sexual harassment on campus:

Speak up. Ignoring sexual harassment does not make it go away. Express your objections clearly, firmly, and in a timely way. There is a chance that the harasser did not realize the behavior was offensive. Also, if you should file charges at a later date, it is sometimes helpful (but not essential) to have objected to the behavior.

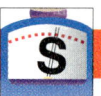

HEALTHWISE CONSUMER

Are Harassing E-Mail Messages Electronic Violations of Stalking Laws?

Institutions might want to examine their harassment policies and state antistalking laws to determine how they will deal with students who threaten other students via e-mail.

A Michigan man has been charged with violating Michigan's anti-stalking law for sending threatening messages via e-mail to a woman he met through a video dating service. After meeting a few times and exchanging messages on their computers, she told him to "get lost."

John Doe then left a message on the woman's answering machine saying that he had secretly watched her leave work. Although he did not threaten her directly, some of his remarks could be construed as putting her safety in jeopardy. The woman called police who told Doe to have no contact with her by telephone or computer. He sent her additional messages, including a threat to e-mail their "story" to America Online and to her parents and friends including the comment "This letter is the LEAST of the many things I could do to annoy you."

Dave Bansar, a policy analyst with the Electronic Privacy Information Center in Washington, D.C., says that electronic stalking should not be treated any differently than physical stalking. "If it's considered stalking when you send mail through the U.S. Postal Service or over the phone, the same kind of rationale should be used for electronic networks."

Although many institutional sexual harassment policies could be interpreted to cover electronic harassment, few if any do so specifically.

Source: "Are Harassing E-Mail Messages Electronic Violations of Stalking Laws?" *About Women on Campus,* Fall 1994. Reprinted by permission of NAWE (National Association for Women in Education) Advancing Women in Higher Education)

Keep records. Include in your records any notes or letters received from the harasser. Write down dates, times, places, witnesses, what happened or what was said, and what you said or did in response.

Tell someone. You may get a clearer perspective on what is happening, or you may find out whether the harasser is a previous offender. You may also establish witnesses who can vouch for your distress.

Get help. The university cannot take steps to solve the problem if you do not report it. It takes courage to confront a harassment problem, but you may keep another person from having the same problem later.

Take it seriously. A sexual harassment allegation has a considerable impact on the individual accused. Do not make allegations that are without foundation, as disciplinary action may result.

The Crime of Rape

Rape is one of the most misunderstood of violent crimes in terms of who it happens to, who commits it, and why it is done. Many women think, "It could never happen to me." But a recent survey indicates that about one of eight women has been raped.

It is also popularly believed that women are "asking for it" with their dress and actions. Research shows that rapists look for targets they perceive as vulnerable, not for women who dress in a particular way. No one asks to be raped, just

rape An act of violence in which a person is forced to engage in unwanted sexual intercourse.

as no one asks to be robbed. Perhaps the most misunderstood aspect of rape is the myth that it is driven by sexual desire, when, in reality, it is driven more by the compulsion to control.

Rape is widely believed to happen only to young women. Although many rape victims are young, rape victims range in age from four months to ninety-two years. It can happen to women of all ages and to boys and men. Males are victims of about 5 percent of all sexual assault cases.

One reason there are so many misconceptions concerning rape is that it is a crime that is difficult to talk about. Although more than 130,000 rapes and attempted rapes are reported each year, perhaps more than 100,000 more go unreported. In fact, police research suggests that less than half of all rapes and attempted rapes are reported.

Factors that may keep people who have been raped from telling about their experience include embarrassment, fear of reprisal, fear of not being believed, and not realizing that a sexual assault by a friend is actually rape. However, reporting information about a rape, or an attempted rape, may prevent another person from being raped.

Defining Rape

By legal definition, **rape** is obtaining sexual intercourse through physical force or the threat of physical force. It is motivated more by the desire or need to control or dominate someone than by sexual desires.

Rape is clearly a nighttime crime. Two thirds of all rapes and rape attempts take place at night, mostly between 6 P.M. and midnight. Most rapes take place in the home, and most rape attempts take place on the street or in a park, field, playground, parking lot, or garage (see Figure 11.6).

As with victims of other violent crimes discussed in this chapter, rape victims tend to be young (sixteen to twenty-four years old) and from low-income families. Most are white, reflecting the racial composition of the general population. African American women, however, have a significantly greater chance of being raped than do white women owing to the higher number of African American women living in low-income/high-crime areas.

Rapists, according to the Bureau of Justice Statistics, generally are married, are over twenty-one years old, are unarmed, and are of the same race as the victim. A rapist will rape and rape again, usually in the same area of town and in the same manner, for example, by blindfolding the victim, wearing a ski mask, or other trademarks. Studies of rapists indicate that these individuals are often

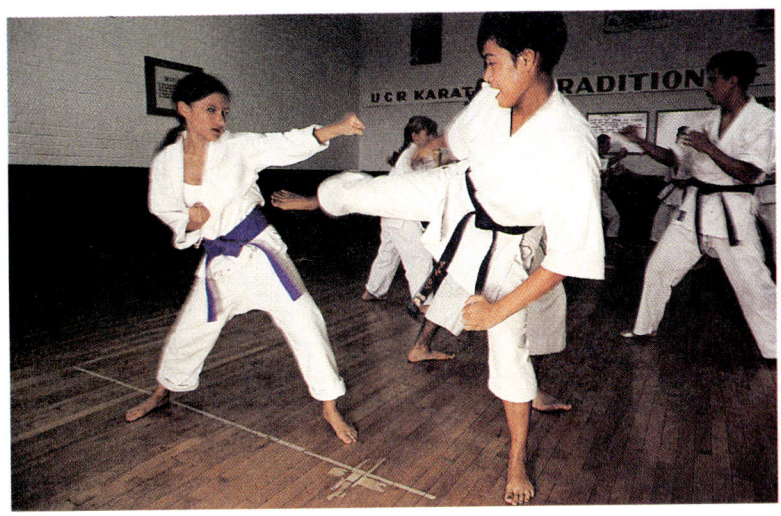

As a measure of self-protection, a growing number of women are signing up for karate or other self-defense techniques. (Source: Photo Researchers, Inc./© Andy Levin)

Characteristics of incident	Rape/sexual assault
Total	100%
Victim/offender relationship	
Relatives	11
Well-known	35
Casual acquaintance	21
Stranger	33
Time of day	
6 A.M. to 6 P.M.	31
6 P.M. to midnight	37
Midnight to 6 A.M.	32
Location of crime	
At or near victim's home or lodging	37
Friend's/relative's/neighbor's home	21
Commercial places	7
Parking lots/garages	6
School	3
Streets other than near victim's home	8
Other	17
Victim's activity	
At work or traveling to or from work	8
School	5
Activities at home	38
Shopping/errands	2
Leisure activities away from home	32
Traveling	6
Other	8
Distance from victim's home	
Inside home or lodging	34
Near victim's home	10
1 mile or less	12
5 miles or less	14
50 miles or less	23
More than 50 miles	6
Weapons	
No weapons present	84
Weapons present	16
Firearm	6
Other type of weapon	10

Figure 11.6 The Anatomy of a Rape: Who Does It, Where, and When. *Most rapes take place at night at or near where the victim lives. The rapist is usually known by the victim. (Source: Bureau of Justice Statistics)*

immature and lack self-respect, self-esteem, and a feeling of responsibility for their own behavior.

Most rape victims offer some kind of resistance. The most common response is to try to yell and get help; to resist physically; to threaten, argue, or reason with the offender; or to resist without force by running away or hiding. However, yelling works only if someone is around to hear. Running away makes sense only if there is a safe place to go to. And active resistance is a good option only when the person being attacked is trained in karate or another self-defense technique. What you should do to try to protect yourself when you feel threatened depends in great part on your assessment of the circumstances before you.

Attacks by Strangers

The most frightening form of rape, assault by a total stranger, is the most commonly reported form of rape. It represents, however, only about one third of all rapes; acquaintance rapes far outnumber stranger rapes. This is because a woman is twice as likely to report being attacked by a stranger as by someone she knows, according to the Bureau of Justice Statistics.

Gang rape is rape done by a group. This is usually a group of males, but gang rape is also done by females. A lot of media attention has been given to gang rapes by teenage males. For example, a twelve-year-old girl was abducted in Los Angeles and raped by dozens of boys over a period of four days; five high school students in suburban New Jersey attacked a seventeen-year-old, mentally retarded girl; and three Houston teens abducted and raped a twenty-six-year-old woman during a three-day crime spree.

Closely related, **sadistic rape** occurs when the rapist is driven to torture or mutilate his victim. This form of rape comprises a very small percentage of reported rapes, less than 1 percent, but obviously is the most dangerous and threatening.

Acquaintance Rape

About two thirds of all rapists are acquainted with the victim in one way or another. They may be the victim's spouse, former spouse, relative, date, neighbor, or coworker. **Acquaintance rape** is the most common and most underreported form of rape.

A common form of acquaintance rape is **date rape.** It is committed on or by a date. The real problem leading to date rape begins with miscommunication. A male might say, "It wasn't rape. She really wanted me to do it." A female might say, "I didn't want to, but he forced me to have sex with him."

Studies show that date rape occurs more frequently among college students, particularly freshmen, than among any other group. In one survey, one in four college women reported being victims of rape or attempted rape. In 84 percent of the cases, the assailant was someone the women knew. Figure 11.7 provides guidelines for making your views clear while on a date.

Another factor contributing to date rape is the so-called date-rape drug, Rohypnol, or Roofies. Slipped into a drink, Roofies dissolve quickly. Their sedative effects are felt within ten minutes, leaving the victim unable to defend her- or himself for up to eight hours. In such a situation, rape without resistance is easy. To avoid the risk of inadvertently taking a date-rape drug, do not accept open drinks from strangers.

Critical Thinking Question

Most laws do not differentiate between stranger rape and date rape. Therefore, date rape, rape by a "friend," is treated by the law with the same severity as rape committed by a total stranger in a dark alley or along a country roadside. Should there be degrees of severity of rape? What do you think is the argument for treating date rape and stranger rape equally under the law?

gang rape A rape committed by a group.

sadistic rape A rape that involves torture or mutilation of the victim.

acquaintance rape Sexual assault committed by a person know to the victim.

date rape Unwanted sexual contact that is committed on or by a date.

Figure 11.7 Dating and Sex: What a Woman Needs to Know and What a Man Needs to Know.

What a woman needs to know

- Be assertive. Polite responses may be misunderstood or ignored. Say, "No," when you mean no. Men often interpret passivity as permission.
- Be aware that your nonverbal actions send a message. If you dress in a sexy manner and flirt, some men may assume you want to have sex. This does not make your dress or behavior wrong, but it is important to be aware of being misunderstood.
- Pay attention to what is happening around you. Do not put yourself in vulnerable situations.
- Trust your intuitions. If you feel you are being pressured into unwanted sex, you probably are.
- Avoid excessive use of alcohol and drugs. Alcohol and drugs interfere with clear thinking and effective communication.

What a man needs to know

- Being turned down when you ask for sex is not a rejection of you personally. Women who say no to sex are not rejecting the person; they are expressing their desire not to participate in a specific act.
- Accept the woman's decision. "No" means no. Don't read other meanings into the answer. Don't continue after she says "No."
- Don't assume that just because a woman dresses in a sexy manner and flirts that she wants to have intercourse with you.
- Don't assume that previous permission for sex applies to the current situation.
- Avoid excessive use of alcohol and drugs. Alcohol and drugs interfere with clear thinking and effective communication.

Another form of unwanted sexual act by an acquaintance is **marital rape**. This takes place when a spouse forces himself or herself on his or her spouse or estranged spouse. It often takes place in an atmosphere of anger, violence, and fear.

The Aftermath

A rape can be over in minutes, but its traumatic effects can last for months, years, or even a lifetime. At a minimum, a person who is raped should go to a physician, clinic, or hospital to deal with the medical problems that may arise, including tissue injury, the potential for HIV and other sexually transmitted diseases, and pregnancy. A victim may or may not wish to prosecute.

Three stages occur in what is called the **rape trauma syndrome**:

1. At first, a person who is raped feels helpless and confused. She is usually in a state of shock, anger, or disbelief and cannot think clearly about what happened to her.
2. The next stage is denial. The woman withdraws from her friends and from her feelings. For a period of time, this reaction serves as a kind of psychological self-protection, as if the woman were saying, "It didn't really happen to me."
3. After a while, the feelings of anger and helplessness come back. The victim often becomes depressed and may avoid having any sex because it reminds her of being raped. Women who have been raped and do not seek psychological counseling may continue to experience these feelings. Rape crisis centers are available in almost every city and county—and also on many college campuses—where women can get help in realizing the impact the rape has had on them.

marital rape A rape that occurs when a spouse forces unwanted sexual contact on his or her spouse or estranged spouse.

rape trauma syndrome A group of symptoms, such as anxiety, sleeplessness, eating disorders, nightmares, guilt, and low self-esteem, that can strike after the occurrence of rape.

A Few Final Words on Violence

A strong probability exists that you will have a close involvement with violence in your lifetime. For some, this means being a victim. For others, it means helping a friend who has been mugged or raped or grieving with the family of a victim of homicide. To help reduce your exposure to violence, as well as to assist victims in need of help, periodically review the skills that you have learned in this chapter. Prevention of violence generally involves precaution and can be incorporated relatively easily into your lifestyle.

Key Concepts

1. Violence is the use of force with the intent to harm oneself or another person.
2. Each year, about 49 million Americans are the victims of a violent crime. This includes homicide, domestic abuse, rape, and other assaults.
3. Although criminals can come from any background, they statistically tend to have a low level of education, be unemployed, have a history of being abused, and come from a single-parent home. Most violent crimes are committed by young men.
4. More than half the victims of all crimes know or have seen the person who committed the crime against them.
5. One of every ten homicides is perpetrated by a relative of the victim. The homicide rate is believed to be related to the availability of handguns, the use of drugs, and the portrayal of violence on television.
6. One method of assuring that conflicts do not escalate into violent encounters is a process known as conflict resolution—negotiation between two individuals facilitated by a third party.
7. Some form of violence occurs in 25 percent of all marriages.
8. In 1996, 3 million children were victims of child abuse. Child abuse includes emotional abuse, physical neglect, physical abuse, and sexual abuse.
9. Rape, sexual intercourse through physical force or the threat of physical force, is motivated by the desire or need to control or dominate someone. Rape is a crime of violence, not a sexual act.
10. Rape can be committed by a stranger, an acquaintance, a date, or a spouse.

Review Questions

1. Describe the "typical" person who commits acts of violence by age, ethnicity, and family background.
2. Describe the "typical" person who experiences violent crime by age, ethnicity, and family background.
3. Describe how the availability of handguns, the viewing of violence on television, and drugs are thought to contribute to the occurrence of violent crime.
4. Define homicide and describe its significance to public health.
5. List and describe three forms of abuse committed on the job, at school or at college, and/or at home. Compare the motives of the abuser in each case.
6. List five guidelines for conducting a conflict resolution session.
7. Write down five questions that help determine whether a relationship is abusive.
8. List several ways to avoid sexual harassment.
9. List four types of abuse that make up what is referred to as child abuse.
10. Name four types of rape and compare each according to by whom, where, and how the crime is committed.

Selected Bibliography

Changes in Criminal Victimization, 1994–95. Washington, DC: U.S. Department of Justice, Bureau of Justice Statistics, 1997.

Journal of the American Medical Association 275, no. 22 (1996) (issue devoted to guns and violence).

Kellerman, A.L., et al. "Gun Ownership as a Risk Factor for Homicide in the Home." *New England Journal of Medicine* 329, no. 15 (1993): 1084–1119.

Report to the Nation on Crime and Justice (2nd ed.). Washington, DC: U.S. Department of Justice, Bureau of Justice Statistics, 1988.

"The Extent and Costs of Crime Victimization: A New Look." *Research Preview,* National Institute of Justice, January 1996.

"Trends in Rates of Homicide Surveillance, United States, 1985–1994." *Morbidity and Mortality Weekly Report* 45, no. 22 (1996): 460–464.

Understanding and Preventing Violence. Washington, DC: National Research Council, National Academy Press, 1993.

Weller, S. "Why Is Date Rape So Hard to Prove?" *Health* (July/August, 1992): 62, 64.

HealthLinks: Web Sites for Violence Prevention

You can access better health as it relates to this chapter by checking out some of the following sites on the Internet. These and sites identified within the chapter can be accessed directly when you visit the *HealthStyles* Web Site located on the Allyn and Bacon homepage at **http://www.abacon.com.**

Community Police Consortium
www.communitypolicing.org
The Community Policing Consortium is a partnership of five of the leading police organizations in the United States. This site contains information about community policing and special training and provides access to numerous curricula, publications, and resources, as well as a chat room on community policing.

Pavnet Online
www.pavnet.org
Pavnet Online is a "virtual library" of information about violence and youth at risk, representing data from seven different federal agencies. The result of a collaboration of the seven agencies, the website for the Partnership Against Violence Network includes information on violence prevention curricula and technical information for states and local communities.

Health Hotlines: Recognizing Violent Behavior

Family Service America (resolution of family problems)
(800) 221-2681
11700 West Lake Park Drive
Milwaukee, WI 53224

National Criminal Justice Reference Service
(800) 851-3420
P. O. Box 6000
Rockville, MD 20849-6000

National Organization for Victim Assistance
(800) TRY-NOVA (879-6682) victims and survivors only
1757 Park Road NW
Washington, DC 20010

National Clearinghouse of Child Abuse and Neglect
(800) FYI-3366 (394-3366)
P.O. Box 1182
Washington, DC 20013

Office for Victims of Crime Resource Center
(800) 627-6872
P.O. Box 6000
Rockville, MD 20849-6000

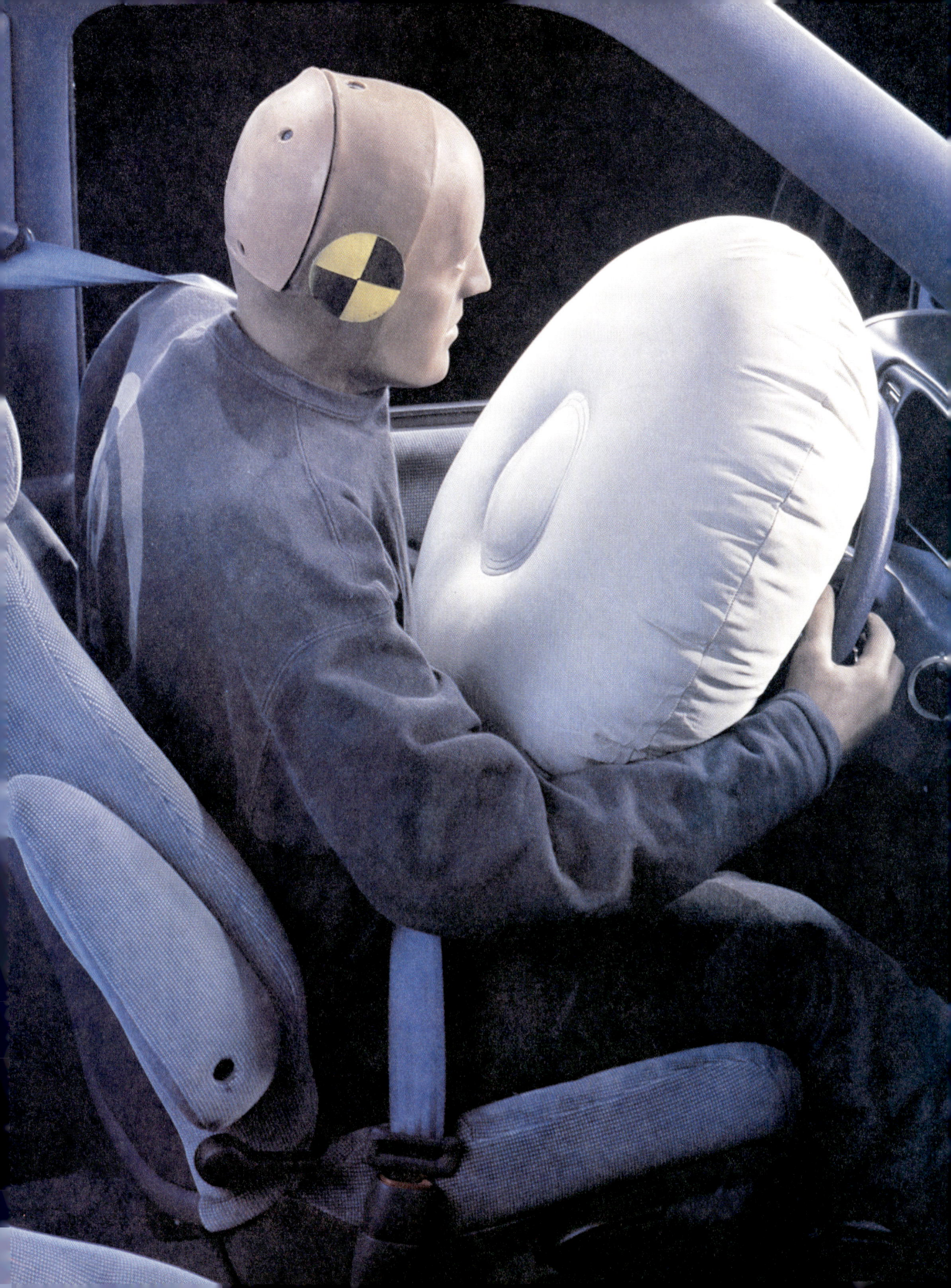

Chapter 12

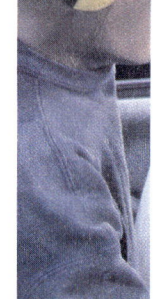
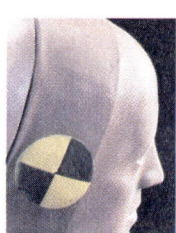
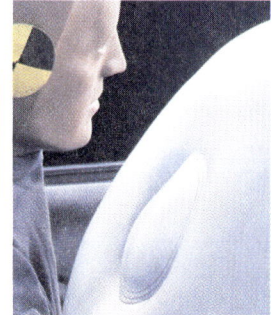

Preventing Unintentional Injuries

Objectives

When you finish reading this chapter, you will be able to:

1. Differentiate between an accident and an unintentional injury.
2. Understand why accidents occur and how they lead to unintentional injury.
3. Describe a person at risk for an unintentional injury.
4. Identify the cost to society, both monetary and in terms of quality of life, of unintentional injuries.
5. Recognize motor vehicle crashes as the primary cause of unintentional injuries in the United States.
6. Identify restraints such as seat belts, child safety seats, and air bags as critical to the reduction of automobile-related injuries.
7. Recognize that alcohol consumption greatly enhances the potential of encountering an unintentional injury.
8. Cite recreational activities that are a source of unintentional injury.
9. List causes of unintentional injuries that occur in the home.
10. Acknowledge that prevention of unintentional injuries involves taking responsibility, taking preventative action, and being prepared to respond when an injury occurs.

What Is Your HealthStyle?

On the eve of her twentieth birthday, Nancy was driving home from college with her roommate. They were going to celebrate Nancy's birthday with some of her high school friends. In addition to the first twenty years of Nancy's life, they intended to celebrate Nancy's next twenty years and the twenty years after that.

A few miles from home, a drunk driver going about forty miles an hour hit Nancy's sports car—not too fast but fast enough to total the car. Nancy and her friend were wearing seat belts, as they always did, and the car had two air bags in the front. Their injuries: bruised faces, arms, and ribs, from the seat belts and air bags.

The other driver had far more extensive injuries and required surgery and several days of hospitalization. In spite of this, she was very lucky even to be alive: she had not been wearing her seat belt and her car did not have an air bag. She told the paramedics who drove her to the hospital that she hardly ever wore a seat belt, although on occasion she did use it when she took long trips on superhighways. She certainly never thought to use her seat belt when driving close to home. But her accident—statistically like many others—took place just a few miles from her house.

In Your Opinion

Nancy and her friend both always buckled up as soon as they sat in a car. Years and years of buckling up finally paid off in one second.

- Have you ever been in an accident in which wearing a seat belt saved your life or saved you from serious injury?
- Has this ever happened to someone you know?
- What skills are needed to maintain the habit of buckling up?
- Do you believe that the driver who caused the accident involving Nancy and her friend will wear a seat belt every time she gets into a car, or do you believe she will continue to take risks with the hope of being lucky again?

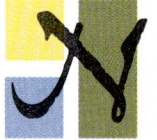

No one intends to have an injury. Nevertheless, unintentional injuries happen every day throughout the country and in your community. But, until they happen to you or someone close to you, you probably give little thought to them. You cross the street against the light, get into the car without putting on your seat belt, ride your bike without wearing a helmet, or stand on a kitchen counter to reach for something. These are all potentially dangerous situations—and each is an unintentional injury in the making.

Unintentional injuries kill more than ninety thousand people a year in the United States and leave millions more with serious disabilities, including quadriplegia and irreversible brain damage. Unintentional injuries are the fifth leading cause of death in the United States for the total population and the leading cause of death for people aged one to thirty-four. For fifteen- to twenty-four-year-olds—the age group that covers most college students—the percentage of deaths due to unintentional injuries is higher than for any other age group (see Figure 12.1).

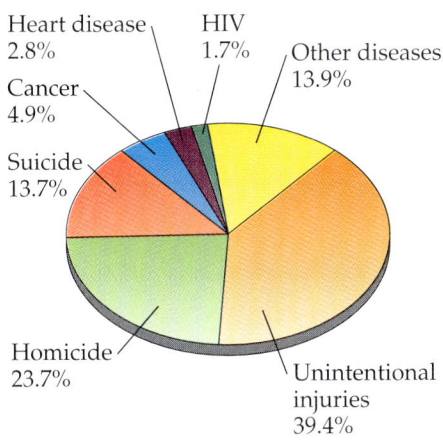

Figure 12.1 Unintentional Injuries Are the Leading Cause of Death in the College Age Group. *Accidents are responsible for more deaths for people aged 15 to 24 than any other cause. (Source: National Center for Health Statistics)*

Unintentional Injuries: Cause and Effect

Unintentional injuries include **trauma** associated with automobile crashes, falls, poisonings, fires, and drownings. These are different from **intentional injuries,** which result from events associated with suicide, homicide, and battery. Intentional injuries are discussed in Chapter 11. Suicide, another form of intentional injury, is discussed in Chapter 3.

The lines between intentional and unintentional injuries are sometimes blurred. For example, a drug overdose could be an unintentional event or it could be a suicide—an intentional event. Although violent events receive more media coverage than do unintentional injuries, the intentional injuries resulting from them represent only about one half of the fatal trauma in this country. Unintentional injuries account for more deaths and an unnecessarily high proportion of emergency room admissions.

Why Unintentional Injuries Take Place

Unintentional injuries may be caused by many different factors. In some cases, one factor alone is not enough to cause an unintentional injury. How many times have you driven too fast without being injured? But when you add several factors together, the chances of being injured are increased—for example, driving too fast *and* failing to obey a traffic signal *and* driving after drinking a few beers or other alcoholic beverages.

In general, unintentional injuries result from the action of one person—the principal actor—who causes the incident simply by not paying attention to something or by not having an adequate level of skill. The driver of a car, for example, needs to pay attention to the road at all times. An injury may occur when the driver's attention is diverted by a passenger or a distraction on the road. Even if a person gives full attention to the task of driving, he or she may lack driving skills or may drive in a thrill-seeking manner, which can greatly increase the possibility of causing injuries.

Risk-taking behavior is a cause of many unintentional injuries. Consider teenagers who, for the thrill of it, jump from a railroad bridge into a river. Drowning occurs more often as a result of such risky behavior—and from falls from docks, bridges, shores, and boats—than from accidents occurring in swimming areas patrolled by lifeguards.

Impaired functioning increases the likelihood of unintentional injuries. Alcohol is the number-one cause of preventable traffic fatalities. Even moderate lev-

unintentional injuries Injuries that are caused by unplanned events, such as automobile crashes, falls, poisonings, fires, and drownings.

trauma A wound or injury, whether intentional or unintentional.

intentional injuries Injuries that result from planned events associated with suicide, homicide, and assault.

risk-taking behavior Actions that intentionally place an individual at risk for personal injury.

els of alcohol in the blood have been found to impair judgment markedly, particularly in teenage drivers and the elderly. Alcohol consumption is also associated with a wide range of nondriving injuries, including those that take place at home, at work, and at play—particularly around the water.

No one knows the full extent of psychological factors related to unintentional injuries. Anger, for example, may be the cause of many fatal automobile injuries. The driver may be preoccupied with his or her anger about something unrelated to driving or may become angered by another driver's action on the road—a case of road rage. It is speculated that many single-vehicle accidents are the result of attempted suicide. Depression, stress, aggressiveness, or belligerence may also contribute to injuries due to a lack of attention on the part of the driver.

Many unintentional injuries are caused by hazards in the environment. Some of these hazards are natural, such as ice on the road. Some are unavoidable or unrecognizable, such as being in or near a building during an earthquake or tornado. Natural events and unavoidable threats like these are difficult to predict, but much can be done to minimize the injuries that result. Studies show that people living in trailer parks have the highest risk of injury and death in a tornado. Seeking shelter in a school or other large public building when a tornado is predicted could significantly reduce these risks.

Other environmental hazards are created by people. For example, a construction site is generally acknowledged to be a hazardous place, yet work must go on there anyway. To protect against injury from falling objects, construction workers and others on the site are required to wear hard hats. Playgrounds can also be hazardous places, yet children continue to play there. Schools put fences around playgrounds so children won't run out into the street, and play equipment is often surrounded by sand or some other soft substance rather than hard pavement as a way to minimize the impact in case a child falls.

Profile of an At-Risk Person

Who is most at risk for unintentional injuries? In an attempt to answer this question, epidemiologists have studied people who have been injured. Although injuries seem to occur randomly, researchers are finding many characteristics shared by people who are injured. As a result, researchers are increasingly able to pinpoint factors that put people at increased risk for injury.

Some factors are unavoidable, such as gender and age. At all ages, men are by far at greater risk for unintentional injury than are women. Moreover, the injuries sustained by men are more serious than those of women. For example, men are twice as likely as women to die from injuries in car crashes. Injury rates vary with age, but the safest time of life is from ages five to sixteen—after the risk of unintentional poisoning is passed and before the risks resulting from driving are a concern among teenagers and young adults.

Some risk factors relating to injury are environmental. Where you live and how much you earn also affect your risk for being injured. Deaths from unintentional injuries are more prevalent in rural areas, especially in the West. This may be due to greater distances to travel and more high-speed driving in these areas and to greater exposure to hazardous equipment, such as farm machinery. The poor in urban and rural areas are at greater risk because they tend to have older, less safe cars and to live in low-quality housing with hazardous products, such as space heaters that can cause fires. Native Americans often have multiple risk factors: They may be poor, live in rural areas, and consume a higher than average amount of alcohol. They have higher death rates from unintentional injuries than do other ethnic groups.

Similarly, injuries on the job do not pose equal risk to all workers. High-risk jobs include mining, construction, agriculture, firefighting, and working on oil

---

HealthLinks
Occupational Safety and Health Administration
www.osha.gov/

Link up with the division of the U.S. Department of Labor dedicated to occupational safety and health. Check out the latest on ergonomics and standards for safe working conditions.

premature death Years of potential life lost; usually measured in terms of years of potential life lost before age 65.

rigs. Even in these risky jobs, the primary reason for on-the-job fatalities is a motor vehicle accident; second is a fall. Working for a bicycle messenger service and riding through downtown traffic and delivering pizza by car or truck are examples of jobs in which motor vehicle accidents might happen to college students. Human error due to alcohol, drugs, inadequate sleep, and other factors causes two thirds of all workplace injuries. Stress is another factor associated with on-the-job injuries. See Figure 12.2 for occupations having large numbers of fatal injuries and for the leading cause of the injury. Note which occupations are associated with unintentional injuries and which ones are associated with intentional injuries.

Collectively, these factors characterize the individual prone to being injured, either by personal attributes or by environmental exposure. People who take care to reduce hazards to which they may be exposed may easily reduce risk and the chances of unintentional injury. Refer to the Here's Looking at You box to explore your own risk level.

What Unintentional Injuries Cost Society

With one exception, the leading causes of death are found most often among older people. That exception is unintentional injuries. As you have just read, even though they are a threat to all ages, children, teenagers, and young adults are at the greatest risk of being injured. After infant mortality, unintentional injuries constitute the leading cause of **premature death** in this country as mea-

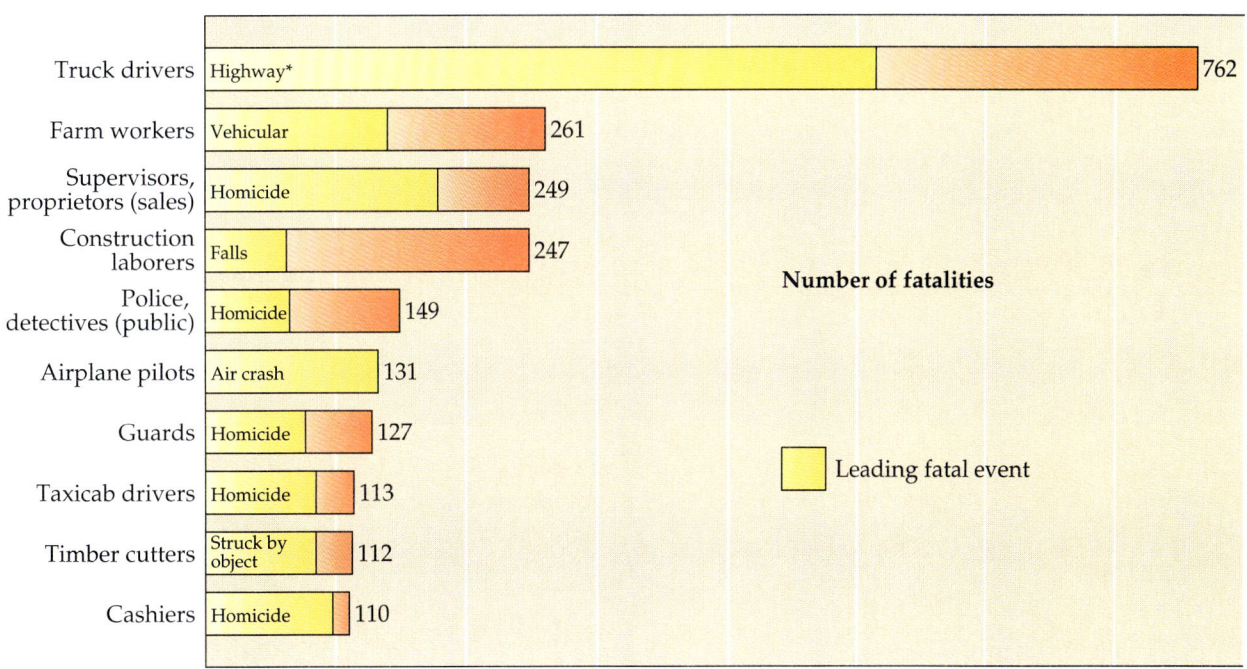

*Highway fatalities include deaths to vehicle occupants resulting from traffic incidents occurring on the public roadways, shoulders, or surrounding areas; excludes incidents occurring entirely off of the roadways (parking lots, industrial premises, farms), incidents involving trains, and deaths to pedestrians or other nonpassengers.

Figure 12.2 **Occupations Having Large Numbers of Fatal Worker Injuries.** *A motor vehicle accident is the number one reason for on-the-job fatalities. (Source: Bureau of Labor Statistics, 1994)*

HERE'S LOOKING AT YOU

Are You at Risk for an Unintentional Injury?

Would you consider yourself an accident waiting to happen? Sometimes injuries can result from common, everyday behaviors such as those listed below. Often the injuries we experience can be avoided simply through better decision making. Take a look at the following list of behaviors and follow the three steps to evaluate your level of risk taking.

STEP #1: Rate your participation in the following behaviors.
1 = frequently   2 = sometimes   3 = never

Step #1 Column		Step #2 Column	Step #3 Column
_____	1. flying in a small private plane	_____	_____
_____	2. flying in a commercial airliner	_____	_____
_____	3. swimming alone	_____	_____
_____	4. driving without safety belts on	_____	_____
_____	5. living on an active earthquake fault	_____	_____
_____	6. living in a "tornado belt" state	_____	_____
_____	7. working in an underground coal mine	_____	_____
_____	8. jay-walking across a street	_____	_____
_____	9. exceeding the speed limit	_____	_____
_____	10. waving away or swatting at a bee	_____	_____
_____	11. tubing on a bumpy downhill course	_____	_____
_____	12. riding double on a bicycle	_____	_____
_____	13. petting or feeding a large stray dog	_____	_____
_____	14. keeping guns and ammunition together	_____	_____
_____	15. sleeping in a house without a smoke detector	_____	_____
_____	16. driving a small compact car	_____	_____
_____	17. taking pills or medicine in the dark	_____	_____
_____	18. talking with food in your mouth	_____	_____
_____	19. stopping incompletely at stop signs	_____	_____
_____	20. driving/riding a motorcycle	_____	_____

STEP #2: For those statements that you marked as 1, try to identify one or more of the following reasons that explain why you participate.

a. save time
b. seek a thrill
c. meet a dare
d. perform a necessary function
e. gain recognition, status, attention
f. eliminate a hazard
g. other reason

STEP #3: For those statements that you marked as 2 or 3 in Step #1, try to identify one or more of the following reasons that explain why you do not participate.

a. It is not economical for me. It might cost me more than the personal benefits derived.
b. It is too inconvenient. The time and hassle are not worth the benefits.
c. It is too dangerous. An injury could happen.
d. It does not provide enough psychological reward (i.e., thrill, recognition, etc.).
e. I do not have enough skill to participate.

Source: Except for opening paragraph, by Alton L. Thygerson, *Safety*, 2d ed., p. 48 (Table 5.2). Copyright © 1991 by Jones and Bartlett Publishers, www.jbpub.com. Reprinted with permission)

sured by years of potential life lost before age sixty-five. Each year, about 2 million potential years of life are lost as a result of unintentional injuries. The next leading causes of premature death, in order, are cancer, heart disease, HIV, homicide, and suicide.

Most unintentional injuries, however, are not fatal. For every injury death, there are about 233 emergency department visits, 19 hospitalizations, and 450 office-based physician visits, according to the Division of Unintentional Injury Prevention of the Centers for Disease Control and Prevention (CDC). The full societal cost of unintentional injuries is difficult to estimate, but according to the National Safety Council, the total cost of unintentional injury and death in 1995 was $434.8 billion. These costs include medical expenses, lost wages and productivity, motor vehicle damage, fire losses, employer costs, administrative expenses

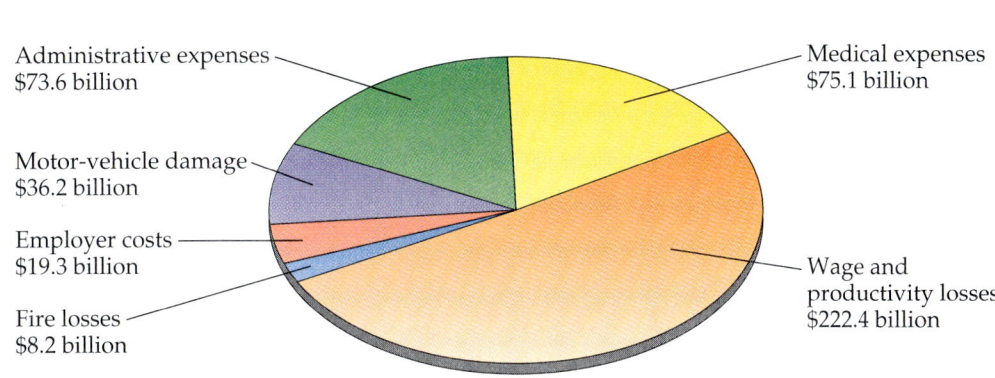

Cost equivalents

The costs of unintentional injuries are immense— billions of dollars. Since figures this large can be difficult to comprehend, it is sometimes useful to reduce the numbers to a more understandable scale by relating them to quantities encountered in daily life. The table below shows how the costs of unintentional injuries compare to common quantities such as taxes, new car prices, or stock dividends.

The cost of...	is equivalent to
...all injuries ($434.8 billion)	...73 cents of every dollar paid in 1995 federal personal income taxes or ...58 cents of every dollar spent on food in the United States in 1995.
...motor-vehicle accidents ($170.6 billion)	...purchasing 730 gallons of gasoline per registered vehicle in the United States or ...a $19,700 rebate on each new car sold in 1995.
...work injuries ($119.4 billion)	...53 cents of every dollar of 1995 corporate dividends to stockholders or ...20 cents of every dollar of 1995 pretax corporate profits.
...home injuries ($95.1 billion)	...an $88,400 rebate on each new single-family home built in 1995 or ...44 cents of every dollar of property taxes paid in 1995.
...public injuries ($63.3 billion)	...a $7.0 million grant to each public library in the United States or ...an $83,700 bonus for each police officer and firefighter.

▬ **Figure 12.3** Cost of Unintentional Injuries, 1995. *(Source: National Safety Council,* Accident Facts, *1996 edition. Reprinted by permission)*

for insurance, and police and legal costs. A single source of injury, the automobile, is estimated to cost society more than $170 billion per year. This is calculated to be the equivalent of getting a $19,700 rebate on each new car sold in 1995. See Figure 12.3 for other cost equivalents of unintentional injuries.

Safety on the Road

The rate of U.S. motor vehicle fatalities has dropped consistently and dramatically over the decades—from a high of 21.65 deaths per 100 million vehicle miles in 1925 to 1.81 deaths per 100 million vehicle miles in 1994. The decline in fatalities in recent years is associated with several factors, including the growing use of seat belts, the introduction of air bags, and an increase in the drinking age to twenty-one. It is illegal in every state and the District of Columbia to sell alcoholic beverages to anyone under the age of twenty-one, and in some states, it is illegal for people in this age group to drive with any alcohol in their blood (see the Cultural View box).

In 1987, states began raising the speed limit from fifty-five miles per hour to sixty-five miles per hour on rural interstate highways, and in 1995, speed limits went even higher—up to seventy-five miles per hour on some interstate highways—when Congress returned the authority to them. Data show that traffic fatalities are rising along with the speed limit. In 1995, the motor vehicle death rate was 1.83 per 100 million vehicle miles—the first increase in the death rate since the mid-1980s.

Motor vehicles account for nearly half of all unintentional deaths in the country. Approximately forty-four thousand individuals die each year as a result of motor vehicle injuries, and more than 2 million others are injured. Others injured on the road are motorcyclists, bicyclists, and pedestrians.

Buckling Up

Seat belts have been standard equipment in automobiles in the United States for many years, but until recently, most Americans did not buckle up. That simple act can save fourteen thousand lives per year. The combined use of a seat belt and a shoulder restraint provides an even greater degree of safety.

To assess the impact of seat belt use on the extent and cost of injuries sustained in automobile injuries, researchers prospectively evaluated more than 1,300 patients who had been taken to one of four Chicago-area hospitals after an accident. Fifty-eight percent of the injured had been wearing a seat belt; 42 percent had not. The benefits of seat belt use were clear: The seat belt wearers had a 60 percent reduction in the severity of injury, a 65 percent decrease in hospital admissions, and a 66 percent reduction in hospital charges compared with injured patients not using a seat belt.

In spite of such overwhelming evidence, most people found one excuse after another not to use seat belts, and usage rates hovered around 10 percent in 1982. During the 1980s, many states passed mandatory seat belt usage laws, and currently all but two states require that at least the people in the front seat wear a seat belt.

As a result of these laws and aggressive education campaigns, about two thirds of the population use seat belts every time they ride in a car. This increase alone translates into significant savings of lives and reduction in injury and expense. Notice in Figure 12.4 that as the rate of seat belt use goes up, the rate of death from motor vehicle crashes goes down.

CULTURAL VIEW

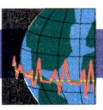

Researchers Identify Who Drinks and Drives, by Age, Sex, and Ethnic Group

Even with increased awareness about the hazards of excessive drinking, happy hours are weekend staples at most college campuses and local bars across the country. And for some people, even one or two drinks could be too much—if they plan to drink and drive.

The National Highway Traffic Safety Administration (NHTSA) and the Insurance Institute for Highway Safety conducted roadside breath-test surveys and have some sobering findings to report about who is drinking and driving.

- *Young adults: a problem group.* College-age people account for half of all driver fatalities involving high blood alcohol concentrations (BACs). In 1996, 7.7 of all drivers participating in the survey were driving with BAC levels of 0.05 or higher, and 2.8 percent were driving with BAC levels of 0.10 or higher. But for drivers ages twenty-one to thirty-four, these percentages were significantly higher: 11.3 percent had BAC levels of 0.05 or higher, and 3.8 percent had BAC levels of 0.10 or higher.

  According to Jim Fell, chief of the research and evaluation division for traffic safety programs at NHTSA, "We need to target this age group to discover what works to reduce their alcohol-impaired driving. We're exploring strategic advertising, trying to find out what kind of information influences them. Another tack is what sort of enforcement efforts will get their response. Is it checkpoints? We're also looking at new legislation because apparently laws enacted thus far haven't changed this group's behavior."

- *More women driving.* Women are driving more often on weekend nights than they did a decade ago, and they are doing so after drinking. In 1996, 5.8 percent of female drivers had 0.05 or higher BACs, compared with 3.9 percent in 1986. Men are still far more likely to drink and drive, but the proportion of male drivers with 0.05 or higher BACs fell to 8.7 percent in 1996 from 9.9 percent a decade earlier.

- *Trends among ethnic groups.* Alcohol-impaired driving among Hispanics has risen noticeably over the past decade. In 1996, 14.9 percent of Hispanic drivers had BACs of 0.05 or higher, versus 13.0 percent in 1986, and 7.5 percent had BACs of 0.10 or higher, versus 4.4 percent in 1986. In contrast, drinking and driving has declined among whites and African Americans.

Overall, the decline in people having high BAC levels drinking and driving isn't statistically significant. "The lack of detectable change in driving at high BACs between 1986 and 1996 is disappointing," says Robert B. Voas, the study's principal investigator. "We have a long way to go in addressing this problem on U.S. roads. Despite progress made, alcohol-impaired driving still is a big problem."

Critical Thinking Question

The *Healthy People 2000* objectives include the following: "Increase use of safety belts and child safety seats to at least 85 percent of motor vehicle occupants." In 1994, the rate was 67 percent. Given the overwhelming evidence that safety belts and child safety seats reduce injury, why are Americans so reluctant to buckle up?

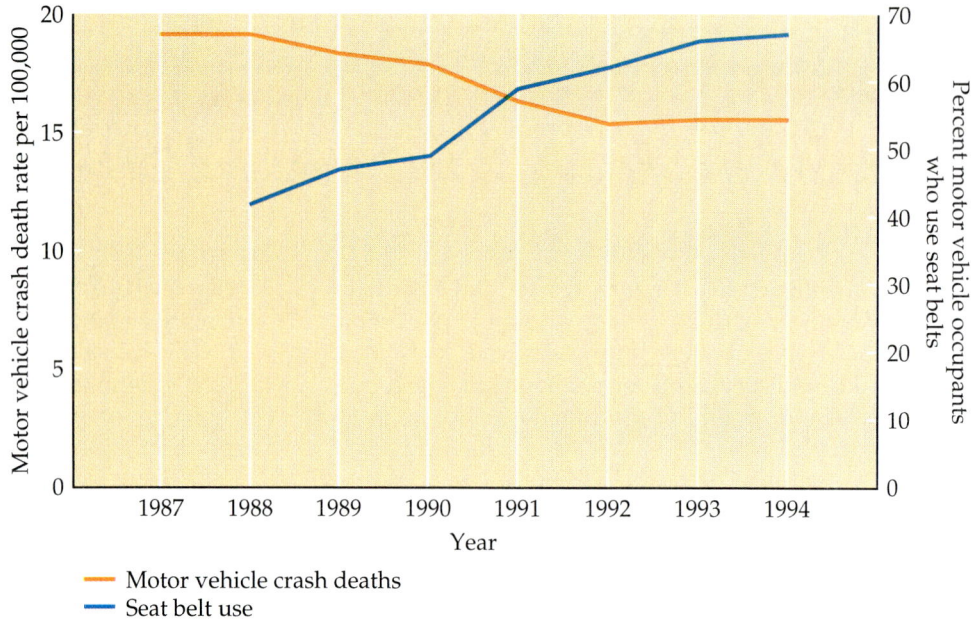

Figure 12.4 **Motor Vehicle Crash Deaths and Seat Belt Use.** *As the rate of seat belt use goes up, the rate of death from motor vehicle crashes goes down. (Source: National Highway Traffic Safety Administration)*

	1987	1988	1989	1990	1991	1992	1993	1994
Motor vehicle crash deaths	19.2	19.2	18.4	17.9	16.4	15.4	15.6	15.6
Seat belt use	—	42	47	49	59	62	66	67

Passive seat belts provide added protection to at-risk drivers who still do not want to buckle up. These belts automatically place a shoulder restraint around both driver and front seat passenger upon their entering the car. Unfortunately, these passive restraints are easy to disengage, making seat belt use still a matter of choice. Also, in some automobiles, passive restraints are not effective unless a lap belt is also used. Drivers and passengers may have a false sense of security if they rely only on the passive systems.

Children are at particular risk when traveling in an automobile. Without some form of restraint, they are likely to stand up, roll over, climb into the front seat, crawl into the well of a station wagon, or otherwise act in an unsafe manner. Even though every state requires child safety belt use, laws cannot solve the problem entirely. One recent survey showed that 75 percent of child safety seats were attached to the car incorrectly or not at all.

Air Bags

Air bags are another safety feature in cars used to protect the driver and front-seat passenger in case of an accident. Introduced as an optional feature in 1990 cars, dual air bags are required for all passenger cars starting with model year 1998 and light trucks beginning with model year 1999. Since they have been in use, air bags have saved the lives of an estimated eighteen hundred people, according to the National Highway Traffic Safety Administration (NHTSA).

Here is how an air bag works. An inflatable bag is concealed in the steering wheel or dashboard of a car until it is activated by a frontal or side crash. Within

---

HealthLinks
National Safety Council
www.nsc.org

Access to resources, statistics, and publications related to public safety.

one tenth of a second after impact, a sensor activates the bag and inflates it, thus creating a protective cushion between the driver and the steering wheel or the front seat passenger and the dashboard and windshield. The bag quickly deflates after absorbing the shock of the forward force of the people in the front seat. This inflate–deflate cycle is completed in less than one second. If all cars were equipped with air bags, it is estimated that automobile crash fatalities would be reduced by 30 percent.

Air bags are not without their problems, and nearly two thirds of the drivers involved in crashes examined in one study suffered some kind of air-bag-related injury. Their lives were saved and most of the injuries were minor—bruises and scratches—but some people suffered broken bones in their arms and hands and face lacerations, including eye injuries. However, more than eighty people have died from air bag injuries.

Short adults (under five feet two inches tall) and children are particularly at risk for air bag injuries. Short people tend to sit with their faces or chests close to the steering wheel, and they can sometimes get in the way of the inflating air bag. Many of the children involved in air bag injuries are believed to have been riding without a safety belt, so they moved forward—into the path of the inflating air bag—during the braking just before the impact. As a result, children, just like short adults, can be too far forward when an air bag is deployed.

Safety experts recommend that everyone in the car wear lap and shoulder belts and that children always sit in the back wearing a belt or placed in a safety seat. Over the long term, "smart" air bags will be designed that can distinguish between adults of varying heights and a child—or even a bag of groceries placed on the front seat—and will tailor protective deployment according to the occupant's specific characteristics. In the meantime, motorists can apply to NHTSA for a certificate that will allow a mechanic to install a switch that will deactivate the air bag system in their cars only for safety reasons—for example, for a small adult, who must sit within 12 inches of the point of potential deployment, or when routine passenger loads require that at least one child sit up front.

Critical Thinking Question

> Air bags were designed to save lives and reduce the incidence of injury in car crashes. Current laws require air bags in cars starting with the 1998 model year and that children be in safety restraints; yet, according to a 1996 report released by the National Transportation Safety Board, at least a dozen children were killed by air bags that year, compared with one in 1993. Many of the children injured and/or killed were not wearing safety restraints. Do you think transportation safety laws are conflicting in terms of the safety of children? What more can the government do to protect children from injury in motor vehicle crashes? What more can parents do?

Motorcycles

Motorcycle riding can be fun, challenging, and exciting. But it can also be dangerous and deadly. The stereotype of an injured motorcyclist, according to the manager of an emergency room in a general hospital, is a young male in his early

passive seat belts Seat belts that automatically place a shoulder restraint around the driver and the front seat passenger upon their entering the car.

air bags Safety devices located behind the steering wheel and/or the dashboard that automatically inflate on impact during a frontal or side crash.

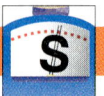

HEALTHWISE CONSUMER

What to Look for in Helmet Safety

There is no question that bicycle and motorcycle helmets save lives. Studies have shown that fatal injuries of bicyclists are at least 60 percent more likely to occur to a rider who is not wearing a helmet. Head injuries are the leading cause of death in motorcycle accidents. They are 40 percent more likely to be fatal to the rider who is not wearing a helmet, according to the National Highway Traffic and Safety Administration. Good helmets are a sound investment; they cost less than a trip to the emergency room.

What Should You Look for in a Bicycle Helmet?

- *A sticker certifying that it meets safety standards* from either the American National Standards Institute or the more stringent Snell Memorial Foundation.
- *Maximum coverage*—the more head area it covers, the more protection it offers.
- *A good fit*—this is the single most important thing a consumer can determine on his or her own. The helmet should be comfortable enough to wear for a long time.
- *Multiple straps with three or four attachment points* inside the helmet will provide a more secure, stable feel. Position the helmet to sit level on your head. Buckle up, fastening the chin strap snugly. If you can fit a finger between the strap and your chin, it is too loose.

Try to pull off the helmet, or have a friend try. If it remains secure, it will probably not fall off during impact. Replace the helmet after a fall. It is sometimes difficult to tell how hard you hit the ground because the helmet's expanded polystyrene foam liner cushions the impact. Damage to the helmet may not be apparent, but the helmet may be weakened. One manufacturer has recently come out with a helmet that uses expanded polypropylene as a liner material. That material can withstand repeated impacts, but it is not widely used.

What Should You Look for in a Motorcycle Helmet?

- *The Department of Transportation (DOT) emblem* on the back. All helmets made after 1988 are required to meet DOT safety standards, but there are some novelty helmets on the market that still do not comply. Only 10 percent of all motorcycle helmets on the market have earned the DOT emblem.
- *A helmet providing full head and face coverage.* Motorcycle helmets come in two basic styles—one offers partial head coverage, the other offers full head coverage without a visor. All three styles can meet federal standards, but it is the full helmet with visor that will protect you the best.

---

twenties who was not wearing a helmet, was doing 60 to 100 miles per hour, and has alcohol in his blood. In this case, the statistics parallel the stereotype. More than 60 percent of motorcycle deaths occur among sixteen- to thirty-four-year-old men. The leading cause of motorcycle injuries is alcohol and drugs. More than fifty thousand alcohol-related motorcycle injuries occur each year, and of the twenty-one hundred motorcyclists who die each year in crashes, 46 percent have alcohol concentrations at or above 0.10 percent, according to the Insurance Institute for Highway Safety.

Other causes of injuries are lack of operator skill—more than 90 percent of motorcycle riders who are injured either taught themselves or learned to ride from a friend—and not wearing a helmet. Motorcycles are more likely than cars to be involved in crashes, and when they do crash, motorcycle riders lack the protection of an enclosed vehicle.

States have had difficulty mandating safety helmet use among motorcyclists, even though data show that an unhelmeted motorcyclist is 40 percent more likely to suffer a fatal head injury than is a helmeted rider. In 1975, most states required helmet use, but under pressure from bikers, many either repealed their helmet laws or weakened them so that they cover only motorcyclists under age eighteen. Clear evidence that the number and severity of injuries are reduced when a helmet is worn has resulted in the reinstatement of laws, and now about half the states require helmet use by all motorcycle riders. In these states, helmet use rates approach 100 percent. However, in the states that mandate helmet use only by those under age eighteen, use rates are only about 50 percent. For tips about what to look for in bicycle and motorcycle helmets, see the Healthwise Consumer box.

Taking another approach to motorcycle safety, some states require that motorcycles have headlights on at all times to increase their visibility. Estimates vary considerably, but headlights are believed to reduce the risk of a daytime motorcycle crash by 50 percent. Most motorcycle injuries, however, take place between 6 P.M. and 3 A.M.

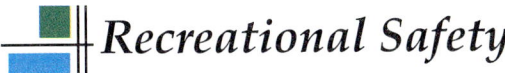
Recreational Safety

Recreational activities are for fun, but unfortunately, a lot of unintentional injuries take place when people are participating in them. A classic injury is a broken nose from contact sports, such as basketball and soccer. Two sports in which injuries occur often are bicycling and swimming.

Safety Issues for Bicyclists

As much fun and good exercise as biking is, it is one of the top causes of recreational injuries. Each year, biking results in about twenty thousand hospitalizations and nine hundred deaths. Children are at particularly great risk of injury from bicycle use. Each year, more than 2 million children receive bicycles as gifts, but only about 5 percent are also given helmets. Tragically, one child dies every day and about two hundred are treated in emergency rooms because of cycling-related head injuries. In fact, nearly one fourth of all significant brain injuries in children fourteen years or younger are bicycle related.

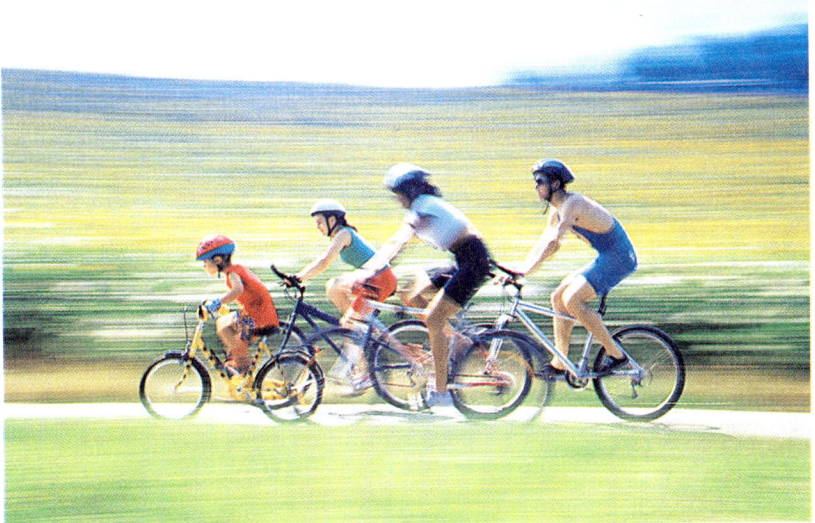

Bike helmets significantly reduce the risk of head and brain injury. You still may get hurt wearing a helmet, but broken bones and bruises will heal while brain damage may be permanent. (Source: © Tony Stone Images/Frank Orel)

Studies show that bike helmets significantly reduce the risk of head and brain injury, and everyone—not just children—should wear a helmet when biking. Even experienced bikers crash every 4,500 miles on average, according to the Bicycle Helmet Safety Institute. Road rash and broken bones will heal; brain damage may be permanent.

A related cause of biking injury is alcohol. Studies show that in about one third of all fatal bike injuries, the biker had been drinking. Bikers aged twenty to twenty-nine are most at risk: 55 percent of those in this age group who died were intoxicated. In addition to impaired judgment from alcohol, bikers who drink are less likely to wear a helmet. A study of bikers who were treated in the University of Maryland Shock Trauma Center found that injured persons whose blood alcohol levels were below 0.10 percent were five times as likely to have worn helmets as those who were legally drunk.

Based on the reduction in injuries after seat belt use and child restraints were mandated, states and local communities are enacting legislation to require helmet use while biking. Such laws are considered so important that a new objective was added to the *Healthy People 2000: National Health Promotion and Disease Prevention Objectives,* to extend to fifty states laws requiring helmets for bicycle riders. As of 1996, only thirteen states had such laws.

On the Waterfront

Going for a swim on a hot day sounds like a pleasant activity, whether it is at the beach, a public or private pool, or the old swimming hole in the country. Yet each year, about forty-five hundred people drown while trying to cool off. Most vulnerable of all are children under age four and males aged fifteen to thirty-four.

The primary cause of drowning among young adult men is alcohol use in conjunction with boating and other water-related activities. It is against the law in every state to operate a boat while under the influence of alcohol, but enforcement is relatively weak. Restricting the sale of alcoholic beverages in boating and swimming areas might reduce the number of teenagers and adults drowning.

Most deaths due to drowning in young adults are alcohol-related, hypothermia-related, or both. **Hypothermia** refers to the loss of body heat. Under the influence of alcohol, for example, two college students might challenge each other to swim across a river, not realizing that their swimming skill is impaired

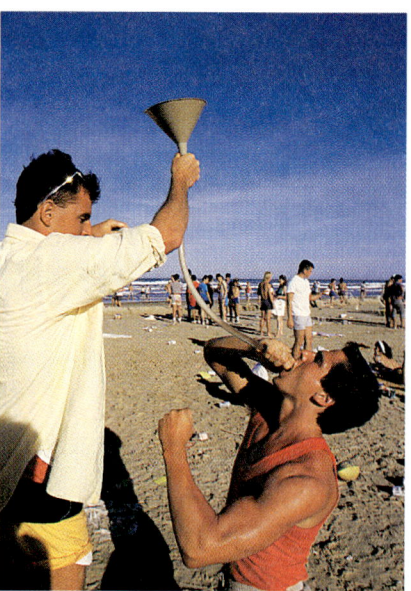

Beach parties have been romanticized in movies and on television, but a word of warning: alcohol in conjunction with boating and other water-related activities is the leading cause of drowning among college-age men. (Source: Stock, Boston/© Bob Daemmrich)

by the alcohol and that the temperature of the water is low enough that their chances of surviving, even if they were sober, are limited.

Sometimes the setting itself causes the problem, and it is estimated that 20 percent of drownings could be prevented by modifying the physical environment. Effective strategies include posting signs at the beach concerning depth and undertow and requiring fences, gates, and proper locking devices around home swimming pools.

Critical Thinking Question

Have you noticed something about injuries discussed in this chapter? The risk of encountering virtually all unintentional injuries seems to be increased by the consumption of alcohol. Car injuries, motorcycle injuries, bicycle injuries, diving injuries, and drowning all occur more often when alcohol is present. If alcohol is such a critical risk factor, why is it so difficult to encourage people not to drink when driving an automobile or when taking part in potentially dangerous recreational activities such as boating, biking, or swimming?

Diving Safety Tips

An estimated five hundred to seven hundred swimmers are seriously injured each year by diving into shallow areas of swimming pools and other bodies of water. Diving injuries can damage the spinal cord and result in **quadriplegia**—paralysis from the neck down affecting both arms and legs—to divers who hit the bottom or side of a pool. The typical victim of a diving injury is a male between the ages of thirteen and twenty-three. Almost 50 percent of all people with diving injuries have been drinking prior to being hurt.

The Consumer Product Safety Commission offers the following advice about safe diving:

- Never dive into above-ground pools. They are too shallow.
- Don't dive from the side of an in-ground pool. Enter the water feet first.
- Dive only from the end of the diving board and not from the sides.
- Dive with your hands in front of you and always steer up immediately upon entering the water to avoid hitting the bottom or sides of the pool.
- Don't dive if you have been using alcohol or drugs because your reaction time may be too slow.

Improper use of pool slides presents the same danger as improper diving techniques. Never slide down head first; slide down feet first only.

HEALTH SKILLS

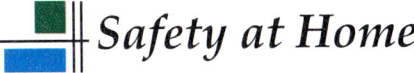
Safety at Home

Many injuries occur at home, from falling down the stairs to falling asleep smoking and starting a fire to exposing children to poisonous cleaning fluids. As with

hypothermia Loss of body temperature to subnormal levels; can result in mental confusion, unconsciousness, and death.

quadriplegia Total paralysis of the body from the neck down, affecting arms and legs.

most unintentional injuries, many injuries at home can be avoided by changing the environment to make it safer.

When a Simple Fall Is Not Simple

When was the last time you fell? How badly were you injured? Most likely you had a scraped knee, a wrenched shoulder, perhaps a broken collar bone, but nothing particularly life threatening. Unfortunately, this is not the case for everyone. Falls are the second leading cause of fatal injuries, resulting in 12,600 deaths and 780,000 hospitalizations a year. The actual number of deaths related to falls may be much higher. While most falls do not result in death, they may result in a decrease in confidence, restriction of physical activity, or other reductions in independence—all of which can negatively affect the quality of life.

Fall-related injuries occur at every age, but the elderly are particularly vulnerable. One third of all elderly people fall each year, and most of these incidents take place at home during usual activities such as walking or using the bathroom. Much can be done in the home to help prevent falls, including installing better lighting and handrails on stairs and in the bathroom, covering slippery floors with skid-free rugs, and wearing shoes with firm soles instead of slippers.

Unfortunately, less can be done to prevent arthritis, cataracts, strokes, dementia, and other neurological impairments that may be precursors to falls. Falls are the leading cause of death from injury for people aged sixty-five and older and one of the primary reasons why an elderly person enters a nursing home. Fear of falling may lead the elderly to limit their activities, thereby causing them to become less independent. See Chapter 18 for more information about promoting a safe home environment for an elderly individual.

Although children die less often from their falls than do the elderly, the injuries children sustain as a result of falls are a significant problem. Children fall most often during play—for example, on the playground or in the back yard. The injuries associated with such falls are usually minor scrapes or broken bones, but in some cases falls result in more serious problems, such as concussions and even brain damage from head injuries.

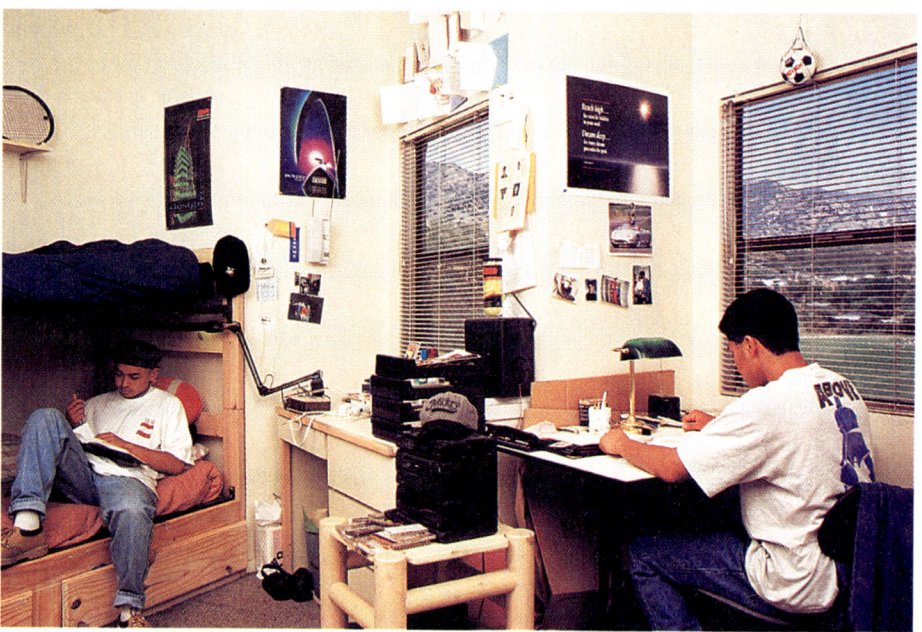

A smoke detector in your dorm room will sound an alarm at the first "sniff" of trouble. Make sure you have a working detector in your room. (Source: © Tony Stone Images/Rene Sheret)

DEVELOPING HEALTH SKILLS

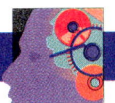

First Aid for Burns

When a person is burned, look at the burn carefully. Is the skin either very white or charred? Is it a big or deep burn? If the answer is yes to either of these questions, it is a *third-degree burn*. One cause of third-degree burn is fire. A *second-degree burn* has blisters. Scalding with hot water can cause a second-degree burn. A *first-degree burn* causes the skin to turn red. A sunburn that does not blister is a first-degree burn.

What to Do for Third-Degree Burns

- Have the victim remain calm while you assist with propping up the burned limb or body part until it is above his or her head, if possible.
- Call 911 immediately.

What to Do for Second-Degree Burns

- Cool the burn immediately. Use an ice pack or a series of towels soaked in cool water.
- When the pain has subsided, which should take about 15 minutes, cover the burn with a gauze pad for protection.
- Unbroken blisters heal faster, so do not break the blister deliberately. If the blister breaks, treat it as a cut by keeping it clean and applying topical antibiotic cream.
- If infection occurs, contact a physician or go to the emergency room.

What to Do for First-Degree Burns

- Do not apply oils, ointments, or sprays to the burn.
- Run cool water at low pressure over the burned area.
- Avoid exposure to additional heat or the sun until the burn heals and the redness is gone.

Up in Smoke

Reading in bed becomes a hazard when you are smoking as you read. Cigarettes cause twenty-three hundred house fires a year and are responsible for the largest percentage of home fires that kill or seriously injure children. Most cigarettes contain additives in both the tobacco and the surrounding paper that can cause them to burn for as long as twenty-eight minutes. Without these additives, a cigarette would self-extinguish after four minutes, which is likely not enough time for furniture to catch fire.

In a typical scenario, an adult falls asleep while smoking and reading or smokes carelessly in bed so that a speck of burning tobacco falls on top of the blanket, where it may smolder for hours. By the time a fire breaks out, the whole household may be asleep. Most fires in the home take place between 10 P.M. and 6 A.M.

Approximately thirty-six hundred people die each year in home fires, and more than six hundred thousand residential fires are serious enough to be reported to fire departments. Residential fires account for about 80 percent of all fire deaths. In general, more deaths are due to inhaling smoke and other poisonous gases than to burns. Burns, however, are the leading cause of childhood injury-related deaths in the home. One of the dangers associated with burns is the subsequent infection of a burn injury, which is complex to treat and carries high risks. See the Developing Health Skills box to learn how to identify and treat the three types of burns.

A primary reason for the decline in the number of fire deaths is greater use of **smoke detectors.** These electronic devices monitor the air in your home or dorm and sound an alarm at the first "sniff" of trouble. In most cases, this is

smoke detectors Smoke-sensitive devices designed to alert occupants of a room or space in the event of a fire.

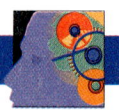

DEVELOPING HEALTH SKILLS

Smoke Alarm Tips

A smoke alarm can save your life in case of a fire. Here are four points to consider for your protection:

- *Install a smoke alarm outside each bedroom or sleeping area in your home.* If you sleep with your door closed, relying on a smoke alarm in the hall may not be safe for you. In such a case, make sure you have a smoke alarm in your bedroom. If you live in a house having more than one level, install a smoke alarm on each level. An additional alarm above the staircase will detect a fire early if it breaks out on the first story.
- *Properly maintain your smoke alarms.* Test your smoke alarms at least once each month to make sure they are working properly. Change the batteries in battery-operated alarms at least once a year or before if the alarm goes off. To help you remember, change the batteries on a notable date—for example, on your birthday or when daylight saving time starts or ends each year.
- *If smoke from cooking causes the alarm to sound, do not remove the batteries or disconnect the power source.* You may have a real need for the alarm before you remember to replace the batteries. Instead of disconnecting the alarm, fan the smoke away from the alarm until it stops sounding. If this happens frequently, it may be necessary to relocate the alarm or install a different type of alarm.
- *Develop an escape plan and review the plan frequently with all members of the family.* Be sure to store keys for deadlocks in an easily accessible location. Be aware that children and elderly people may need some special assistance should a fire occur. To ensure that everyone escapes safely, establish a meeting place outside the house—perhaps by the mailbox—for all members of the family. When a fire occurs, get out of the house immediately and use a neighbor's telephone to notify the local fire department by calling 911. Do not return to the house until a firefighter says it is safe.

---

before you even see the first trace of smoke. What the detector is responding to is the production of gases that precedes a full-blown fire. According to a recent study, smoke detectors can reduce the potential for death in 86 percent of fires and the potential for severe injuries in 88 percent. Smoke detectors range in price from less than $15 to more than $100, depending on the type. Read the Developing Health Skills box to learn more about smoke alarms.

Another reason for the reduction of residential fires is that homes today are built with **flame-retardant materials** in the walls and floors and in heating and electrical systems. Older housing, particularly substandard housing in inner cities, is more at risk for fires. Fabrics, too, are less flammable today, especially materials designed for sleep wear. Ignited clothing used to be a major cause of burns in children and the elderly, but it now accounts for only 5 percent of all burn deaths.

Other Burns

Burns aren't caused just by fire. Another kind of burn that occurs at home frequently seriously injures both children and the elderly: burns from hot—actually, scalding—water from the faucet. The culprits are water heaters that are adjusted to heat water as high as 150 degrees to 160 degrees Farenheit. It takes only a one-second exposure to 160-degree water to develop a burn. A similar burn would take 30-seconds to develop from direct exposure to 130-degree water.

For all their patriotic associations, fireworks present another very serious hazard, particularly to children. About nine thousand people are treated each year in emergency rooms for injuries associated with fireworks. More than half of these injuries are burns, many of them involving the head and face. Fireworks may also cause the victim to be permanently blinded or to lose fingers, arms, and legs. Nearly half of the victims of fireworks injuries are less than fifteen years old.

Laws restricting the sale and use of fireworks are among the strongest ways to prevent fireworks-related injuries. Most cities have at least some restrictions on fireworks, and many have mandatory fines if the regulations are violated. General education about the dangers of fireworks also provides a major prevention option.

Poison Alert

Children are inquisitive by nature, and when they find pretty-colored pills or bottles with bright liquids, they want to know what is in them. And so they open them up, put the pills or liquid in their mouths, and become accidental poisoning statistics.

Each year, some seven hundred thousand children under five years of age swallow poison unintentionally and 90 percent of these encounters take place in the home. Children are particularly vulnerable because their body mass is so small that it takes only a few swallows for the damage to be done.

Deaths associated with unintentional poisoning dropped significantly with the introduction of **child-resistant packaging** of prescription medicines in 1974. But child-resistant packaging does not mean child-proof packaging, and the National Safety Council reports that child-resistant containers are designed to keep out 80 percent of children less than four years old. This leaves 20 percent of the children unprotected.

Adults are also victims of unintentional poisoning. Review the following list of poisonous materials that may be in your dorm or home:

Ammonia	Lamp oils
Antifreeze	Liniment
Bleaches	Mouthwash
Colognes and perfumes	Nail polish remover
Detergents	Paint thinner
Fertilizers	Pesticides
Furniture polish	Pet medications
Home permanent solutions	Toilet bowl cleaners

All of these substances should be stored in tamper-proof containers and out of reach of children. Do not store them near food or in food containers; someone may unintentionally get a food and a poison product mixed up and swallow the poison. Never place kerosene, antifreeze, paints, or solvents in cups, glasses, or milk or soft-drink bottles customarily used for food or drinks; a mix-up might occur. Some injuries occur when cleaning agents are combined. Always follow directions when using household cleaners. Finally, do not put medications in containers other than the ones they came in; flush all medications down the toilet when they are out of date.

In case of poisoning, call your local poison control center, rescue squad, hospital, or physician immediately, and follow these procedures:

flame-retardant materials Substances designed to resist or retard burning.

child-resistant packaging Product packaging designed to discourage or prevent children from gaining access to the contents.

- If poison is inhaled, move the victim into fresh air as quickly as possible.
- If poison gets on skin, remove contaminated clothing and wash the area immediately with soap and water.
- If a poison has splashed into the eyes, immediately flood the eyes with cool water from a container held above the eyes. Continue flooding for fifteen minutes.
- The most important item to have in every home in case of accidental poisoning is *syrup of ipecac,* a liquid that helps to induce vomiting. Syrup of ipecac is inexpensive, is a valuable time saver, and can be bought in a drugstore without a prescription. It should be used only upon the recommendation of a poison control center or physician. Although vomiting is not normally considered a first aid measure when petroleum distillates have been swallowed, this procedure may be recommended by the poison control center or physician. Activated charcoal might be recommended by the poison control center as first aid when a corrosive poison or petroleum product has been swallowed.

HEALTH SKILLS

A Structure for Preventing Unintentional Injuries

Prevention of unintentional injuries is a primary concern of several federal agencies:

- The Consumer Protection Safety Commission (CPSC) is responsible for protecting the public from unreasonable risks for injury posed by consumer products. It has jurisdiction over 1 million manufacturers, distributors, and retailers, and the more than fifteen thousand products that they produce and sell. The CPSC protects the public in a number of ways, ranging from providing safety information and warnings to drafting safety standards. One specific activity of the CPSC is to recall a product when it is found to present a risk to the consumer. The commission estimates that its various activities prevent more than 1 million injuries annually.
- The Occupational Safety and Health Administration (OSHA), an arm of the Department of Labor, establishes safety and health standards for the workplace. It regulates noise and ambient toxic levels, sets standards for the operation of equipment, and enforces procedures for inspection in plants and other places of business.
- The CDC's Division of Unintentional Injury Prevention monitors trends in unintentional injuries in the United States, conducts research to better understand risk factors, and evaluates interventions to prevent these injuries.

These governmental agencies, however, can only do so much to help prevent unintentional injuries. Prevention begins by every person taking responsibility for safety. A safe health style begins with you *taking responsibility* for your own safety. Second, a safe health style requires *taking preventive action* to reduce your risk for suffering an unintentional injury. Finally, because accidents cannot be totally avoided, a safe health style requires *being prepared to respond* when something does happen.

Take Responsibility

Injury prevention is a partnership, but it is only as effective as each partner. There are several things that you can do on the personal level and on the community level to prevent injuries. For example, you are responsible for fastening your seat belt when you ride in an automobile and you are responsible for following traffic laws. Your community is responsible for passing laws concerning safe driving speeds. You are responsible for not depending on a drunk driver to give you a ride home. Your community is responsible for enforcing laws related to drinking and driving.

At home, you are responsible for providing a safe home environment for your children, including child-resistant cabinet latches, electrical outlet covers, and barriers at the top of stairways. Your community requires that medicines be packaged safely so that children are not likely to take them unintentionally, but you are responsible for where those medications are stored.

Take Preventive Action

Many unintentional injuries could have been prevented or made less serious. The reduction of injury begins with practicing safe day-to-day living. Here is a list of safe-living principles that can help you reduce your risk of unintentional injury. Space is provided for you to add to the list.

On the road

- Wear your seat belt.
- Use child safety seats properly.
- Remain within posted speed limits.
- Drive at a safe speed, regardless of the legal limit.
- Wear helmets when riding a bike or motorcycle.
- Never drive after drinking.
- Never ride with someone who has been drinking.
-
-
-

During recreational activities

- Wear reflective clothing.
- Maintain equipment in good repair.
- Never operate boats under the influence of alcohol.
- Wear personal flotation devices.
- Respect the power of nature by avoiding swimming in dangerous surf or driving in a blinding snowstorm.
-
-
-

At home

- Install smoke detectors in or near every bedroom.
- Have a fire escape plan.
- Maintain slip-resistant floor coverings.
- Use poison labels on containers.
- Use child protective latches.
- Discard dangerous chemicals and drugs.
- Install handrails in bathtubs and showers.
- Use lighting to reduce the hazards in yards and hallways.
-
-
-

Critical Thinking Question

> In *Healthy People 2000*, the following objective is listed: "Provide academic instruction on injury prevention and control, preferably as a part of comprehensive school health education, in at least 50 percent of public school systems." Given the threat of unintentional injuries to the school-age population, why would *Healthy People 2000* set a goal of only 50 percent? Why is it so difficult to provide academic instruction on injury prevention?

Be Prepared to Respond

Not all injuries can be prevented, but their impact can be minimized by proper and prompt action taken by men and women like yourself who come to the aid of injury victims. Although there is no substitute for complete first aid training through an accredited course of study, everyone—even the untrained—needs to understand a few basic principles of first aid and emergency medicine.

The following are seven basic recommendations from the American Red Cross and the National Safety Council:

1. In an emergency situation, first protect yourself. Avoid approaching an automobile with downed electric power lines around it. Do not attempt to save a drowning person if you are not trained in water rescue. The situation can become worse if you become a victim, too.
2. Do not move the victim unless it is necessary to prevent further injury. Keep the victim in the position best suited to his or her condition or injury. Sometimes this means having the victim lie down; in other cases, he or she can sit. In general, it is not recommended that the victim get up or walk around.
3. Avoid or overcome chilling by using blankets or some other means of covering the victim's body. If the victim is exposed to cold or dampness, place blankets or additional clothing under him or her as well. Keeping warm is especially important for victims who are experiencing **shock**—a condition of reduced circulation to the vital organs.
4. Find out what happened. Ask witnesses about the situation. Was there an incident that caused the injury? Did the victim suddenly get ill and fall down on the street? This information could reveal a great deal about the nature of injuries. Look for emergency medical identification such as a Medic Alert bracelet or necklace, which may provide some clues about the victim's health and the possible cause of the injury.
5. Seek help immediately by calling 911 for emergency or 0 for the operator or by sending a bystander to call for medical assistance. When you call, talk clearly and directly, and tell the operator what happened in one sentence. For example, "I have just witnessed an automobile crash and someone is injured badly." The person on the other end of the phone will give you instructions on what to do. You will be asked where the incident happened. If you do not know the address, look for a street sign or landmark that will give the rescue team an idea of where to go. The operator might ask you for other information, including the extent of injuries. Answer these questions as best you can. When the operator has no more questions, he or she will tell you to hang up and go back to the scene of the accident to wait for assistance. Do not hang up until the operator tells you to.

shock A condition of reduced circulation to the vital organs.

cardiopulmonary resuscitation (CPR) A combination of mouth-to-mouth breathing and chest compression used during cardiac arrest to keep blood flowing to the heart muscle and brain; an emergency procedure.

6. If you are trained in **cardiopulmonary resuscitation (CPR)**, survey the victim following your ABC training. *A* refers to the airway: Is the air passage open? *B* refers to breathing: Is the victim breathing? *C* refers to circulation: Can a pulse be detected? This is an indication that the person's heart is beating and blood is circulating. If the victim is not breathing, has an open air passage and no pulse, it is time to start CPR. CPR involves rescue breathing (mouth-to-mouth resuscitation) as well as compressing the chest to get the victim breathing and blood circulating. *Cardio* refers to the heart, and *pulmonary* refers to the lung.
7. Check to see if the victim is bleeding severely. If so, control the bleeding by applying direct pressure over the wound and elevating it, if possible. Many people incorrectly believe that tourniquets—devices such as a handkerchief, neck tie, or scarf bound tightly above the wound to stop circulation—are necessary to stop severe bleeding. In fact, their use is no longer recommended.

Contact your local chapter of the American Red Cross, American Heart Association, or other group for information on classes in first aid, CPR, and additional emergency techniques.

Key Concepts

1. The percentage of deaths due to unintentional injuries is higher for fifteen- to twenty-four-year-olds—the age group that covers most college students—than for any other age group.
2. Unintentional injuries include trauma associated with automobile crashes, falls, poisonings, fires, and drownings. They are different from intentional injuries associated with suicide, homicide, and battery.
3. The line between unintentional and intentional injuries is sometimes blurred. For example, a drug overdose could be an unintentional event or it could be a suicide—an intentional event.
4. Unintentional injuries usually result from the action of one person—the principal actor—who causes the incident simply by not paying attention to something or by not possessing an adequate level of skill.
5. When several risk factors are compounded, the chances of being injured are increased.
6. The single largest cause of unintentional injuries is the automobile.
7. Even moderate levels of alcohol in the blood have been found to impair judgment markedly. Alcohol is the number-one cause of traffic fatalities and swimming and boating deaths.
8. Men are by far at greater risk for unintentional injury than are women, and this holds true at all ages.
9. Prevention of unintentional injuries involves taking personal responsibility, taking preventive action, and being prepared to respond when unexpected events occur.
10. Proper and prompt first aid can help injury victims.

Review Questions

1. Explain why unintentional injuries represent a significant public health concern.
2. Explain why unintentional injuries occur.
3. How would you characterize a person at risk for an unintentional injury?
4. Calculate the monetary cost of unintentional injuries to society.

5. What is the primary cause of unintentional injuries in the United States? List secondary causes.
6. Explain the impact of seat belts, child safety seats, and air bags on the rate of unintentional injuries.
7. Explain how alcohol consumption greatly enhances the potential of encountering unintentional injuries.
8. List unintentional injuries that result from recreational activities and day-to-day living in the home and on the road.
9. List steps to take to prevent diving injuries, poisonings, and automobile crashes—all sources of unintentional injuries.
10. Explain how taking responsibility, taking preventive action, and being prepared to respond when an injury occurs can reduce the number and severity of unintentional injuries.

Selected Bibliography

Accident Facts. Chicago, IL: National Safety Council, (updated annually).

Burt, C.W. "Injury-Related Visits to Hospital Emergency Departments: United States, 1992." *Advance Data, Number 261.* Hyattsville, MD: National Center for Health Statistics, 1995.

National Electronic Injury Surveillance System. Washington, DC: National Consumer Product Safety Commission, 1995.

National Summary of Injury Mortality Data, 1988–1994. Atlanta, GA: Centers for Disease Control and Prevention, National Center for Injury Prevention and Control, 1996.

Safety and Health. Chicago, IL: National Safety Council, (published monthly).

"Setting the National Agenda for Injury Control in the 1990s." *Morbidity and Mortality Weekly Report* 41, no. RR-6 (1992):1–38.

Singh, G.K., Kochanek, K.D., and M.F. MacDorman. "Advance Report of Final Mortality Statistics Reports, 1994." *Monthly Vital Statistics Report* 45, No. 3, Supplement. Hyattsville, MD: National Center for Health Statistics, 1996.

Traffic Safety Facts 1995: Alcohol. Washington, DC: National Highway Traffic Safety Administration, 1996.

HealthLinks: Web Sites for Preventing Unintentional Injuries

You can access better health as it relates to this chapter by checking out some of the following sites on the Internet. These and sites identified within the chapter can be accessed directly when you visit the *HealthStyles* website located on the Allyn and Bacon home page at **http://www.abacon.com**.

CDC National Center for Injury Prevention and Control (NCIPC)
www.cdc.gov/ncipc
Home page for the lead federal agency for injury prevention. It provides a link to statistical data, information on publications and resources, and links to related Web Sites for the three general areas of acute care; rehabilitation and disabilities, unintentional injury prevention, and violence prevention.

Consumer Products Safety Commission
www.cpsc.gov
CPSC, an independent federal regulatory agency, helps keep American fam-

ilies safe by reducing the risk of injury or death from consumer products. Contains methods for reporting unsafe products.

National Fire Protection Association
www.nfpa.org
This site contains the latest information about the National Fire Protection Association (NFPA), its departments, publications, seminars, and educational programs.

National Highway Transportation Safety Administration
www.nhtsa.dot.gov
NHTSA is responsible for reducing deaths, injuries, and economic losses resulting from motor vehicle crashes and is responsible for setting and enforcing safety performance standards for motor vehicles and motor vehicle equipment. Through this site you can access information on vehicle compliance testing, buying a safer car, recalls, technical service bulletins, and consumer complaints.

Health Hotlines: Preventing Unintentional Injuries

Aquatic Injury Safety Foundation
(800) 342-0330
1310 Ford Building
Detroit, MI 48226

Consumer Product Safety Commission
(800) 638-2772
Washington, DC 20207

National Fire Protection Association
(800) 344-3555
Batterymarch Park
Quincy, MA 02269

National Head Injury Foundation
(800) 444-6443
1176 Massachusetts Avenue NW, Suite 100
Washington, DC 20036-1904

National Highway Traffic Safety Administration, Auto Safety Hotline
(800) 424-9393
400 7th Street SW, Room 5319
Washington, DC 20590

National Institute for Occupational Safety and Health
(800) 356-4674
4676 Columbia Parkway
Cincinnati, OH 45226

Office of Navigation Safety and Waterway Services, Coast Guard Hotline
(800) 368-5647
7323 Telegraph Road
Alexandria, VA 22310

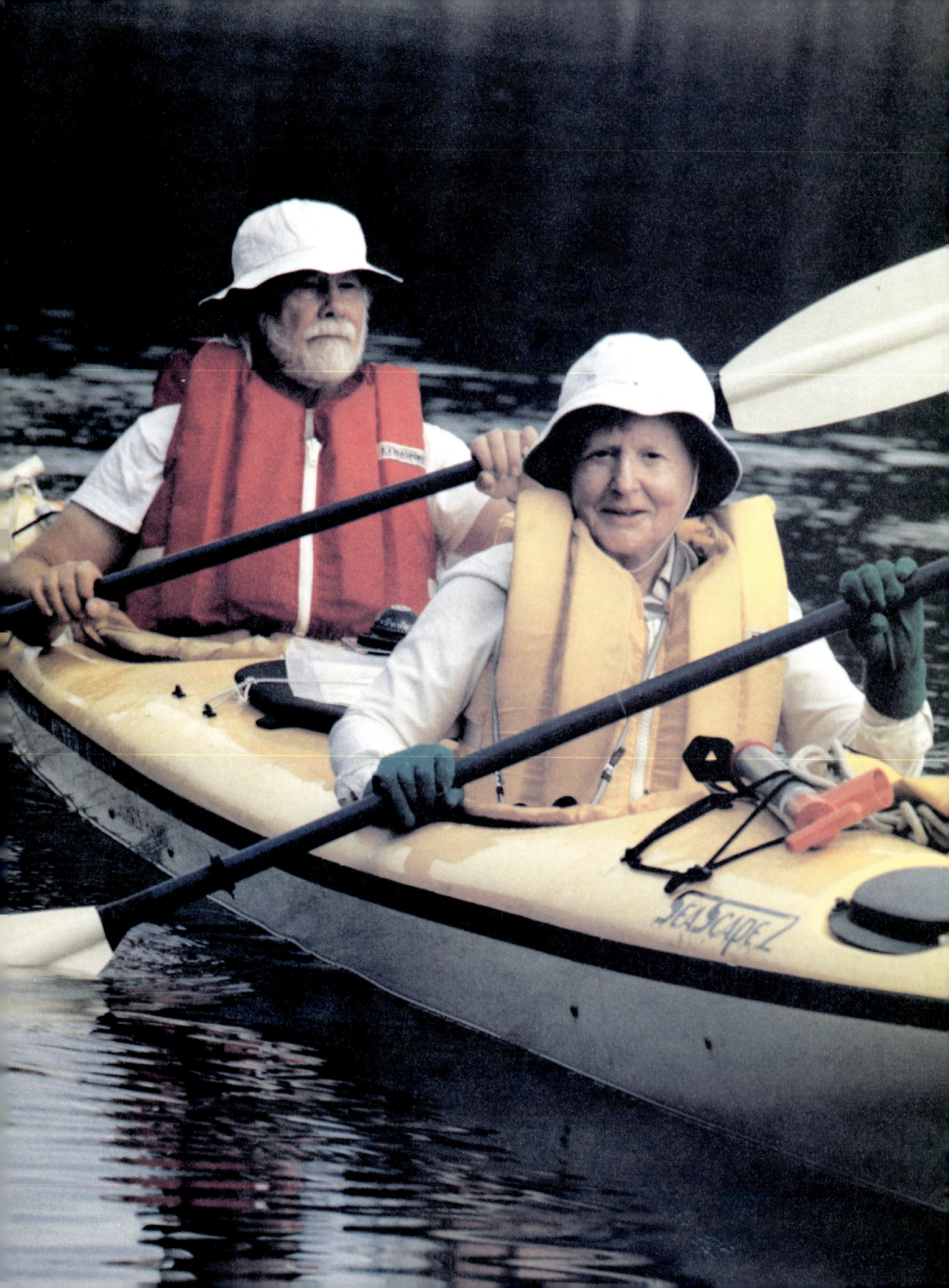

Chapter 13

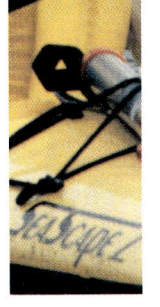
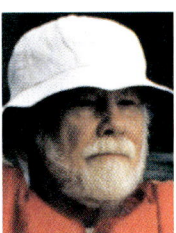
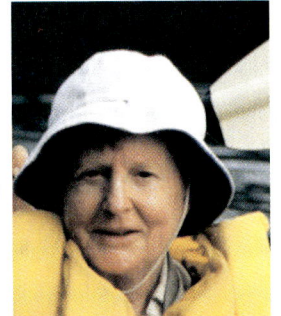

Reducing the Risk for Chronic Disease

Objectives

When you finish reading this chapter, you will be able to:

1. Differentiate between chronic illness and infectious illness.
2. Explain the natural history of a chronic illness, including the asymptomatic and symptomatic periods.
3. Relate lifestyle choices to the occurrence of chronic illness.
4. Describe the risk factors associated with cardiovascular disease and determine your personal risk for cardiovascular disease.
5. Name several cardiovascular diseases and describe the symptoms and treatment modalities for each.
6. Describe the risk factors associated with cancer.
7. Name several types of cancer and describe the prevalence of each.
8. Explain the importance of early detection of cancer and name several screening procedures that can lead to early detection.
9. Compare dental disease with more life-threatening forms of chronic illness.
10. Examine ways of helping individuals who have chronic illness, including psychological support and pain management.

What Is Your HealthStyle?

Louise was in a state of panic: She had discovered what she thought could be a lump in her left breast. But her breasts were lumpy, so she wasn't sure. She had read a lot about breast cancer in the newspaper and in women's magazines, and the thought of it made her very anxious.

As the months went by, Louise's anxiety increased, and unfortunately, so did the size of the tumor. Eventually, she could no longer deny its existence. She went to a physician who, after running the proper tests, confirmed Louise's worst fears—the tumor was malignant. Because she had waited until the tumor had grown larger, Louise needed more extensive surgery than she might have if she had seen her physician when she first detected the lump. In addition, there was concern that the cancer may have spread. Louise had a partial mastectomy, a course of chemotherapy, and a breast reconstruction. Five years later, she remains cancer-free and is happy to be alive.

When Mariana felt a lump in her breast, she, too, was in a state of panic. But she channeled that panic into swift action. She made an appointment to see her physician the next day, and her physician immediately ordered a mammogram and an ultrasound. When the results indicated the lump was malignant, she directed Mariana to a breast cancer specialist.

After a series of tests, including biopsies, and a second opinion from another breast cancer specialist, Mariana underwent a lumpectomy. Her doctors were confident that the cancer had been detected and treated early enough to prevent it from spreading to other tissue. Mariana's mental and physical scarring were minimal, but five years later, she remains vigilant and faithfully examines her breasts every month.

In Your Opinion

Louise avoided treatment; Mariana sought it immediately. Even so, both are living five years later.

- What health skills did Mariana practice in making her decision to seek early diagnosis and treatment?
- Given that both women survived their breast cancer, how important is early detection and treatment?
- What advice would you give to a man or woman who had detected a lump or otherwise suspected that he or she had cancer?
- Would you respond differently if that person had early signs of heart disease?

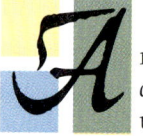

A chronic problem is one that is marked by long duration or frequent recurrence. In fact, the term *chronic* comes from the Greek word *chronos*, which means "time." In a social sense, think of chronic unemployment, chronic homelessness, or chronic urban decay. It is not a pretty picture. So, too, it is not pleasant to think of chronic diseases with their accompanying progressive pain and increasing disability. In some cases, however, there are ways to interrupt and even reverse the course of a disease—just as unemployment, homelessness, and urban decay can be reversed.

Millions of Americans have survived heart attacks or cancer. Many of these survivors lead healthier lives as a result. A heart attack survivor may once have eaten cholesterol-rich foods that clogged his arteries or perhaps led a sedentary lifestyle, but now he follows a low-fat diet and exercises regularly. A woman who has had basal cell cancers removed from her face once spent hours in the sun without protection from cancer-producing ultraviolet rays, but now when she goes out on sunny days, she wears sunscreen and a wide-brimmed hat.

Everyone knows someone who suffers from heart disease, cancer, diabetes, arthritis, asthma, tooth decay and gum disease, or a host of other chronic conditions. Chronic diseases are the leading cause of death and disability in the United States and a major source of pain and discomfort. Nearly 100 million Americans—46 percent of the country's population—have chronic diseases or disabilities, and the proportion of people who have to limit their activities due to chronic illness is increasing. African Americans disproportionately face these limitations (see Figure 13.1).

Chronic diseases develop over a long period of time, in part as a result of lifestyle choices. Smoking alone is associated with an increased incidence of the leading chronic diseases—heart disease, cancer, and lung disease. Still other chronic diseases develop through the process of living in a highly industrialized country at the end of the twentieth century. Certain cancers and lung diseases, for example, are associated with polluted air and chemicals in the workplace. Another important factor associated with chronic diseases is that people are living longer and so are subject to diseases that usually do not present themselves until the later years of life, such as osteoporosis and Alzheimer's disease. To read about both osteoporosis and Alzheimer's disease, see Chapter 18.

Not surprisingly, rates of chronic conditions are high among the elderly, and about 88 percent of people over age sixty-five have at least one chronic condition. It may be difficult for young adults to appreciate the relevance of chronic diseases in their life because they may think it will be many years before they have symptoms of one. However, people of all ages are at risk for chronic conditions. Researchers at the University of California, San Francisco, recently reported that one quarter of the children under age eighteen and more than one third of young adults aged eighteen to forty-four had at least one chronic condition.

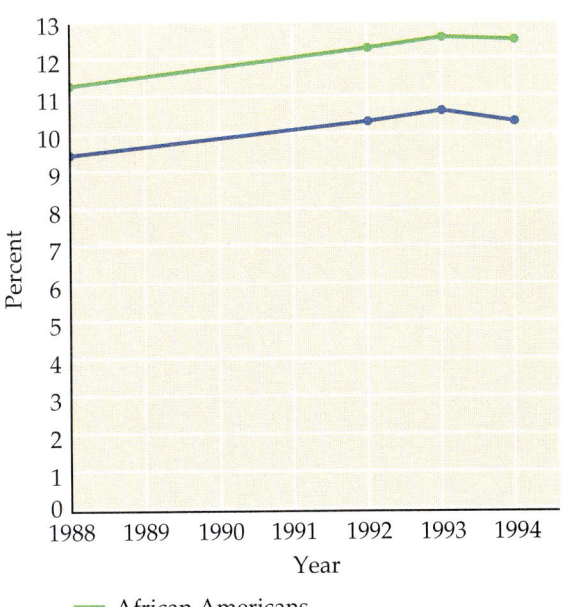

Figure 13.1 **Percentage of Americans Facing Limited Activities Due to Chronic Conditions.** *An increasing number of Americans have to limit their activities due to chronic illness. (Source: National Center for Health Statistics)*

Characteristics of Chronic Illness

Chronic illness is a generic term for diseases, such as atherosclerosis, cancer, asthma, diabetes, multiple sclerosis, schizophrenia, or arthritis. Chronic illness may result from a genetic condition, such as cystic fibrosis, or from poor hygiene, such as tooth decay. A chronic illness can affect the individual physically, mentally, or both. Sometimes, a chronic illness only minimally interferes with daily functioning; at other times, it requires round-the-clock medical attention.

Even given these differences, chronic illnesses have several common characteristics:

- They involve some degree of permanence.
- They result in some form of disability.
- They are progressive—that is, they get increasingly worse or become more debilitating.
- They require a long period of care or supervision.

Chronic versus Infectious Diseases

Chronic diseases differ from infectious diseases in three key ways. First, the two disease groups differ in their causes. For the most part, infectious or communicable diseases are a result of microorganisms and are contagious. (Infectious diseases are covered in Chapters 14 and 15.) Chronic diseases, in contrast, are generally not contagious. They are mostly a result of inherited factors or lifestyle factors, such as diet, personal hygiene, tobacco use, or exposure to toxic chemicals. (New research shows that microorganisms may play a role in chronic conditions, including stomach ulcers.)

Second, infectious diseases usually develop quickly and last for a comparatively brief period—sometimes only a matter of hours or days. Chronic diseases develop over a period of years and usually linger for a lifetime.

Third, chronic and infectious diseases differ concerning outcome. Persons who have infectious diseases may recover completely. Healthy people generally do not die of the common cold. As with many infectious diseases, they may feel miserable for a while, but in time, they usually recover completely. (There are exceptions to this rule, including malaria, hepatitis, the human immunodeficiency virus (HIV), and other virulent infectious diseases.) It is just the opposite with chronic diseases. People who have chronic diseases tend to remain ill for a long period of time. Again, there are exceptions. People have recovered from cancer, heart disease, and other chronic conditions.

Critical Thinking Question

> Two reasons cited for the rising mortality due to chronic disease are (1) medicine's success in dealing with infectious diseases and (2) medicine's success in extending life expectancy. Therefore, it could be said that successful medical intervention does not prevent death, it just changes the causes of death. Suppose cures for cardiovascular disease and cancer were discovered. What chronic disorder might then emerge as the next leading cause of death?

Changing Patterns of Mortality

Americans are living longer—nearly seventy-six years on average versus fifty in 1900—but when they die, death is due mostly to chronic diseases. At the beginning of the twentieth century, infectious diseases were the leading cause of death. Over the past half century, medical and social changes have led to detection and treatment of infectious diseases, numerous drugs to control disease, and an expanded understanding of the behavioral causes of many health threats.

Thanks to medical interventions and healthier lifestyles, infants, children, and young adults now survive what once were fatal illnesses and often live long enough to incur chronic illnesses. At a time when adults could anticipate living only about fifty or sixty years, chronic diseases were proportionately less common. But the proportion of population over age sixty-five has grown from 4 percent in 1900 to more than 12 percent today. An estimated one third of this older population has fair or poor health status, and the severity of chronic illness among this population is likely to rise as the elderly themselves get older (see Chapter 18).

Natural History of Chronic Diseases

Because chronic diseases occur over a long period of time, a period often occurs when the disease exists without any outward signs or clinical symptoms. This is called the **asymptomatic period.** In most cases, people with asymptomatic chronic conditions live normal lives without knowing that they have a chronic disease.

In the case of cardiovascular disease, for example, the presence of **plaque,** or fatty deposits, in the arteries is a clear signal of disease. Yet until the symptoms of disease appear, most people do not know that they have been accumulating plaque in their arteries.

More dramatically, a college basketball player might not know that he or she has an enlarged heart until collapsing during a game, or an elderly woman might not know she has osteoporosis until she falls, compresses her spine, and is left crippled and in chronic pain.

At some point during the course of a disease, clinical symptoms appear. This is called the **symptomatic period.** These signs, such as a lump, lesion, or other abnormal growth, may be apparent to the trained eye or touch. But many of the symptoms of chronic diseases are nonvisual, such as an increase in blood pressure.

It is usually up to a physician to determine when signs and abnormalities suggest the presence of a disease. This determination is called the **diagnosis.** Given the complexity of medical practice, diagnosis has become an extensive focus of medical training. A lump in the breast, for example, may or may not indicate the presence of a malignant tumor. Only through a **biopsy** of the lump tissue, a medical diagnostic procedure, can the lump be evaluated properly to determine whether it is cancerous.

Most chronic diseases, if left unrecognized and untreated, eventually lead to major impairment or even death. For this reason, early detection is highly important. Early signs, although not proof, should be taken as serious warnings and reasons to see your physician. One consistent fact concerning nearly all chronic diseases is that early detection through recognition of signs and symptoms leads to an increased chance of survival.

Lifestyle Choices and Disease

Lifestyle choices are important factors not only in chronic disease but also in overall personal health. Many such behaviors are presented in greater detail in other chapters of this book. The most common lifestyle causes of chronic diseases are smoking, poor diet, failure to exercise, and heavy consumption of alcohol.

chronic illness An illness marked by gradual onset, long duration, or frequent recurrence.

asymptomatic period A period in which a disease exists without any outward signs or clinical symptoms.

plaque A deposit of fatty material in a blood vessel wall.

symptomatic period A period during the course of a disease in which symptoms appear.

diagnosis A physician's opinion of the nature or cause of a disease based on observation and laboratory tests.

biopsy The removal of bits of living tissue and fluid from the body for diagnostic examination.

TABLE 13.1 Common Chronic Diseases and Risk Factors

Disease	Nonbehavioral risk factors	Behavioral risk factors	Symptoms	Preventive measures
Asthma	Allergies; family history; young age; viral infections; bronchitis	An attack may be triggered by: cigarette smoking; perfumes; exercise; aspirin; industrial/occupational exposures to air pollution; emotional anxiety	Coughing; shortness of breath; tightness in chest; wheezing; itchy or sore throat; increased breathing rate	Stay away from triggers; take allergy medications; exercise; recognize and treat symptoms early
Breast cancer	Genetic predisposition; cancer in one breast; uterine cancer; age; Caucasian race; early menstruation—late menopause	Women who have delayed child-bearing; women over 35; increased use of alcohol; increased fat content in diet; never having given birth	Lump in breast, armpit; breast pain; nipple discharge; itching, enlargement, retraction of nipple; change in breast contour or symmetry	Self-examination of breast every month; mammography; physical examination by gynecologist annually
Cervical cancer	Genetic predisposition; age	Intercourse at early age; multiple partners; smoking; papilloma virus infection	Abnormal vaginal bleeding; abnormal Pap smear	Avoid early sexual intercourse; avoid multiple partners; avoid cigarette smoking; annual gynecological exam
Cirrhosis of the liver	Genetic predisposition	Heavy alcohol/drug consumption; hepatitis	Weakness, fatigue; weight loss; nausea; abdominal pain; jaundice; amenorrhea; impotence; male breast increase	Discontinue use of alcohol/drugs
Dental disease	Age; fluoride-deficient drinking water; poverty	Fear of professional care; excessive between-meal snacks; failure to brush and floss regularly	Stained teeth; bad breath; tooth cavities; tooth loss; painful gums and tongue	Well-balanced nutritious diet; limit between-meal snacks; brush and floss regularly; have regular professional dental care

TABLE 13.1 Common Chronic Diseases and Risk Factors (continued)

Disease	Nonbehavioral risk factors	Behavioral risk factors	Symptoms	Preventive measures
Diabetes	Genetic predisposition	Obesity or being overweight; trauma to trigger onset	Increased urination; excessive thirst; rapid weight loss; high blood glucose levels; increased ketones in blood glucose	Well-balanced nutritious diet; maintain proper weight; exercise
Heart disease	Genetic predisposition; age; high blood pressure; diabetes	Poor physical exercise; cigarette smoking; obesity; poor stress management	Chest pain; breathing difficulty; spitting up blood; weight loss; lung collapse	Discontinuance of smoking; maintain low cholesterol levels; healthy diet (low in saturated fat, low amounts of junk food); regular exercise program; medical checkup
Lung cancer	Genetic predisposition; age	Cigarette smoking; environment (air, industrial pollution)	Cough; breathing difficulty; spitting up blood; weight loss; lung collapse	Discontinuance of smoking; elimination of environmental risks; education; medical checkup
Lung disease	Genetic predisposition; age	Environment (air, industrial pollution); cigarette smoking	Breathlessness; persistent cough; crowing sound during breathing; wheezing; spitting up blood; weight loss; lung collapse	Discontinuance of smoking; elimination of environmental risks; education; medical checkup
Stroke	Genetic predisposition; previous stroke; heart attack; age; high blood pressure	Cigarette smoking; heavy alcohol consumption; high-fat diet	Brief loss of vision; slurred speech; nausea; vomiting; sensory loss; weakness or paralysis	Discontinuance of smoking; control blood pressure; maintain low cholesterol levels; healthy diet (low in saturated fat, low amounts of junk food); regular exercise program; medical checkup

Chapter 13 Reducing the Risk for Chronic Disease

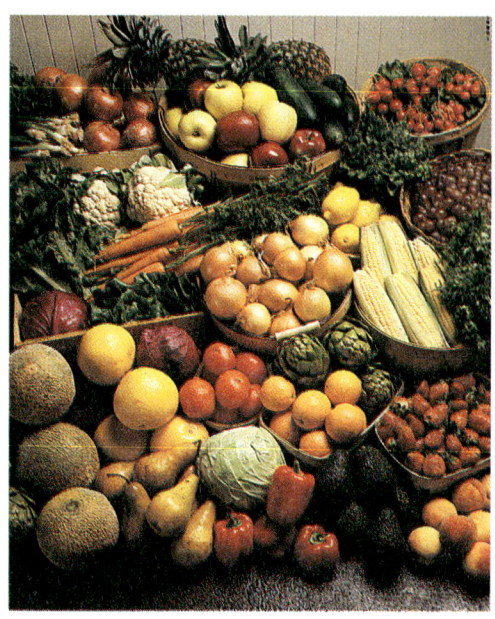

Eating a healthy diet is an important factor in preventing chronic diseases such as heart disease and some cancers. (Source: FPG International/© Ralph Pleasant)

Other factors contribute to the occurrence of chronic disease: not taking advantage of available health screening techniques, such as mammography to detect breast cancer and sigmoidoscopy to detect colon cancer, or not taking medication for hypertension. Genetic predisposition, gender, and advancing age are recognized factors that contribute to chronic and degenerative diseases over which you have little control.

Given the current state of knowledge about chronic diseases, it is important to control the modifiable factors about which you are aware, monitor those you cannot avoid, and take steps to minimize the negative health impact of all lifestyle choices. Although prevention does not guarantee that you will not develop a chronic disease, it could improve your odds in favor of better health.

Chronic diseases are far too numerous to provide complete information about each one in this chapter. Table 13.1 provides a brief overview of the common chronic diseases. The remainder of this chapter focuses on two of the most common and most life-threatening chronic diseases, heart disease and cancer, as well as on one of the least life-threatening yet most common chronic health problems, dental disease.

From the Heart: Cardiovascular Diseases

Diseases of the heart and blood vessels—collectively called **cardiovascular diseases**—are the leading cause of death in the United States. They claim the lives of 42 percent of the 2.3 million Americans who die every year. To illustrate how great a toll cardiovascular diseases take, the National Center for Health Statistics estimates that if all forms of cardiovascular disease were eliminated, life expectancy would rise by almost ten years. If all forms of cancer were eliminated, in contrast, the gain would be three years.

Heart Disease Facts

Heart disease remains the number-one killer despite the fact that over the past twenty years, the death rate from cardiovascular disease has declined dramati-

cardiovascular disease Disease of the heart and blood vessels.

hypertension High blood pressure; generally means the heart is working harder than normal.

cally—by more than 46 percent for all cardiovascular diseases, 51 percent for coronary heart disease, and more than 60 percent for stroke. This decline is due in great part to better surgical techniques, improved drugs, more effective medical management, and a better understanding of the risk factors for heart disease.

The picture is not as bright for African Americans. Although the number of fatalities from heart attacks for African Americans has dropped over the years, too, there are significant disparities between African Americans and whites. Heart attack death rates are nearly 5 percent higher for African American males than for white males and more than 30 percent higher for African American females than for white females. Researchers at the National Center for Health Statistics gave three possible explanations for this:

- Whites have more consistently reduced their risks for heart diseases than have African Americans. Whites are more likely to quit smoking and to change their diets to include low-fat and low-cholesterol food.
- African Americans have a higher prevalence of **hypertension,** or high blood pressure, than whites, and high blood pressure is one of the risk factors for heart disease.
- The health gap between African Americans and whites reflects the fact that a greater proportion of African Americans are poor and live in areas where health care is less than adequate.

Even though women report that the health risk they are most concerned about is breast cancer, far more women die of heart disease than of breast cancer (see Figure 13.2). Of 2,000 postmenopausal women in a year, 20 get heart disease and 12 die of it, whereas 6 develop breast cancer and 2 die of it. Overall, heart disease is the leading killer of women over age forty. Women typically lag ten years behind men in developing heart disease because of protection offered by the female hormone estrogen. Estrogen production, however, drops significantly after menopause.

Recent research findings document the relationship between estrogen and heart disease:

- Premenopausal women rarely have a heart attack.
- Women who have a hysterectomy (surgical removal of the uterus and sometimes the ovaries) before natural menopause have an increased risk for cardiovascular disease.

HealthLinks
American
Heart Association
www.amhrt.org
The leading private organization dedicated to heart health, providing press releases, statistical data, and resources regarding cardiovascular care.

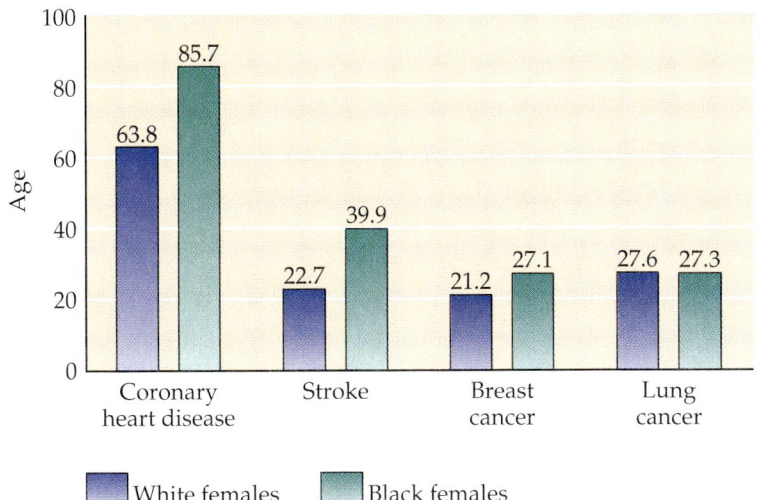

■ **Figure 13.2 Age-Adjusted Death Rates of Leading Killers of Women.** *Even though they are more concerned about dying of breast cancer, far more women die of heart disease. (Source: National Center for Health Statistics and the American Heart Association. Reproduced with permission of the American Heart Association from 1997 Heart and Stroke Fact Statistical Update, 1996. Copyright American Heart Association)*

- Women who take replacement estrogen after menopause have less coronary disease than do women who do not take estrogen.

Critical Thinking Question

The *Healthy People 2000* objectives include the following: "Increase to at least 60 percent the proportion of adults with high blood cholesterol who are aware of their condition and are taking action to reduce their blood cholesterol to recommended levels." In 1992, the proportion was 44 percent. The relationship between high cholesterol and cardiovascular disease is well established, yet most Americans don't even know their blood cholesterol level. How might this situation be changed? Do you think the entire U.S. population should be required to take a cholesterol screening? Would such an extensive program be cost-effective?

Who Is at Risk?

The major risk factors associated with cardiovascular disease are related to lifestyle and include smoking, hypertension, elevated cholesterol, elevated iron in the blood, overweight, adult-onset diabetes, and sedentary lifestyle. Non-lifestyle risk factors for cardiovascular disease include family history of the disease, age, and sex.

Smoking is the single most important risk factor associated with heart disease. Cigarette smokers have a 70 percent greater risk of dying of heart disease than do nonsmokers. Moreover, smoking is estimated to account for more than 20 percent of all coronary heart disease deaths and 40 percent of such deaths in people under age sixty-five. Smoking cessation, however, can substantially reduce this death rate, even only two years after quitting. Quitting can also significantly reduce the risk for stroke.

Data from the Framingham Heart Study—the longest ongoing study in the United States of heart disease—show that people who have high blood pressure have three to four times the risk for developing coronary heart disease and as much as seven times the risk for a stroke as do those who have normal blood pressure. Obesity is a risk factor by itself, but it also contributes to high blood pressure levels. A 10 percent weight loss in an overweight, hypertensive person can significantly reduce his or her blood pressure. Obesity also contributes to adult-onset diabetes, which in turn is a risk factor for heart disease because it may speed the rate at which fat is deposited on the artery wall, thus clogging the flow of blood to the heart.

The Framingham Study has also found that the incidence of heart disease increases as blood cholesterol levels rise and drops as blood cholesterol levels fall. People who received a cholesterol-lowering diet and medication reduced their cholesterol levels by 9 percent and had a 19 percent lower incidence of heart disease than did those not on the diet or receiving medication.

Sedentary lifestyle is another major contributor to heart disease, and recent data from the CDC show that people who are not physically active are twice as likely as physically active people to die of coronary heart disease. Much has been written about athletes who drop dead from heart disease while competing, but it is important to note that healthy people usually do not die while exercising. The athletes in the news tend to have either serious heart defects (which are usually present from birth) or advanced but undetected coronary artery disease.

Diagnosing Heart Disease

Heart disease is diagnosed in two ways: screening and detection. **Screening** for heart disease involves an analysis of risk factors associated with the disease. Such procedures are done on individuals assumed to be healthy. Although screening tests do not provide absolute proof of the existence of an abnormal heart condition, so much is known about the relationship of specific risk factors to the incidence of heart disease that by identifying them early, a physician can prescribe the appropriate behavior change—for example, stop smoking, adjust your diet, or begin blood pressure medication. Should a screening test or a combination of apparent risk factors raise suspicion of the existence of heart disease, a physician is more likely to detect heart disease at a very early stage.

Detection of heart disease is done on individuals suspected of having some form of cardiovascular abnormality. In many cases, detection involves the same procedure as screening; the difference is mainly in the physician's purpose.

An **electrocardiogram (ECG)** is used for both screening for and detecting heart disease. To perform an ECG, a medical technician attaches electrodes to the body. As the heart beats, these electrodes transmit the electrical impulses that cause the heart to contract to a device that records them. After a series of impulses is recorded, a trained technician or physician interprets the ECG and can identify any abnormalities.

An ECG is the principal test for screening asymptomatic individuals, those who have yet to experience chest pains or have a heart attack. The American Heart Association recommends that a baseline ECG be taken at age twenty, again at age forty to forty-five, and then only as suggested by other risk factors. An ECG can also detect heart disease at an early stage. When used for detecting heart disease, an ECG should not be the only diagnostic tool used.

Some people, in addition, undergo a **stress electrocardiogram (ECG),** also known as a maximal exercise tolerance or treadmill test because a treadmill is used to produce an elevated heart rate. Reliable testing protocols have also been developed using walking, running, a stationary bicycle, or going up and down steps. The stress ECG might be compared with a high-speed road test of a car. The results reveal how the heart performs under pressure—more precisely, under high-intensity exercise. A stress ECG is a better diagnostic procedure than a resting ECG. It is also an effective means of determining fitness level.

Stress tests are recommended for people who have a history of cardiac risk factors and for sedentary individuals who wish to begin an exercise program. This is because strenuous exercise may result in severe heart problems and even death for at-risk persons. Stress tests are also required in certain occupations that involve unusual endurance and strength and affect public safety, such as police work and fire fighting.

Forms of Heart Diseases

The term *cardiovascular disease* actually refers to many diseases. Some are directly related to the heart; others are related to the circulatory system, including veins and arteries. **Atherosclerosis,** the most common form of hardening of the arteries (also called arteriosclerosis), is the single biggest cause of heart and blood vessel disease. It is a slow, progressive disease that may start in early life. Atherosclerosis is characterized by thick deposits of fatty substances (plaque) such as cholesterol on the inner walls of the arteries. As a result of these deposits, the

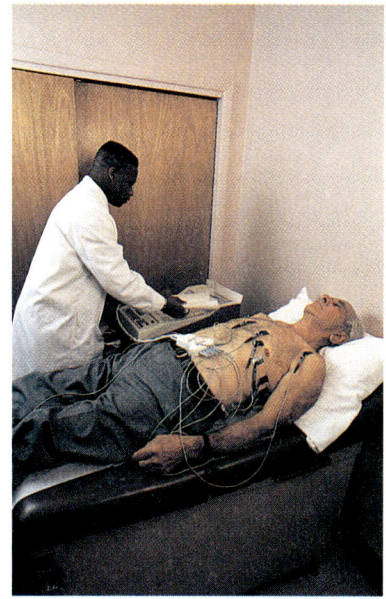

An electrocardiogram (ECG) can detect abnormalities in the heart at an early stage of disease. You should have a baseline ECG at age 20 and again at age 40 to 45. (Source: FPG International/© Terry Qing)

screening Analysis of risk factors done on a person thought to be well for the purpose of preventing disease or making an early diagnosis.

electrocardiogram (ECG) A screening procedure used to detect heart disease; a graphic record of the heart's action obtained from an instrument that records heart activity.

stress electrocardiogram (ECG) A maximal exercise tolerance test using a treadmill to produce an elevated heart rate in order to reveal how the heart performs under pressure and high-intensity exercise.

atherosclerosis A thickening and loss of elasticity of the inner walls of the arteries.

internal channels of the arteries become narrow, and blood moves through them with great difficulty. This makes it easier for a clot to form, which can block the artery and thus deprive the heart, brain, or other organs of blood.

Heart attack (myocardial infarction), the number-one killer in the nation (about five hundred thousand deaths a year), usually results from atherosclerosis. Heart attacks are fatal for about 36 percent of the people who have them, so there are far more people who have had a heart attack and lived to tell the story than there are people who have died of them. However, those who survive a heart attack are at a significantly increased risk of having a second heart attack and of developing angina and other heart-related conditions.

People have heart attacks when the heart does not get enough oxygen. A heart attack is also called a *myocardial infarction.* (*Myocardium* is the heart muscle; *infarction* is death from lack of oxygen.) Although a heart attack appears to be sudden, it is usually the result of long-standing conditions that gradually deprive the heart of the oxygen it needs. When blood flow to an area of the heart muscle stops or is insufficient because of a blockage in the arteries, a heart attack occurs.

With the blood supply blocked, cells in the heart muscle die and the muscle cannot function properly. Victims typically feel a crushing chest pain or a tingling sensation down the left arm or left side of the face. The American Heart Association lists the following as warning signals of heart attack:

- Uncomfortable pressure, fullness, squeezing, or pain in the center of the chest lasting more than two minutes
- Pain spreading to the shoulders, neck, or arms
- Severe pain, lightheadedness, fainting, sweating, nausea, or shortness of breath

A person can have a heart attack without having all of these symptoms.

Angina pectoris, a condition that results in a temporary reduction in the blood supply to the heart, can cause feelings of discomfort similar to but not as strong as those of a heart attack. Although an angina attack is not a heart attack, its symptoms should be taken seriously because they could be a forewarning of other heart problems. An angina attack usually takes place during physical activity or periods of emotional upset. Nitroglycerin or some other medication can prevent or reduce the pain of angina.

Arrhythmia is an erratic beating of the heart that can cause a heart attack. Nearly everyone experiences an occasional skip of a heartbeat due to too much excitement, too much caffeine, or for no reason at all. There is nothing dangerous about this. Arrhythmia becomes life threatening when a chain of beats is missed so that the heart muscle does not contract effectively. As a result of this, the brain does not get enough oxygen-containing blood and the victim loses consciousness and can go into cardiac arrest and die. Arrhythmias may be caused by a damaged heart muscle or by extreme emotional distress. Common forms of arrhythmia include **tachycardia** (excessively rapid heart rate), **bradycardia** (abnormally slow heart rate), and **fibrillation** (irregular, convulsive movements of the heart muscle resulting in a failure to pump blood).

Stroke, also called a cerebrovascular accident (CVA), is the third leading cause of death in the country. Each year, about one hundred and fifty thousand people die of stroke. It is also a major cause of morbidity, with about five hundred thousand Americans suffering nonfatal strokes each year. A stroke results when the supply of blood pumped by the heart to the brain is cut off or when bleeding occurs in the brain. When the damage takes place in the right side of the brain, sensory and motor function is lost on the left side of the body. This is known as left **hemiplegia.** When the damage occurs on the left side of the brain,

heart attack (myocardial infarction) A condition that occurs when the blood supply to part of the heart muscle (the myocardium) is severely reduced or stopped. Normally circulating blood brings oxygen and other nutrients to the heart.

angina pectoris Chest pain; a symptom of a condition in which the heart does not get as much blood as it needs.

arrhythmia An erratic heartbeat.

tachycardia Excessively rapid beating of the heart.

bradycardia Abnormally slow beating of the heart.

fibrillation Irregular convulsive movement of the heart muscle.

stroke A clot or break in a blood vessel in the brain that disrupts blood flow to the brain.

hemiplegia The loss of sensory and motor function on one side of the body.

transient ischemic attack (TIA) A stroke that causes minimal damage but signals the possibility of a more severe stroke.

systolic pressure The pressure measured in the arteries when the heart contracts.

diastolic pressure The pressure measured in the arteries when the heart relaxes.

loss of function occurs on the right side of the body, affecting communication skills, including speaking, writing, reading, and listening. This condition is known as right hemiplegia.

Transient ischemic attacks (TIAs) are little strokes that cause minimal damage but are warning signals of a possibly more severe stroke. Men are more likely to suffer all kinds of strokes than are women and African Americans are more likely to suffer strokes than are whites. Women who take oral contraceptives are more at risk for stroke than are those who do not. The risk for stroke increases with age for both sexes.

Often, the body gives warning signals of an impending stroke. The following are warning signals for stroke, according to the American Heart Association:

- A sudden, temporary weakness, clumsiness, or numbness of the face, arm, or leg
- Temporary difficulty with or loss of speech or trouble understanding speech
- Sudden, temporary dimness or loss of vision, particularly in one eye, or an episode of double vision
- Unexplained headaches
- Temporary dizziness, unsteadiness, staggering, or difficulty walking
- A recent change in personality or mental ability

Hypertension (high blood pressure) is called the silent killer because it has few symptoms but affects about 50 million Americans and can lead to heart attack, stroke, and heart and kidney failure. High blood pressure adds to the workload of the heart and arteries and can cause them not to function as well as they should. Approximately 25 percent of adults have high blood pressure, defined as blood pressure greater than a **systolic pressure** of 140 or a **diastolic pressure** of 90. This is written as 140/90, and is referred to as 140 over 90. Systolic pressure represents a contraction of the heart muscle; diastolic pressure represents a relaxation of the heart muscle. Normal blood pressure is about 120/80 for young adults.

Hypertension occurs more frequently after age thirty-five and among African Americans more often than among whites. It is associated with obesity, high-sodium diets, and other controllable risk factors, but by far the most important factor predicting hypertension is genetic predisposition. If one of your parents has or had hypertension, you have a 50 percent chance of having it too. This risk rises to 90 percent if both parents are or were affected. Blood pressure can be lowered successfully through salt restriction, weight control, and exercise. If these treatments fail to lower blood pressure, medication is indicated.

Repairing the Heart

From $50 for a good pair of walking shoes to $50,000 for a coronary artery bypass to more than $250,000 for a heart transplant, there are many ways to prevent and treat heart disease. Regular aerobic exercise, the kind that raises the heart rate and is done for 20 minutes three or more times a week, can help prevent and correct high blood pressure. As little as a five- to ten-pound weight loss can also help decrease blood volume and the amount of blood pumped by the heart, which in turn reduces pressure in the arteries.

Medications have proven successful in lowering blood pressure, stabilizing mild to moderate heartbeat irregularities, relieving angina, raising cardiac output, and lowering the heart's demand for blood. Some of these drugs can reduce heart attack deaths by more than 25 percent if administered within the first few hours after the onset of heart attack symptoms and can cost up to $2,000 per dose.

Far cheaper is common aspirin. Extensive tests on more than twenty-two thousand male physicians over age forty show that healthy men can cut their risk

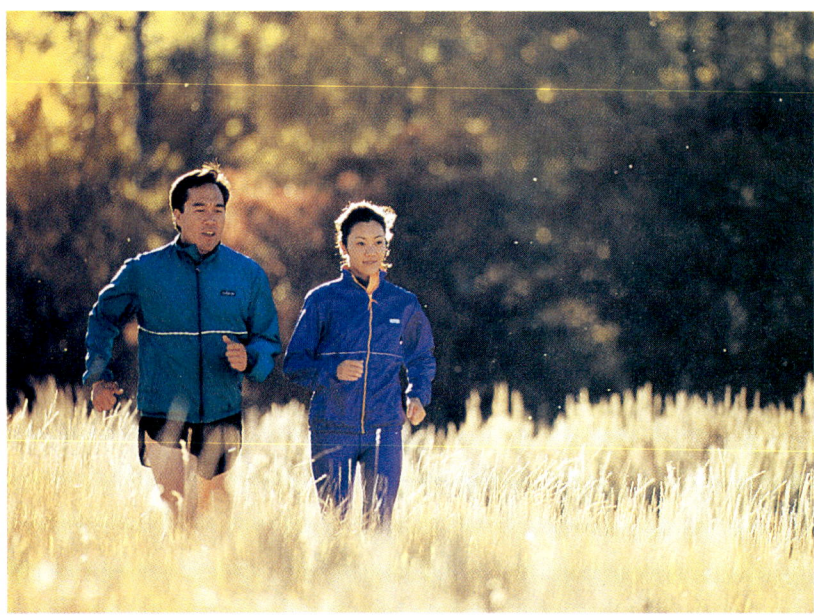

Exercise is a good way to maintain a healthy heart. It is also cost-effective: You can buy a good pair of walking shoes for $50; a heart transplant costs more than $250,000. (Source: © Tony Stone Images/Lori Adamski Peek)

of a heart attack nearly in half by taking one aspirin every other day. Recent studies on female nurses suggest similar results. Aspirin can also significantly reduce second heart attacks. The medical community has not totally adopted this preventive concept, however, because aspirin is not without risk.

Drugs usually have side effects, and heart drugs are no different. Some side effects of heart drugs include fatigue, nausea, impotence in men, and depression. Even aspirin can cause nausea and internal bleeding when taken on a regular basis. If medications are successful in reducing the cardiac problem, however, more risky surgery can be avoided.

A low-cost lifesaving technique for heart attack victims is **cardiopulmonary resuscitation (CPR).** CPR, which involves rescue breathing (mouth-to-mouth resuscitation) alternating with pressure applied to the chest, is a basic life skill that is used in emergency situations. It has been estimated that if one of every three Americans were trained in CPR, more than one hundred thousand lives a year could be saved.

For people who have severely clogged arteries, surgical options (see Figure 13.3) include **coronary angioplasty,** in which the coronary artery is widened with an inflated balloon catheter; **coronary artery bypass,** in which the blood flow is rerouted from the blocked part of the artery using a length of vein taken from another part of the body; and a **heart transplant,** in which a normally functioning heart from a person who has recently died is implanted in place of the diseased one. Each of these procedures has limited success, but collectively, they have improved the quality of life and in many cases have extended the lives of millions of heart patients.

Artificial hearts have been used to extend the life of otherwise terminal patients until transplant donors can be found. The artificial heart gets its power to operate from a source outside the body, so it is not an effective long-term replacement for the original organ. Even with incredible advances such as an artificial heart, the best advice is to take care of the organs you have and not count on medicine to provide replacement parts when they malfunction.

cardiopulmonary resuscitation (CPR) A combination of mouth-to-mouth breathing and chest compression used during cardiac arrest to keep blood flowing to the heart muscle and brain; an emergency procedure.

coronary angioplasty A surgical procedure to widen the coronary artery with an inflated balloon catheter.

coronary artery bypass A surgical procedure to reroute blood flow from the blocked part of an artery by using a length of vein taken from another part of the body.

heart transplant A surgical procedure in which a normally functioning heart from a person who has recently died is implanted into a person with a diseased heart.

Getting Help for Mental Health Problems | **329**

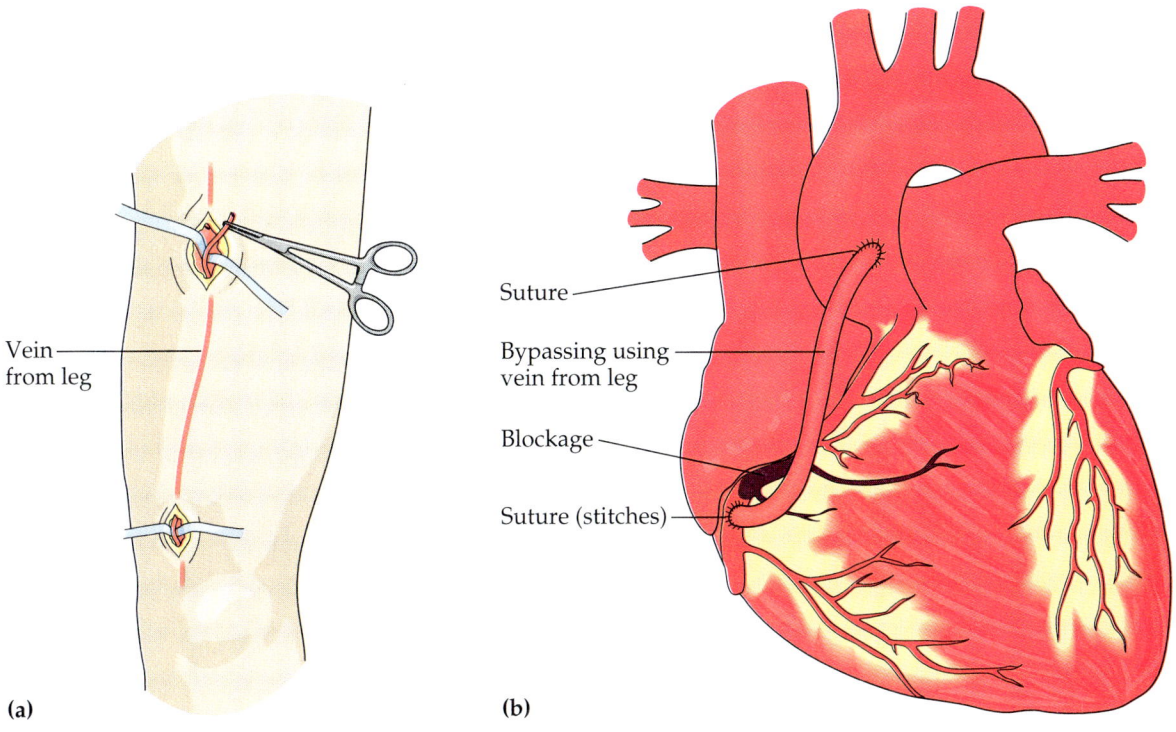

In a coronary artery bypass, the blood flow to the heart is rerouted from the blocked part of the artery using a length of vein taken from another part of the body. In effect, it bypasses the clogged area.

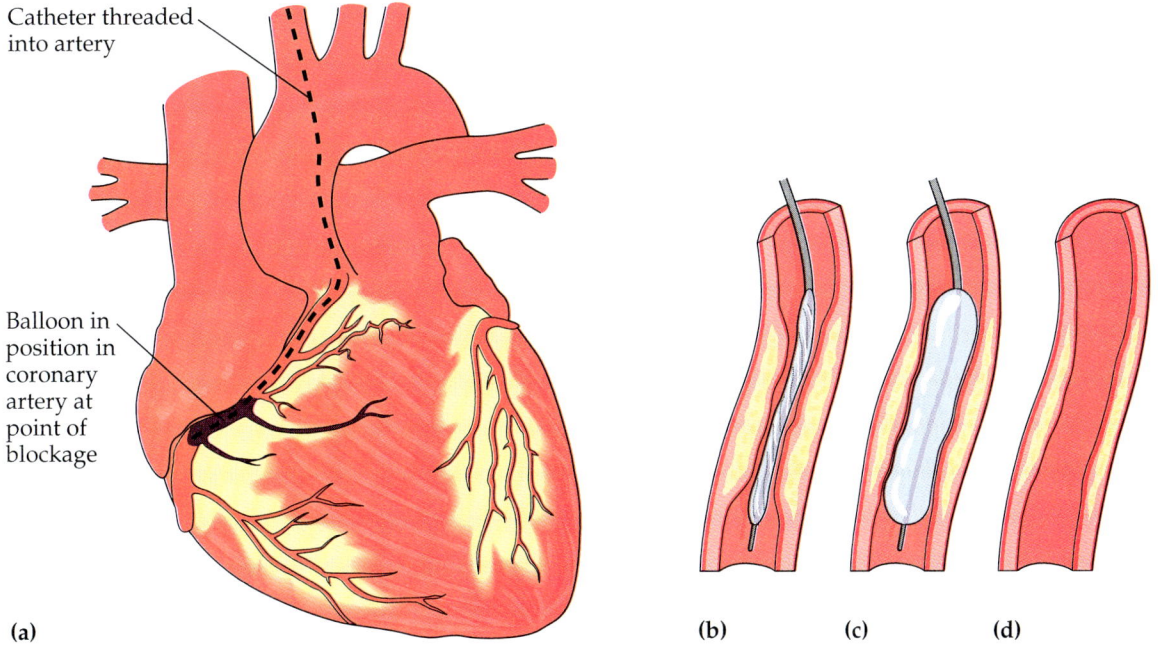

Coronary angioplasty involves widening the coronary artery with an inflated balloon catheter. It is one way to help people with severely clogged coronary arteries survive.

Figure 13.3 *Coronary Artery Bypass (top) and Coronary Angioplasty (bottom)*

The Big C: Cancer

One of the most feared of all diseases, cancer, strikes people of all ages—in childhood, adolescence, the prime of life, and old age. Cancer is the second leading cause of death in the United States. It accounts for about one of every four deaths from all causes in the United States, and it kills more children than any other disease. It is estimated that 1,382,000 Americans were diagnosed with cancer in 1997 and approximately 560,000 died of cancer that year. Because of exposure to **carcinogens** (cancer-causing substances) in the environment, the longer a person lives, the greater the chance of developing cancer.

In time, 30 percent of Americans now living will develop cancer, and it will affect approximately three out of four families. This is not encouraging news. Some people are so fearful of cancer that they put off having routine examinations so they do not have to be confronted with a diagnosis of cancer. Ironically, early detection could save them from the ravages of the disease.

Over the past thirty-five years, the incidence of cancer in the population has increased, mainly because of increases in lung cancer (see Table 13.2). To illustrate this point, lung cancer recently replaced breast cancer as the leading cause of cancer death among women. Overall, there has been a more rapid increase in the incidence of cancer among men than among women and among African Americans than among whites. At the same time, pockets of decrease in the incidence of cancer have occurred, particularly in cancer of the cervix, testicle, and stomach and in Hodgkin's disease. Because of improvements in early detection and treatment, the five-year survival rates are in the 90 percent range for many types of cancers that have not spread.

The good news is that perhaps 50 percent or more of cancer incidence can be prevented through smoking cessation and changed dietary habits. By not smoking and by eating carefully, including less fat and more fruits and vegetables, you can greatly reduce your risk of acquiring this often-deadly disease.

The Basics of Cancer

Cancer is not actually one disease. It is a group of more than 100 diseases, all characterized by uncontrolled growth and spread of abnormal cells. Normally, cells reproduce in an orderly manner following the genetic rules of growth. But some cells become abnormal and fail to follow these rules. They continue to divide and grow and eventually band together into **tumors,** or masses of tissue.

Not all tumors are cancerous. In fact, most are **benign,** or harmless. Benign tumors do not invade other cells or spread to other parts of the body. They are different from cancerous tumors in their very structure, and they cannot change into cancerous tumors. Benign tumors, however, can cause problems if they block some crucial part of the body and prevent it from functioning.

Only **malignant** tumors are cancerous. If left untreated, malignant tumors spread into nearby tissues and organs, crowding out healthy cells and replacing them with cancer cells. The most dangerous characteristic of malignant tumors is that they **metastasize,** or spread to other parts of the body through the bloodstream or lymph system. In this way, a single cancer cell can spread the disease throughout the entire body.

No one knows exactly what causes a normal cell to become a cancer cell. Scientists believe that most cancers develop through repeated or long-term contact with cancer-causing agents. There are two basic kinds of carcinogens: **initiators** and **promoters.** Initiators start the cell damage that can lead to cancer. Examples of initiators are cigarette smoking, X rays, and certain chemicals. Promoters do not actually cause cancers, but they help them to grow. Alcohol, for example, promotes mouth, throat, and possibly liver cancer when combined with an initiator such as tobacco.

carcinogen A cancer-causing agent or factor.

tumor A mass of tissue that accumulates in the body.

benign tumor A tumor that is usually harmless and does not invade other cells or spread to other parts of the body.

malignant tumor A cancerous tumor that spreads to nearby tissues and organs, crowding out healthy cells and replacing them with cancer cells.

metastasize To spread to other parts of the body through the bloodstream or lymph system.

initiator A carcinogen that starts cell damage that leads to cancer.

promoter A carcinogen that helps cancer to grow.

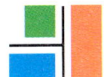

TABLE 13.2 Twenty-Year Trends in Cancer Death Rates* (per 100,000 Population)

Sites	Sex	Rates in 1971–1973	Rates in 1991–1993	Percent changes
All sites	Male	204.5	219.0	7%
	Female	132.0	142.0	8%
Brain	Male	4.7	5.1	9%
	Female	3.2	3.5	9%
Breast	Male	0.3	0.2	-33%
	Female	26.8	26.4	-1%
Cervix	Female	5.6	2.9	-48%
Colon and rectum	Male	25.3	22.3	-12%
	Female	20.0	15.1	-25%
Corpus uteri	Female	4.7	3.4	-28%
Esophagus	Male	5.0	6.2	24%
	Female	1.4	1.5	7%
Hodgkin's disease	Male	1.9	0.7	-63%
	Female	1.1	0.4	-64%
Kidney	Male	4.3	5.1	19%
	Female	1.9	2.3	21%
Larynx	Male	2.8	2.5	-11%
	Female	0.3	0.5	67%
Leukemia	Male	8.9	8.4	-6%
	Female	5.3	4.9	-8%
Liver	Male	3.4	4.6	35%
	Female	1.8	2.1	17%
Lung	Male	61.3	73.5	20%
	Female	12.7	32.9	159%
Melanoma	Male	2.0	3.2	60%
	Female	1.3	1.5	15%
Multiple myeloma	Male	2.8	3.8	36%
	Female	1.9	2.6	37%
Non-Hodgkin's lymphoma	Male	5.8	8.1	40%
	Female	3.9	5.3	36%
Oral cavity	Male	5.9	4.4	-25%
	Female	1.9	1.6	-16%
Ovary	Female	8.6	7.8	-9%
Pancreas	Male	11.1	10.0	-10%
	Female	6.7	7.3	9%
Prostate	Male	21.4	26.8	25%
Stomach	Male	10.4	6.6	-37%
	Female	5.0	3.0	-40%
Testis	Male	0.7	0.2	-71%
Thyroid	Male	0.4	0.3	-25%
	Female	0.5	0.4	-20%
Urinary bladder	Male	7.2	5.7	-21%
	Female	2.2	1.7	-23%

*Adjusted to the age distribution of the 1970 U.S. census population.

Note: Even though death rates declined or remained stable, the number of deaths increased because the population over 65 has become larger and older. The U.S. population increased 22% from 1973 to 1993. American Cancer Society Surveillance Research, 1997.
Data source: Vital Statistics of the United States, 1993

Source: Reprinted by the permission of the American Cancer Society, Inc., Cancer Facts and Figures 1997)

HealthLinks
National Cancer Institute
www.nci.nih.gov

Link up with this federal agency dedicated to cancer research for the latest in cancer findings and recommendations

Who Is at Risk?

Although the basic causes of cancer are unknown, scientists have discovered several conditions often connected with abnormal cell growth. In some—but not all—cases, you can do something to reduce your risk for getting cancer.

The single behavior that most often results in death from cancer is smoking. People who smoke two or more packs of cigarettes a day are fifteen to twenty-five times more likely to die of cancer than are nonsmokers. Put another way, cigarette smoking accounts for 87 percent of lung cancer deaths and 29 percent of all cancer deaths. It also increases the risk for developing other cancers, particularly those of the mouth, pharynx, larynx, esophagus, pancreas, and bladder. Studies also show that cancer can be caused by passive smoking in healthy nonsmokers, by smokeless tobacco, and by the tar produced by smoking marijuana.

Repeated exposure to sunlight over a long period of time is a major cause of skin cancer. The sun's ultraviolet rays harm the skin. Fair-skinned people have less of a pigment called **melanin** in their skin to block some of the sun's damaging rays, and they are at greater risk of getting skin cancer than are dark-skinned people. The amount of time spent in the sun or in a tanning booth determines the extent of damage.

Large doses of X rays or ionizing radiation can cause cancer, depending on both the dose and the duration of exposure. The most common sources of ionizing radiation for medical reasons are diagnostic procedures and radiation therapy. Medical equipment is now designed to deliver the lowest possible dose without sacrificing the beneficial effects. Most of the information about the effects of radiation comes from studies of survivors of the atomic bombs dropped in Japan in 1945. The studies show increased rates among survivors of several types of cancer, including breast, thyroid, lung, and stomach cancer and acute leukemia.

Excessive amounts of alcohol are linked to a number of cancers. Heavy drinking is associated with cancers of the mouth, throat, esophagus, and liver. The cancer risks of alcohol are increased even more in drinkers who also smoke cigarettes.

Foods are linked to the risk of certain cancers, both positively and negatively. On the down side, cancers of the esophagus and stomach are common where large quantities of smoked, salt-cured, and nitrite-cured foods are eaten. Salami, bologna, and ham are examples of these foods. A high-fat diet not only is full of calories but also increases your risk for developing breast, colon, and prostate cancer. On the protective side, foods high in fiber—whole grain breads, rice, broccoli, carrots, apples—appear to dilute intestinal contents and reduce the amount of time carcinogens spend in the intestine. A high-fiber diet may reduce your risk for developing colon cancer. Vitamin A protects against cancers of the esophagus, larynx, and lung, and vitamin C protects against cancer of the esophagus and stomach. Fresh fruits and vegetables are good sources of both of these vitamins.

Many occupations expose workers to toxic fumes, gases, airborne particles, and liquids. Occupational carcinogens include asbestos, vinyl chloride, formaldehyde, and arsenic. In addition to the worker being at risk, his or her family may also be in jeopardy. Exposed workers significantly multiply their risks if they smoke.

Certain families are no doubt cancer-prone, and up to 10 percent of all cancers may be hereditary. Specific examples of genetically linked cancers are retinoblastoma (an eye cancer that causes blindness) and familial polyps of the colon (which lead to colon cancer). In addition, two genes were found recently to play a role in breast cancer. If a woman has both genes, which are known as BRCA1 and BRCA2, she has a lifetime risk of 56 percent for developing breast cancer, regardless of family history. A woman is also at increased risk for getting

melanin Brownish-black skin pigment.

breast cancer if her mother, aunts, sisters, or other close female relatives have had the disease. Overall, familial breast cancer accounts for about 5 percent to 10 percent of all breast cancers.

Recent research has shown that certain viruses cause cancer in laboratory animals and that they also may cause several types of cancer in humans. These include leukemias, lymphomas, and cancers of the cervix and liver. In addition, the acquired immune deficiency syndrome (AIDS) has been linked to a type of cancer known as Kaposi's sarcoma and to certain lymphomas and leukemias. AIDS is caused by HIV.

Types of Cancer

Cancer comes in many shapes and forms. It can affect your lungs or your limbs. It can affect your bones or your skin. All of the body's tissues and organs are susceptible to cancer (see Table 13.3). The following descriptions of several common cancers include statistics on incidence, risk factors, symptoms, and survival rates.

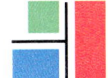

TABLE 13.3 Where Cancer Strikes

Leading Sites of New Cancer Cases and Deaths—1997 Estimates*

Cancer Cases by Site and Sex		Cancer Deaths by Site and Sex	
Male	**Female**	**Male**	**Female**
Prostate 334,500	Breast 180,200	Lung 94,400	Lung 66,000
Lung 98,300	Lung 79,800	Prostate 41,800	Breast 43,900
Colon & rectum 66,400	Colon & rectum 64,800	Colon & rectum 27,000	Colon & rectum 27,900
Urinary bladder 39,500	Corpus uteri 34,900	Pancreas 13,500	Pancreas 14,600
Non-Hodgkin's lymphoma 30,300	Ovary 26,800	Non-Hodgkin's lymphoma 12,400	Ovary 14,200
Melanoma of the skin 22,900	Non-Hodgkin's lymphoma 23,300	Leukemia 11,770	Non-Hodgkin's lymphoma 11,400
Oral cavity 20,900	Melanoma of the skin 17,400	Esophagus 8,700	Leukemia 9,540
Kidney 17,100	Urinary bladder 15,000	Stomach 8,300	Corpus uteri 6,000
Leukemia 15,900	Cervix 14,500	Urinary bladder 7,800	Brain 6,000
Stomach 14,000	Pancreas 14,200	Liver 7,500	Stomach 5,700
All sites 785,800	All sites 596,600	All sites 294,100	All sites 265,900

*Excluding basal and squamous cell skin cancer and in situ carcinomas except bladder. American Cancer Society Surveillance Research, 1997.

Source: Reprinted by the permission of the American Cancer Society, Inc., from Cancer Facts and Figures 1997

LUNG CANCER Lung cancer is the number-one cause of cancer death. Each year, an estimated 178,000 new cases are diagnosed and some 160,000 people die of it. In recent years, the incidence of lung cancer in men has been declining, but it is rising in women. The main risk factors for lung cancer are cigarette smoking, sidestream smoking, and occupational exposures to asbestos and other agents.

Symptoms include excessive coughing, chest pain, shortness of breath, chronic bronchitis, sputum containing blood, and difficulty in swallowing. Early detection may be difficult because these symptoms do not usually appear until the disease is at an advanced stage and has metastasized or spread.

The outlook for lung cancer patients is bleak: Most die within a year, and only 14 percent survive for five years after diagnosis.

BREAST CANCER Breast cancer is the second-leading cause of death from cancer for women (after lung cancer), killing about forty-four thousand women a year. The incidence of breast cancer increased about 4 percent a year between 1982 and 1987 and has recently leveled off. The increase is due in great part to screening programs that can detect tumors before they become clinically apparent. It is estimated that about one in eight women will develop breast cancer in their lifetimes. (A small percentage of men get breast cancer, and about three hundred males a year die from it.)

The main risk factors for women are being over age fifty, a family history of breast cancer, never being pregnant or having a first pregnancy after age thirty and estrogen therapy. (Estrogen is often taken by postmenopausal women to treat discomforts sometimes associated with the cessation of menstruation. Studies suggest that it can protect against heart disease and osteoporosis but that it can promote the growth of existing breast cancer and contribute to cancer of the uterus.)

Symptoms of breast cancer include a lump, thickening or swelling of the breast, discharge from the nipple, or retraction of the nipple. Early detection by breast self-examination or mammography can significantly increase survival rates.

When the disease is localized at the time of diagnosis, five-year survival rates are as high as 97 percent. If the cancer has spread regionally to adjacent lymph nodes, survival rates drop to 76 percent, and for distant metastases, to 20 percent.

PROSTATE CANCER Prostate cancer is the second-most-common cause of cancer death in men (after lung cancer). The prostate is a small gland that surrounds the urethra and produces much of the liquid in semen. Each year, nearly 350,000 new cases are diagnosed, and about 42,000 men die of it. Approximately one in five men will develop prostate cancer. Risk factors are being over age fifty, workplace exposures to cadmium and other carcinogens, and a high-fat diet. The rate of prostate cancer in African American men is 32 percent higher than in whites. African American men also develop the disease about three years earlier than do whites. The increased incidence is thought to be due to lifestyle rather than to genetics, because this high rate developed in African Americans only in recent decades.

Symptoms include problems with urination, blood in the urine, and persistent pain in the back, hips, and pelvis. Prostate cancer grows slowly and in the early stages, there are often no symptoms. Early detection can increase survival rates.

The outlook is excellent when the disease is confined within the prostate. These men are just as likely to be alive fifteen years later as men in the general population. If the disease is still localized, the five-year survival rate is 87 percent.

COLON AND RECTUM (COLORECTAL) CANCERS Colon and rectum (colorectal) cancers have declined in recent years, probably because of increased sigmoidoscopic screening and polyp removal (which helps prevent progression of polyps to invasive cancers). This decline is seen largely among whites; the incidence rates for African Americans have stabilized but have not yet begun to decline. The colon is the last five or six feet of the digestive tract. Each year, there are about ninety-four thousand new cases of colon cancer and thirty-seven thousand new cases of rectal cancer, and about forty-six thousand and eight thousand deaths, respectively. Major risk factors are being over age forty, family history of polyps of the colon, inflammatory bowel disease and a high-fat diet.

Symptoms include rectal bleeding, blood in the stool, change in bowel habits (constipation or diarrhea), and general abdominal discomfort. When colorectal cancer is detected at an early localized stage, the five-year survival rate is 91 percent. However, only about one third of cases are discovered at this stage. After it has spread regionally to adjacent organs or lymph nodes, survival rates drop to 63 percent and to 7 percent if the disease, has spread to distant parts of the body.

SKIN CANCER Skin cancer falls into two broad classes: **basal cell** and **squamous cell** cancers, which are more common and highly curable, and **melanomas**, which are relatively rare but more serious. The epidermis, or outer layer of the skin, contains both basal and squamous cells. Basal cells are small, round cells found in the lower part, or base, of the epidermis; squamous cells are flat cells that look like fish scales and make up most of the epidermis. More than nine hundred thousand cases of basal and squamous cell cancers are diagnosed each year. Most are discovered so early and are so readily cured that only about twenty-two hundred people die from basal or squamous cell cancers.

Melanomas, in contrast, are far more fatal. Each year, more than forty thousand new cases are diagnosed and some seventy-three hundred people die of melanoma. The incidence of melanoma is increasing at the rate of 4 percent a year. In 1980, about 1 in 250 persons developed melanoma; today, this risk is 1 in 120, and in the year 2000, it is expected to be 1 in 90.

Critical Thinking Question

The *Healthy People 2000* objectives include the following: "Increase to at least 60 percent the proportion of people of all ages who limit sun exposure, use sunscreens and protective clothing when exposed to sunlight, and avoid artificial sources of ultraviolet light (e.g., sun lamps, tanning booths)." Currently, only about 30 percent of the U.S. population take such precautions. Given the clear evidence that associates sun exposure with cancer, why do you think so few Americans use sunscreens and protective clothing? If it took more than forty years to change public opinion about the hazards of smoking, how long do you think it will take to change public opinion about sun exposure?

General risk factors associated with skin cancer are extensive exposure to the sun, fair complexion, and freckling (see the Your Environmental Neighborhood box). The incidence of skin cancer is very low among African Americans because of heavy skin pigmentation. For basal and squamous cell cancers specifically, additional risk factors include X-ray treatments for skin conditions, burn scars, occupational exposure to certain chemicals, and a precancerous change of the

basal cell A small, round cell in the lower part (base) of the epidermis.

squamous cell A flat cell that makes up most of the epidermis.

melanoma A skin cancer that often starts as a mole-like growth and grows in size and changes color; the most serious of the various types of skin cancer.

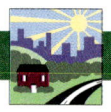

YOUR ENVIRONMENTAL NEIGHBORHOOD

The Sun and Skin Cancer

Wealthy Victorians admired fair skin. But in the 1920s Coco Chanel helped to change that ideal when she returned from a vacation on the Duke of Windsor's yacht sporting a deep tan. Soon her "look" became the rage.

Bronzed skin became a status symbol, and generations of sunbathers cultivated tans in backyards and on beaches. In recent years, however, medical research has proven that the sun can be dangerous to your skin, and now tans are considered a badge of ignorance, foolhardiness, or both.

The sun is the leading cause of cancer in the United States. Skin cancer rates are up 50 percent since 1980. One in six Americans can expect to develop some form of skin cancer, and for those who live in the Sunbelt states, the prediction is one in three. Skin cancer is the most prevalent form of cancer in women aged twenty-five to twenty-nine, and it is the number-two cancer among women aged thirty to thirty-four (after breast cancer). The death rate from melanoma in men over age fifty is now increasing faster than that of any other cancer.

Unfortunately, the most serious damage from overexposure to the sun occurs to children. Eighty percent of the skin damage that will eventually lead to cancer affects children and teenagers. A bad burn before age eighteen heightens the chance of developing malignant melanoma later in life. But it is dif-

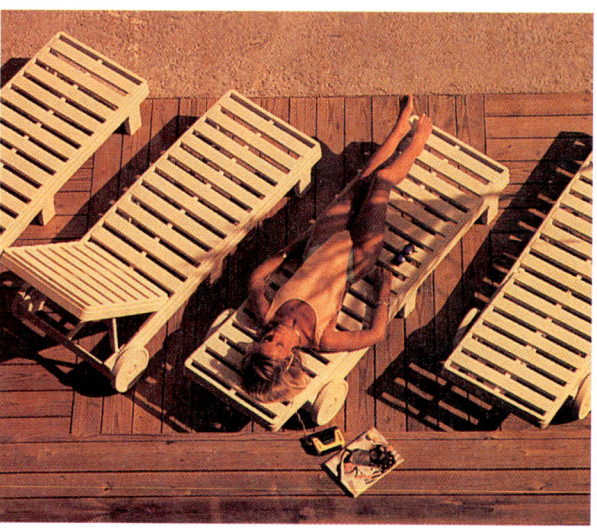

The sun is the leading cause of cancer in the United States. Don't bask in the sun, and when you go out wear a wide-brimmed hat and a sunscreen with a sun protection factor (SPF) of at least 15. (Source: Tony Stone Images/© Chip Henderson)

skin known as actinic **keratosis.** For melanomas, additional risk factors are brown moles and three or more blistering sunburns during adolescence.

Symptoms of skin cancer include a mole, birthmark, or beauty mark that changes color, size, or texture or an open sore that does not heal correctly. Early diagnosis is critical. For basal and squamous cell cancers, cure is likely if they are detected and treated early. Catching melanomas before they spread can result in a 95 percent five-year survival rate. Rates drop to 61 percent and 16 percent, respectively, when melanomas have spread regionally and to distant parts of the body. About four fifths of melanomas are diagnosed at the early stage.

Other common sites of cancer are the cervix, testicles, colon, and stomach. Some cancers are clearly linked to specific behaviors, such as oral cancer to smokeless tobacco use. Other cancers, such as leukemia (a cancer of the white blood cells), arise from unknown origins.

Screening for Cancer

As the statistics clearly illustrate, the best line of defense against a cancer spreading is early detection. Studies show that screening for cancer of the breast, cervix, colon, rectum, uterus, and other areas can significantly reduce cancer mortality.

ficult to convince teenagers to wear sunscreen, and only one in five uses it.

The increased incidence of skin cancer is due in part to the gradual depletion of the ozone layer, which protects the earth from the sun's ultraviolet rays. In 1985, scientists discovered a hole in the ozone layer over the Antarctic and have since noted erosion in other areas, including over Australia and the United States. The intensity of the sun's ultraviolet rays is greater than anything previous generations were exposed to.

Experts agree that the best way to combat the increased risk of cancer is to concentrate prevention efforts on the young. The good news is that nine out of ten women interviewed in a Gallup Poll said they were more careful with their children than they were with themselves when they were younger. And in Hollywood, California, none of the celebrities has a tan, says a prominent dermatologist there. The same ultraviolet rays that cause skin cancer cause premature aging of the skin, and the actors and actresses know they will be ineligible for parts if they look old.

What Can You Do to Protect Yourself?

- Avoid peak sun hours whenever possible. Peak hours are 10 A.M. to 2 P.M., or 11 A.M. to 3 P.M. during daylight saving time.
- Wear a wide-brimmed hat and other protective clothing if sun exposure will be prolonged or occur during peak hours.
- Be aware that sand, snow, water, and even concrete can reflect up to 85 percent of the sun's rays.
- Do not assume that a tan protects against the sun. It is a sign of skin damage. Keep using sunscreen to avoid further damage.
- Keep babies under six months old out of direct exposure to the sun; their delicate skin is especially vulnerable to damage.
- Remember that it is never too late to be careful. Adults who stay out of the sun or use sun protection will reduce their risk of cancer and reverse existing skin damage; skin will become smoother, sunspots will begin to fade, and wrinkling will be less obvious.
- Examine yourself monthly for any changes in your skin, especially a mole or beauty mark, and make sure that a physician looks at any spot that has changed in color, texture, or size.
- Research about the benefits and possible side effects of sunscreen is still being done. Proponents of sunscreen advise liberal application 20 minutes before going into the sun; that you use about one ounce per whole body application; that the sunscreen have a sun protection factor (SPF) of 15 or greater; and that if you live in the Sunbelt, use a sunscreen daily, year-round.

A **Pap smear** involves scraping and analyzing some cells from the cervix and is effective in reducing death from cancer of the cervix by as much as 75 percent. The American Cancer Society recommends that women who are or have been sexually active or have have reached age eighteen should have an annual Pap test and pelvic examination. After three consecutive normal annual examinations, the test may be performed less frequently.

Mammography, which is a low-dose breast X ray, and clinical breast examination reduce death from breast cancer by 30 percent. Women should get a baseline mammogram at age thirty-five to have for comparison, have a new one every year or every other year from age forty to age forty-nine, and then one every year thereafter. In 1997, the American Cancer Society began recommending yearly mammograms for women under age fifty, but some studies still question the validity of regular mammograms for women in this age group.

Although most women get a Pap smear routinely, only about 36 percent of women over age forty have ever received a mammogram and clinical breast examination. Some of the reasons for not having these examinations are ignorance, fear, discomfort, and cost: A mammogram can cost $100. Check your health insurance policy to see if you are covered for this. It is required to be covered for women over age fifty in some states.

keratosis A rough patch or horny growth of the skin.

Pap smear A test for identifying cervical cancer that involves scraping and analyzing cells from the cervix.

mammography A screening technique used to detect breast cancer.

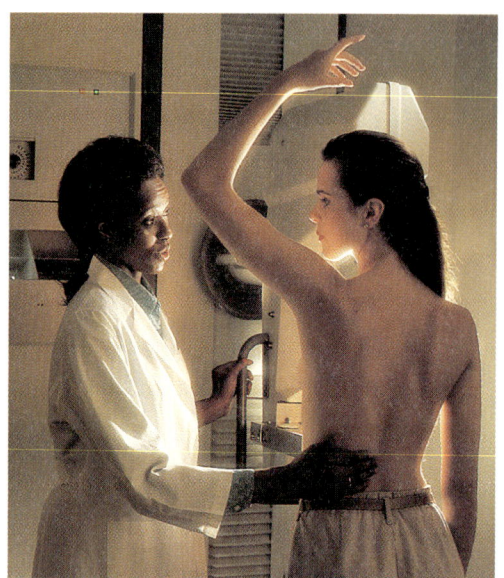

A mammogram—a low-dose breast X ray—and a clinical breast examination can detect breast cancer early and reduce death from this disease by 30 percent. (Source: FPG International/© Jeff Kaufman)

A yearly **prostate-specific antigen (PSA) test** is recommended by the American Cancer Society for men over age fifty. A higher level of PSA in the blood can be a sign of prostate cancer. Men over age forty who have a family history of prostate cancer or who are African American should also have this test every year. The value of early detection of prostate cancer is controversial. Many prostate tumors are slow growing and no rigorous study has demonstrated that men who are treated early with surgery and radiation survive longer.

HEALTH SKILLS

Self-Tests for Cancer

A free test, which is being done by a growing percentage of women, is **breast self-examination (BSE).** The American Cancer Society recommends that all women over age twenty do a BSE every month. Because BSE is not nearly as effective as mammography or examination by a physician, women are encouraged not to depend solely on it for early detection. Figure 13.4 gives the sizes of breast lumps according to how and when they are typically discovered. See the Developing Health Skills box to learn how to do a breast self-exam.

Although testicular cancer is relatively rare—it accounts for only 1 percent of all cancers among men—the risk for dying from it can be reduced with a self-examination. The best time to do this is after a warm bath or shower, when the skin is most relaxed. Roll each testicle between the thumb and fingers of both hands. See your physician promptly if you find any hard lumps. This self-examination should be conducted monthly by adult men—particularly young men, because it is the most common form of cancer among men between the ages of twenty and thirty-five. This procedure is especially important for men who have a history of undescended testicles. A testicular examination by a trained physician is recommended as a routine part of all periodic health examinations.

To check for colon and rectum cancers, the American Cancer Society recommends a digital rectal examination every year after age forty, a stool blood test every year after age fifty, and **sigmoidoscopy** every three to five years after age fifty. A digital rectal examination is also recommended each year for men over forty years old as a means of detecting prostate cancer. In sigmoidoscopy, a physician uses a hollow lighted tube to inspect the rectum and lower colon.

In addition, a cancer-related checkup is recommended every three years for people twenty to forty years of age and every year after age forty. This checkup includes looking for cancer of the thyroid, mouth, skin, lymph nodes, testes,

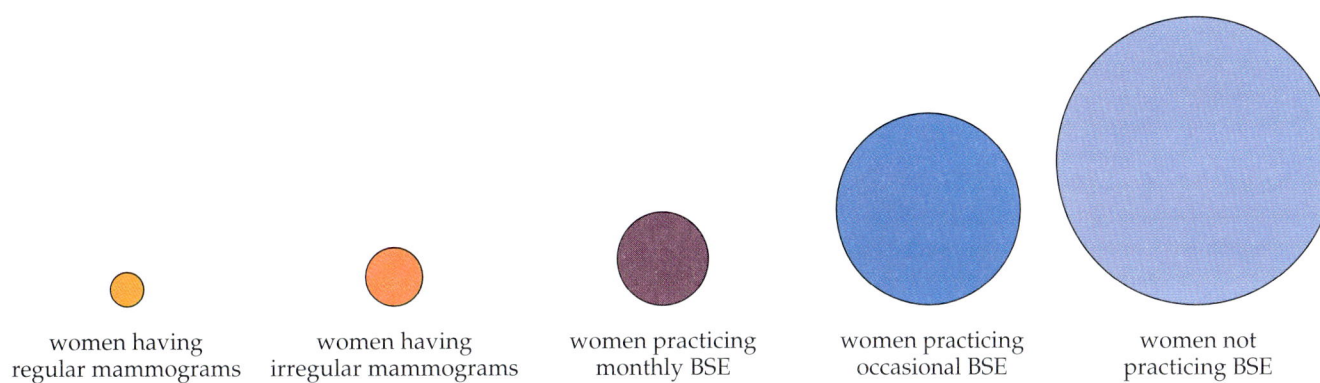

Figure 13.4 Breast Lumps: Sizing Them Up. *(Source: Reprinted by permission from the* National Women's Health Report *17 (no. 5), October 1995, published by the National Women's Health Resource Center, Washington, DC))*

prostate, and ovaries. Your physician should also review good health habits, including tips on eating a healthy diet, quitting smoking, and other lifestyle choices that relate to cancer. This is because an unhealthy lifestyle is the cause of two thirds of all cancers. Your dentist, too, should check regularly for signs of oral cancer, most of which are associated with smoking.

You should be aware of any changes in your own body and be alert to the American Cancer Society's seven warning signals:

Change in bowel or bladder habits

A sore that does not heal

Unusual bleeding or discharge

Thickening or lump in breast or elsewhere

Indigestion or difficulty in swallowing

Obvious change in wart or mole

Nagging cough or hoarseness

The American Cancer Society recommends that you see your physician if you have any of these warning signals.

Benefits and Risks of Treatment

Surgery, radiation, and chemotherapy are the principal forms of cancer treatment. Although each carries risks, the benefits, as documented in survival rates, more often outweigh the risks.

The primary treatment for cancer is surgical removal of the malignant growth. This is particularly effective when the cancer has not metastasized. Over the years, surgical techniques have improved so that removal causes less bodily disfigurement. For example, in 1970, most mastectomies done in the United States involved the complete removal of the breast and the surrounding tissue, particularly the lymph nodes. This is called a **radical mastectomy.** Today, such radical surgery is very seldom done. Alternatives include **lumpectomy,** a procedure that involves removal of the cancerous lump only; **partial mastectomy,** which involves removal of only the part of the breast containing the lump; and **modified radical mastectomy,** which involves selective removal of the breast and surrounding tissue.

For some kinds of cancer—notably cancers of the blood and lymph system—radiation and chemotherapy are the primary forms of treatment. With those treatments, the survival rates for patients who have the lymph node cancer known as Hodgkin's disease are around 75 percent. Men who have prostate can-

prostate-specific antigen (PSA) test A blood test that can identify signs of prostate cancer.

breast self-examination (BSE) An examination done by a woman to herself to identify abnormal breast tissue.

sigmoidoscopy A screening procedure in which a physician uses a hollow lighted tube to inspect the rectum and lower colon.

radical mastectomy The complete surgical removal of the breast and surrounding tissue, particularly the lymph nodes.

lumpectomy The surgical removal of only the cancerous lump from the breast.

partial mastectomy The surgical removal of only the part of the breast containing the cancerous lump.

modified radical mastectomy A selective removal of the breast and surrounding tissue.

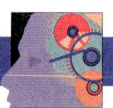

DEVELOPING HEALTH SKILLS

How to Do a Breast Self-Exam

The best time to do breast self-exam is right after your period, when breasts are not tender or swollen. If you do not have regular periods or sometimes skip a month, do it on the same day every month. Use the following procedure to perform your breast self-exam.

1. Lie down and put a pillow under your left shoulder. Place your left arm behind your head.

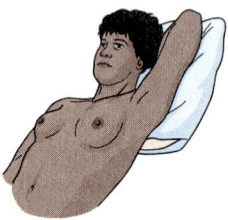

2. Use the finger pads of your three middle fingers on your right hand to feel for lumps or thickening. Your finger pads are the top third of each finger.

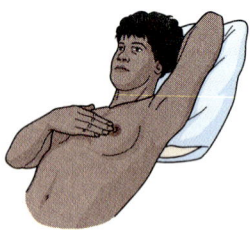

3. Press firmly enough to know how your breast feels. If you're not sure how hard to press, ask your health dare provider. Or try to copy the way your health care provider uses the finger pads during a breast exam. Learn what your breast feels like most of the time. A firm ridge in the lower curve of each breast is normal.

4. Move around the breast in a set way. You can choose either the circle (A), the up and down (B), or the wedge (C). Do it the same way every time. It will help you to make sure that you've gone over the entire breast area, and to remember how your breast feels.

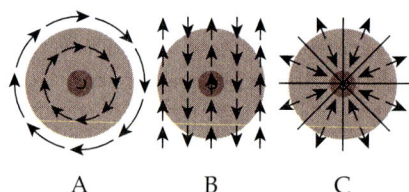

A   B   C

5. Now examine your right breast using left hand finger pads. If you find any changes, see your doctor right away.

For Added Safety: You should also check your breasts while standing in front of a mirror right after you do your breast self-exam each month. See if there are any, changes in the way your breasts look: dimpling of the skin, changes in the nipple, or redness or swelling.

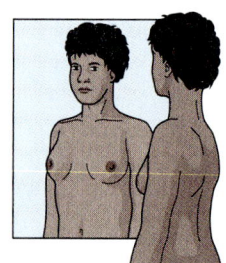

You might also want to do a breast self-exam while you're in the shower. Your soapy hands will glide over wet skin making it easy to check how your breasts feel.

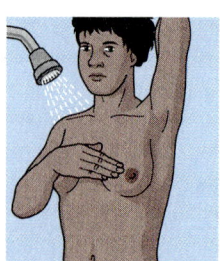

Source: Reprinted by the permission of the American Cancer Society, Inc.

cer often choose radiation as the primary therapy because traditional prostate surgery can cause impotence.

For most other cancers, radiation and chemotherapy are used following surgery to prevent metastases, shrink growths that cannot be removed, and relieve pain. The side effects of radiation and chemotherapy are both dangerous and dramatic and may include anemia, severe nausea, uncontrollable infections, and baldness. In each case, the benefits of treatment, as documented in survival rates, need to be weighed against the risks.

There are, in addition, alternative cancer treatments, many of which have proven to be quackery. One popular therapy, laetrile, or apricot pit therapy, was proven to be a hoax. Other "treatments" include devices that give off warmth and vibrations and are said to detect and destroy cancer cells. These treatments may provide a ray of hope to the otherwise hopeless cancer patient, but little evidence supports their effectiveness in delaying the effects of the disease. In fact, traditional medicine remains greatly concerned that patients who avail themselves of such ineffective approaches run the risk for greater suffering and may miss opportunities for treatment that could prolong life.

Another kind of cancer treatment—mind–body care—is moving from the fringes of medicine into the mainstream. According to this approach to treatment, the mind can actually cure the body. The field is officially called **psychoneuroimmunology**—*psycho* for the mind and emotions, *neuro* for the brain and central nervous system, and *immunology* for the body's natural defense against abnormal cells or external invaders such as bacteria or viruses. This chapter discusses mind–body treatments for cancer. Chapter 14 discusses their use in treating AIDS patients.

In one study of people treated for the early stages of colon cancer or malignant melanoma whose cancers were in remission, thirty patients received an eight-week course in relaxation and cognitive therapy, a technique that focuses on changing a person's self-defeating beliefs. Researchers found that patients who took the course had more active natural killer cells, which protect the body against tumor growth, than did patients who did not take the course.

Another example of a mind–body treatment for cancer is imagery. Clinical studies show that cancer patients can reduce their level of pain through imagery—for example, thinking of something pleasant. This helps promote relaxation, which, in turn, can ease the pain. A more controversial use of imaging is to shrink a cancer by focusing the mind on an image of it being attacked by the body and visualizing the cancer getting smaller. To learn more about mind–body treatments and cancer, see the Cultural View box.

Smile Please: Dental Disease

Fortunately, the most prevalent of the chronic diseases affecting both children and adults is not life threatening, but it is often an overlooked source of discomfort, pain, and possibly disfigurement: dental disease. Diseases of the gums and teeth affect virtually all people to some extent. As with other chronic diseases, your family history can play a role here. No matter how thoroughly you brush and floss, you have a good chance of getting cavities or inflamed gums if they run in your family. However, even for people in such families, dental disease can be held in check if preventive hygiene measures are taken.

The two major families of dental disease are **dental caries,** or tooth decay, and **periodontal disease,** or gum disease. More than 95 percent of the U.S. population has experienced some form of dental disease.

psychoneuroimmunology A mind–body approach to treatment. It involves the mind and emotions *(psycho)*, the brain and central nervous system *(neuro)*, and the body's natural defense system *(immunology)*.

dental caries Tooth decay.

periodontal disease Gum disease.

CULTURAL VIEW

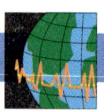

Mind–Body Treatments Moving into the Mainstream

There are still believers and nonbelievers, but mainstream medicine is increasingly accepting some of the principles of mind–body treatments. Side-by-side with chemotherapy and radical surgery to remove tumors, doctors are "prescribing" meditation and mental exercises to breathe in good healthy air and exhale bad cancer cells. "The people who do the best are the people who say to themselves, 'I am going to beat this thing,'" says a California breast cancer patient who meditates, prays, and attends support groups.

Each year at just one Kaiser hospital in Sacramento, California, about 800 cancer and other patients listen to a tape while they are unconscious during surgery. What they hear is a soothing voice guiding their bodies through relaxation and then recovery. In addition to imagery, other techniques used in mind–body treatment include:

- Hypnosis: During a state that resembles sleep, the therapist can use the power of suggestion to help reduce perceptions of pain. Some studies show that hypnosis can prolong the lives of breast cancer patients; other studies do not confirm this.
- Meditation: Using this technique, a cancer patient can "breathe away" cancer, or "relax away" pain by relaxing all the muscles in the body, starting with the face and moving downward.
- Art therapy: Cancer patients use art therapy as a way to express themselves, particularly about their illness. One breast cancer patient, who used art therapy after surgery and chemotherapy, was asked to trace her hand on a piece of paper. When she looked at it, she realized her feeling of losing control.
- Prayer: This is perhaps the oldest form of mind–body therapy. One study from a San Francisco hospital found that heart patients who did not know they were being prayed for suffered fewer heart attacks and needed fewer drugs than did similar patients who were not being prayed for.

What is the science behind these treatments? Studies published in mainstream journals, including the *Journal of the American Medical Association*, suggest that mind–body techniques reduce stress, which can hamper the response of the immune system. A more controversial theory considers mind–body techniques to be potent medicines in themselves. According to this theory, imagery, meditation, or prayer, for example, can trigger the body's endocrine or immune system to counterattack disease. Controlled clinical studies are under way to examine the effectiveness of several of the mind–body techniques being used.

So mind–body treatments may—or may not—cure cancer, but can they harm patients? Some doctors say yes. They are concerned that patients may rely more on their own healing powers and not seek traditional, proven treatments for cancer, such as chemotherapy. Summing up what many nonbelievers think, one New York psychiatrist says: "Going to a psychosocial support group may help cancer patients emotionally, but it isn't going to help their cancer."

Critical Thinking Question

It probably seems unusual to consider dental disease in the same textbook chapter as heart disease and cancer. Why do you think we chose to do so? How are these three diseases similar? How are they different? What prevention strategies are effective in reducing the occurrence of all three?

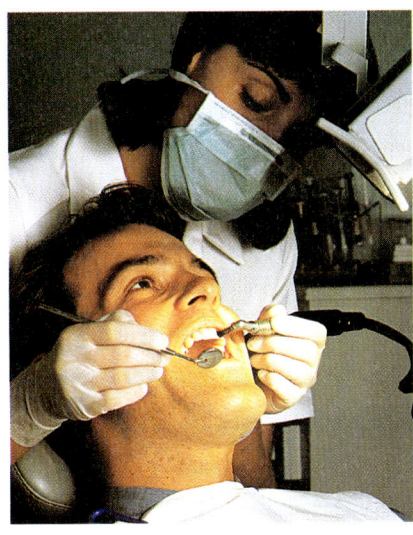

Regular professional dental care, brushing, and flossing can help prevent the most prevalent chronic diseases: dental caries and periodontal disease. (Source: © Tony Stone Images/Tim Brown)

Tooth decay, the most prevalent dental condition, develops when the acids in plaque attack the teeth. **Dental plaque** is a colorless film of bacteria that forms on the teeth and gums. (Dental plaque is not related to arterial plaque, which is a buildup of fatty deposits on arterial walls that can lead to heart disease.) If not removed, dental plaque becomes concentrated colonies of bacteria. These colonies mix with sugars and starches to form acids that attack the enamel of the tooth, break it down, and lead to a cavity—a single location of decay in a tooth. A dentist can identify areas of tooth decay, either visually or with X rays, and remove the decayed area of the tooth and replace it with a filling, a metal alloy designed to become a functional part of the tooth in place of the area lost to decay. Many people fear going to the dentist and put off routine dental care. In such circumstances, a single cavity can lead to complete loss of a tooth and perhaps several teeth.

Plaque affects the gums as well, causing them to become red, tender, and swollen. This is called **gingivitis,** and it is the first stage of periodontal disease. More than half of all adults aged thirty-five and over have the early stages of this disease. If left untreated, periodontal disease can result in a degeneration of the gum tissue that holds the teeth in place. This is called **periodontitis,** or pyorrhea. Although this usually begins as a painless condition, it can result over time in painful loss of the supporting bone and ultimately in loss of teeth.

The good news about dental diseases is that they are preventable with routine brushing and flossing and regular professional dental care. The maintenance of healthy teeth requires regular brushing with a soft brush to remove plaque. This should be done after eating, at least two times per day. Brushing is most effective when

- Enough time is spent brushing to ensure that all teeth and gums and the tongue are brushed adequately (some dentists recommend brushing for as long as three minutes)
- Brushing patterns are adequate to clean all surfaces
- Brushing is frequent enough to stay ahead of the buildup of plaque (two or three times per day, especially after eating)

Brushing alone, however, cannot clean between the teeth. In order to clean these surfaces, it is necessary to use dental floss—a specially designed thread for cleaning between the teeth. Flossing should be done once per day. To see how well you are preventing dental problems, see the Here's Looking at You box.

HealthLinks

American Dental Association
www.ada.org

A link with the leading organization dedicated to dental health, containing pertinent information on research and clinical issues, as well as information on continuing education courses and programs.

dental plaque Noncalcified accumulation of microorganisms that attach to the teeth.

gingivitis A condition in which the gums are red, tender, and swollen.

periodontitis Degeneration of the gum tissue that holds the teeth in place.

HERE'S LOOKING AT YOU

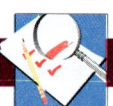

How Well Do You Know Your Teeth?

Of course we're supposed to brush every day. But how many of us know why? Take this test to find out if you're truly treating your teeth well.

1. You can catch gum disease from
   a. kissing
   b. sharing a toothbrush
   c. both
   d. neither
2. Toothbrushing prevents
   a. detached gums
   b. root decay
   c. stained teeth
   d. none of the above
3. You're least likely to get cavities from eating
   a. raisins
   b. pure sugar
   c. an English muffin
4. Who's especially susceptible to getting gum disease?
   a. pregnant women
   b. menopausal women
   c. teetotalers
5. If you can't brush your teeth after a meal, what's the best thing to do?
   a. eat a banana
   b. chew gum
   c. use a toothpick
6. The minimum time for a thorough toothbrushing is
   a. one minute
   b. three minutes
   c. four minutes
7. Which will relieve toothache pain fastest?
   a. aspirin
   b. clove oil
   c. saltwater

Answers: **1. c.** By age thirty-five, three in four Americans have at least the beginnings of gum disease, an

---

Dental care is not complete without a regular appointment with a dentist, usually once or twice a year, to examine your teeth and gums. Early detection of tooth decay or gum disease is critical to arresting the effects of plaque buildup. Your dentist will take baseline X rays of your teeth and jaws and occasional follow-up X rays to detect any abnormalities. A dental hygienist will remove **calculus,** or tartar, which is plaque that has hardened on the tooth surfaces, and may apply topical fluoride, a substance that hardens enamel and makes teeth more resistant to the acid that causes dental decay. Fluoride occurs naturally in water or is added to the water supplies in most municipalities in the United States. It is also in most toothpastes. Fluoride may be the real tooth fairy: Research shows that it reduces cavities by as much as 40 percent in children and 35 percent in adults.

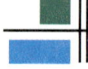

Living with Chronic Disease

When you ask people how they feel, most respond, "Fine, thank you." But for people who have chronic diseases, and especially for those who have degenerative diseases such as arthritis, life can be difficult. Chronically ill people may never regain the full level of health they enjoyed before the onset of their illnesses, and they may face a continuing loss of function and the constant threat of ever more serious medical problems as their illnesses progress. As medical advances help people who have chronic diseases live longer, they are left with the human challenge of coping with their disability. This may affect not only the person who has the disease but also his or her family and friends.

calculus Dental plaque that has hardened on tooth surfaces; also called tartar.

irritation and infection below the gum line caused by certain bacteria in dental plaque. But occasionally bacteria transmitted via the saliva of someone with gum disease can bring on gum disease in someone who doesn't even have plaque. So, if your partner isn't taking care of his teeth, take the problem seriously. Your own gums may be at risk. **2. d.** Toothbrushing removes plaque and prevents cavities above the gum line, but not below. When plaque isn't cleaned out, the gums fall away, allowing germs to get at your roots and even at the bone anchoring the teeth. Gum disease is the nation's leading cause of tooth loss. To prevent it, you have to floss regularly. **3. b.** Sugary foods, including candy and chocolate, are cleared from the mouth more quickly than starchy foods. Raisins are a special case because they stick between teeth so tenaciously. **4. a.** Nearly all pregnant women get some signs of gum disease because hormones associated with pregnancy increase swelling, bleeding, and tiny infections in the gums. There's an old saw: lose a tooth for every child. To keep it from coming true, brush after every meal, floss daily, and see a dentist at the beginning of your pregnancy. **5. b.** Chewing gum stimulates copious secretions of saliva, and saliva's chemicals neutralize tooth decaying acids. Pop in a piece when you finish a meal. Sugarless gum works much better than regular, and gum containing xylitol works best of all, reducing tooth decay by as much as 85 percent. (The sweetener keeps bacteria from mass-producing.) The gum's sold mostly in health food stores. **6. b.** To make this task less daunting, try dividing your mouth into ten sections. (Include a section each for the roof of your mouth, tongue, and the inside of your right and left cheeks, all places where bacteria congregate.) Then count to twenty alligators as you brush each section. The average American spends about thirty seconds brushing. **7. b.** If your dentist can't see you right away for a painful cavity or infection, saturate a cotton ball in oil of clove (sold at many pharmacies) and put it on the aching tooth. The anesthetic oil should ease the pain in a couple of seconds.

Source: "How Well Do You Know Your Teeth?" *Health*, January–February 1995, p. 20. Reprinted by permission of Time Inc. Health

Psychological Adjustment

One of the most difficult adjustments for someone who has a chronic disease to make is modifying the view of him- or herself from a healthy, fully abled person to one who is not fully able. Think of how sick you view yourself when you are fighting a bout of influenza or are weak from mononucleosis. Yet your role as a sick person is likely to last only a few weeks at most. For people who have chronic diseases, being sick or in pain becomes a lifelong state. There is assault on self-esteem, and a period of depression is not uncommon. In fact, psychiatrists find that depression—not the threat of another attack—is one of the most formidable problems in getting heart attack patients through convalescence and rehabilitation.

Realistic adjustments in lifestyle often need to be made at school or work to accommodate a chronic disease. A college student recently diagnosed as a diabetic, for example, might have to allow some extra time during the day for monitoring blood glucose or administering insulin. With the same diagnosis, someone who has an extremely strenuous job—a police officer or firefighter, for example—might need to consider some job or career modifications.

Similarly, leisure activities might change as a result of chronic disease. Continuing with the diabetes example, an avid rock climber newly diagnosed with diabetes may find at some point that rock climbing carries too high a risk for foot injury. (People who have diabetes are at high risk for serious foot injuries because the disease compromises the body's circulatory system.) A safer alternative for exercise might be swimming or riding a stationary bike.

As with other health conditions, positive steps can be taken. For example, cancer patients who believe that they have some control over their health status are less likely to experience severe depression than are patients who give up. In addition to using basic coping skills (see Chapter 4), there are specific things that researchers have identified that chronically ill patients and their families can do to help themselves cope with the illness:

- Learn as much as possible about the disease and treatment options.
- Accept and readjust to physical changes in the body.
- Learn how to express feelings about having the disease.
- Express a personal sense of empowerment and control, particularly as related to health care decisions.
- Seek out support groups and other resources in the community.
- Develop meaningful relationships with family, friends, and members of the health care team (physician, nurse, social worker, and others).
- Maintain a sense of hope.

The Reality of Pain

For many people who have chronic illness, pain is a reminder that they are not well. At some point in the illness, between 60 percent and 90 percent of patients who have life-threatening cancer have pain severe enough to warrant receiving narcotics such as morphine. The pain can come from the primary tumor or a far-flung metastasis or from the treatment itself—surgery, radiation, or chemotherapy.

Medication works in 90 percent of cases in reducing or controlling the physical component of pain. For 10 percent of patients who have advanced cancer, pain becomes intractable. Even so, they can often benefit from the combined efforts of a pain-control team, which includes anesthesiologists, psychiatrists, surgeons, cancer specialists, nurses, psychologists, and social workers. Looking at nonpharmacological ways of controlling pain, the National Cancer Institute reports that there is a role for a wide range of supports, including deep breathing exercises, massage, biofeedback, imagery, and music therapy. A recent study showed that the nonthreatening qualities of listening to music put cancer patients at ease and enabled them to relax. Humor or laugh therapy has proven successful in some cases. Distractions such as watching television can also take a person's mind away from the pain.

Concluding Thoughts

The best medical advice concerning chronic diseases is to keep them in the proper perspective for your life. For the most part, they tend to act slowly and provide years of warning. Preventive measures—most particularly, not smoking and following a healthy diet—along with early detection and medical intervention have proven effective in the treatment and cure of many chronic diseases that only a few years ago were considered death sentences.

Key Concepts

1. A chronic disease is marked by long duration or frequent recurrence.
2. Nearly 100 million Americans—46 percent of the country's population—have chronic diseases or disabilities, and the proportion of people who have to limit their activities due to chronic illness is increasing.
3. Over the past fifteen years, the death rate from diseases of the heart and

blood vessels has declined dramatically due in great part to better surgical techniques, improved drugs, more effective medical management, and a better understanding of the risk factors for heart disease.
4. Smoking is the single most important risk factor associated with heart disease. Smokers have a 70 percent greater risk than nonsmokers for dying of heart disease.
5. Hypertension is called the silent killer because it has few symptoms but can lead to heart attack, stroke, and heart and kidney failure.
6. Cancer is a group of more than 100 diseases, all characterized by uncontrolled growth and spread of abnormal cells.
7. Benign tumors do not invade other cells or spread to other parts of the body. Malignant tumors spread to nearby tissues and organs, crowding out healthy cells and replacing them with cancer cells.
8. A mammography, a low-dose breast X ray, and clinical breast examination reduce death from breast cancer by 30 percent.
9. The most prevalent chronic diseases are dental caries and periodontal disease—both preventable by means of brushing, flossing, and regular professional dental care.
10. Coping with a chronic illness includes making realistic adjustments in your lifestyle.

Review Questions

1. Compare and contrast chronic illness and infectious illness.
2. List lifestyle choices that lead to chronic illness. List lifestyle choices that reduce the risk for chronic illness.
3. Describe controllable risk factors associated with cardiovascular disease. Describe noncontrollable risk factors that increase the potential for cardiovascular disease.
4. Identify the symptoms and treatment modalities for atherosclerosis, myocardial infarction, angina pectoris, arrhythmia, stroke, transient ischemic attacks, and hypertension.
5. Describe controllable risk factors associated with cancer. Describe noncontrollable risk factors that increase the potential for cancer.
6. Identify the symptoms and treatment modalities for lung cancer, breast cancer, prostate cancer, colon and rectum cancer, and skin cancer.
7. Explain the importance of early detection of cancer and name several screening procedures that can lead to early detection.
8. Explain the importance of good dental hygiene as a means of reducing the risk for dental disease.
9. List similarities and differences between cardiovascular disease, cancer, and dental disease.
10. List specific strategies for coping with chronic illness and describe how you would help someone implement these strategies.

Selected Bibliography

Burt, V., et al. "Prevalence of Hypertension in the U.S. Adult Population." *Hypertension* 25 (1995): 305–313.

Cancer Facts and Figures. Atlanta, GA: American Cancer Society, (updated annually).

Clinical Practice Guidelines, Management of Cancer Pain. Rockville, MD: Agency for Health Care Policy and Research, Public Health Service, 1994.

"Coronary Heart Disease Attributable to Sedentary Lifestyle." *Morbidity and Mortality Weekly Report* 39, no. 32 (1990): 541–544.

Heart and Stroke Facts Statistics. Dallas, TX: American Heart Association, (updated annually).

Hoffman, C., et al. "Persons with Chronic Conditions: Their Prevalence and Costs." *Journal of the American Medical Association* 276, no. 18 (1996): 1473–1479.

HealthLinks: Web Sites for Reducing the Risk of Chronic Diseases

You can access better health as it relates to this chapter by checking out some of the following sites on the Internet. These and sites identified within the chapter can be accessed directly when you visit the *HealthStyles* Web Site located on the Allyn and Bacon home page at **http://www.abacon.com**.

CDC National Center for Chronic Disease Prevention and Health Promotion
www.cdc.gov/nccdphp/nccdhome.htm

The home page for the division of the Centers for Disease Control and Prevention dedicated to the prevention of chronic diseases and maternal and infant health. Access the latest information on cancer, cardiovascular disease, diabetes, oral diseases and conditions, and other serious chronic diseases and conditions and discover what is and can be done to prevent these disorders.

ChronicNet
www.chronicnet.org

Developed jointly by The Robert Wood Johnson Foundation and the National Institute for Computer-Assisted Reporting, ChronicNet provides an easily accessible electronic Rolodex of national and local experts, as well as statistics relating to chronic care at the local level, and contacts to caregivers in your state who are pioneering innovative projects.

American Cancer Society
www.cancer.org

Private organization dedicated to cancer prevention, including information, statistics, and resources regarding cancer.

National Heart, Lung, and Blood Institute
www.nhlbi.nih.gov/nhlbi/nhlbi.htm

Access information about cardiovascular disease, blood disorders, lung disorders, sleep problems, as well as the latest information on the Women's Health Initiative.

Health Hotlines: Reducing the Risk for Chronic Disease

American Academy of Allergy and Immunology
(800) 822-2762
611 East Wells Street
Milwaukee, WI 53202

American Cancer Society
(800) ACS-2345 (227-2345)
National Office
1599 Clifton Road NE
Atlanta, GA 30329

American Dental Association
(800) 947-4746
Public Information and Education
211 East Chicago Avenue
Chicago, IL 60611

American Diabetes Association
(800) 232-3472
1600 Duke Street
Alexandria, VA 22314

American Heart Association
(800) 242-8721
P.O. Box 17025
Baltimore, MD 21203

Arthritis Foundation
(800) 283-7800
1330 West Peachtree Street
Atlanta, GA 30309

National Cancer Institute
Cancer Information Services
(800) 4-CANCER (422-6237)
550 North Broadway, Suite 300
Baltimore, MD 21205

National Heart, Lung and Blood Institute
Education Programs Information Center
(800) 575-WELL (575-9355)
P.O. Box 30105
Bethesda, MD 20824-0105

National Institute of Neurological Disorders and Stroke
(800) 352-9424
Building 31, Room 8A-06
Bethesda, MD 20892-2540

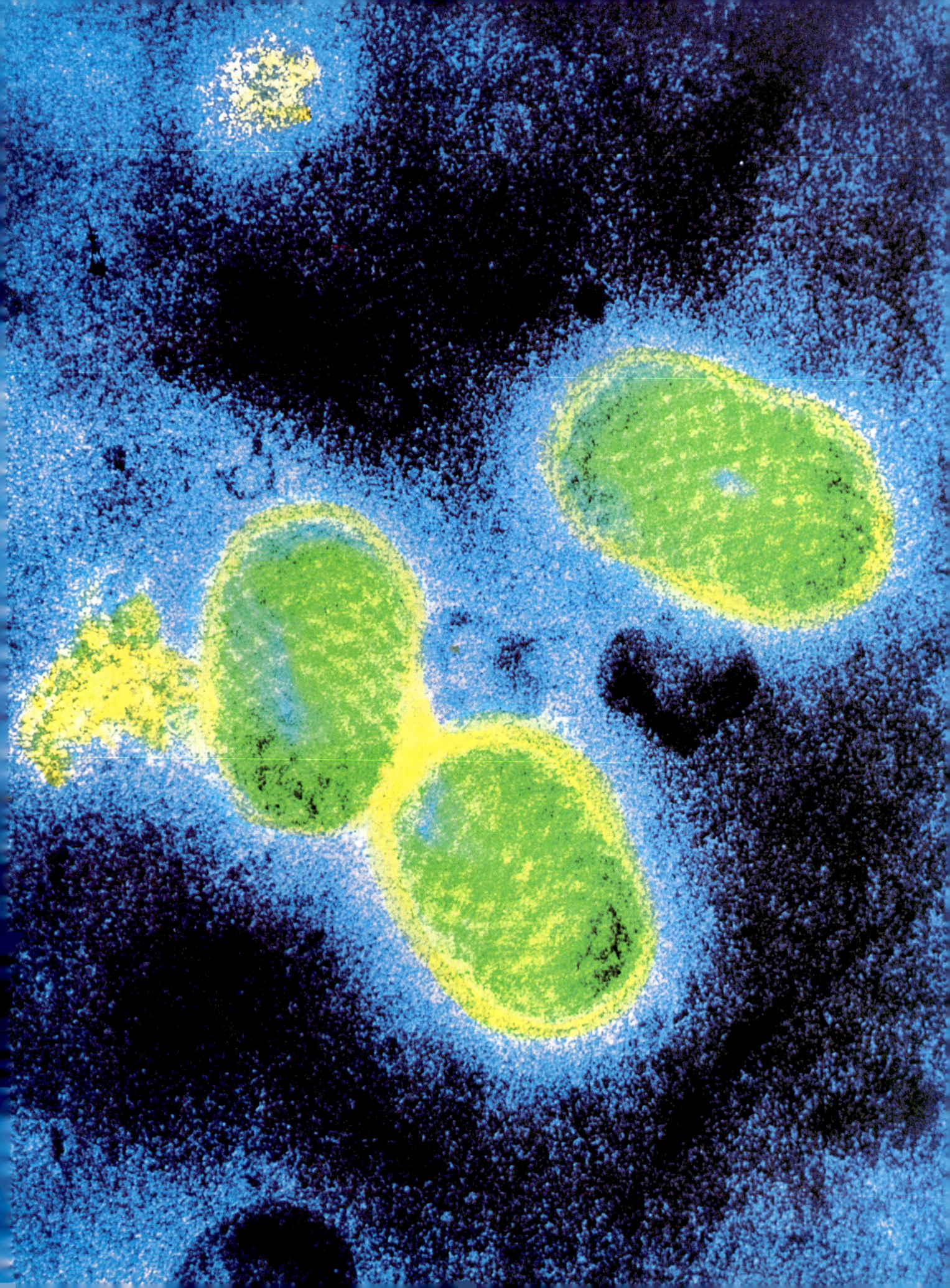

Chapter 14

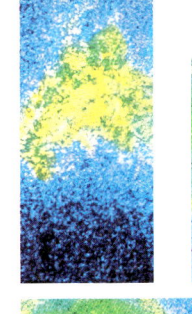
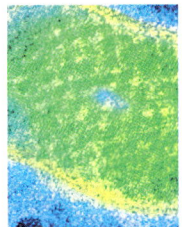
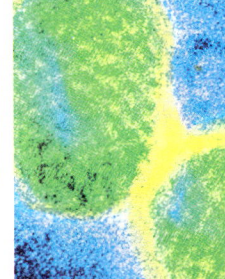

Reducing the Risk for Infectious Disease

Objectives

When you finish reading this chapter, you will be able to:

1. Describe how infectious diseases spread from one person to another.
2. Name seven families of pathogens and the characteristics of each.
3. Understand the body's defense against infections, including nonspecific and specific defense mechanisms.
4. Identify four ways pathogens get into a person's body.
5. Explain how virulence, dosage, and resistance influence the spread of infectious disease.
6. Understand immunity and its function in the maintenance of good health.
7. Differentiate between active immunity and passive immunity.
8. Describe the progress of a disease once infection has occurred.
9. Identify common infectious diseases and briefly describe the symptoms of each.
10. Suggest actions that an individual can take to reduce the risk for acquiring an infectious disease.

What Is Your HealthStyle?

Beth had a bad sore throat and went to the student health service to get some medicine. She had an important term paper to write and didn't want a "stupid" sore throat to get the better of her. The physician did a throat culture and when she found that Beth had strep throat, she gave her a prescription for an antibiotic medicine. Beth began as a compliant patient, taking her medicine as prescribed. But when the antibiotic made her feel better in two days, she stopped taking it. Unfortunately for Beth, treatment of bacterial infections with antibiotics requires a full course of treatment. Soon after she discontinued her medication, Beth had a relapse—and in fact felt even worse.

Kim lives down the hall from Beth, and she also paid a visit to the student health services to follow up on her flu-like symptoms—achy joints and fatigue. Like Beth, she had a paper to write but was feeling so tired that she couldn't work on it. Kim's problem was diagnosed just as she feared it would be: the flu. She knew that the flu is caused by a virus, and that antibiotics cannot help a viral disease. Her best bet for recovery was to build up her health with plenty of rest, liquids, and a good diet. A weakened system would only lead to a relapse—and there were enough infectious diseases going around the dorm that she didn't want to take any chances on catching something else.

In Your Opinion

Both Beth and Kim had an infectious disease, but they followed different routes to recovery. They both started to do the right thing, seek medical attention, but only one followed through correctly.

- What do these two scenarios tell you about infectious diseases?
- What health skills did Kim use that Beth did not?
- Did health knowledge influence the outcome? What about health-related attitudes?
- What would you have done in either of their cases?

---

infectious disease Also known as *communicable* or *contagious* disease. A disease caused by pathogens, such as bacteria or viruses, that spread from someone who is infected to someone who is not yet infected.

chain of infection A metaphor for infectious disease transmission in which each link in the chain represents a single factor necessary for disease to spread.

pathogen A microorganism, such as a bacterium, virus, protozoan, parasitic worm, fungus, or rickettsia, that causes disease.

Infectious diseases are a part of human history. Smallpox, a highly contagious, disfiguring, and much feared disease, dates back at least to ancient Egypt, with evidence of the typical scarring preserved on mummies. It lasted as a major health threat until 1977, when a worldwide effort to eradicate the disease finally succeeded. In fourteenth century Europe, bubonic plague, carried by infected rats, killed millions of people and decimated entire cities. The plague still exists and there are occasional outbreaks, but with antibiotic treatments, deaths from it are rare.

What has changed over the centuries is a better understanding of how diseases are spread, how to control them and, in the case of smallpox, how to eradicate them completely. In spite of these advances, infectious diseases remain a public health concern in the United States. Sexually transmitted diseases (STDs), such as *chlamydia* and *gonorrhea* are increasing at an alarming rate. (STDs are covered in Chapter 15.) New diseases continue to be discovered and new cures sought. Medical researchers are still debating the causes of chronic fatigue syndrome, and the search continues for an acquired immune deficiency syndrome (AIDS) vaccine. In addition, vulnerable populations, the very young and the elderly, are at higher risk of getting infectious diseases and dying. So it is that with infectious diseases we celebrate some of our most important health victories and face some of our most important medical challenges.

How Diseases Are Spread

An **infectious disease,** also known as a *contagious* or *communicable disease,* is the result of agents, such as bacteria or viruses, that spread through a variety of ways from someone who is infected to someone who is not yet infected. Chronic diseases, in contrast, are not contagious. You cannot contract cancer, heart disease, or hypertension from someone else.

Chain of Infection

Several factors influence the spread of disease within a population. These factors are best understood as links in a chain, each critical to the process of disease transmission, yet none alone is capable of causing disease. The six factors that make up the **chain of infection** provide insight not only into the spread of infection but also into ways the spread can be halted. Figure 14.1 shows the chain of infection using tuberculosis as the example.

- The first link in the chain of infection is the causative agent, a microorganism that causes the disease. This microorganism is also called a **pathogen.** There are six traditionally identified groups of pathogens: bacteria, viruses, proto-

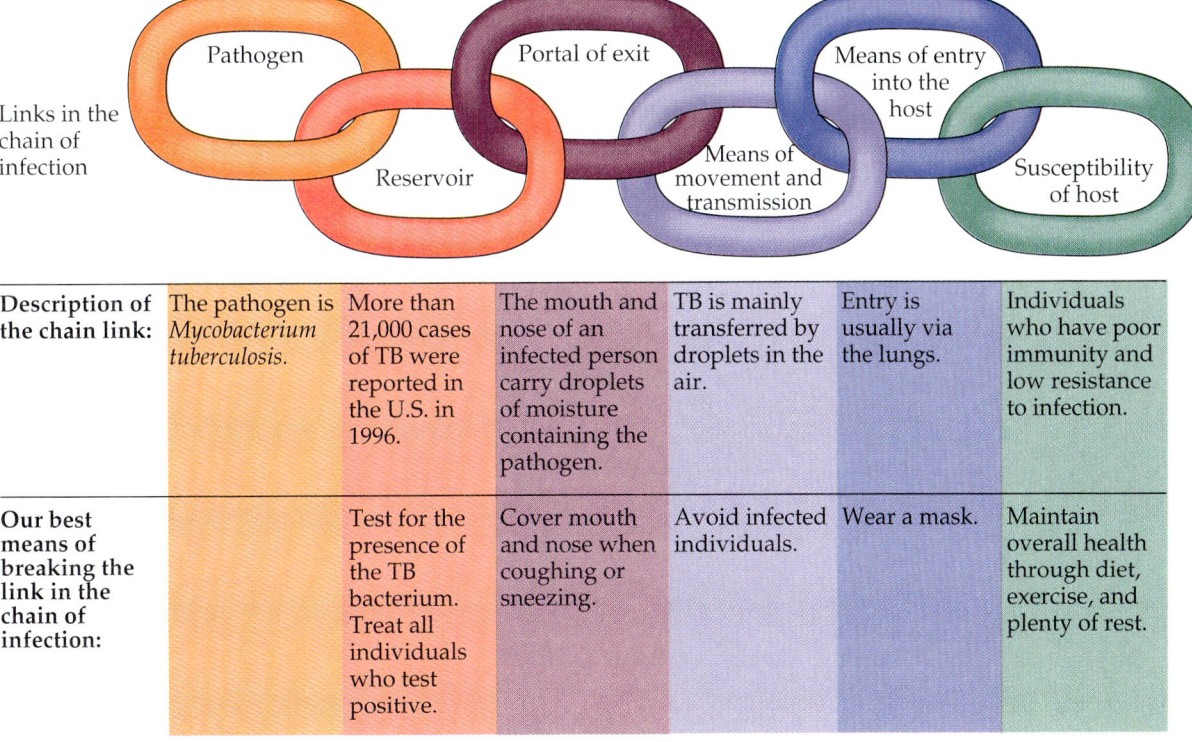

Links in the chain of infection	Pathogen	Reservoir	Portal of exit	Means of movement and transmission	Means of entry into the host	Susceptibility of host
Description of the chain link:	The pathogen is *Mycobacterium tuberculosis*.	More than 21,000 cases of TB were reported in the U.S. in 1996.	The mouth and nose of an infected person carry droplets of moisture containing the pathogen.	TB is mainly transferred by droplets in the air.	Entry is usually via the lungs.	Individuals who have poor immunity and low resistance to infection.
Our best means of breaking the link in the chain of infection:		Test for the presence of the TB bacterium. Treat all individuals who test positive.	Cover mouth and nose when coughing or sneezing.	Avoid infected individuals.	Wear a mask.	Maintain overall health through diet, exercise, and plenty of rest.

Figure 14.1 Chain of Infection. *In the example of tuberculosis, the spread of infection can be stopped if any one of the links in this chain is broken or missing.*

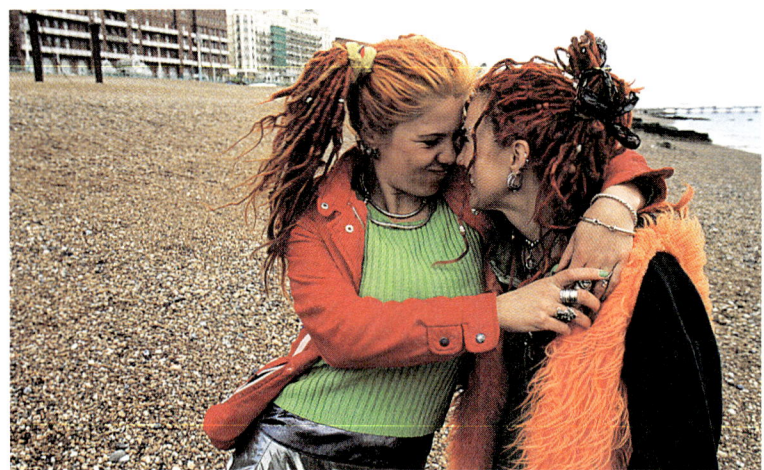

One of the links in spreading an infectious disease is when the infectious agent enters a new host. Body piercing can provide such an opportunity. (Source: © Tony Stone Images/Brendan Beirne)

zoa, parasitic worms, fungi, and rickettsias. In addition, many researchers believe that there is another disease-causing agent, called a prion.

- The second link is the **reservoir of the pathogen,** the place where it resides. The reservoir, or source, is either a human or an animal. When the pathogen lives in a human, that person usually shows signs of the disease. Sometimes, however, that person is a carrier; that is, he or she carries the disease but does not have any symptoms or show any signs of it.
- The next link in the chain is called the **portal of exit.** This is how the pathogen moves from the source to a new host. It can move by means of mucus, spit, blood, semen, feces, or in many other ways.
- The **means of transmission** represents the next link. There are five main means of transmission of a pathogen: the air, direct physical contact, contaminated food and water, **vectors** (insects or animals), and pathogens existing in the body in a controlled state.
- In order for infection to spread, the pathogen now must find a new home. This link in the chain of infection is called **entry into new host.** The pathogen can enter by many of the routes through which it left the reservoir—blood, semen, mucus, or through cuts or other open areas of the body.
- Finally, for the chain of infection to continue, the pathogen has to find a hospitable host. This link is called **host susceptibility.** The presence of a pathogen in the body does not necessarily mean that a person has to get sick from it. When conditions are right, the pathogens multiply and produce disease in the new host.

The chain of infection is a useful analogy for understanding how to prevent the spread of an infectious disease. Any link in the chain of infection represents a possible point of intervention. If any one of the links of the chain is broken or missing, the spread of infection can be stopped. For example, even before infectious diseases were fully understood, people used a method of quarantine to limit the spread of disease. By preventing noninfected persons from coming into contact with infected persons, the act of quarantine successfully cut the chain of infection by restricting the reservoir of the pathogen, one of the early links in the chain.

Most modern efforts at controlling infectious disease have been directed at breaking the last link in the chain, host susceptibility, through immunization. Scientists believe that through adequate immunization, the pool of people who are susceptible to infection can be reduced and eventually eliminated. Smallpox was controlled and eventually eradicated through this process. **Eradication** means that the first link in the chain, the pathogen, no longer exists in adequate amounts to cause disease. In the case of AIDS, there currently is no vaccine, so the focus of control is on the means of transmission—semen, vaginal secretions, and blood. By promoting abstinence, condom use for sexually active people, clean needles for injecting drug users, and a safe blood supply, the chain of infection can be broken.

Causes of Infection

Everything has to be caused by something, and infection is no different. There are six basic pathogens, or causative agents of infection.

Bacteria are single-celled, plant-like microbes that act in a variety of ways to produce symptoms of infection. For example, they produce **toxins,** or poisons, in the body. Although bacteria reproduce inside the body, they do so outside the human cell as well and thus can be killed or inhibited by **antibiotics.** Strep throat, tuberculosis, pneumonia, gonorrhea, cholera, and whooping cough are examples of infections caused by bacteria.

Viruses, chains of nucleic acid surrounded by a protein coat, are the most primitive form of life and cannot reproduce on their own. However, when they invade the human cell, they use the cell's reproductive capabilities. They are the tiniest and toughest of infectious pathogens. Antibiotics have no effect on viruses, and in most cases no drugs exist that can kill them. Some physicians prescribe antibiotics for patients who have influenza to prevent **secondary infection,** but they have no effect on the influenza itself. **Interferon,** a protective substance made by the body, is one of the main means of attacking viruses. Some viral infections have been successfully prevented with vaccines. Examples of infections caused by viruses include the common cold, influenza, measles, rabies, herpes, smallpox, and AIDS.

Protozoa are single-celled parasites that produce toxins and release enzymes that interrupt the body's ability to function normally. Protozoa-caused infections, such as malaria, sleeping sickness, and amoebic dysentery, are generally associated with a tropical environment and poor sanitation and are not a public health problem in the United States. The one major exception is giardiasis, which can be caught by drinking contaminated water. Hikers and travelers to countries where giardia is prevalent, such as Russia and other former Soviet bloc countries, are especially at risk for getting giardiasis. Protozoan infections can be treated with drugs.

As the name indicates, **parasitic worms** are multicelled animals usually shaped like flat or round worms. They release toxins inside the body and feed off blood and compete for food with the host. As a result, people infected with worms, for example, tapeworms, are often anemic and malnourished. Most worm infections can be treated successfully with drugs and can often be prevented with good hygiene and proper cooking of food. Trichinosis is an example of a parasitic infection caused by not cooking pork thoroughly.

Fungi are either single-celled or multicelled plant-like organisms that usually grow on the surface of the skin. They release enzymes that in turn digest cells. Antifungal topical ointments and drugs can kill fungi. Athlete's foot is an example of an infection caused by a fungus. Fungi are also **allergens** and in some parts of the country cause considerable discomfort.

A microorganism that is often described as somewhere between viruses and bacteria is **rickettsia.** It is much larger than a virus, is treated with antibiotics, and is parasitic in nature (it requires living cells for growth). Rickettsias are usually transmitted by insects, such as ticks. Common rickettsial diseases are Rocky Mountain spotted fever and typhus.

Prions are made of protein and do not contain any genes or genetic material. This feature distinguishes them from the other kinds of infectious agents discussed above. It is believed that these nonliving proteins can reproduce themselves, and thereby spread disease. Some scientists question the soundness of the prion hypothesis, but the scientist who discovered them, Stanley B. Prusiner,

reservoir of the pathogen A place (either a human or an animal) where a pathogen resides.

portal of exit The means by which the pathogen moves out of the source into a new host.

vectors Insects or animals that carry disease.

host susceptibility The ease with which a person is exposed to and becomes infected by a pathogen.

eradication The removal of a disease by the elimination of all reservoirs of the disease-causing pathogen. Smallpox was eradicated.

bacteria Single-celled, plant-like microbes that act to produce symptoms of infection.

toxin A poisonous substance produced by a microorganism; can cause certain infectious diseases.

antibiotic A chemical substance that destroys or inhibits the growth of bacteria.

virus A chain of nucleic acid surrounded by a protein coat that invades cells and uses the cells' reproductive capabilities.

secondary infection An infection that occurs in conjunction with, or as a result of, another infection but arises from a different pathogen.

interferon A chemical substance produced by white blood cells that "interferes" with growth of a virus and also inhibits the virus's ability to infect cells; also made synthetically.

protozoa Single-celled parasites that produce toxins and release enzymes that interrupt the body's ability to function normally.

parasitic worms Multicelled animals that release toxins inside the body, feed on blood, and compete with the host for food.

fungi Single-celled or multicelled plant-like organisms that usually grow on the surface of the skin.

allergen A substance that is perceived by the body as an irritant; induces an allergic or hypersensitive state or reaction.

rickettsia A rod-shaped microorganism that is transmitted by vectors and causes a variety of diseases, such as typhus.

prion A mutated, three-dimensional protein that changes the shape of surrounding prions, causing pockets of diseased and dying brain cells.

was awarded the Nobel Prize for his work in 1997, thus granting it institutional validity.

Prions reside naturally in the brain cells of people and animals and normally do no harm. When they mutate into an abnormal shape, however, they change the surrounding prions into defective three-dimensional forms as well. These newly shaped prions multiply throughout the brain like a spreading infection, and pockets of the affected brain tissue gradually die. There is strong evidence that diseases characterized by poor muscle coordination and memory loss, such as mad cow disease and Creutzfeldt-Jakob disease, are caused by prions. See Table 14.1 for a comparison of common infectious diseases.

Critical Thinking Question

> The *Healthy People 2000* objectives include the following: "Reduce the following indigenous cases of vaccine-preventable diseases to zero in the United States: Diphtheria among people aged 25 and younger; tetanus among people aged 25 and younger; and polio among all age groups." Given the fact that no cases of diphtheria were recorded in 1995, and no cases of indigenous polio have been recorded since data have been collected for the national objectives, why should this particular objective be maintained? Shouldn't we declare that we have eradicated these three diseases in the United States?

How Infections Get into Your Body

When an infected person coughs or sneezes, microorganisms may be carried *through the air* on droplets of moisture and breathed in by another individual. Mumps, measles, and chickenpox are spread through the air. Until recently, it was thought that this was the primary means of spreading colds and influenza, but research now shows that they spread more *through direct physical contact*, such

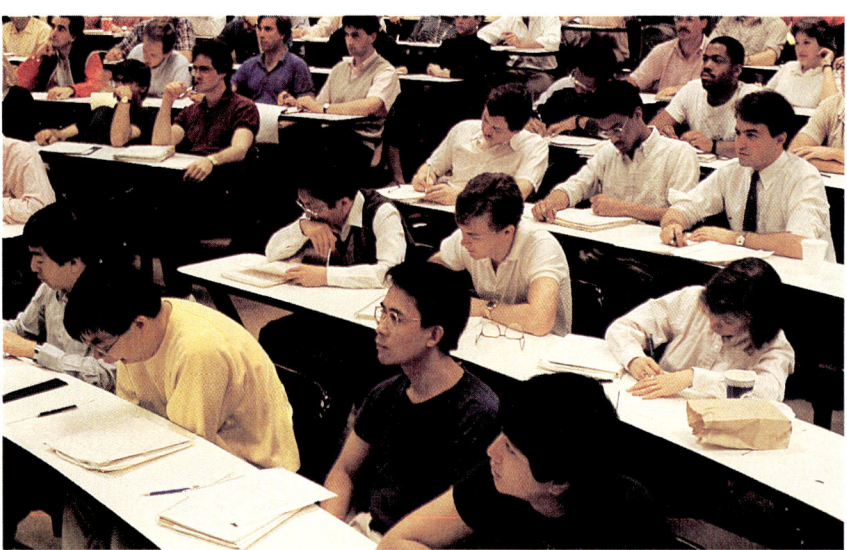

Infectious agents that can cause illnesses such as mumps and measles are spread through the air. This is why some diseases can quickly spread around a college campus. (Source: © Tony Stone Images/Joseph Nettis)

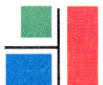

TABLE 14.1 Common Infectious Diseases by Cause

Cause	Disease	Cause	Disease
Bacteria	Botulism		Mumps
	Cholera		Papilloma
	Dental caries		Polio
	Diphtheria		Smallpox
	Gonorrhea	**Protozoa**	Amoebic dysentery
	Legionnaires' disease		Giardiasis
	Lyme disease		Malaria
	Meningitis		Sleeping sickness
	Pertussis (whooping cough)		
	Pneumonia	**Parasitic worms**	Tapeworm disease
	Scarlet fever		Trichinosis
	Staph infection		Pinworm
	Strep throat		Hookworm
	Toxic shock syndrome	**Fungi**	Athlete's foot
	Tuberculosis		Valley fever
Viruses	AIDS		Ringworm
	Chickenpox		Histoplasmosis
	Common cold	**Rickettsias**	Rocky Mountain spotted fever
	Hantavirus		Typhus
	Hepatitis		
	Herpes	**Prion**	Creutzfeldt-Jakob
	Influenza		Bovine spongiform encephalopathy (mad cow disease)
	Measles		
	Mononucleosis		

as through shaking hands, hugging, and kissing. Cold viruses can also be transmitted from inanimate objects through direct physical contact, for example, from a glass used by a person who has a cold. Examples of other infectious diseases carried through direct physical contact include sexually transmitted diseases and leprosy. See the Developing Health Skills box to learn how important hand washing is.

Another means of transmission is *by contaminated food and water*. Hookworm can come from eating contaminated food, and giardiasis and cholera from drinking or swimming in contaminated water. Still other diseases are carried *by vectors,* insects or animals that carry diseases. Plague is carried by fleas that live on rats, malaria is carried by mosquitoes, and Lyme disease is carried by deer ticks.

Some diseases are not carried at all; they are simply *already there,* living in a controlled state within a person's body. That person develops symptoms of disease only when something upsets the body's normal state, which allows the infecting organism to begin reproducing. For example, women normally have yeast growing in their vaginas. Taking antibiotics, however, can change the environment of the vagina so that yeast growth takes place at a greater-than-normal pace, which in turn can result in yeast infection. Yeast infection is discussed in Chapter 15.

Why Everyone Doesn't Get Sick

Not everyone gets sick when exposed to a disease-causing pathogen. This is because the conditions associated with getting sick can vary widely. First, the

DEVELOPING HEALTH SKILLS

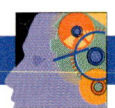

Do You Wash Your Hands?

A recent survey of people in public rest rooms confirmed that the spread of at least some infectious diseases could be curbed if greater attention was spent on hand washing after going to the bathroom. Dirty hands can spread diseases ranging from colds to diarrhea to other intestinal problems.

A report to medical researchers and epidemiologists attending a American Society of Microbiology meeting confirmed that:

- Only 60 percent of people using the rest rooms at Pennsylvania Station in New York City washed up. Other cities have higher rates: 71 percent washed up at a casino in New Orleans, 69 percent at the Golden Gate Park in San Francisco, and 64 percent at a Braves game in Atlanta.
- Women wash up more than men: 74 percent of women washed their hands, but only 61 percent of men did. However, men used soap more often than women did.

virulence, or strength, of the causative agent may vary even among pathogens causing the same disease. You might be exposed to a highly virulent strain of a virus, for example, while your neighbor is exposed to a weaker strain of the same virus. You would most likely show symptoms, but your neighbor might never know he or she had been exposed to an infectious disease.

Second, dosages or the amount of pathogens present during disease transmission, can vary widely. Your roommate might be exposed to a large dosage of the bacterium that causes strep throat, perhaps from kissing a person who is infected. Another classmate might be exposed to only a small dosage, perhaps from breathing the droplets of moisture exhaled by an infected person. Your roommate stands the better chance of becoming infected.

Finally, the **resistance** of individuals to infection varies. Resistance is the capacity of the immune system to handle the invasion of an organism. Some people have a strong resistance to disease; others have a low resistance. It is possible that too much stress can lower your resistance. People who have a high resistance to disease are less likely to get sick even when exposed to infections. No one, however, goes through life infection-free, and even the hardiest of people have bouts of illness over a lifetime.

Nonspecific Lines of Defense

Given that we are constantly surrounded by disease-causing organisms, our bodies have developed highly successful ways to prevent pathogens from entering the body, and, in the event that they do, to prevent them from causing illness. **Nonspecific defense mechanisms** include the skin, the mucous membranes, cilia, and a general chemical defense mechanism called phagocytes. The skin, for example, serves as a mechanical barrier as long as it remains intact. The **mucous membranes** that line the passageways leading into the body trap foreign material in their sticky secretions. And the cilia of the mucous membranes in the upper respiratory tract sweep impurities out of the body.

Body secretions, such as digestive juices and tears, may contain acids or enzymes that destroy invading organisms. Finally, certain reflexes aid in preventing foreign matter, including microorganisms, from entering the body; sneezing, vomiting, and diarrhea are reflexes that expel pathogens.

If a pathogen successfully passes these physical barriers, it will encounter one of the nonspecific chemical defense mechanisms of disease prevention: phagocytes, interferon, and inflammation. **Phagocytes** are white blood cells that attack foreign invaders such as bacteria. For example, when an injury occurs, such as a cut in the skin, phagocytes are attracted to the area, where they surround invading bacterial cells and render them harmless. As the phagocytes do their work, large numbers of them are destroyed, so eventually the area around the cut becomes filled with dead white blood cells, a substance often referred to as pus.

The body produces another line of defense against viruses: interferon, a chemical substance produced by white cells that "interferes" with the growth of a virus and inhibits the viruses' ability to infect cells. Interferon works against all viruses, so it is considered a nonspecific defense mechanism. This substance is actually produced by virus-infected cells, yet provides protection for uninfected cells, thus preventing the spread of viral infection. Interferon represents great promise in the search for a cure for viral infection. Unfortunately, producing interferon in the laboratory is extremely expensive, meaning that it cannot be routinely used by medical science. Synthetic versions of interferon, made by genetic engineering, have been used to treat viral infections and some types of cancer.

Throughout the time that phagocytes and interferon are fighting infection, inflammation occurs. **Inflammation** is the heat, redness, swelling, and discomfort that results from increased blood flow and secretions of histamine and other substances in the infected tissue. Often, inflammation is the first symptom of infection.

Immunity: The Final Line of Defense

Immunity is the most complex, most specific, and final line of defense against disease. **Immunity** is best understood as the body's ability to destroy pathogens that it has encountered in the past, before they are able to cause disease. Whereas the defenses against disease we have presented thus far are nonspecific (they act to prevent or reduce the harm of all invaders), immunity is specific not only to each disease, but also to each strain of organism that causes disease. Because of its specificity, the human body's immune system provides a remarkable line of defense against disease-causing and noxious substances.

Active and Passive Immunity

Immunity to an infectious disease means that the body is resistant to a particular organism that produces infection. There are two kinds of immunity: active and passive. In **active immunity,** the body develops its own resistance to disease. For example, once you've had measles, your body develops a lifelong immunity to the disease. In **passive immunity,** resistance to disease initially comes from an external source. Infants who are breast-fed carry passive immunity to certain diseases because they receive protective antibodies from their mothers' milk. This immunity usually lasts only about as long as the mother breast-feeds.

The key factor in both active and passive immunity is the presence of antibodies. **Antibodies** are specific proteins that are produced principally in the blood in response to foreign substances in the body called **antigens** (for antibody generators). The antibodies react specifically with the antigen that produced them. To return to the example of measles, if you are infected with the measles virus, your body first recognizes the measles antigen, then begins to produce antibodies unique to the measles virus. It takes several days for the body to produce enough antibodies to get rid of the measles virus and to build up an immunity to measles. If you are exposed to measles a year later, the antibodies already in your blood protect you from getting the disease.

virulence The strength of pathogens present during disease transmission.

resistance The capacity of the immune system to fight the invasion of an organism.

nonspecific defense mechanisms The body's various barriers to all disease; as opposed to those defense mechanisms intended to prevent one particular disease.

mucous membranes The moist, protective lining that covers some of the openings to the body and the air passages.

phagocytes White blood cells that attack and consume foreign cells.

inflammation The body's response to injury; it fights infection and promotes healing.

immunity The body's ability to destroy pathogens that it has once encountered, before they are able to cause disease.

active immunity The body's development of its own resistance to disease.

passive immunity Resistance to disease that initially comes from an external source.

antibodies Specific proteins that are produced principally in the blood in response to foreign substances in the body.

antigens Foreign substances in the body that cause the production of antibodies.

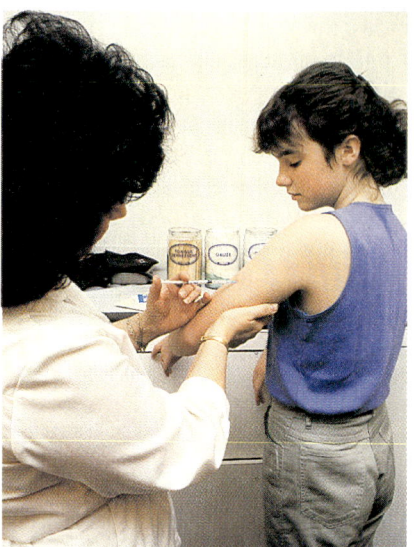

To make sure your immunizations are up-to-date, check with the college health service. A shot in the arm is good protection against infectious diseases. (Source: © Tony Stone Images/John Riley)

A Shot of Protection

A single measles vaccine can provide the immunity you need to protect yourself from this potentially damaging disease. Once vaccinated against measles or a number of other diseases, the immune system is prepared to produce the appropriate antibodies. Thus, when exposed to measles, you do not get the disease. Some vaccinations provide lifetime immunity and others require periodic updates. For example, you need to get a vaccination against mumps only once in your life, but you need a new tetanus shot every ten years or when treated for a puncture wound if more than five years have elapsed since the last booster (see the Here's Looking at You box).

Vaccinations are made in four different ways: with a live but weakened virus, with a dead virus, with a virus closely related to but weaker than that for which immunity is sought, or with a nonpoisonous version of a toxin produced by a bacterial agent.

Critical Thinking Question

> Many parents fail to make sure that their children are immunized. Perhaps this is due to parental fear that their children will contract polio or pertussis from a vaccination. Or perhaps this is due to simple negligence. One of the most successful means of assuring immunizations, however, is to ask schools to require that entering students provide evidence that they have "had their shots." What might be other means of assuring immunization, particularly among non-school-aged populations?

For example, the polio vaccine developed by Dr. Jonas Salk and approved for mass use in 1955 uses a killed virus, and the one developed by Dr. Albert Sabin and approved for mass use in 1961 uses live but weakened polio viruses. There are other differences between the two vaccines. The Salk vaccine is injected into

HERE'S LOOKING AT YOU

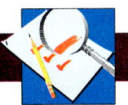

Keep Your Immunizations Up-to-Date

Keep a record of your immunization history. You will need this for enrollment in school and travel to exotic places, and to show another physician if you move or change physicians. The following list identifies the vaccinations that you may need, as an adult.

Type of immunity	Frequency of booster doses	Your status
Cholera	Every 6 months while exposed	_____
Diphtheria	Every 10 years	_____
Hepatitis B	Every 5 years for high-risk individuals	_____
Influenza	Every year for people 65 or older and those with chronic illnesses	_____
Measles	In late adolescence or early adulthood	_____
Mumps	Lifetime immunity	_____
Plague	Every 3 to 6 months while exposed	_____
Pneumococcal pneumonia	Once for people 65 or older and those with chronic illnesses	_____
Polio	Only when exposure is anticipated	_____
Tetanus	Every 10 years or when treated for a puncture wound if more than 5 years have elapsed since last booster	_____
Typhoid fever	Only if traveling to a location where this disease is prevalent	_____
Typhus	Every year if exposed	_____
Yellow fever	Only if traveling to a location where this disease is prevalent	_____

the body; the Sabin vaccine is taken by mouth, usually on a lump of sugar. Prior to these vaccines, more than thirty thousand cases of polio a year occurred in the United States. When the polio virus attacks the spine, paralysis of the legs results; when the virus gets into the brain, it paralyzes muscles needed for breathing, swallowing, and other body functions. Because of the widespread use of the vaccine, the United States has been nearly free of polio for more than a decade. In fact, the only recorded cases are related to the vaccine itself, not because there is any polio virus in the environment.

This illustrates a major controversy about the safety of vaccines: Is it better to have the dead Salk vaccine or the live Sabin one? The benefits and risks of immunization are being weighed heavily in the cases of diphtheria, pertussis, and tetanus. (A combined vaccine for these three diseases is known as the DPT vaccine.) Pertussis, also called whooping cough, is one of the most virulent of the traditional childhood diseases, and it can kill 1 of every 100 affected children. On the benefit side of the vaccine ledger, fewer than 10 babies out of 3.5 million immunized in the United States die each year from pertussis. On the risk side, about 35 children develop brain damage each year from the effects of the pertussis part of the DPT vaccination. Some parents who are worried about the pertussis vaccine risks have their children immunized with a DT shot—it vaccinates against diphtheria and tetanus only. As a result, the incidence of pertussis infection has increased in recent years.

Protecting yourself or your family against an infectious disease by keeping immunizations up-to-date is only one aspect of immunity. Another is protecting the community by reducing the overall incidence through **herd immunity**. With herd immunity, a large proportion of the population is vaccinated against a par-

herd immunity The vaccination of a large proportion of a population against a particular disease to significantly reduce the chances of spread of infection.

ticular disease, thus significantly reducing the chances of infection in any one individual. Mass immunization against smallpox is an example of using the concept of herd immunity.

Critical Thinking Question

> The economic benefits of the Smallpox Eradication Program have been substantial for all of the world's countries, as preventive measures and treatment facilities for smallpox are no longer needed. According to the CDC, the cost to the United States for the successful thirteen-year campaign to eradicate smallpox throughout the world was about $30 million. Since smallpox was eradicated in 1977, this total investment is returned to the United States every twenty-six days in the form of medical expense savings. What other diseases do you think might be eradicated through an effective education campaign coupled with immunization? Why do you think the United States has failed to "invest" in such a campaign?

Disorders of the Immune System

The immune system is not perfect, and there are several ways in which it can break down. **Autoimmune diseases** are particularly difficult because they cause the body to attack itself. In essence, the antibodies attack the body's own cells as if they were invading infections. Examples of autoimmune diseases are lupus erythematosus, which affects mainly women aged eighteen to thirty-five, causes pain and anemia, and can result in death; multiple sclerosis, a crippling central nervous system disease; myasthenia gravis, a nerve conduction disease that causes weakness of the muscles, especially in the face and neck; and rheumatoid arthritis, a debilitating joint disease.

Allergies are the result of the body's overzealous response to an allergen, a substance perceived as an irritant. Allergens can be dust, ragweed, pollen, dog hair, or foods, even chocolate. In allergic people, the allergen produces a high level of antibodies that in turn release histamine, a chemical in the skin, respiratory passages, and digestive tract. Depending on the allergic response, a person can experience intense itching, difficulty breathing, or diarrhea and vomiting.

Allergies are very complex, and histamine is but one component. In addition, there is more to allergies than an overactive immune response. Allergies are often tied to a person's psychological or emotional state. Many allergies decline during adolescence, but a significant number of people do not have allergic symptoms until they are adults. The mechanism and timing of allergies are still poorly understood.

Immune deficiency diseases may be inherited. This is the case with *agammaglobulinemia*, a rare genetic autoimmune disease that results in the body's inability to produce any antibodies. It is, in essence, the breakdown of the immune system. A youth identified only as David, who was born with this deficiency, lived his entire life in a germ-free bubble in a Texas hospital, waiting for medical researchers to discover a way for his body to develop antibodies. David died at age twelve when he chose to lead a life outside the bubble. He lived only a few months.

autoimmune disease A disease in which antibodies attack the body's own cells as if they were an invading infection.

allergy The result of the body's overzealous response to an allergen.

immune deficiency disease Any of a variety of diseases or syndromes that compromise the immune system.

incubation The stage during which there are no symptoms of disease and, in most cases, the infected person is not contagious.

prodromal stage A highly contagious period in a disease in which some symptoms may be apparent but the infected person does not feel ill.

Finally, immune deficiency may be acquired, as is evident by the full name of the disease AIDS—acquired immune deficiency syndrome. AIDS is caused by the human immunodeficiency virus (HIV), which destroys one of the key elements in the immune response, T-lymphocytes, and results in a compromised immune system. HIV is often transmitted sexually and therefore is covered in more detail in Chapter 15.

Can You Boost Your Own Immunity?

You've read about how psychoneuroimmunology is used as a treatment for cancer. Is it really possible to laugh away a cold or to think positively and fight back the AIDS virus or other infectious agents? Psychologists and immunologists are working together on this mind–body connection and tentatively report that it may be possible to boost your own immunity with positive thinking.

In one study involving homosexual men at risk for AIDS, training in aerobics, relaxation, and stress management resulted in an increase of more than 10 percent in levels of the immune system's T-4 cells, which usually decline in number as infection with HIV progresses. According to the researchers, the goal of this training is to delay the onset of AIDS itself. Although these findings are tantalizing, work on the mind–body connection is still in its infancy, and more needs to be known before we know whether you can actually laugh away a disease.

Stages of Infectious Disease

Although communicable diseases differ in how they are caused, there is a general pattern to the course of infectious diseases (see Figure 14.2). After the causative agent finds a hospitable host and begins multiplying, there is a period of **incubation**. During this time, there are no symptoms of disease, and in most cases, the infected person is not contagious. Incubation usually lasts a few days to two weeks.

Next comes the **prodromal stage,** which is a highly contagious period. Some symptoms are usually apparent, but the person does not feel sick enough to stay at home. Sometimes during the prodromal stage, an infected person has no symptoms and does not even know he or she is infected. Disease is easily and unknowingly spread during this time.

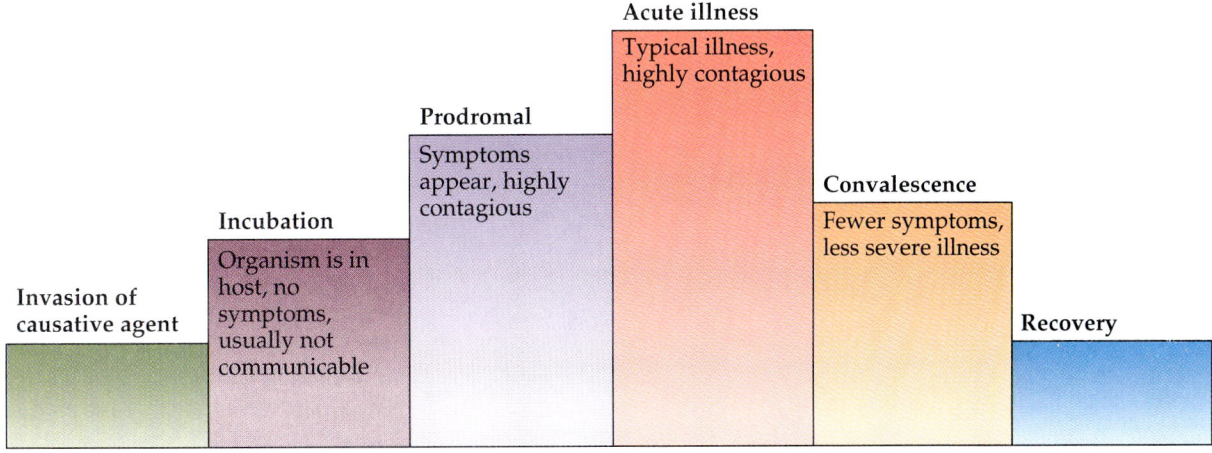

Figure 14.2 Stages of Disease. *Infectious diseases follow a course of action beginning with incubation, progressing through the prodromal stage, acute illness, convalescence, and finally, recovery.*

The **acute stage** of illness occurs when symptoms are fully developed. These differ for each disease. Chickenpox looks different from measles. A cold manifests itself differently from tuberculosis. During the acute stage, the infected person remains highly contagious.

The final stages of an infectious disease are **convalescence,** a decline in the severity of symptoms, and **recovery,** when the infection is successfully defeated and the body returns to its healthy state. During these stages, the infection leaves the body through mucus, pus, blood, feces, tears, sweat, and other flushing processes. In some infectious diseases, such as AIDS, a person may remain in the acute stage, never reaching convalescence or recovery.

Critical Thinking Question

One of the most common mistakes made when treating a bacterial disease is to take enough prescribed antibiotic to treat the symptoms of the disease but not enough to fully treat the disease itself. This can "knock out" the least virulent strain of the bacteria and leave the harder-to-treat strains still in the body. Such a practice not only leads to a relapse but also can contribute to the development of a more virulent strain of the infectious agent. What kinds of implications can this practice have on public health? What might public health officials do to change such behaviors?

Common Infectious Diseases

Each year, Americans lose 2 billion days from school, work, and other major activities because of illnesses from infectious diseases (see Table 14.2). Given the enormity of the problem, it is reassuring to know that most of us recover from these illnesses. Upper respiratory infections, colds, and influenza cost $5 billion in direct medical costs for visits to physicians and for medication but cause little mortality. The killer infectious diseases include AIDS, pneumonia, meningitis, and hepatitis B. Furthermore, because people who have AIDS have severely compromised immune systems, they are also more susceptible to infectious diseases such as pneumonia and tuberculosis. Table 14.3 illustrates trends in selected infectious diseases. The incidence of some diseases has declined markedly since 1950 and 1960, and some rose. Some of today's diseases hadn't even been discovered then.

Common Cold

The cold is indeed common. The average adult in the United States has at least two colds a year, and children have as many as twelve. Colds are caused by more than 120 rhinoviruses (*rhino* is the Greek word for "nose") as well as by adenoviruses, influenza viruses, and other viruses. Put them all together and you have more than 1 billion colds a year, which means a lot of runny noses, watery eyes, sore throats, headaches, fevers, aches, and pains.

DEVELOPING HEALTH SKILLS

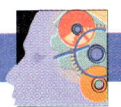

How to Cope with a Common Cold

Although a cold is not life threatening, getting one is annoying and always seems to come at the wrong time—just before final exams or during a vacation. Although there is no cure, common sense and the following tips will help you get through a cold, which typically runs seven to nine days.

- Get plenty of rest.
- Drink extra fluids—water, fruit juices, tea, and, yes, chicken soup—to loosen the phlegm. Hot liquids of any sort are likely to soothe the sore throat that often accompanies a cold.
- Add humidity with a humidifier or vaporizer. The moist air helps your lungs get rid of germs and can relieve the pain of a sore throat. You can also get relief from the steam rising off a bowl of chicken soup.
- To help ease a cough, gargle with warm, salty water or take cough suppressant medicine.
- For a stuffed nose, try a decongestant nasal spray or drops. Be sure to follow recommended dosages.
- Take aspirin or acetaminophen to reduce fever and muscular aches.

Cold viruses are highly contagious. They contaminate the air and surfaces such as telephones and doorknobs and can survive in these environments for several hours or even days. You are likely to get a cold if you (1) breathe air filled with cold viruses, (2) shake hands with someone who has a cold virus on his or her hands, or (3) touch a virus-laden surface and then touch your own eyes or nose. Recent research indicates that more colds are spread by hand-to-hand contact than through the air and that families who wash hands frequently have significantly fewer colds.

Although washing your hands frequently during the winter months can reduce your risk of catching a cold, it is virtually impossible not to be exposed to cold viruses and ultimately to succumb to them. This means that you can count on getting a cold again and again and again. In 1970, Nobel Prize-winning chemist Linus Pauling began promoting large doses of vitamin C as a way to prevent colds, but his research has been controversial.

The bad news is that there is no cure for a cold. But the good news is that once you get a cold, it lasts for only about a week (see the Developing Health Skills box).

Influenza

Influenza, sometimes called the flu, has many of the same symptoms as a cold—congestion, sore throat, fever, aches, and pains—but they are more severe and last longer. For example, it is not uncommon for adults who have the flu to have temperatures as high as 103 degrees Fahrenheit or for temperatures to rise as high as 105 degrees Fahrenheit in children.

Flu viruses are transmitted much the same way cold viruses are, except that flu viruses are more contagious. Moreover, the flu can be deadly, particularly for young children, the elderly, and those in ill health. A worldwide influenza epidemic that took place in 1918 and 1919 killed 20 million people.

Vaccines are available against some flu viruses, but because strains mutate, or change, and new ones emerge, vaccination cannot provide full immunity. The flu vaccine, which must be taken annually, is recommended for the elderly, those with chronic illnesses, and other people at high risk. Influenza is treated the same

acute stage The stage at which symptoms of a disease are fully developed.

convalescence A state characterized by a decline in the severity of disease symptoms.

recovery A period in which infection is successfully defeated and the body returns to its healthy state.

influenza A severe viral infection involving the respiratory tract.

TABLE 14.2 Common Infectious Diseases

Disease name	Pathogen	How transmitted	Symptoms	Preventive measures	Treatment
AIDS	Virus	By direct contact with infected person, usually during sexual intercourse (anal, vaginal), and by exchange of blood	Often no symptoms exist; combination of weight loss, night sweats, cough, new skin rashes, changes in bowel function; unexplained chronic fever	Avoid sexual contact and blood exchange with infected person; use a condom; do not share needles	No known cure; protease inhibitors, AZT, and other drugs taken orally can decrease symptoms; treat opportunistic diseases associated with AIDS
Athlete's foot	Fungus	By contact with organism, usually on shower floors, towels, or by direct contact with infected person	Rash, peeling of skin; severe itching	Keep feet dry, change socks frequently, use antifungal foot powder	Antifungal creams/powders
Chickenpox	Virus	By air, through inhalation of droplets exhaled from infected person	Rash develops 2–3 days after inhalation of virus; fever and itching of lesions over the body, perhaps mouth or throat	Immunization	Trim fingernails closely; oral acyclovir; calamine lotion, oral antihistamines for itching; acetaminophen or ibuprofen (not aspirin) for fever
Cold	Virus	By air, through inhalation of droplets exhaled from infected person; by direct contact	Runny nose; itchy eyes; generally uncomfortable feeling; nasal congestion; sore throat; cough	Avoid contact with infected individuals	Treat with bed rest, plenty of fluids, and aspirin, acetaminophen, or ibuprofen for relief of pain; pseudoephedrine for congestion
German measles (rubella)	Virus	By air, through inhalation of droplets exhaled from infected person; by direct contact	Rash; swelling of lymph nodes; fever (mild)	Immunization	Gamma globulin may block symptoms; fluids; rest

TABLE 14.2 Common Infectious Diseases (continued)

Disease name	Pathogen	How transmitted	Symptoms	Preventive measures	Treatment
Influenza	Virus	By air, through inhalation of droplets exhaled from infected person; by direct contact	Fever for 1–7 days; nausea; sudden tiredness; vomiting; aching muscles; headache; sore throat; bronchitis	Immunization for high-risk persons (especially the elderly)	Fluids; aspirin (not young children), acetaminophen or ibuprofen to control fever; rest
Measles (rubeola)	Virus	By air, through inhalation of droplets exhaled from infected person; by direct contact	Red spotty rash; off-and-on high fever; unpleasant cough	Immunization	Aspirin, acetaminophen, or ibuprofen to avoid temperature variation; bland oral fluids
Mononucleosis	Virus	By direct contact	Severe sore throat; swollen lymph glands; tiredness; white spots on tonsils, tongue, and soft palate; enlarged spleen	Avoid contact with infected individuals	Confirm disease via blood count test for unusual white blood cells, positive mono-spot test; treat with bed rest; oral rinse for throat
Whooping cough (pertussis)	Bacterium	By air, through inhalation of droplets exhaled from infected person; by direct contact	Cough, sometimes creating a loud "whooping" sound; fever; vomiting	Immunization; antibiotic to household contacts of infected individuals	Antibiotics, corticosteroids in specific stages; frequent small feedings; cough medicines are of only slight benefit; careful observation

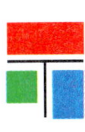

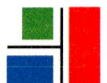

TABLE 14.3 Selected Infectious Disease Trends: Reported Cases in the United States

Disease	1950	1960	1970	1980	1990	1996
Acquired immune deficiency syndrome (AIDS)	—	—	—	—	41,595	66,885
Diphtheria	5,796	918	435	3	4	2
Hepatitis A	NA*	NA	56,797	29,087	31,441	31,032
Hepatitis B	NA	NA	8,310	19,015	21,102	10,637
Hepatitis C	—	—	—	—	2,553	3,716
Legionellosis (Legionnaires' disease)	—	—	—	475	1,370	1,198
Malaria		72	3,051	2,062	1,292	1,800
Measles (rubeola)	NA	NA	47,351	13,506	27,786	508
Measles, German (rubella)	NA	NA	56,552	13,506	1,125	238
Measles, combined	319,124	441,703	NA	NA	NA	NA
Mumps		NA	104,963	8,576	5,292	751
Pertussis (whooping cough)	120,718	14,809	4,249	1,730	4,570	7,796
Poliomyelitis, paralytic	33,300	2,525	31	8	7	5
Smallpox	Last documented case occurred in 1949					
Toxic shock syndrome (TSS)	—	—	—	—	322	145
Tuberculosis	121,742	55,494	37,137	27,749	25,701	21,337

Source: U.S. Centers for Disease Control and Prevention
*NA = Not available.
Note: AIDS and TSS data reflect post-1980 discovery of an infectious agent; legionellosis data reflect post-1970 discovery of an infectious agent.

way as a cold, except that children and adolescents should not take aspirin when they have the flu. Youngsters have a significantly increased risk for Reye's syndrome, a potentially fatal condition associated with taking aspirin. Instead, to reduce symptoms, children should take nonaspirin pain relievers.

Pneumonia

Pneumonia, an inflammation of the lung tissue, is among the leading causes of death in the United States. Pneumonia has more than fifty known causes, including viruses, bacteria, and chemical irritants. Although people over age sixty-five account for most of the deaths from pneumonia, the mortality rate is rising among young adults. This is due to an increase in the number and types of pneumonia-causing bacteria that are resistant to antibiotics; a worsening of air pollution, which can make the lungs more susceptible to bacterial infection; and a rise in the number of pneumocystic pneumonia cases, especially among people infected with HIV.

Bacterial pneumonia is the main type of pneumonia that follows an attack of influenza. It is also the most frequent type of pneumonia in older people. The pneumonia bacteria normally live in the mouth or throat. The immune system usually provides protection, but pneumonia develops when the bacteria invade the lungs. One pneumonia-causing bacterium is *Legionella pneumophila,* also known as Legionnaires' disease because fifty-eight people became ill from it following a meeting of the American Legion in Philadelphia in 1976. A vaccine that protects against the most common pneumonia-causing bacterium lasts five years

pneumonia An inflammation of the lung tissue.

bacterial pneumonia Pneumonia that develops as a result of invasion of the lungs by bacteria.

mycoplasma A tiny microorganism and causative agent of many diseases of the joints and lungs.

fungal pneumonia Inflammation of the lungs caused by a fungus.

mononucleosis A disease of unknown cause; symptoms include fever, headache, nausea, extreme fatigue, and swollen spleen and lymph nodes.

chronic fatigue syndrome A group of symptoms that result in a prolonged state of fatigue.

or longer and is recommended for people over age sixty-five and others with chronic illnesses.

Mycoplasmas and viruses, which are spread through droplets in the air or by contaminated hands, cause pneumonia primarily in children and young adults. The influenza virus is a deadly cause of pneumonia, particularly for pregnant women and people who have heart or pulmonary disease. **Fungal pneumonia** is rare, but a pneumonia called valley fever caused by fungi in the soil is more prevalent in Southern California and other places where people are already sensitized by smog in the air.

A chest X-ray gives the clearest evidence of lung inflammation and pneumonia. Antibiotics are used for treating bacterial pneumonia; other forms are treated by rest and the body's natural healing capabilities.

Mononucleosis

A disease caused by the Epstein-Barr virus and transmitted in saliva by kissing or other person-to-person contact, **mononucleosis,** or "mono," strikes primarily adolescents and young adults. It is most common among fifteen- to nineteen-year-olds, followed by those in the twenty- to twenty-four-year-old range. Symptoms include fever, headache, nausea, extreme fatigue, and swollen spleen and lymph nodes. The disease is debilitating, and recovery requires several weeks and sometimes months. Although most of the symptoms usually last only two to three weeks, a person recovering from mononucleosis can expect to feel fatigued for several more weeks.

Mononucleosis can be detected by a blood test. The only treatment is rest and drinking plenty of liquids.

Chronic Fatigue Syndrome

Most people suffer from periods of fatigue, but people who have **chronic fatigue syndrome** suffer for prolonged periods—for six months and longer. In addition, they have several other symptoms, including muscle and joint pain, sore throat, impaired short-term memory or concentration, headaches, unrefreshing sleep, and lingering tiredness after exercise.

Chronic fatigue syndrome is a relatively new condition—it was first defined in 1988—and its cause is still unknown. Some physicians, in fact, doubt that it is a distinct disease. It was initially linked to the Epstein-Barr virus (EBV), which can cause a chronic active infection that results in persistent fatigue. However, subsequent research has indicated that people who have chronic fatigue syndrome are no more likely to be infected with EBV than people not suffering from the disease.

A current hypothesis is that a virus, stress, or other transient traumatic condition may chronically activate the immune system. According to this hypothesis, the immune system, which ordinarily gears down after an infection has been eliminated, remains activated after the initiating condition has passed. The result is that unusually high concentrations of immune activating factors, some of which are known to cause fatigue at high doses, remain in the bloodstream.

Given that its causes are not known, treating chronic fatigue syndrome is difficult. General advice from physicians specializing in the disease include being as active as possible. Doctors sometimes prescribe low-dosage antidepressants to help patients sleep and feel better and other drugs to treat body pains. With these combined treatments, patients often improve.

Estimating how many people have chronic fatigue syndrome is also difficult. Based on surveillance data, the CDC estimates that it occurs in 4 to 10 adults in every 100,000, which means that 100,000 to 250,000 people nationwide suffer from it. But since many people who have this condition do not seek medical help

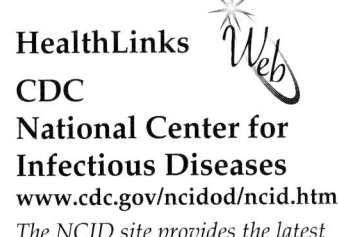

HealthLinks
CDC
National Center for Infectious Diseases
www.cdc.gov/ncidod/ncid.htm
The NCID site provides the latest information on emerging and re-emerging infectious diseases in the United States and throughout the world.

for it, it is possible that the incidence is considerably higher—and that between 0.5 million and 1.25 million people actually suffer chronic fatigue syndrome.

Tuberculosis

An airborne bacterial disease, **tuberculosis** (TB) is spread by inhaling germs called tubercle bacilli that come from someone who has a contagious form of TB. It is most easily spread in a crowded, poorly ventilated environment, which is why it is often associated with poverty.

TB initially affects the lungs, but it can also settle in almost any organ in the body, including the kidneys, brain, heart, liver, and bones. It causes patients to lose weight and energy. In the nineteenth century, it was called consumption because of the way it ate away, or "consumed," its victims.

The leading killer at the beginning of the twentieth century, TB was most often treated in sanitariums in the mountains in hope that breathing fresh country air would induce a remission. Mortality from it declined sharply in the United States with the introduction of antibiotics (as well as of improvements in sanitation, nutrition, and general standards of living). Now, however, TB has reemerged as a public health problem for several reasons. One is that many strains of TB have become resistant to the antibiotics used to treat the disease. Having more people infected with active TB contributes to the spread of the disease. Another is that people who have HIV are unusually prone to it and are an added reservoir for the infection. A third reason is the growing number of immigrants from Southeast Asia and Central America, regions where TB is prevalent. Other crowded areas where TB is spreading are homeless shelters and prisons.

TB can be detected by a simple skin test, and most forms are effectively treated by taking antituberculosis drugs for a period of six months or longer.

Hepatitis

Hepatitis is an inflammation of the liver usually caused by a virus. It is most often identified as three distinct diseases: hepatitis A, hepatitis B, and hepatitis C (formerly called non-A, non-B hepatitis). The **hepatitis A** virus is shed in the bowel movements of infected persons and is often spread in child care centers and other places filled with young children, mostly because of poor hand-washing habits. The incubation period ranges from fifteen to fifty days. During this time, there are no signs of disease, and it is possible for an infected person to spread hepatitis unknowingly before he or she develops symptoms. Hepatitis A symptoms vary widely in severity, ranging from mild, flu-like illnesses in young children to serious liver inflammation in the elderly. Some hepatitis patients become jaundiced (yellow). Gamma globulin can provide short-term immunity.

The **hepatitis B** virus circulates in the bloodstream and is excreted in the infected person's body fluids, including blood, saliva, semen, and vaginal secretions. It is seen mainly among men who have sex with men, injecting drug users, people with tattoos, dialysis patients, health care workers, and employees of institutions for the mentally retarded. The incubation period is two to six months, and during the latter part of this period the infected person is contagious. Symptoms are fever, chills, nausea, loss of appetite, enlarged liver, jaundice, cirrhosis of the liver, and liver cancer. There is a vaccine against hepatitis B, which is recommended for people at risk. Employers must offer the vaccine to employees who might handle blood in their work. This includes all health care workers, firefighters, and police.

The **hepatitis C** virus, is spread primarily by blood-to-blood contact. About 50 percent of all cases are related to injecting drugs. It is also seen among dialysis patients, people who have hemophilia and others receiving blood transfusions, and health care workers. There is also some concern that it may be spread through sexual contact.

---

tuberculosis An airborne bacterial disease spread by inhaling germs called tubercle bacilli; symptoms include fever, wasting, and cheesy formations in the lungs.

hepatitis An inflammation of the liver, usually caused by a virus.

hepatitis A A form of hepatitis transmitted in human wastes and contaminated food and water.

hepatitis B A form of hepatitis transmitted by blood and sexual contact.

hepatitis C A type of hepatitis, previously known as non-A, non-B hepatitis, that resembles other forms of hepatitis but cannot be classified as either.

MMR vaccine A vaccine that provides immunity to measles, mumps, and rubella.

Lyme disease A bacterial infection transmitted by deer tick bites.

nosocomial infection A hospital-acquired disease; most are caused by bacteria.

The hepatitis C virus was identified in 1988, and a test for its presence was developed in 1990. Because of the way it attacks the body, hepatitis C is an infectious disease that results in a chronic disease. It causes an infection of the liver that is usually lifelong and incurable. This sets the stage for cirrhosis and liver cancer. The infection is most common among people aged thirty to forty-nine, most of whom contracted it at least a decade earlier. Because most infected people have few if any symptoms, they can carry the disease for years without knowing it. The recommended course of treatment is interferon injections three times a week for a year, but this defeats the virus in only 20 percent of the people treated. Without effective interventions, a National Institutes of Health Consensus Conference recently predicted the emergence of a hepatitis C epidemic over the next few decades.

Childhood Diseases

Although they can affect adults as well, several viral infectious diseases are called childhood diseases because they are usually contracted during childhood. These diseases include mumps, rubella (German measles), and measles. Mumps is generally a mild disease, causing some discomfort in children, but it may cause painful swelling of the testicles in men. Rubella, too, is a mild disease in childhood, but it can cause birth defects such as deafness, blindness, mental retardation, and behavioral problems if a woman contracts it during early pregnancy. Measles is a severe disease and can lead to inflammation of the brain.

A combined measles, mumps, and rubella vaccine, the **MMR vaccine**, provides immunity from these diseases. In a 1964–1965 outbreak of rubella, the last epidemic before a vaccine was developed in 1969, twenty thousand babies were born with birth defects.

Lyme Disease

Lyme disease is a bacterial infection caused by tick bites. It commonly occurs during the summer months. Named after the town of Lyme, Connecticut, where it was first described in 1976, Lyme disease has spread across the United States and is rapidly spreading through Europe, Russia, and Japan. The dominant mode of transmission is the bite of an infected deer tick. Scientists link the growth of the disease to the increase in the deer population in temperate climates of the world.

Lyme disease causes flu-like symptoms, a rash, joint pains that can develop into chronic arthritis, irregular heartbeat, and neurological problems such as double vision, numbness, irritability, difficulty concentrating, and poor memory. During the early stages of the disease, its progress can be halted with antibiotics. However, it is a difficult disease to diagnose, and early symptoms, such as a bull's-eye halo around the bite, a rash, and fever, are sometimes absent, and blood tests of infected humans can be negative. Preventive measures include keeping pets free of fleas and ticks and wearing clothing that is tight around the ankles and wrists when walking in high grasses or gardening in tick-infested areas.

Nosocomial Infections

Most people go to the hospital with the anticipation of getting better, but at least 5 percent of all patients develop an infectious disease while they are hospitalized, and 3 percent of those infected actually die of the infection. These hospital-acquired diseases, which are caused mostly by bacteria, are called **nosocomial infections.** Ironically, intensive care units (ICUs), which house the sickest of patients, have the highest rate of nosocomial infection of any hospital area. Although ICU patients may account for only 15 percent of hospital admissions, they account for 50 percent or more of nosocomial infections. These patients

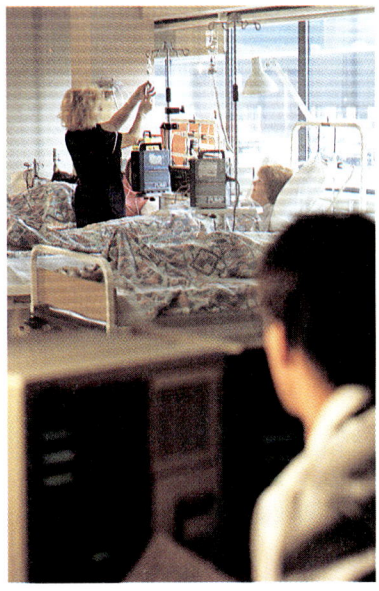

Intensive care units, which house the sickest patients in the hospital, are also the riskiest place to be. They have the highest rate of hospital-acquired bacterial diseases called nosocomial infections. (Source: © Tony Stone Images/I. Burgum/P. Boorman)

CULTURAL VIEW

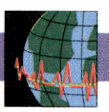

Heart Disease, Cancer, and Mental Disorders... It May Be a Virus

When two Australian researchers first proposed that a bug was to blame for most peptic ulcers, challenging the accepted wisdom that too much acid was the culprit, they were widely ridiculed. Fifteen years on, it is now accepted that *Helicobacter pylori* not only causes many ulcers, but also increases the risk of gastric cancer.

This is not an isolated example of infectious agents causing illness in hitherto unsuspected ways. At the same time as the world experiences a resurgence of infectious diseases, new technology is helping provide evidence they may play a role in everything from some cancers to chronic conditions such as heart disease, arthritis, and psychiatric disorders.

Just a few decades ago, diet and toxins were blamed for most liver cancers. Now it is estimated that, globally, more than 95 percent are due either to hepatitis B or C. Cancers develop as a result of these viruses replicating in the liver, as well as the damage they cause to cells and the body's own immune response.

Cervical cancer is another common malignancy largely due to infection, with strains 16 and 18 of the human papilloma or genital warts virus (HPV) implicated in up to 85 percent of cases. Different strains of the virus have also been implicated in some head, neck, and skin cancers.

Other viruses are associated with rare cancers, such as Epstein-Barr virus with Burkitt's lymphoma and possibly Hodgkin's disease; and HTLV-1 and -2 with some leukemia. Kaposi's sarcoma was once known only as a rare cancer mainly affecting elderly men of Jewish or Mediterranean origin. Now it is the most common cancer in AIDS patients. Research has strongly linked Kaposi's sarcoma with a newly identified infectious agent dubbed human herpes virus 8. The virus is believed to prolong the life of cells so it can stay alive longer, but in so doing increases the cancer risk, says Professor Tony Cunningham, director of the Westmead Institute of Health Research. He says there's also speculation that human herpes virus 6 has a role in multiple sclerosis.

Whether infections have a role in psychiatric disorders is one of the more fascinating areas of emerging research interest. There has been ongoing debate about whether viral infections contribute to schizophrenia, mood disorders, and chronic fatigue syndrome. But Professor Ian Hickie, professor of community psychiatry at the University of New South Wales, says there's also mounting evidence that depression can somehow result directly from the body's own immune response to viral infections, suggesting that illness can be depressing for more than just the obvious.

The ulcer saga illustrates that viruses are not only agents popping up in unexpected places. A common bacterial cause of respiratory illness, *Chlamydia pneumonia*, is being investigated as a possible cause of coronary artery disease, and may also play a role in asthma. Many experts remain skeptical, but Associate Professor Peter Timms, a molecular biologist at Queensland University of Technology, believes the evidence on heart disease has rapidly become convincing. Cytomegalovirus (CMV) has also been linked to cardiovascular disease.

But what does this mean, apart from keeping infectious disease researchers in jobs, and reminding us to remain open-minded about the cause of illness? A better understanding of their causes raises the hope of improved methods of treatment and prevention, although many uncertainties remain about the role of infectious agents in some of the diseases mentioned above. A potential vaccine against cervical cancer is now under development. And, studies have recently begun in Scandinavia to determine whether treating *Chlamydia pneumonia* improves outcomes for heart disease patients.

Dr. Peter Collignon, an infectious diseases expert in Canberra, believes that the advent of more sophisticated technology will lead to even more conditions being linked with infections. He notes that tuberculosis was regarded as a hereditary disease 100 years ago because it occurred in families. "It took a long time for people to accept it was due to an infection," he says. "If you had said 20 years ago that peptic ulcer disease was an infection you would have been regarded as crazy."

Source: "Heart Disease, Cancer, and Mental Disorders...It May Be a Virus," *Sydney Morning Herald,* February 15, 1997. Reprinted by permission

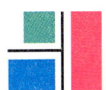

TABLE 14.4 What's New: Examples of Pathogenic Microbes and Infectious Diseases Recognized since 1973

Year	Microbe	Type	Disease
1973	Rotavirus	Virus	Major cause of infantile diarrhea worldwide
1975	Parvovirus	Virus	Aplastic crisis in chronic hemolytic anemia
1976	*Cryptosporidium parvum*	Parasite	Acute and chronic diarrhea
1977	Ebola virus	Virus	Ebola hemorrhagic fever
1977	*Legionella pneumophila*	Bacteria	Legionnaires' disease
1977	Hantaan virus	Virus	Hemorrhagic fever with renal syndrome (HRFS)
1977	*Campylobacter jejuni*	Bacteria	Enteric pathogens distributed globally
1980	Human T-lymphotropic	Virus	T-cell lymphoma-leukemia virus I (HTLV-1)
1981	Toxic producing strains of *Staphylococcus aureus*	Bacteria	Toxic shock syndrome (tampon use)
1982	*Escherichia coli* O157:H7	Bacteria	Hemorrhagic colitis; hemolytic uremic syndrome
1982	HTLV-II	Virus	Hairy cell leukemia
1982	*Borrelia burgdorferi*	Bacteria	Lyme disease
1983	Human immunodeficiency virus (HIV)	Virus	Acquired immunodeficiency syndrome (AIDS)
1983	*Helicobacter pylori*	Bacteria	Peptic ulcer disease
1985	*Enterocytozoon bieneusi*	Parasite	Persistent diarrhea
1986	*Cyclospora cayatanensis*	Parasite	Persistent diarrhea
1988	Human herpes virus-6	Virus	Roseola subitum (HHV-6)
1988	Hepatitis E	Virus	Enterically transmitted non-A, non-B hepatitis
1989	*Ehrlichia chafeensis*	Bacteria	Human ehrlichiosis
1989	Hepatitis C	Virus	Parenterally transmitted non-A, non-B liver infection
1991	Guanarito virus	Virus	Venezuelan hemorrhagic fever
1991	*Encephalitozoon hellem*	Parasite	Conjunctivitis, disseminated disease
1991	New species of Babesia	Parasite	Atypical babesiosis
1992	*Vibrio cholerae* O139	Bacteria	New strain associated with epidemic cholera
1992	*Bartonella henselae*	Bacteria	Cat-scratch disease; bacillary angiomatosis
1993	Sin nombre virus	Virus	Adult respiratory distress syndrome
1993	*Encephalitozoon cuniculi*	Parasite	Disseminated disease
1994	Sabia virus	Virus	Brazilian hemorrhagic fever
1995	HHV-8	Virus	Associated with Kaposi sarcoma in AIDS patients

Source: Centers for Disease Control and Prevention, *Report of NSTC Committee on International Science, Engineering and Technology* (CISET) Working Group on Emerging and Re-Emerging Infectious Diseases, May 1996

often have more compromised immune systems and undergo numerous invasive procedures and catheterizations that present opportunities for the spread of infection. Nosocomial infections are difficult to treat because many of the bacterial strains found in hospitals are resistant to antibiotics.

Emerging Diseases

The diseases presented in brief in this chapter in no way cover the infectious diseases that are about to face humankind. Excitement over what was once thought to be "control" of infectious diseases did not take into account the extraordinary resilience of pathogens, which have a remarkable ability to evolve, adapt, and develop resistance to drugs. Researchers also failed to take into account the fact that disease-carrying insects develop resistance to pesticides in a very short time. Other contributing factors to the increase in new or reemerging infectious diseases are population shifts, increased urbanization and crowding, environmental changes, and worldwide commerce and travel. For a new view of what might constitute infectious disease, see the Cultural View box.

Concerning viruses alone, medical science has identified approximately one per year for the last several decades. And, because of the fact that microorganisms continue to mutate, the diseases known today may represent only a small fraction of those known tomorrow. Consider the list of relatively new infectious diseases in Table 14.4.

New diseases have appeared within the United States, including Lyme disease, Legionnaires' disease, and, most recently, hantavirus pulmonary syndrome (HPS). HPS was first recognized in the southwestern United States in 1993 and has since been detected in more than twenty states and in several other countries in the Americas. By 1997, it had been confirmed in 156 people in the United States and had a 48 percent fatality rate. Other new or reemerging threats in the United States include multidrug-resistant TB; antibiotic-resistant staphylococcal, enterococcal, and pneumococcal infections; and diarrheal diseases caused by the parasite *Cryptosporidium parvum* and by certain strains of *Escherichia coli (E. coli)* bacteria.

Although salmonella, a bacteria found in poultry, eggs, meat, and milk, is a well-known cause of food poisoning, a recent CDC study found that the number-one cause of food-borne illness comes from a relatively obscure bacterium found in poultry, *Campylobacter jejuni*. Campylobacter, which causes bloody diarrhea and abdominal pain, is responsible for about 4 million infections a year. Strains of it are emerging that are resistant to antibiotics. With an increase in antibiotic-resistant strains of bacteria and a decline in the number of new antibiotics introduced into the U.S. market, the resilient bacteria are winning the race between drug-resistant bacteria and new drugs.

Why are infectious diseases reemerging? The reasons for the resurgence of infectious diseases are complex and not fully understood. Perhaps most important, however, is the continual evolution of pathogenic microorganisms.

Critical Thinking Question

At present, HIV is a very delicate organism. It is not passed from one person to another through casual contact. Imagine for a moment that HIV mutates into a resilient virus that could be spread effectively through droplets in the air or through physical contact, much as the common cold is spread. What would be the threat to public health? How would public health authorities need to respond?

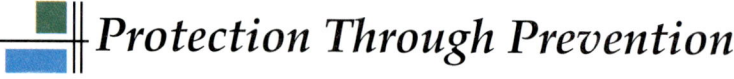
Protection Through Prevention

Reye's syndrome A condition characterized by neurological disorders and swelling of the brain; may result in significant permanent brain damage.

While medical researchers are continuing to expand the arsenal against infectious diseases, the best way to stop the spread of disease is prevention. And the best way to prevent disease is through education and informed action taken by the public at large. Recent events have been encouraging.

Reye's syndrome may affect the brain of children and adolescents after a minor bout with influenza. This condition can result in significant permanent brain damage and death. After an aggressive public health campaign to alert parents to the association between Reye's syndrome and taking aspirin for the symptoms of influenza, the use of aspirin during a flu-like illness in children decreased from 69 percent in 1981 to 16 percent in 1985. Also in 1985, the reported incidence of Reye's syndrome was much lower than in any previous year and has remained low. Public health education was effective.

Campaigns about AIDS have helped slow down the spread not only of HIV but also of other sexually transmitted diseases. The examples of Reye's syndrome illustrate that informed action is possible and that in the case of infectious diseases, some informed action can save your life.

Reducing Your Risk for an Infectious Disease

HEALTH SKILLS

The ultimate responsibility for the prevention of infectious disease remains with you. There are some specific actions that you can take to reduce your risk. Here are several suggestions:

- *Maintain overall good health.* By eating right, exercising, and getting plenty of rest, you can boost your ability to fight off disease if and when you are exposed to an infectious disease. You can also boost your resistance by maintaining a positive mental attitude.
- *Practice basic hygiene.* Basic cleanliness is sometimes taken for granted, yet it is one of the most important aspects of disease prevention. Wash your hands, bathe on a regular basis, and brush your teeth. All of these are effective ways to reduce the spread of infectious diseases.
- *Keep your vaccinations up-to-date.* Your immune system needs your help. By keeping up with all recommended vaccinations, you greatly reduce (prevent in most cases) the spread of specific diseases such as measles and mumps.
- *Treat all minor infections seriously.* A minor cut, a minor cold, or a minor boil presents little threat—until secondary complications set in. It is not uncommon, for example, for a boil to lead to generalized infection, resulting in a life-threatening situation. A minor case of influenza can lead to secondary infections, resulting in pneumonia, one of the most common causes of death.
- *Support your local public health authority.* The state and local public health departments are charged with health promotion and disease prevention. They need your cooperation to prevent disease. That support can be as simple as heeding the advice to get the latest flu shot. It can also mean volunteering to assist with a public education campaign to immunize children. Through working to reduce the threat of infectious disease in your community, you are actually reducing your own risk for disease.

▬ *Key Concepts*

1. An infectious disease is the result of infectious agents, such as bacteria or viruses, that spread from someone who is infected to someone who is not infected.
2. Infectious diseases are caused by pathogenic microorganisms such as bacteria, viruses, protozoa, parasitic worms, fungi, rickettsias, and prions.
3. Infectious diseases follow a course of action beginning with incubation, and progressing through the prodromal stage, acute illness, convalescence, and, finally, recovery.

4. Immunity is resistance to infectious disease. In active immunity, the body develops its own resistance to disease. In passive immunity, resistance to disease initially comes from an external source.
5. Once vaccinated for a disease, your body is prepared to mobilize the appropriate antibodies necessary to fight that disease.
6. Vaccines have been instrumental in wiping out epidemics of serious diseases such as polio and in eliminating smallpox. Nevertheless, the safety of vaccines is still questioned.
7. The average adult in the United States has at least two colds a year. Research suggests that frequent hand washing may reduce your risks.
8. Mononucleosis, caused by the Epstein-Barr virus, is a debilitating disease. Recovery lasts from a few weeks to several months.
9. Tuberculosis, thought to be under control earlier this century, is reemerging as a public health problem.
10. Public education campaigns resulting in informed action have proven to be effective in reducing the spread of infectious diseases.

Review Questions

1. List five links in the chain of infection and give one example of how each link can be cut.
2. Name the seven families of pathogens and give an example of a disease caused by each.
3. Describe four ways pathogens are carried.
4. Explain the importance of virulence and dosage to the spread of disease.
5. Describe the course of a disease beginning with infection through to recovery.
6. List common infectious diseases and briefly describe the symptoms and severity of each.
7. Explain the concept of immunity and how it protects the body against infection.
8. Explain the relationship between a positive mental attitude and disease prevention.
9. Identify two examples of successful public health campaigns to prevent disease and briefly describe each.
10. List several actions that you can take to personally prevent the spread of infectious disease.

Selected Bibliography

Freed, G.L., et al. "Safety of Vaccinations." *Journal of the American Medical Association* 276, no. 23 (1996): 1869–1872.

Lederberg, J., et al. *Emerging Infections: Microbial Threats to Health in the United States.* Washington, DC: The National Academy Press, 1992.

"Summary of Notifiable Diseases, United States." *Morbidity and Mortality Weekly Report.* Published annually. See also ongoing weekly coverage of selected notifiable disease reports.

The Race against Lethal Microbes. Chevy Chase, MD: Howard Hughes Medical Institute, 1996.

Health HotLinks: Web Sites for Reducing Your Risk of Infectious Disease

You can access better health as it relates to this chapter by checking out some of the following sites on the Internet. These and sites identified within the chapter can be accessed directly when you visit the *HealthStyles* Web Site located on the Allyn and Bacon home page at **http://www.abacon.com.**

American Academy of Pediatrics
www.aap.org
Web site committed to the attainment of optimal physical, mental, and social health for all infants, children, adolescents, and young adults. Contains such pertinent information as the latest immunization schedule, as well as helpful tips for parents.

CDC National Immunization Program
www.cdc.gov/nip/home.htm
The NIP provides leadership for the planning, coordination, and conduct of immunization activities nationwide. At this site, you can access the latest information on adult and child immunization needs, as well as press releases about emerging infectious diseases.

Health Hotlines: Reducing the Risk for Infectious Disease

Chronic Fatigue and Immune Dysfunction Syndrome
(800) 442-3427
P.O. Box 220398
Charlotte, NC 28222

Hepatitis Hotline
(800) 223-0179
American Liver Foundation
1425 Pompton Avenue
Cedar Grove, NJ 07009

Lyme Disease Foundation
(800) 886-5963
One Financial Plaza
Hartford, CT 06103-2610

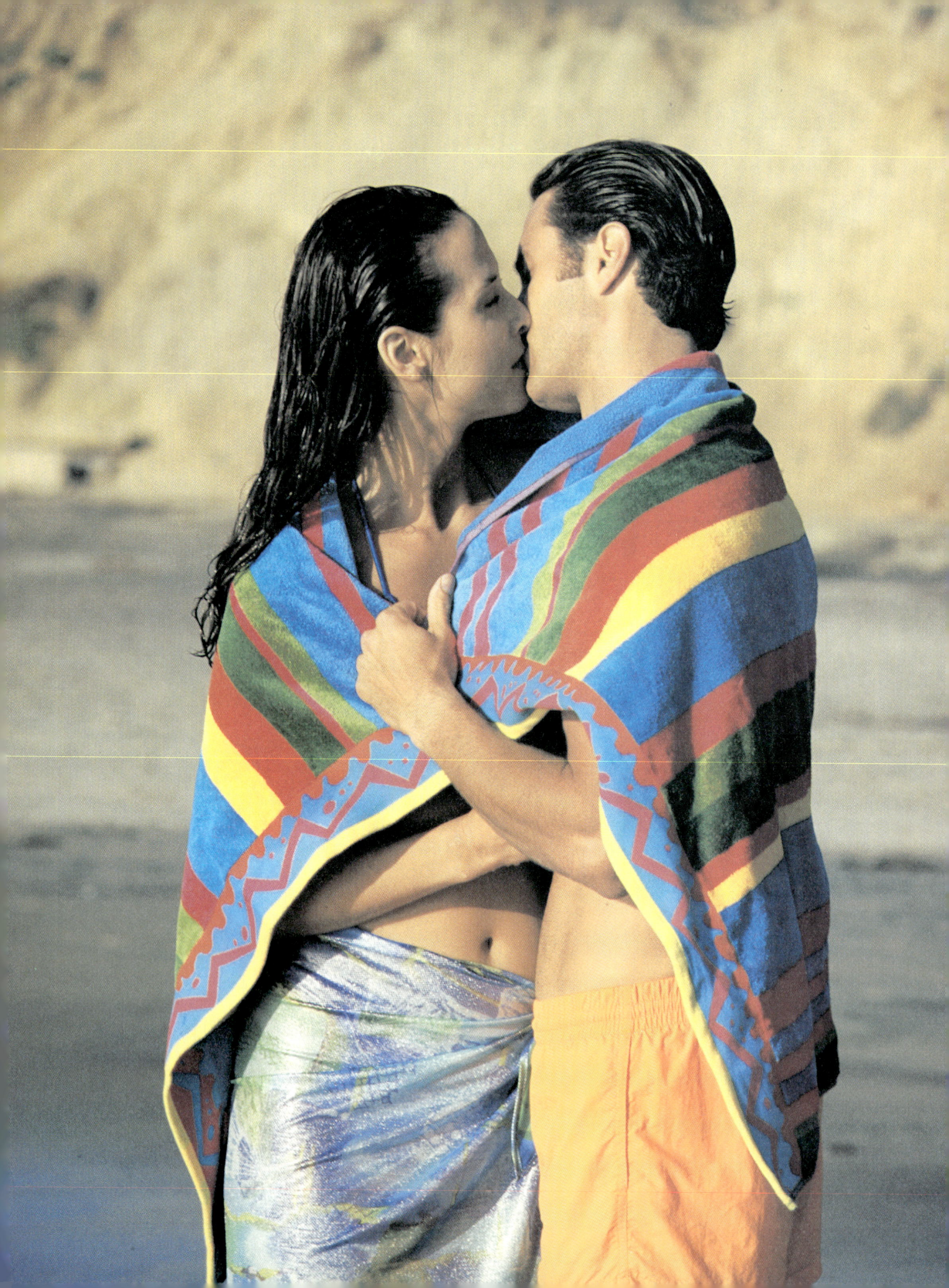

Chapter 15

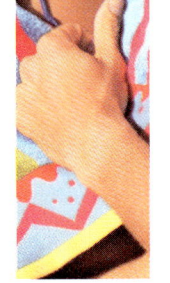
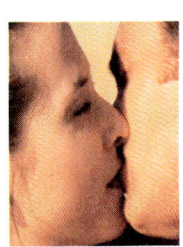
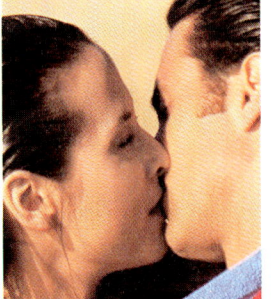

Reducing the Risk for Sexually Transmitted Diseases

Objectives

When you finish reading this chapter, you will be able to:

1. Recognize sexually transmitted diseases (STDs) as a major public health problem in the United States.
2. Explain why many STDs can be cured but have not been brought under control.
3. Describe the significance of asymptomatic carriers to the overall STD epidemic.
4. Identify how most STDs are spread.
5. List primary prevention measures that reduce the potential for contracting an STD.
6. Name and describe several viral STDs including HIV/AIDS, hepatitis B, human papilloma virus, and genital herpes.
7. Name and describe several bacterial STDs including chlamydia, gonorrhea, and syphilis.
8. Name and describe other STDs, including vaginitis as well as pubic lice and scabies.
9. Explain the concept of safer sex and list measures that assure the risk of sexual activity is kept low.
10. Recognize the symptoms of STDs, and know when to seek an STD examination from a physician.

What Is Your HealthStyle?

John thought he knew a lot about diseases—all diseases. His mother is a physician, and they often discussed some of the interesting cases she treated. John is sexually active, but given his "knowledge" about diseases, he was not concerned about getting any of the sexually transmitted diseases that some of the people he knew at school had. After all, John knew whom he slept with, and they were what he would call "nice girls" who were sure to be "clean." Although he usually practiced safer sex because he was concerned about the possibility of pregnancy, on occasion he didn't take the time to buy condoms.

On one such occasion, John contracted herpes from a date, who had contracted it from a previous partner. The disease is in remission now for John, but it is not gone from his system. It is a lifelong reminder of bad decision making.

Leon is not as knowledgeable as John about all diseases, but he had read materials about AIDS that were distributed by the student health service and knew that each time he had sex without a condom, he was taking a risk for HIV infection. The few times Leon had had sex, he had known the person pretty well, but he had recognized that he didn't know anything about the person's previous partners or whom those partners had slept with. So Leon always used a condom.

When Leon met Inge, it didn't take long for him to recognize that Inge was more special than anyone else he had dated. After dating for a while, they became sexually involved. Although Leon was sure it wasn't necessary, he still made a point to have condoms with him before they went out. In a pinch, he could stop by the student union and buy some from the condom vending machine in the men's room. Or Inge could purchase them from the machine in the women's room. In any event, he felt it was important—using a condom was the responsible thing to do.

In Your Opinion

John and Leon were both responsible young men and wanted to have good sexual relations but also to protect themselves. John was more concerned about protecting himself from becoming a father; Leon was concerned about that, too, but was more aware of the risks for contracting STDs, particularly the HIV infection.

- What values were influencing John's action? Personal gratification? Personal protection? Personal health?
- What decisions did John and Leon make that related to their health and to the health of others?
- What health skills did Leon use that John didn't?
- How would you handle a situation in which you wanted to have sex but were concerned that appropriate precautions weren't being taken to protect you from getting an STD?

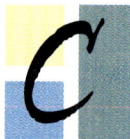

College students: Beware of sexually transmitted diseases.

- Of the ten most frequently reported infectious diseases in the United States, five are STDs.

- Of the total reported cases of STDs, 86 percent occur to people aged fifteen to twenty-nine.
- Approximately one of every five young people has received treatment for a sexually transmitted disease.
- Single people are more likely to have had more than one sex partner in the last year, to have had sex partners whose sexual history they don't know, and to get an STD than are married people.
- At current rates, at least one person in four will contract an STD at some point in his or her life.

Clearly, STDs are a major health concern for college-aged populations, which is why they deserve special consideration. A recent survey found that almost half of U.S. adults say they know at least one person who has had an STD. There are effective treatments to combat many of the STDs, but these curable diseases continue to threaten the health of Americans largely because they go unrecognized and untreated.

What Are STDs?

Collectively, more than twenty-five infectious organisms that are transmitted through sexual activity are classified as **sexually transmitted diseases.** These, along with the dozens of clinical syndromes that they cause, make up the group of infectious diseases and syndromes called STDs. Although STDs are caused by a variety of organisms, they all share one common factor: They have an affinity for the moist, warm genital areas.

STDs can result in mild discomfort, infertility, lifelong pain, or death. Some STDs facilitate the spread of other STDs and are highly correlated with serious chronic diseases such as cancer. Pregnant women who have STDs can pass along

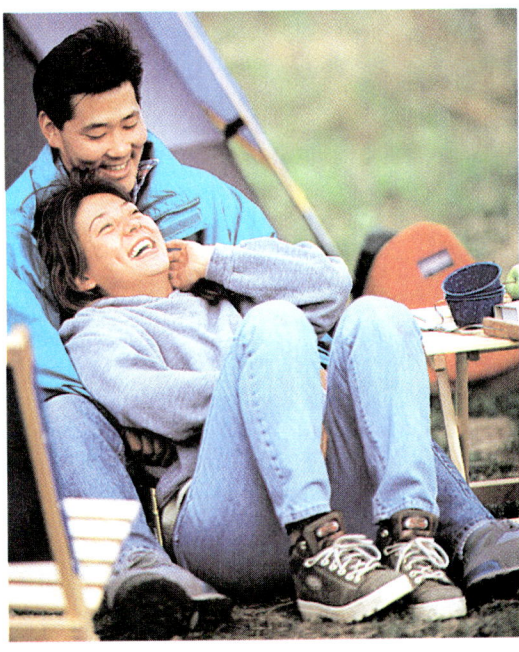

College students are at high risk of getting an STD, but this risk is significantly reduced among mutually monogamous couples. (Source: © Tony Stone Images/Lori Adamski Peek)

sexually transmitted diseases (STDs) Infectious diseases and syndromes that are spread primarily through sexual activity.

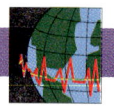

CULTURAL VIEW

MTV Makes Health Hip

Music Television (MTV), the network that has been taking the youth culture's electronic pulse since the early 1980s, surprised many in 1995 by offering several innovative programs that explored health issues sandwiched between music videos and its standard 20-somethingish fare. Most notably "Out of Order: Rock the Vote Targets Health Care" comprised six half-hour installments that dramatized issues such as drug and alcohol abuse, hospitalization crises, child abuse, eating disorders, and sexually transmitted diseases. Among other things, the network championed safe sex with a "no glove, no love" admonishment. Even MTV's interview/home-shopping program, "The Goods" (normally a clearinghouse for Rolling Stones tour jackets and the like), presented a program—called "Think Positive"—that marketed a package of popular consumer items, with profits going to the AIDS cause.

In a more dramatic and personal way, MTV viewers were confronted with the harsh realities of AIDS during the 1994–95 airing of the series "The Real World." This popular, if somewhat contrived, documentary focused on seven young people brought together under one San Francisco roof and the unrelenting scrutiny of MTV's cameras. One member of the group, Pedro Zamora, was charming, gay, and HIV-positive. He was also a nationally known activist who, after learning at age 17 that he was HIV-positive, carried his plea for AIDS awareness to young people across the United States and to Congress.

As viewers witnessed Zamora's interactions with his roommates, his marriage, and his AIDS activism, they came to care about a young man whose life would be claimed by his disease in November 1994. Indeed, "The Real World" was never more illuminating than in the programs in which Zamora was most prominent.

Source: "MTV Makes Health Hip," reprinted with permission from *Medical and Health*, 1996. © 1995 Annual Encyclopedia Britannica

---

a range of disorders to their children, including mental retardation and blindness, as well as the disease itself. Women are especially vulnerable to STDs and associated complications because they are more biologically susceptible to certain sexually transmitted infections than men are and are more likely to have asymptomatic infections that commonly result in delayed diagnosis and treatment. While not all college students are sexually active, those who are active are at an unusually high risk for STDs because they frequently have unprotected sexual intercourse and are often sexually involved with multiple partners.

Spread of STDs

STDs are a significant health problem for a variety of reasons. First, they are difficult to control because there is a period of time following exposure before symptoms appear. This is called an **incubation period.** It can range from hours to years, but it usually lasts for days or weeks. During this time, **asymptomatic carriers** (infected people who have no symptoms) provide a source of infection or reinfection for others. Asymptomatic people usually do not know they have a disease. One study suggests that 71 percent of the cases of primary genital herpes are acquired from a partner who had no symptoms at the time of exposure. On average, fewer than 25 percent of patients who have genital herpes infections have symptoms.

Second, ways to provide immunity against STDs continue to evade medical science, with the sole exception of immunity to hepatitis B. Not only is there no vaccine but also some of the long-standing methods of treatment no longer work. This is best illustrated by the appearance of penicillin-resistant gonorrhea.

TABLE 15.1   Incidence of STDs in the United States

Common STDs	Estimated or actual annual incidence, 1996	Effective treatment available
Chlamydia	4 million	Yes
Trichomoniasis	3 million	Yes
Pelvic inflammatory disease (PID)	1 million	Yes
Human papilloma virus (HPV)	0.5–1 million	Yes
Gonorrhea	390,000	Yes (but antibiotic-resistant strains exist)
Genital herpes	200,000–500,000	No
AIDS	66,900	No
Syphilis	11,400	Yes
Hepatitis B	10,600	No

Source: Centers for Disease Control and Prevention, Division of STD/HIV Prevention

Third, the incidence of STDs is directly linked to increased sexual activity in general and to the use of the birth control pill in particular. The pill eliminated pregnancy prevention as a motive for using a condom or diaphragm, both of which can often prevent the transmission of some STDs. In addition, the pill encourages the rapid growth of gonorrheal and other organisms because it increases alkalinity and moisture in the female genital tract. (Vaginal jellies and foam, in contrast, are acidic and create an environment that does not promote the growth of infectious organisms.) At about the same time that the pill gained popularity in the 1960s (some would say *because* of the pill's popularity), the sexual revolution became a reality. This contributed to the STD problem because the leading risk factor related to the spread of STDs is multiple partners. As the number of sexual partners increases, the risk of exposure to STDs increases.

Fourth, impaired judgment about sexual behavior often accompanies the use of alcohol and other drugs. Under the influence of these drugs, inhibitions are reduced, which can lead to less safe sexual practices and the spread of STDs (see Chapters 9 and 10).

Fifth, because there is social stigma associated with having such diseases, many people who are diagnosed as having an STD do not identify their contacts because of fear of social embarrassment. If infected, these unnotified contacts can unknowingly pass the disease along to others. Also, carriers are often reluctant to come forward for treatment, so they remain infected and at risk for infecting others (see the Cultural View box).

The true incidence of STDs is difficult to pinpoint because only four diseases are officially reported: AIDS, gonorrhea, hepatitis B, and syphilis. The other STDs are more difficult to track precisely. Table 15.1 shows the estimated annual incidence of STDs in the United States and whether there is an effective treatment available for each. See Figure 15.1 for an illustration of how STDs spread.

Prevention and Treatment

The best hope for controlling STDs rests in a combination of prevention and treatment. STD prevention is best accomplished by practices that reduce risk. The risk factors related to STDs are reasonably well understood. No matter who

incubation period The period of time following exposure to an infectious disease before symptoms appear.

asymptomatic carrier A person who has a disease but no symptoms.

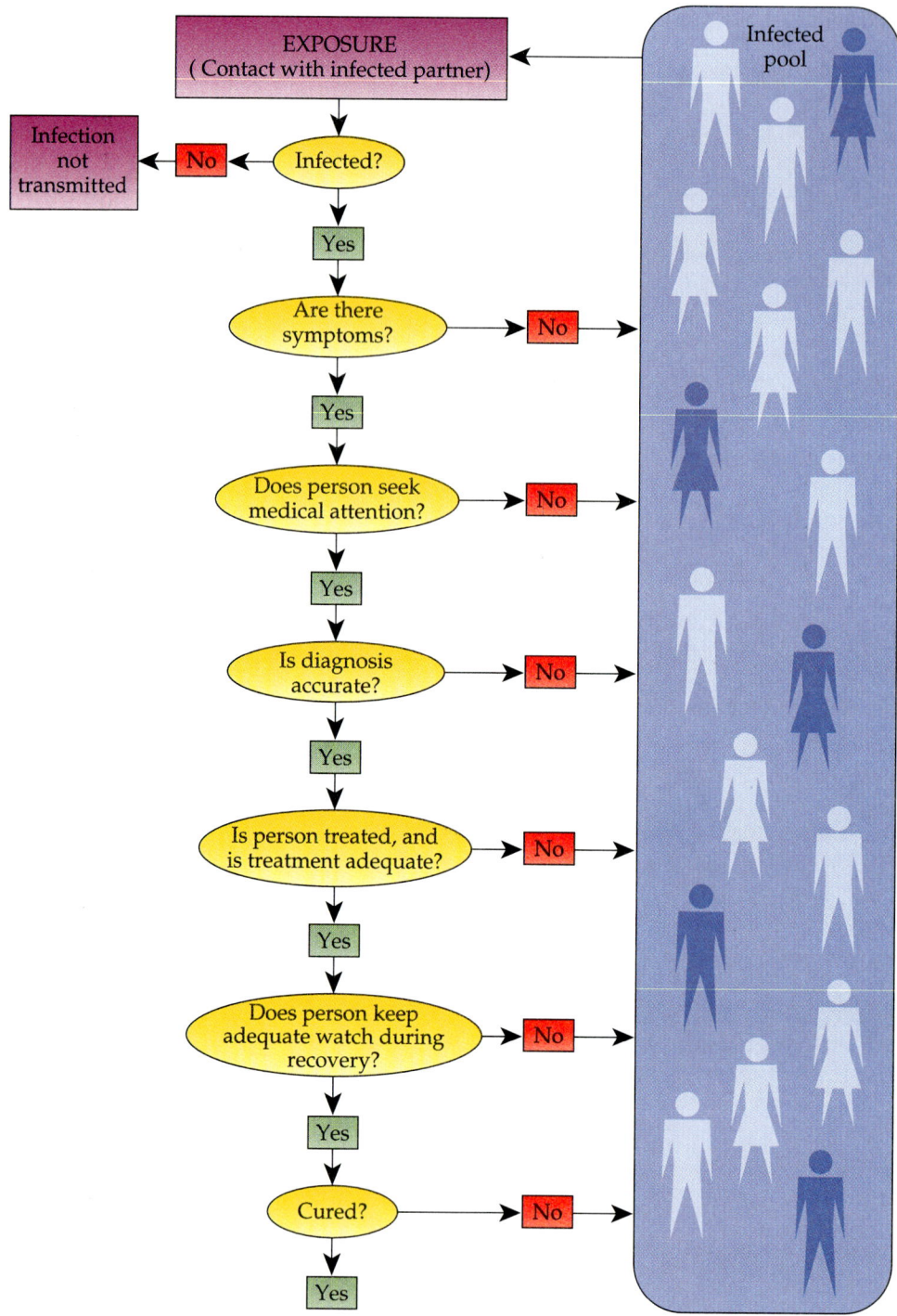

Figure 15.1 The Cycle of STD Transmission among Sexually Active Individuals. *Asymptomatic carriers provide a constant pool that is a source of infection or reinfection for others. This diagram shows other sources that contribute to the pool of infected people.*

you are—a teenager, a college student, a business executive—there are generally three ways to get one of these diseases.

First, in almost all cases, only sexually active people are exposed to STDs. Exceptions include congenital syphilis, yeast, pubic lice, and scabies, but for the most part, to be exposed to an STD, a person must participate in an activity that allows the movement of pathogens from one individual to another through the genitalia or other tissue, such as the mouth or anus. Persons who abstain from sexual contact seldom contract STDs.

Second, to contract an STD, an individual must have sex with a person who is infected with the disease. (Remember, infection is not the same as having symptoms. One of the main problems with STDs is that many of those infected show no visible symptoms.) In a mutually monogamous relationship in which neither partner carries an STD, the risk for acquiring a disease is slight. When one or both members of the relationship have sexual contact with other partners, the risk rises.

Finally, the risk for being exposed to an STD increases when no prophylactics are used. The condom is not a guarantee of protection against STDs, but its use can greatly reduce the risk for transmitting or contracting most diseases. Until recently, only a male condom was available. A new condom designed for use by women provides protection similar to that of the male condom. (See Chapter 17 for more information about the female condom.) In both cases, additional protection can be gained with the use of condoms containing the spermicide nonoxynol-9.

When an STD is suspected, what then? Steps can be taken to further prevent the spread of disease:

- Have a medical examination as soon as signs of an STD appear so that the correct diagnosis is made and appropriate treatment begins in a timely fashion.
- Have follow-up examinations after treatment to confirm that the disease has been cured.
- To prevent others from acquiring the disease, inform all sexual contacts of the problem. Their contacts should be notified as well.

The following are suggestions for reducing the risk for getting an STD. Note that there are two phases—before you decide to have sex and when you have sex.

HEALTH SKILLS

Before you decide to have sex:

Assess your risk. What type of behavior are you interested in or willing to engage in? Does that behavior place you at risk? If so, what precautions can you take?

Assess your potential partner's risk. If your partner has had sex with someone else, there is a possibility that he or she has contracted an STD. You cannot tell whether someone has an STD simply by looking at or even by asking him or her. Surveys show that both men and women lie about their previous sexual encounters (see the Here's Looking at You box).

Communicate your feelings about safer sex to your potential partner. If he or she is not willing to respect your wishes to have safer sex, you should insist on postponing having sex.

Have a checkup. If you suspect that you or your partner may be at risk for having an STD, postpone having sex until both of you have been checked by a physician. Although a checkup does not guarantee that a person is disease-free, it is the best means available for checking for the presence of STDs.

When you have sex:

Use a condom. The proven method for reducing risk is to wear a condom during sexual activity. This does not guarantee protection against the transmission of all diseases, but it is the most important risk-reducing behavior for sexually active people. For added protection, use condoms containing nonoxynol-9.

Select your sexual activity. Not only does the act of sexual intercourse place you at risk, so too does the type of activity in which you engage. For example, anal intercourse often results in tearing of tissues and some bleeding. People having anal intercourse are at high risk for contracting HIV. Vaginal intercourse carries risks as well, but not nearly as high.

Visually examine your partner's genitals. Prior to engaging in sexual intercourse, take the time to look for a sore or any discharge. Any obvious sore is a warning sign. If you find such a sign, postpone sexual contact. Examining your partner's genitals can be difficult, but you can make it part of lovemaking and the open communication between you.

Wash your genitals before and after sexual contact. The risk of transmission can be reduced somewhat by simple hygiene. Washing the genitals with warm water and soap before and after intercourse can decrease risk of transmission of STDs.

Critical Thinking Question

Secondary virginity is a term that has become common when speaking of the practice of returning to abstinence after being sexually active. *Serial monogamy* refers to the practice of having sexual intercourse with only one sexual partner for a period of time but having a series of partners in close succession. Many people, however, feel that both these terms suggest an oxymoronic condition, or contradictory messages. What are the disease risks of each practice? Is either a real possibility? Does such terminology promote healthy behavior or confound it?

acquired immune deficiency syndrome (AIDS) A combination of symptoms caused by the human immunodeficiency virus (HIV).

human immunodeficiency virus (HIV) The virus that causes AIDS.

helper T-cells White blood cells that are needed by the body's immune system to fight a variety of disease-causing organisms.

opportunistic diseases Diseases common to individuals infected with HIV that under normal conditions would be defeated by the body's immune system.

Pneumocystis carinii **pneumonia** A rare form of pneumonia that is often present in persons living with AIDS.

Kaposi's sarcoma A rare, deadly cancer characterized by reddish-purple blotches on the skin; one of the symptoms of AIDS.

Viral Diseases

Viral diseases represent one of the continuing challenges to medical science. This is because, for the most part, virally caused diseases cannot be cured. The mystery of how to cure the common cold, for example, has evaded researchers to date. Fortunately, the body recovers from the common cold in a matter of time. This is not the case with viral STDs. Time does not cure them. We discuss four common viral STDs here: HIV infection and AIDS, papilloma virus, hepatitis B, and genital herpes. Table 15.2 outlines selected STDs.

HIV Infection and AIDS

Acquired immune deficiency syndrome (AIDS) is caused by the **human immunodeficiency virus (HIV),** a virus that causes a lifelong infection that usually weakens the body's immune system. AIDS is a late manifestation of infection with HIV. AIDS was first reported in the United States in 1981, and since then, the number of cases has grown rapidly. By the end of 1996, more than 580,000 people in the United States had been diagnosed with AIDS, nearly 300,000 were

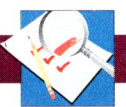

HERE'S LOOKING AT YOU

Should You Believe What You Hear?

Your sexual partner says he or she has been tested for STDs and is "clean." Should you believe him or her? A recent survey conducted for the Kaiser Family Foundation asked more than 700 men and women aged eighteen to sixty-five if they would do the following and got some disturbing answers.

	Yes	No	Don't know
Ask a new sexual partner if he or she is infected with any STDs	12%	85%	3%
Tell a new sexual partner if they are infected with an STD	11	86	3
Use condoms each time they have sex with this new sexual partner	22	75	3
Use protection, such as a condom, when they have oral sex	4	89	7
Get tested for STDs before they have sex for the first time or stop using condoms	11	85	4
Use condoms to prevent STDs if they are already using a different kind of birth control to prevent pregnancy	31	65	4

Do you think these findings are accurate? If you are sexually active, would your answers to each of these questions fall with the majority or the minority? If you are not sexually active, how accurately do you think these results reflect people you know?

Given the results of this survey, should you believe what you hear? Based on what you are likely to hear, what can you do to protect yourself from getting STDs?

---

living with HIV infection and with AIDS, and more than 360,000 persons who had had AIDS had already died of the disease (see Figure 15.2). Worldwide, about 30.6 million people—roughly 1 in every 100 people of reproductive age on earth—are infected with HIV, according to the United Nations AIDS Program.

HIV kills a specific kind of white blood cell that is needed by the body's immune system to fight a variety of disease-causing organisms. Without these white blood cells (called **helper T-cells**), the body is vulnerable to infections. The early symptoms of AIDS, as well as the causes of death, are **opportunistic diseases,** or diseases that would otherwise be defeated by the body's immune system. The most common of such opportunistic diseases is *Pneumocystis carinii* **pneumonia,** which occurs in more than half of AIDS patients. **Kaposi's sarcoma,** an otherwise rare skin cancer, is also common among people living with AIDS.

Under the original CDC definition, people infected with HIV were diagnosed as having AIDS when they developed blood infections, Kaposi's sarcoma, or any of twenty-one other indicator diseases. In 1993, the definition was revised to include pulmonary tuberculosis, recurrent pneumonia, invasive cervical cancer, and a T-cell count of 200 or below. (Normal T-cell count is 1,000 to 1,200.) The new definition takes into account what has been learned about the course of the disease and also its spread among females.

Initially, HIV and AIDS in the United States spread largely among men who have sex with men and then among people who inject drugs. In 1985, women accounted for only 7 percent of the cases. By 1996, women living with AIDS made up 20 percent of the cases, and AIDS was the third leading cause of death among women aged twenty-five to forty-four. Although more white adults have AIDS than do African American or Hispanic adults, minority groups have a

HealthLinks
Centers for Disease Control and Prevention (CDC)
www.cdc.gov/
Home page for the government agency dedicated to disease intervention and prevention. This address links you with the CDC research database, Wonder; the National Center for HIV, STD, and TB Prevention; and the National AIDS Clearinghouse; as well as all the latest data and publications put out by the CDC, including the MMWR and the HIV/AIDS Surveillance Report.

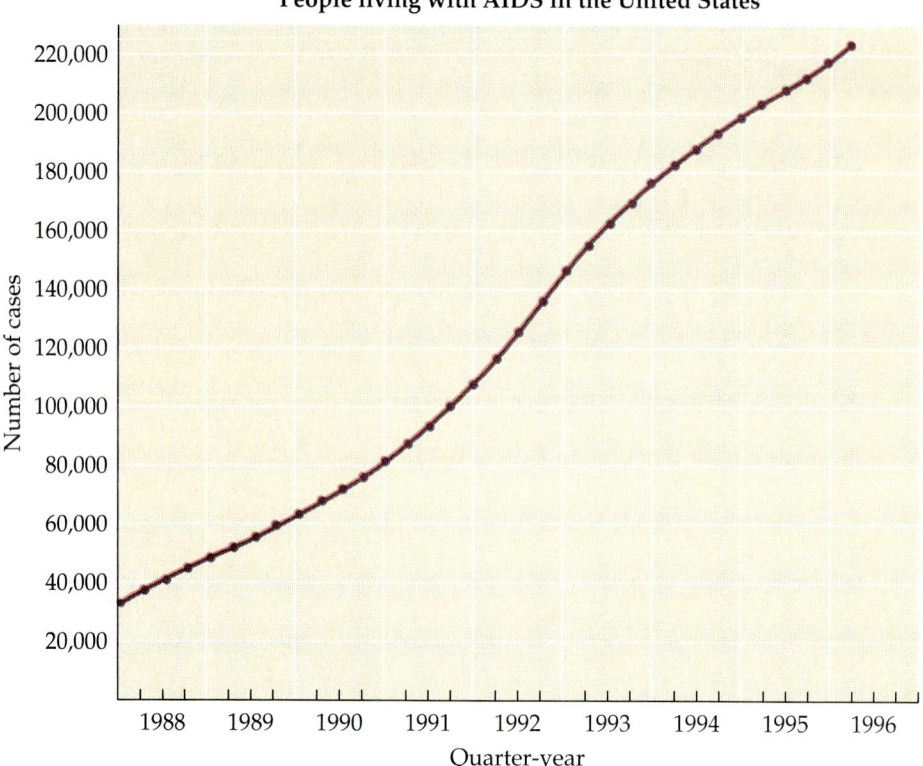

Figure 15.2 People Living with AIDS in the United States. *The number of people living with AIDS in the United States continues to rise dramatically. (Source: Centers for Disease Control and Prevention, HIV/AIDS Surveillance Report, 1996)*

higher incidence of the disease, especially minority group women and children. It is the leading cause of death among African American women aged twenty-five to forty-four, and more than half of the pediatric AIDS cases in 1996 occurred in African Americans. See Figure 15.3 to see who gets AIDS today.

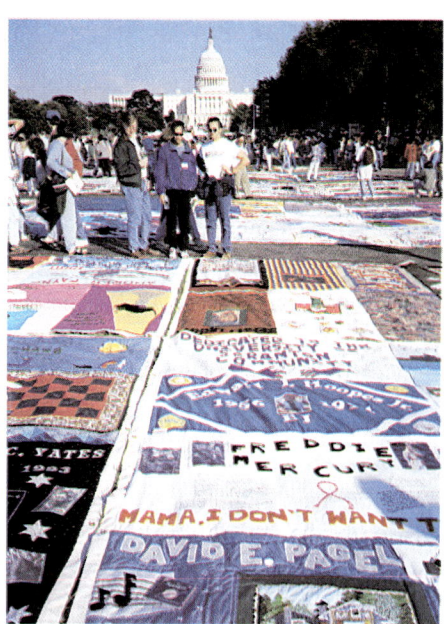

The AIDS Quilt, a personal memory of people who have died of AIDS, serves as a reminder of the serious consequences of unhealthy decisions. People with AIDS are living longer today, thanks to new combinations of drugs. (Source: The Image Works/ © Sondra Dawes)

By exposure category	Adult males	Adult females
Men who have sex with men	50%	
Injecting drug use	23%	34%
Men who have sex with men and inject drugs	5%	
Hemophilia/coagulation disorder	1%	
Heterosexual contact	5%	40%
Receipt of blood transfusion, blood components, or tissue	1%	2%
Other/risk not reported or identified	15%	24%

By exposure category	Annual rates per 100,000 adults		
	Males	Females	Total
White	29.9	3.5	16.2
Black	177.6	61.7	115.3
Hispanic	88.9	22.7	55.8
Asian/Pacific Islander	13.6	2.1	7.5
American Indian/Alaska Native	23.2	5.4	14.1

Figure 15.3 Who Gets AIDS. *Same-sex intercourse is the leading cause of infection among men. Heterosexual intercourse with someone infected with HIV is the main cause of infection among women. (Source: Centers for Disease Control and Prevention, HIV/AIDS Surveillance Report, 1996)*

HIV is transmitted during unprotected sexual contact with an infected person through body fluids such as blood, semen, and vaginal fluid. It is also spread in nonsexual ways, such as through needle sharing among injecting drug users and, less commonly and now very rarely, through transfusions of infected blood or blood clotting factors. The risk for getting HIV by receiving blood for medical reasons has been significantly reduced since donated blood began to be tested for the virus in 1985. Babies born to mothers who are HIV-infected may become infected themselves before birth, during the birth process, or through breastfeeding.

Critical Thinking Question

The *Healthy People 2000* objectives include the following: "Increase to at least 50 percent the proportion of sexually active, unmarried people who used a condom at last sexual intercourse." The last time data were collected on this objective, the proportion was 19 percent. Why has the use of condoms met with such resistance? Do you feel that the condom presents a barrier to sexual responsiveness? Or do you think the "it-couldn't-happen-to-me" attitude overrules the motive to use protection? Which reason do you think most represents the attitude of college students?

These are the only ways to get HIV infection. You cannot get it through everyday contact. It is not transmitted through mosquito bites, sweat, tears, or saliva. You cannot get AIDS from clothes, a telephone, a drinking fountain, or a toilet seat. And you cannot get it by going to class or working with someone living with AIDS. In general, you cannot get AIDS through kissing. However, the CDC reported the first case of HIV transmission through a kiss in 1997, when a woman apparently became infected from a deep kiss with a man who had bleeding gums and canker sores. According to the CDC, the virus was transmitted through the man's blood, not his saliva. The CDC recommends against "French" kissing or open-mouthed kissing with an infected person because of the possibility of contact with blood.

There have been some positive developments in the effort to combat HIV. For example, epidemiologists have discovered that some persons exposed to HIV become infected and others do not. They believe this is most likely because of the means of exposure. For example, more than 90 percent of persons who were exposed through an HIV-infected unit of blood became infected. So we know that blood-to-blood contact is a very efficient way that HIV is spread. On the other hand, many health care workers are splashed with blood or bloody body fluids and this type of exposure has caused very few occurrences of HIV infection.

When HIV was first discovered, a positive diagnosis meant a prognosis of death within about ten years. Recent research, however, has produced a handful of drug treatments, which focus on different stages of HIV and the biology of the disease. Most promising are protease inhibitors. These drugs stop—or inhibit— the replication of HIV by preventing the enzyme protease from making copies of itself and infecting cells. In effect, protease inhibitors lower the amount of HIV in a person's blood and can reduce the likelihood that the person will transmit the virus to others. Reducing the viral load (the amount of HIV in the body) can substantially increase the life span of people living with AIDS. A test to detect viral load is now being used. It is common to use combination therapy—protease inhibitors and other drugs, including azidothymidine (AZT). Work is progressing on a vaccine to control HIV in already infected persons as well as to prevent uninfected persons from getting the disease.

The new drug treatment has led to a dramatic decline in AIDS deaths—a 44 percent decline in the United States in 1997, compared with the first half of 1996. Ironically, the very success in treating HIV has led to riskier behavior among young gay men. Researchers at the University of California at San Francisco surveyed fifty-four gay men seeking HIV testing and found that about one quarter of them said they were "less concerned about becoming HIV positive" because they believed they could benefit from the new therapies.

Blood tests are available to detect the presence of HIV antibodies. Only people who have participated in high-risk behaviors should be concerned. These tests can be provided through anonymous means at some local health departments and campus health centers. At an anonymous site, you do not give your name or other identifier; instead you give a made-up name or number so you can call for the test result without having it reported to others or tracked back to you. You can also get a test from your private physician. An increasing number of states are requiring the reporting of people who test positive for HIV infection. See the Developing Health Skills box to see whether you should get an AIDS test.

Home HIV collection kits are also available at some drugstores and by calling toll-free phone numbers. The procedure is simple: prick your finger, put some drops of blood on a card labeled with an identification number, and mail it to a certified lab. In about a week, you call the toll-free number using your ID number. If you test negative (you are not infected), you will get the results by a recorded message. If you test positive (you are infected), a trained counselor will

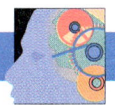

DEVELOPING HEALTH SKILLS

Should You Get an AIDS Test?

You have probably heard about the "AIDS test." The test doesn't actually tell you if you have AIDS. It shows if you have been infected with HIV. It looks for changes in blood that occur after you have been infected.

The Public Health Service recommends you be confidentially counseled and tested if you have had any sexually transmitted disease or have shared needles; if you are a man who has had sex with another man; or if you have had sex with a prostitute, male or female. You should be tested if you have had sex with anyone who has done any of these things.

If you are a woman who has been engaging in risky behavior and you plan to have a baby or are not using birth control, you should be tested.

Your doctor may advise you to be counseled and tested if you are a hemophiliac or have received a blood transfusion between 1978 and 1985.

Source: U.S. Centers for Disease Control and Prevention

If you test positive and find you have been infected with the AIDS virus, you must take steps to protect your partner.

People who have always practiced safe behavior do not need to be tested.

There's been a great deal in the press about problems with the test. It is very reliable if it is done by a good laboratory and the results are checked by a physician or counselor.

If you have engaged in risky behavior, speak frankly to a doctor who understands the AIDS problem or to an AIDS counselor.

For more information, call your local public health agency. They're listed in the government section of your phone book. Or call your local AIDS hotline. If you can't find the number, call 1-800-342-AIDS. A state-by-state listing of AIDS hotlines is at the end of this chapter.

---

give you the news and refer you to medical treatment and long-term counseling. All conversations are confidential or anonymous.

It takes a minimum of six to twelve weeks for a person infected with HIV to develop enough antibodies to test positive. During that time, it is possible to be infected, to test negative, but to transmit the virus to another person. Because of this time lag, the American College Health Association warns that a negative test result should not be a substitute for safer sex.

Papilloma Virus

The **human papilloma virus (HPV)** causes genital warts, or small bumps on the genitals. In men, these usually appear on the glans penis and in women on the labia or just inside the vagina. Each year, as many as 1 million new cases of papilloma virus infection are diagnosed in the United States. According to the Institute of Medicine, 25 percent of the women in this country are infected with human papilloma virus.

The virus is highly contagious through direct contact with the warts. Thus, sexual intercourse, whether vaginal, oral, or anal, provides an ideal mode of transmission. Depending on the location of the warts, a condom may or may not provide protection against this disease. The most severe complication related to the incidence of genital warts is cervical cancer. Women who are infected or who have male partners who have genital warts are ten times more likely to develop cervical cancer. The papilloma virus is present in about 90 percent of cervical cancers tested. The virus may also play a role in cancer of the vagina, vulva, penis, and anus.

human papilloma virus (HPV)
The agent responsible for an STD characterized by warts, usually on the genitalia; also called genital warts.

Currently, no test is available to determine the presence of the papilloma virus, so diagnosis is made by visual confirmation. One of the primary difficulties in controlling the incidence of genital warts is the number of asymptomatic carriers of the disease. Both men and women often have no visible genital warts yet are infectious. Treatment involves removal of the warts by freezing or surgery.

Because there is no cure, primary preventive measures are critical in controlling this virus. Preventive measures include the use of condoms, bathing with warm soapy water before and after intercourse, and carefully selecting sexual partners.

Hepatitis B

Of the several types of hepatitis, only **hepatitis B** is considered an STD, although there is some concern that hepatitis C is also spread through sexual contact. Hepatitis B is transmitted in the same manner as HIV, through body fluids such as blood and semen. Injecting drug users, men who have sex with men, family members of hepatitis B carriers, and health care professionals involved with blood work are particularly at risk for infection with hepatitis B. In 1996, nearly eleven thousand new cases of hepatitis B were reported.

Hepatitis causes mild fever, fatigue, sore muscles, headache, upset stomach, joint pains, and dark urine. The characteristic sign is yellowing of the whites of the eyes. The skin may become jaundiced, a condition characterized by a yellow color.

The disease may be diagnosed by a blood test. Its most severe complications include cirrhosis of the liver and liver cancer. About one thousand people a year in the United States die of hepatitis B-related diseases.

An effective vaccine has been available since 1981. This preventive measure makes hepatitis B the only viral STD for which a vaccine is available. Persons in high-risk groups are encouraged to become immunized, and health care workers in many places are required to be vaccinated. As with most other STDs, use of a condom can reduce the chances of contracting the disease. Hepatitis B, however, is transmitted through nonsexual means as well, and therefore the condom is not foolproof.

Genital Herpes

Nearly half a million people each year in the United States acquire genital herpes infection, and 20 million Americans who already have the disease suffer recurrences. It is a lifelong disease that has no cure.

Genital herpes, usually called **herpes simplex type 2,** is a viral infection. Herpes sores, which resemble blisters, occur in men on the penis or near the anus. In women, sores may be on the labia majora, labia minora, inside the vagina, or around the anus. Genital herpes **lesions** may also be found in the mouth but are not to be confused with cold sores, a type of herpes simplex caused by a related pathogen.

When first infected, an individual may experience high fever and in some cases **meningitis** (inflammation of the membranes surrounding the spinal cord and brain). In addition, the infected person may feel fatigued and achy and have enlarged lymph nodes. Herpes sores are often painful. An examination by a physician, sometimes involving a swab taken from the blisters or ulcers, is the best means of diagnosing herpes simplex type 2.

About two weeks after the initial infection, the symptoms disappear. The disease is far from cured, however. The virus has simply retreated. It usually resides in nerve tissue and awaits some triggering mechanism that again causes it to produce symptoms. Recurrences are generally less severe than the initial herpes outbreak.

The most serious consequence of genital herpes infection involves its transfer from mother to baby, either across the placenta or during the birth process. About two thirds of the infants infected with herpes virus at birth have **systemic infection**, and the rest have more localized infections, usually involving sores around the mouth or infection of the eyes. Babies born with herpes infection suffer severe neurological and vision difficulties, and nearly half of those with systemic infection die.

The best that medical science has to offer is relief of the symptoms of genital herpes infection during an outbreak. The primary drug used to relieve the symptoms of genital herpes infection is **acyclovir.** Usually prescribed in ointment form, acyclovir prevents the herpes virus from reproducing itself. This, in turn, reduces the amount of virus shed from the affected skin. It also reduces the length of time during which symptoms are present and the severity of the symptoms themselves. Acyclovir does not prevent recurrence of the infection.

Prevention is the best way to deal with an incurable disease like herpes. The preventive measures we discussed previously apply here.

Bacterial Diseases

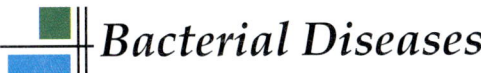

Bacterial diseases, as opposed to viral diseases, can usually be cured with some form of antibiotic therapy. The difference between the two infections is due not only to the different pathogens causing them but also to the location of the microorganism in the infected individual. In the case of a viral infection, the microorganism is located inside the cell; in the case of a bacterial infection, the microorganism is located outside the cell wall. This is one reason why bacterial diseases can be cured.

Chlamydia

Chlamydia, which infects four million Americans each year, is the most common STD in the country. It is estimated that about 10 percent of college students are infected with this disease. Women are infected with chlamydia nearly six times more often than are men. College-age women are at highest risk for chlamydia. Of infected women, 46 percent are aged fifteen to nineteen years and one third are aged twenty to twenty-four.

The symptoms of chlamydia infection in men include a whitish discharge from the penis and some discomfort. In women, there is some discomfort in the genitalia, itching, and burning. It is generally believed that 80 percent of women have no symptoms in the early stages of chlamydia infection and therefore do not seek treatment. Chlamydia is diagnosed through an examination by a physician using a swab from affected sites. Results are known in a few days.

For pregnant women, the risk of premature delivery is much greater with chlamydia infection, and many babies of infected mothers develop the eye disease conjunctivitis. Because of this, some medical researchers believe that chlamydia infection is the greatest cause of preventable blindness throughout the world. HIV transmission is apparently aided by the presence of chlamydia infection.

If left untreated, chlamydia can cause irreparable damage to the reproductive organs. In men, inflammation from the infection can cause scar tissue on the vas deferens, which can result in sterility. In women, inflammation of the fallopian tubes can also result in sterility and, in some cases, an increased risk of tubal pregnancy.

Women are at risk for a serious complication from chlamydia infection. That complication is **pelvic inflammatory disease (PID).** In the early stages of PID, chlamydia infection is generally located in the vagina. As the disease progresses,

hepatitis B A viral disease characterized by inflammation of the liver that is often transmitted through sexual intercourse.

herpes simplex type 2 A virus usually transmitted by sexual contact and causing open sores on the genitals.

lesions A change in tissue, or sores.

meningitis An inflammation of the membranes surrounding the spinal cord and brain.

systemic infection An infection affecting the body as a whole.

acyclovir A drug used to relieve the symptoms of genital herpes infection.

chlamydia A common bacterial STD, which, if untreated, can cause serious, painful infections of the urinary tract in men and infection of the reproductive organs in women.

pelvic inflammatory disease (PID) An infection in the pelvic area usually involving the uterus, fallopian tubes, and/or ovaries; half the cases are caused by chlamydia.

however, it spreads to the lining of the uterus and into the fallopian tubes. Infection in the fallopian tubes involves the inner walls of the tubes and creates pus, which may leak into the pelvic cavity and onto the ovaries. Symptoms of PID include severe abdominal pain and fever.

Frequently, the tubes affected by PID are left partially or totally blocked by scar tissue. A partial block contributes to the increased risk of tubal pregnancy. A total block results in sterility. Early treatment may prevent permanent tube blockage but cannot repair damage already done. PID is a leading cause of sterility among women. Chlamydia may account for as many as half of the 1 million cases of PID that are recorded each year in the United States.

Tetracycline and other antibiotics are used to treat chlamydia. Pregnant women should not use tetracycline because of its effects on the developing fetus.

Gonorrhea

Gonorrhea is caused by the bacterium *Neisseria gonorrhoeae.* Each year, four hundred thousand cases of gonorrhea are reported. Symptoms of gonorrhea in a man include a burning sensation when urinating and a whitish discharge from the penis. Because few men are asymptomatic, treatment for gonorrhea in men often begins in the early stages of the disease. Without treatment, the disease can cause urinary obstruction, inflammation and abscesses of the prostate, and sterility. Recent research has found that gonorrheal infection contributes to the transmission of HIV.

As with a chlamydia infection, 80 percent of women with gonorrhea are commonly believed to be asymptomatic and therefore do not seek treatment early in the course of the disease. Those who do show symptoms often experience abnormal vaginal discharges, some discomfort in the vaginal area, and pain during urination. Unfortunately, these signs are unreliable indicators of gonorrhea because they may be caused by a range of other STDs as well as by other nonsexually related conditions. Diagnosis of gonorrhea is done by a test of secretions from the cervix, throat, rectum, or penis (depending on the kind of intercourse). Some test results are available immediately; some take a few days.

The most severe complications of gonorrheal infection in women include PID, blindness in infants, and gonococcal arthritis. Infantile blindness due to gonococcal infection was brought under control with the mandatory use of eye drops following birth.

Once diagnosed, gonorrhea is treated with antibiotic therapy, usually in the form of penicillin. In recent years, strains of gonorrhea have developed that are resistant to penicillin. In these cases, other antibiotic agents are used.

Syphilis

Syphilis, once the most feared STD, infected more than 50,000 people in 1990 but only 11,400 in 1996. This decline from a new infection rate of 20.3 cases per 100,000 persons in 1990 to 4.4 cases per 100,000 in 1996 shows that it is possible to significantly reduce the incidence of an STD through prevention and treatment. Penicillin has been the main treatment since 1947. Health officials are cautiously optimistic about the possibility of eliminating new cases of syphilis in the United States. However, the current U.S. syphilis rate is ten times the Canadian rate.

Caused by the *Treponema pallidum* spirochete, syphilis infection progresses through predictable stages. **Primary syphilis** is characterized by a painless sore at the site of the infection. The sore is usually round with raised edges and is called a **chancre.** Syphilis is highly contagious while a chancre is present. If left untreated, the chancre heals by itself, often leaving the infected person with the misconception that the disease is gone and there is no reason for concern.

Actually, the healing of the initial chancre is only an indication that the disease has progressed into **secondary syphilis,** which is characterized by a general

---

Neisseria gonorrhoeae The bacterium that causes gonorrhea.

syphilis A bacterial STD that spreads through the bloodstream and causes a systemic infection.

primary syphilis Characterized by painless sores, called chancres, at the site of the infection.

chancre A painless, round sore with raised edges indicative of syphilis.

secondary syphilis A highly contagious disease characterized by a general rash on the body, sore throat, fever, and pains in the joints and muscles.

late syphilis A disease characterized by generalized infection that can produce heart failure, blindness, loss of muscle control, brain damage, and death.

vaginitis A vaginal infection usually caused by yeast or protozoa.

yeast infection A condition characterized by itching; burning during urination; a white, thick, odorless discharge; painful intercourse; and general discomfort. Caused by *Candida.*

rash on the body, sore throat, fever, and pains in the joints and muscles. As in primary syphilis, secondary syphilis is highly contagious.

A period of latency follows secondary syphilis, during which time no outward symptoms are present. This latent period can last from one to forty years and is usually not a period of contagion. Again, the infected individual may be fooled into thinking that the syphilis infection is gone. In fact, the disease is spreading to other parts of the body, including the brain and spinal cord.

The final stage of the disease is referred to as **late syphilis.** This stage of generalized infection can produce heart failure, blindness, loss of muscle control, brain damage, and death.

At any stage, syphilis can be diagnosed by visual observation and/or confirmed with a blood test. Treatment is effective and involves a penicillin regimen. The body does not develop immunity to syphilis, so a person treated for the disease can contract it again and again. If a pregnant woman has syphilis, treatment is critical to avoid damage to both mother and fetus. The spirochete crosses the placenta and in most cases causes either a miscarriage or stillbirth or congenital syphilis, which often results in malformations of body parts and partial blindness and deafness. Like chlamydia and gonorrhea, syphilis contributes to HIV transmission.

Critical Thinking Question

> The *Healthy People 2000* objectives include the following: "Reduce congenital syphilis to an incidence of no more than 40 cases per 100,000 live births." In 1994, the incidence was 55.6 per 100,000 live births. Given the recent major decline in primary syphilis, the rates for congenital syphilis are predicted to drop as well. What might account for the decline in this disease: An effective public health campaign? The occurrence of another, more feared disease? Social change?

Other STDs

Organisms other than viruses and bacteria can cause STDs in both men and women. These are not especially life threatening but can cause discomfort and require diagnosis and treatment.

Vaginitis

Virtually every woman experiences **vaginitis,** a vaginal infection, at some point in her life. In fact, vaginitis is a common reason for a woman to see a physician. It is usually caused by either a yeast or a protozoal infection.

One prevalent form of vaginitis is a **yeast** (fungus) **infection** caused by *Candida* (sometimes called *Monilia*). *Candida* is present in the vaginal area of many women. Under normal conditions, the presence of *Candida* causes no problems because the environment of the vagina is usually acidic enough to ward off infections. However, certain conditions can alter this, including antibiotic therapy, use of contraceptive pills, menstruation, wearing panty hose and nylon underwear, douching, and even lack of sleep. Symptoms occur when the fungus grows fast enough to produce symptoms such as itching; burning during urination; a

TABLE 15.2 Common Sexually Transmitted Diseases

Disease name	Pathogen	How transmitted	Symptoms	Preventive measures	Treatment
AIDS	Virus (human immunodeficiency virus)	By direct contact with infected person, usually during sexual intercourse (anal, vaginal), and by exchange of blood	Often no symptoms exist; combination of weight loss, night sweats, cough, new skin rashes, changes in bowel function, unexplained chronic fever	Abstinence; avoid sexual contact and blood exchange with infected person; use a condom; do not share needles	No known cure; protease inhibitors, AZT, and other drugs taken orally can decrease symptoms; treat opportunistic diseases associated with AIDS
Chlamydia	Bacterium (*Chlamydia trachomatis*)	By contact with infected person, usually during sexual intercourse	Whitish pus discharge from the penis; frequent, painful urination; often no symptoms exist	Avoid sexual contact with infected person; use a condom	Azithromycin, tetracyclines, or erythromycin
Crabs	Parasite (pubic lice)	By contact with infected person, usually during sexual intercourse	Intense itching on genital area; nits on hair shafts	Avoid sexual contact with infected person; scrupulous cleaning after intercourse	Various topical ointments, shampoos, lotions prescribed by physician (e.g., lindane lotion)
Genital warts	Virus (papilloma virus)	By contact with infected person, usually during sexual intercourse	Pinky-brown raised areas with tendency to form a cauliflower-shaped mass on external genitalia	Avoid sexual contact with infected person; use a condom	Washing with soap and water twice daily; painting lesions with podophyllin; surgical removal

TABLE 15.2 Common Sexually Transmitted Diseases (continued)

Disease name	Pathogen	How transmitted	Symptoms	Preventive measures	Treatment
Gonorrhea	Bacterium (*Neisseria gonorrhoeae*)	By contact with infected person, usually during sexual intercourse	Burning on urination; milky discharge from penis; urgency to urinate; in women, inflammation of vagina; often no symptoms	Education; use a condom; early diagnosis; avoid sexual contact with infected person	One intramuscular dose of ceftriaxone plus seven days of oral doxycycline
Herpes simplex type 2	Virus (herpes virus)	By contact with infected person, usually during sexual intercourse	Small groups of blisters on a reddened base of external or internal genitalia; painful urination	Avoid sexual contact with infected person, especially during outbreaks; use a condom	No known cure; normal saline solution to help prevent infection; apply antiviral agents (e.g., acyclovir) to skin
Syphilis	Bacterium (*Treponema pallidum*)	By contact with infected person, usually during sexual intercourse	Primary—painless chancre on external genitals. Secondary—skin rash, achiness. Tertiary—lesion, problems with nervous system and cardiovascular system	Avoid sexual contact with infected person; use a condom	Penicillin or tetracycline
Yeast infection	Fungus (*Candida albicans*)	By direct contact with infected person or normal flora overgrowth with hormonal changes, diabetes, oral antibiotics, or immunodeficiencies	Vaginal discharge of thick, whitish, cheesy substance; skin may be bluish-red, scaly; intense vulval and vaginal itching	Identify early and treat early to reduce severity of symptoms	Nystatin suppositories in the vaginal canal for 2 weeks; axole antifungal creams in vaginal canal for 7–10 days; diflucan orally

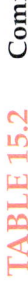

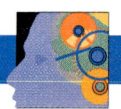

DEVELOPING HEALTH SKILLS

The Proper Use of a Condom

1. Latex condoms should be used because they may offer greater protection against HIV and other viral STDs than natural membrane condoms.
2. Condoms should be stored in a cool, dry place out of direct sunlight.
3. Condoms in damaged packages or those that show obvious signs of age (e.g., those that are brittle, sticky, or discolored) should not be used. They cannot be relied on to prevent infection or pregnancy.
4. Condoms should be handled with care to prevent puncture.
5. The condom should be put on before any genital contact to prevent exposure to fluids that may contain infectious agents. Hold the tip of the condom and unroll it onto the erect penis, leaving space at the tip to collect semen, yet ensuring that no air is trapped in the tip of the condom.
6. Only water-based lubricants should be used. Petroleum- or oil-based lubricants (such as petroleum jelly, cooking oils, shortening, and lotions) should not be used because they weaken the latex and may cause breakage.
7. Use of condoms containing spermicides may provide some additional protection against STDs. However, vaginal use of spermicides along with condoms is likely to provide still greater protection.
8. If a condom breaks, it should be replaced immediately. If ejaculation occurs after condom breakage, the immediate use of spermicide has been suggested. However, the protective value of postejaculation application of spermicide in reducing the risk of STD transmission is unknown.
9. After ejaculation, care should be taken so that the condom does not slip off the penis before withdrawal; the base of the condom should be held throughout withdrawal. The penis should be withdrawn while still erect.
10. Condoms should never be reused.

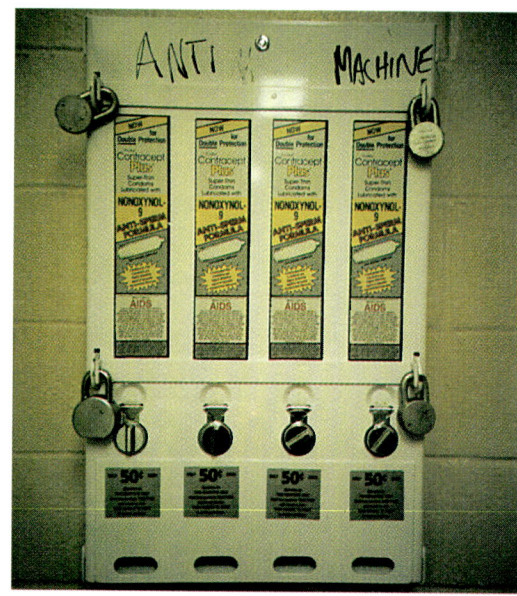

Condoms containing the spermicide nonoxynol-9 provide additional protection from STDs and are conveniently available in vending machines. (Source: The Image Works. © M. Antman)

Source: U.S. Centers for Disease Control and Prevention

white, thick, odorless discharge; painful intercourse; and general discomfort. Diagnosis is through personal observations, which may be verified by a culture taken by a physician. Treatment is usually an antifungal drug in the form of suppositories or ointment. Antifungal drugs are now available over the counter, thus facilitating self-diagnosis and treatment.

One fact that is often overlooked by women who suffer from yeast infections is that their sexual partner can carry the infection without symptoms and reinfect them even after treatment is successful. This process of one partner infecting the other after treatment is called the ping-pong effect. It can be avoided simply by treating the male sexual partner with an antifungal cream regardless of whether any symptoms are present.

Protozoal vaginitis, unlike yeast infections, is transmitted primarily by sexual means. Sexually active women run an increased risk of this infection, which is called **trichomoniasis.** The symptoms include a foul or fishy odor, accompanied by itching, a burning sensation, and sometimes pain in the vaginal area.

The most effective treatment involves the antiprotozoal drug metronidazole. There are no serious complications resulting from trichomoniasis. As with other forms of vaginitis, men can carry the disease organism and transmit it to a woman, so both partners should be treated at the same time.

Here are some suggestions for avoiding vaginitis:

- Wear loose cotton underwear and avoid tight pants or jeans. This is especially important when wearing pantyhose or tights.
- Always wipe from the front (vagina) to the back (anus) after urinating.
- Use condoms, especially if having anal sex.
- If your sexual partner is an uncircumcised man, he should wash (with water only) and dry under his foreskin daily.
- Avoid excess soap, vaginal deodorants, deodorized panty shields, or bubble bath solutions.
- Minimize the use of antibiotics or request *Candida* treatment when prescribed antibiotics.
- Keep healthy. When people are stressed or run down, they are more prone to infections.

Pubic Lice and Scabies

Another form of STDs, pubic lice (crabs) and scabies, is caused by spider-like parasites that live in the genital area of both men and women. They are highly contagious and are common among college students. Both are spread by close physical contact, and also by sheets, towels, and the infamous toilet seat. Diagnosis is usually a simple matter of checking pubic hair in a good light. The nits (eggs) or lice are visible to the naked eye. Symptoms include extreme itching and other skin discomfort. Because people who have lice and scabies tend to scratch their skin severely, secondary infection is a concern.

Treatment for lice and scabies usually involves an insecticide shampoo, topical creams, and overall good hygiene. Once diagnosis is confirmed, it is recommended that all bed linens, towels, and clothes be washed in hot water. What happens if these infestations are left untreated? Such a possibility is highly unlikely because the itching is so severe that help is almost always pursued. The presence of pubic lice or scabies may be a warning to have a complete STD checkup.

How Do You Know If You Have an STD?

HEALTH SKILLS

Sometimes it is hard to tell if you have an STD or not. With some infections, a lot of people do not get symptoms. They may look and feel healthy but still have an STD. It is also possible that a little knowledge can be hazardous to your health. For example, the information contained in this chapter provides a brief description of the symptoms of some STDs but does not contain adequate information for you to make a confirmed diagnosis. To take care of yourself properly, you need to know what the symptoms are of different STDs and when to see a physician.

If you are sexually active and suspect that you have been in contact with an infected person (or even if you have just changed sexual partners), it is important to have a checkup just in case, even when you feel fine. (Also, remember that some STDs can be transmitted from one person to another even without having sexual intercourse. Remaining abstinent is not an absolute guarantee of protec-

protozoal vaginitis A condition transmitted sexually and characterized by a foul or fishy odor, accompanied by itching, burning sensations and pain in the vaginal area.

trichomoniasis A protozoal vaginitis transmitted primarily through sexual means.

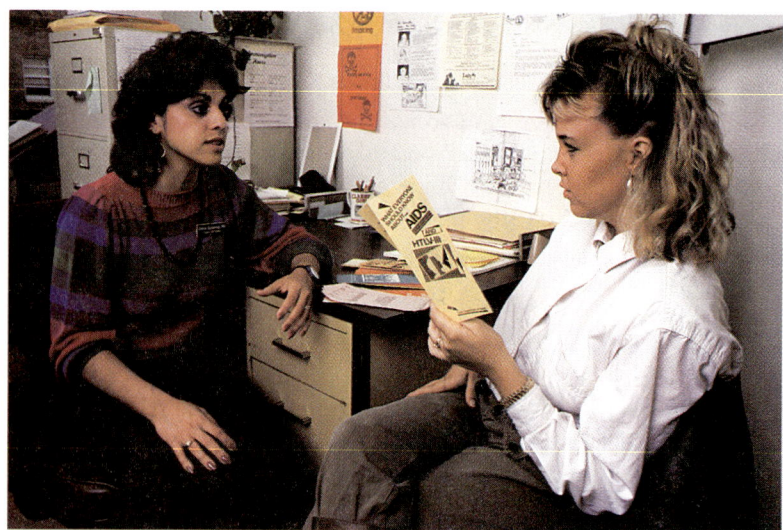

You should get an STD checkup if you are sexually active and suspect that you have had unprotected contact with an infected person. Remember: you can feel fine and still be infected. (Source: Stock, Boston/© Bob Daemmrich)

tion against STDs.) If you are concerned at all, see your physician. Do not feel you are wasting his or her time. Making sure shows that you are being responsible about your health.

If you have any of the following symptoms, a checkup is vital:

- Unusual discharge from the vagina or penis
- Burning pain, stinging, or irritation when passing urine
- A sore, blister, ulcer, warts, or break in the skin, or rash in the genital area
- A low abdominal pain or pain during intercourse

Do not make the mistake of waiting to see if a rash or a pain "clears up." The fact that discomfort disappears does not mean you no longer have a disease. If you or your sexual partner has any of the above symptoms, discuss them together and do not have sex until you have had a checkup by a physician.

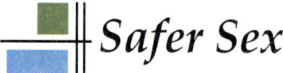 Safer Sex

The different diseases described in this chapter may threaten your health to a greater or lesser extent, depending on your sexual practices. Precautions are not guaranteed to result in total protection from STDs. But you can substantially reduce your risk by establishing a pattern of behavior that results in **safer sex.** This involves:

- *A willingness to prepare ahead for sex.* Make a decision now about your sexual behavior. If you are considering having sex, preparation means knowing the facts and discussing them with your partner. Do not be embarrassed to talk about STDs. And do not be embarrassed to insist on protecting yourself.
- *A commitment to using condoms with nonoxynol-9 is the only proven risk-reducer other than abstinence.* Although not perfect, a condom with spermicide is the best known protection against most STDs. Safer sex includes the use of a new condom every time you have sex (see the Developing Health Skills box).
- *Truly understanding that if you are sexually active you can get STDs.* One of the most dangerous attitudes relative to STDs is denial—to pretend that "it" will not happen to you. If you are sexually active, "it" *can* happen to you. Acting responsibly means accepting the reality of risk, then taking action to reduce the risk. And if symptoms do appear, see a physician for early treatment.

safer sex A pattern of responsible sexual behavior characterized by reduced risk for disease.

Critical Thinking Question

The term *safe sex* has been used for years to suggest that, by using condoms and taking other precautions, sexual intercourse can be made risk-free. A more recent term, *safer sex*, has been used to acknowledge that no amount of precaution can render sexual activity totally risk-free. Do you think either of these terms accurately depicts the actual risk of sexual activity? Do you feel most people your age practice safer sex? What are the trends on your campus?

Key Concepts

1. Modern medicine can cure some STDs but cannot control them.
2. Asymptomatic carriers provide a constant infected pool that is a source of infection or reinfection for others.
3. The leading risk factor related to the spread of STDs is multiple partners. Indirectly, the sexual revolution has contributed to the STD problem.
4. The risk for being exposed to an STD increases when no preventive prophylactics (i.e., condoms) are used.
5. The most serious health complications caused by STDs are infertility, tubal pregnancy, infant blindness, mental retardation, cancer, and death.
6. Viral STDs include AIDS, human papilloma virus, hepatitis B, and genital herpes. Papilloma virus infection is currently the fastest growing STD.
7. The most dangerous STD is AIDS. It is transmitted through body fluids such as blood, semen, and vaginal fluid.
8. Bacterial STDs include chlamydia, gonorrhea, and syphilis.
9. The two most common causes of vaginitis, an inflammation of the vagina, are a yeast infection and a protozoal infection.
10. The best hope for controlling STDs rests in prevention rather than treatment.

Review Questions

1. List evidence that STDs represent a major public health problem in the United States.
2. Of the STDs presented in this text, list those that can be cured with antibiotics, those that can be prevented with vaccination, and those that must be controlled through personal and social action.
3. Describe the significance of asymptomatic carriers to the overall STD epidemic.
4. Describe risk factors for the spread of STDs.
5. Make a list of measures that you can take to reduce your potential for contracting an STD.
6. Describe how HIV/AIDS, hepatitis B, human papilloma virus, and genital herpes are diagnosed and treated.
7. Describe how chlamydia, gonorrhea, and syphilis are diagnosed and treated.
8. Describe how vaginitis, pubic lice, and scabies are diagnosed and treated.
9. Explain the concept of "safer sex" and list measures that assure the risk of sexual activity is kept low.
10. List the symptoms of STDs that should prompt a visit to a physician.

Selected Bibliography

Benson, A.S., (ed.). *Control of Communicable Diseases in Man*, 15th ed. Washington, DC: American Public Health Association, 1990.

Centers for Disease Control and Prevention. "The HIV/AIDS Epidemic: The First 10 Years." *Morbidity and Mortality Weekly Report* 40 (1991): 357–369.

Centers for Disease Control and Prevention. *HIV/AIDS Surveillance Report*. Published twice a year.

Eng, T.R., and W.T. Butler, eds. *The Hidden Epidemic: Confronting Sexually Transmitted Diseases.* Washington, DC: Institute of Medicine, National Academy Press, 1997.

Hatcher, R.A., et al. *Contraceptive Technology.* New York: Irvington, 1990.

The CDC's Case Definition of AIDS: Implications for the Proposed Revisions. Washington, DC: U.S. Congress, Office of Technology Assessment, 1992.

HealthLinks: Web Sites for Reducing the Risk of Sexually Transmitted Diseases

You can access better health as it relates to this chapter by checking out some of the following sites on the Internet. These and sites identified within the chapter can be accessed directly when you visit the *HealthStyles* Web Site located on the Allyn and Bacon home page at **http://www.abacon.com.**

American Social Health Association

http://sunsite.unc.edu/ASHA

ASHA is dedicated to stopping STDs and their harmful consequences to individuals, families, and communities. Find information on STDs, women's health, the latest research, and link up with national organizations dedicated to STD prevention.

HIV/AIDS Treatment Information Service

www.hivatis.org

The HIV/AIDS Treatment Information Service (ATIS) provides information about federally approved treatment guidelines for HIV and AIDS. ATIS is staffed by bilingual (English and Spanish) health information specialists who answer questions on HIV treatment options and refer individuals to an extensive network of federal information services and national and community-based organizations for treatment-related information.

Health Hotlines: Reducing the Risk for Sexually Transmitted Diseases

American Social Health Association, Herpes Resource Center
(800) 230-6039
P.O. Box 13827
Research Triangle Park, NC 27709

CDC National AIDS Clearinghouse
(800) 458-5231
P.O. Box 6003
Rockville, MD 20849-6003

CDC National AIDS Hotline
(800) 342-AIDS (342-2437)
P.O. Box 13827
Research Triangle Park, NC 27709

CDC National STD Hotline
(800) 227-8922
P.O. Box 13827
Research Triangle Park, NC 27709

HIV/AIDS Treatment Information
(800) HIV-0440 (488-0440)
P.O. Box 6303
Rockville, MD 20849-6303

National Association of People with AIDS
(800) 808-8060 (pharmacy)
1413 K Street NW, 8th Floor
Washington, DC 20005

State HIV/AIDS Hotlines

Alabama	(800) 228-0649
Alaska	(800) 478-2437
Arizona	(800) 334-1540
Arkansas	(800) 364-2437
California	(800) 367-2437 (northern)
	(800) 922-2437 (southern)
Colorado	(800) 252-2437
	(303) 782-5186 (only Denver)
Connecticut	(800) 203-1234
Delaware	(800) 422-0429
District of Columbia	(202) 332-2437
Florida	(800) 352-2437
Georgia	(800) 551-2728
Hawaii	(800) 321-1555
Idaho	(800) 677-2437
Illinois	(800) 243-2437
Indiana	(800) 848-2437
Iowa	(800) 445-2437
Kansas	(800) 342-AIDS
Kentucky	(800) 840-2865
Louisiana	(800) 992-4379
Maine	(800) 851-2437
Maryland	(800) 638-6252
Massachusetts	(800) 235-2331
Michigan	(800) 872-2437
Minnesota	(800) 248-2437
Mississippi	(800) 826-2961
Missouri	(800) 533-2437
Montana	(800) 233-6668
Nebraska	(800) 782-2437
Nevada	(800) 842-2437
New Hampshire	(800) 752-2437
New Jersey	(800) 624-2377
New Mexico	(800) 545-2437
New York	(800) 541-2437
North Carolina	(800) 342-AIDS
North Dakota	(800) 472-2180
Ohio	(800) 332-2437
Oklahoma	(800) 535-2437
Oregon	(800) 777-2437
Pennsylvania	(800) 662-6080
Puerto Rico	(800) 981-5721
Rhode Island	(800) 726-3010
South Carolina	(800) 322-2437
South Dakota	(800) 592-1861
Tennessee	(800) 525-2437
Texas	(800) 299-2437
Utah	(800) 366-2437
Vermont	(800) 882-2437
Virginia	(800) 533-4148
Washington	(800) 272-2437
West Virginia	(800) 642-8244

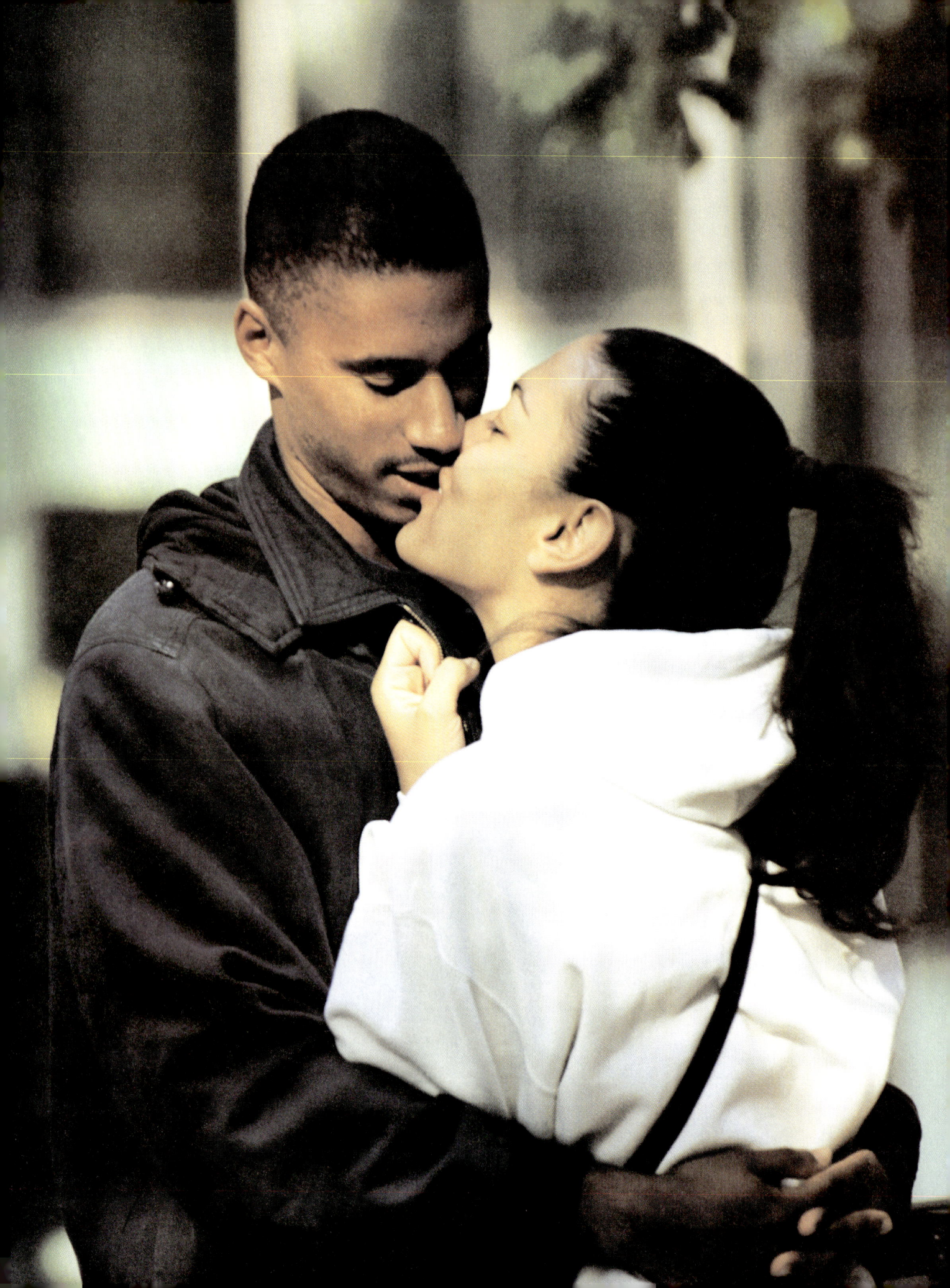

Chapter 16

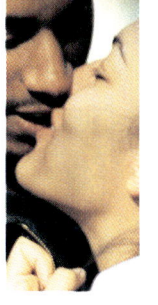
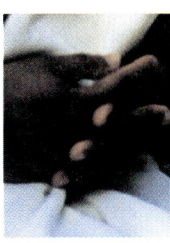
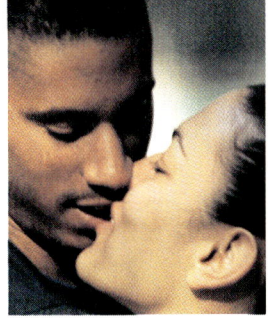

Sexuality

Developing Healthy Relationships

Objectives

When you finish reading this chapter, you will be able to:

1. Recognize that sexuality is a complex collection of qualities that make up a person's sexual attitudes, influence a person's sexual behaviors, and affect relationships with others.
2. Explain the importance of gender identity and sex role relative to sexuality.
3. Acknowledge the differences in sexual practice and attitudes between cultures and between individuals within a particular culture.
4. Recognize the hormones that most influence sexual development and secondary sex characteristics.
5. Differentiate between three sexual orientations: heterosexual, homosexual, and bisexual.
6. Recognize that when verbal and nonverbal languages conflict, miscommunication about sexual desires can result.
7. Define love in terms of intimacy, passion, and commitment.
8. Understand that sexual pleasure may take the form of masturbation, outercourse, or intercourse.
9. Understand the pattern of human sexual response, including its four phases: excitement, plateau, orgasm, and resolution.
10. Identify sexual dysfunctions that occur in both men and women, in men alone, and in women alone.

What Is Your HealthStyle?

Jorge was putting pressure on Marisa to have sex, but she wasn't sure she wanted to. She liked him, and they had a good time together going to the movies, but she felt the relationship was superficial. They laughed and had fun together, but they never had a serious discussion about how they felt about things that were important to each other. "Maybe he's immature," thought Marisa, "or maybe we just aren't right for each other." Whatever the reason, it was holding Marisa back from further involvement; and because communication between them was so poor, Marisa wasn't sure that would change. Marisa decided that she was going to say no to Jorge—and to a relationship that never seemed to develop fully.

Alan and Nadia had been going together for a few months, and they both felt very comfortable with each other. They had so much in common, and they loved talking with each other and sharing ideas. When Nadia was upset over a poor mark on a paper, Alan knew just what to say to make her feel better; and when either of them got an A, they celebrated together. Even though Alan was reluctant at first to talk about himself and what some of his dreams were for life after college, Nadia made him feel comfortable. Because of the trust they shared in each other, Nadia and Alan were able to discuss their fears and needs openly as their relationship grew and became more intimate.

In Your Opinion

Being able to communicate your feelings is an important component in the decision to say yes or no to having sex. Marisa and Nadia had different communication experiences—and different outcomes.

- Most people who are sexually active have said yes to sex sometimes and no on other occasions. What factors go into such a decision?
- What health skills were evident in Marisa's decision to say no to Jorge?
- What health skills were evident in Nadia's and Alan's relationship?
- What are the hazards of becoming sexually involved with someone who is difficult to talk with?

Sexuality means something different to almost every person. Over the course of time, it can also mean different things to the same person. Love, lust, intimacy, attraction, and infatuation are some of the feelings that are associated with sexuality. Just as personality is the embodiment of a collection of qualities that make up a person and his or her relationship with others, **sexuality** is the embodiment of a collection of qualities that make up a person's sexual attitudes and behaviors and influence his or her relationships with others.

The term *sexuality* is a broad term encompassing biological, psychological, sociocultural, and ethical components of behavior. Healthy sexuality suggests a number of conditions:

- A state of comfort with your gender and sex role
- An ability to form positive interpersonal relationships

sexuality A collection of qualities that make up a person's sexual attitudes and behaviors and influence his or her relationships with others.

gender identity A sense of comfort with one's gender; an acceptance of one's maleness or femaleness.

sex role Overt behaviors that disclose ourselves as male or female to others.

- An ability to respond to erotic stimulation with pleasure
- An ability to make mature judgments about sexuality

A sense of comfort with your gender suggests an acceptance of your maleness or femaleness. This is sometimes referred to as **gender identity.** Your gender identity is evident in your **sex role** behavior, what you do to disclose yourself as male or female to others.

The ability to form positive interpersonal relationships (with persons of the same or opposite sex) suggests a desire to be close to someone else, the ability to empathize with another person's feelings, and the ability to commit to the importance of a relationship.

The ability to respond to erotic stimulation with pleasure suggests a healthy functioning sexual response, both biological and psychological.

Finally, an ability to make mature judgments about sexuality suggests a clear understanding of personal values and beliefs, an ability to make sex-related decisions that respect the dignity of others while acknowledging personal desires and drives, and the ability to restrain from sexual behavior when conditions suggest risk to personal health or to the health of others. Basic to all is honest and effective communication, particularly about sexual feelings.

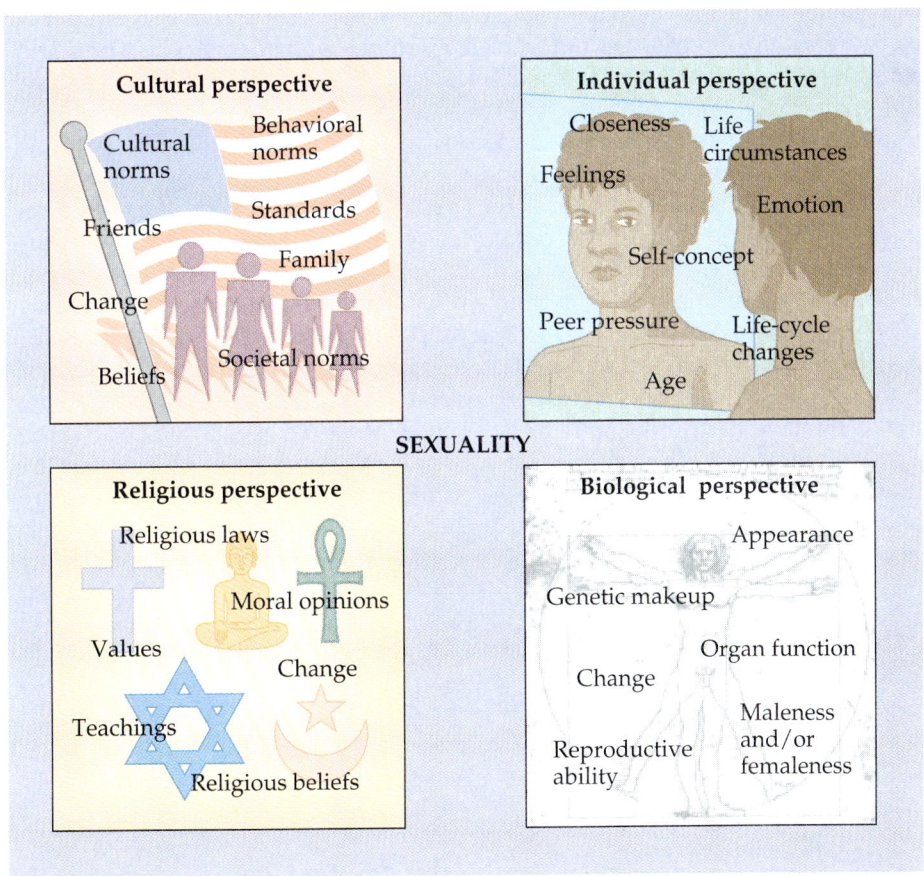

▬ **Figure 16.1 Cornerstones of Sexuality.** *Your sexuality has been shaped by at least four perspectives: biological, cultural, individual, and religious. These four orientations will continue to shape your sexuality throughout your life.*

Points of View about Sexuality

To further understand sexuality, it is helpful to consider different points of view. Consider the following four perspectives: cultural, religious, personal, and biological. These four points of view have shaped your sexuality to date and will continue to do so throughout your life (see Figure 16.1).

Your Culture

Sexual values, attitudes, and practices differ from culture to culture. On one Irish island, normal frequency of sexual intercourse is best measured in terms of times per year. Times per week is the best measure for one Polynesian group, whereas times per day is the measure used by one African tribe, even for men and women well into their sixties.

Behaviors and attitudes can also differ within a culture and can change within a culture over time. In the United States, for example, some of the pioneers in the birth control movement were jailed in the 1920s because of their beliefs. Today, various methods of birth control are widely available in drug stores and college health clinics, and most adult American women report using some form of birth control.

The application of different standards of sexual conduct to men and women (the double standard) also illustrates how behaviors and attitudes can differ within a culture. For example, in the Victorian era, well-to-do men regularly sought the companionship of prostitutes but wanted a virtuous woman for a wife. The double standard exists today. Many men still view sex as a conquest and find that multiple sex partners are acceptable. Most women, however, are not so accepting of multiple sex partners. The double standard can be particularly troublesome for college students attempting to understand sexuality and make decisions about sex.

What has come to be known as the **sexual revolution** is a product of the last third of this century. Increased premarital and extramarital sexual activity and liberalized attitudes toward homosexuality, abortion, masturbation, and pornography are indications of change from earlier standards. As recently as the early 1960s, public opinion polls showed that most Americans believed that sex before marriage was wrong. Today, most unmarried men and women are sexually active. By age nineteen, nearly 90 percent of men and 75 percent of women report that they have had intercourse at least once. Most never-married or divorced men and women in their thirties, forties, and fifties have had at least one, but more often several, sexual encounters, and it is not uncommon for divorced or widowed men and women in their sixties, seventies, and eighties to develop ongoing nonmarital sexual relationships.

Critical Thinking Question

> The sexual revolution was characterized by significant sexual behavioral changes. Based on what you know about the sexual revolution of the 1960s, what social impact do you think it has had on us today—positive and negative? What do you think the next sexual revolution will bring? Whereas the birth control pill played a major role in the last sexual revolution, what technology, drug, or social viewpoint might play the primary role in the next revolution?

sexual revolution A period of time (thought to begin in the 1960s) characterized by a significant liberalization of sexual behavior and attitudes.

Your Religion

Teachings of all the major religions include standards for sexual conduct. As with cultural values, sexual values are subject to change and interpretation. The Old Testament, for example, endorsed sex for procreation. The ancient Jews were told in Genesis to be fruitful and multiply. In fact, a young married couple was encouraged to have sexual intercourse as often as possible. The husband was even exempted from military service for a year to tend to such duties. Adultery, meanwhile, was forbidden and made part of the law in the Ten Commandments: "Thou shalt not commit adultery."

American attitudes about sex were strongly influenced by the Puritans, who considered sex a necessary evil. Again, sex was for procreation, not for pleasure. To reinforce this, rigid dress codes were developed to inhibit sexual thoughts or fantasies and temptations. Not all Puritans, however, were so sexually repressed. Early New England church records include the letters CF after a person's name, which refer to "confessing fornication." Another sign is readily seen in some cross-stitched family trees, where the birth date of the firstborn is well shy of nine months, indicating conception before marriage.

Even today, religion affects society's view of sexual practices and behavior. Much of the controversy surrounding issues such as sex education, abortion rights, and sexual orientation has its roots in religion. Religion often plays a major role in the establishment of personal values, beliefs, and a moral and ethical code of conduct. Values, however, arise not only from religious mandates but also from an individual's interpretation of such teachings.

You as an Individual

As important as culture and religion are to sexual attitudes and behavior, the primary determinant remains you, the individual. No two people are alike. Not only do you differ physically from your best friend but also you differ intellectually, emotionally, and sexually.

In sexual behavior, as in other behaviors, society pressures us to act like everyone else. Many people, both men and women, report that they become sexually active because of peer pressure. They want to appear "normal." Sometimes the desire for social acceptance conflicts with an individual's value system.

The individual perspective on sexuality may change throughout the life cycle. Our lives are made up of stages during which major changes and developments take place. Most broadly, these periods are childhood; adolescence; and early, middle, and late adulthood.

HealthLinks

Sexuality Information and Education Council of the United States (SIECUS)
http://www.siecus.org

Information, guidelines, and materials for advancement of healthy and proper sex education.

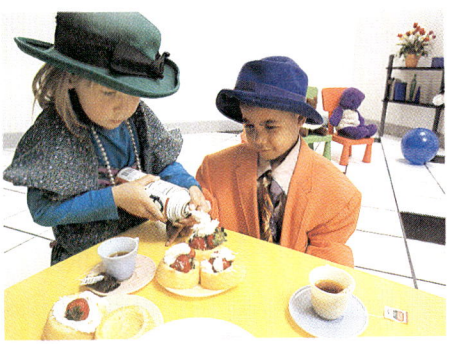
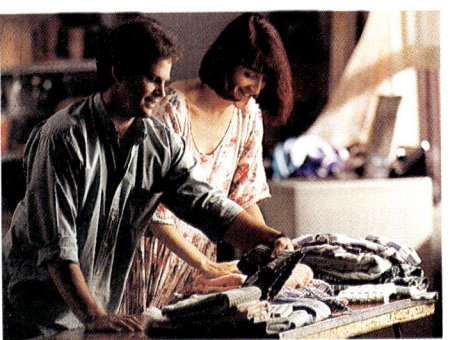

Children learn about sex roles from their family. They progress from playing house as youngsters to keeping house as adults. (Sources: LEFT Tony Stone Images/© Andy Sacks; RIGHT © Tony Stone Images/Bruce Ayres)

In childhood, the family has the most influence on a young person's ideas about sexuality. Sexuality within the family is evident in the sexual interactions of the adults. Also, it is evident in the pattern of same-sex and opposite-sex relationships. It is in childhood that sexual identity is established, sex roles are learned, and beliefs and values about sex and sexuality are established.

Adolescent sexual development is marked by the development of secondary sex characteristics, those physical signs of maturity as one moves from being a child to being a woman or a man. Physical maturity is accompanied by an increased interest in engaging in sexual activity. The physical ability to engage in sexual activity, however, is not always accompanied by the cognitive development needed to understand and to act to prevent the health risks of sexual involvement. Due to the incongruent development states of physical body and mind, adolescents are especially at risk for sexually transmitted diseases and unwanted pregnancy.

For some people, the transition from puberty to adult sexuality is fairly smooth; for others it involves turmoil. Although the changes are predictable, much depends on how each individual perceives them. For example, the experience of pregnancy is significantly different for a married woman in her twenties or thirties who has always wanted to have children than for a teenager whose life is disrupted by the need to drop out of high school, at least temporarily, to deliver and care for her child.

Likewise, changes that take place in late adulthood can bring a renewed sense of intimacy to some people but threaten the sexuality of others. After menopause, some women see themselves as being past their sexual prime. For others, cessation of menstruation sometimes increases sexual interest among older couples because of the altered ratio of hormones and elimination of fear of pregnancy.

Males in their sixties and above typically require longer periods of time to achieve erection and reach orgasm. For some, this slowed sexual response may be distressing. However, this same slowing down can lead to a more relaxed and caring sexual relationship. As a result, older couples often redefine their relationships, focusing on a new sense of intimacy (see Chapter 18).

There is no correct, precise timetable for sexual life-cycle changes. Puberty usually takes place in the early teens, but individuals may mature early as well as late. The timing of first sexual intercourse experience likewise depends on physical as well as emotional maturity. Some sexual milestones are missed completely on purpose or by happenstance or are modified to fit a person's lifestyle. For example, priests and nuns vow to remain celibate; one couple decides not to have children; another couple is infertile and adopts children.

Critical Thinking Question

The *Healthy People 2000* objectives include the following: "Reduce the proportion of adolescents who have engaged in sexual intercourse to no more than 15 percent by age 15 and no more than 40 percent by age 17." Data to date suggest very little movement toward this goal. In fact, about 40 percent of adolescents have had sex by age 15 and more than 65 percent have had sex by age 17. Why might the high level of sexual activity among adolescents be seen as a public health issue? What do you think might be the major barriers to achieving these goals?

androgens Male sex hormones.
estrogens Female sex hormones.

Your Biology

Finally, there is a biological perspective to human sexuality. The functions of the genitalia have not changed for millions of years, yet our understanding of the biological aspects of sex and sexuality has definitely changed. For example, the seminal vesicle was named because it was believed to be a storage site for sperm. Through scientific study, we now know that the seminal vesicle is a gland that secretes a portion of the semen, not a site for storage. (Sperm are stored for two to four weeks in the epididymis, a sac above the testes.) See Your Sexual Body: A Primer on Reproductive Anatomy and Physiology on pp. 429–439.

The primary biological factor establishing sexual identity is your genetic makeup. After conception, the human fetus has the potential to develop into either sex. After about the seventh week of development, however, the sex (male or female) is established. The normal female has two X (female) chromosomes (or XX), and the normal male has one X and one Y (male) chromosome (or XY). The sex chromosome is carried by the sperm. If an X-bearing sperm fertilizes an egg, the resulting XX combination produces a female. If the egg is fertilized by a Y-bearing sperm, the resulting XY combination produces a male (see Figure 16.2).

The development of physical and psychological sex characteristics is influenced by hormones that are secreted in response to genetic makeup. The hormones that most directly affect sexuality are **androgens** for men and **estrogens** for women. Androgens are produced chiefly in the testicles but are also produced by women. Estrogens are produced chiefly in the ovaries but are also present in men. Sexuality is adversely affected by a deficiency in these hormones.

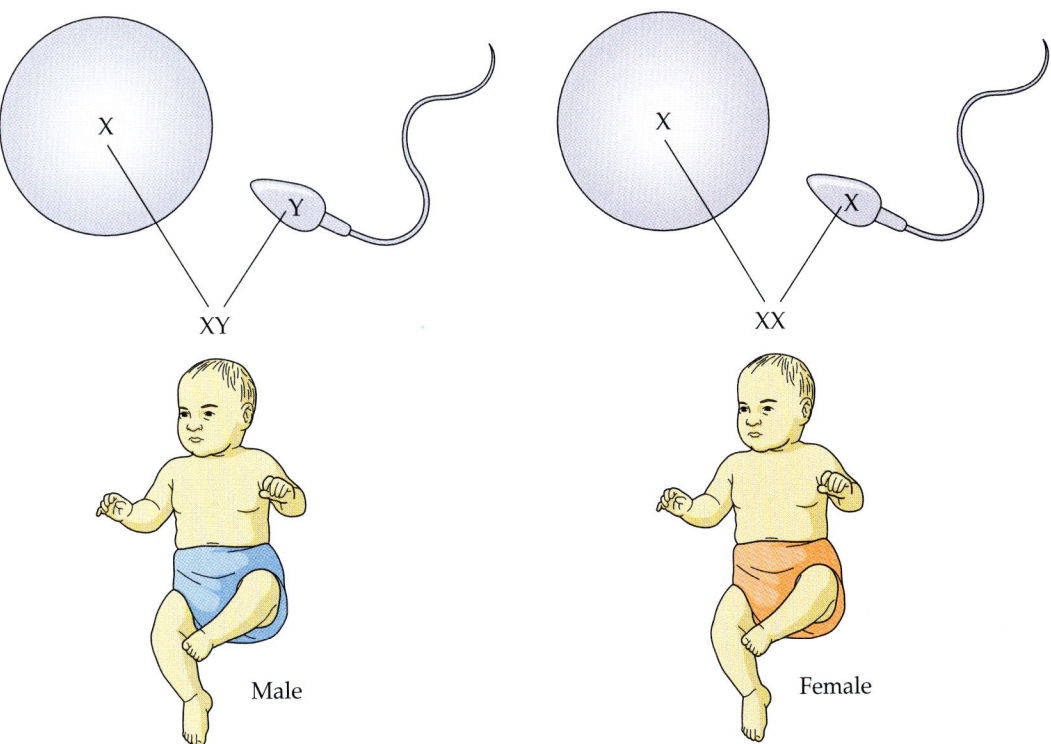

Figure 16.2 When Sperm Meets Egg: Determinants of Sex. *Your sex is determined genetically. A female has two X (female) chromosomes and a male has one X and one Y (male) chromosome.*

Men who have an androgen deficiency have a decrease in sexual responsiveness and sexual drive; for women, an estrogen deficiency can cause infertility and atrophy of the genitalia. All men, whether they are heterosexual, homosexual, or bisexual, produce a small amount of estrogen. Homosexuals do not produce an increased estrogen level, nor can their orientation be changed by doses of androgens. Similarly, all women produce some androgens, and lesbians are no more likely to have increased levels of androgens than are heterosexual women.

Your Sexual Orientation

Sexual orientation refers to a person's enduring attraction to individuals of a particular gender. Attraction can take many forms, emotional, romantic, or sexual. The word *enduring* is important, because a casual interest in the same or opposite gender is normal throughout life, and especially during early adolescence. Such a normal, but passing, attraction should not be considered a definitive sign of sexual orientation.

Three sexual orientations are commonly recognized: **heterosexual,** an attraction to individuals of a different sex; **homosexual,** an attraction to individuals of the same sex; and **bisexual,** an attraction to individuals of both sexes. Individuals who have a homosexual orientation are often referred to as **gay** (both men and women) or as **lesbian** (women only).

Despite extensive research, scientists have yet to explain the origin of sexual orientation. Some researchers suggest that genetic or inborn hormonal factors determine sexual orientation. Others believe that life experiences during early childhood are most important. Most scientists do agree, however, that sexual orientation is shaped for most people at an early age through the interaction of biological, psychological, and social factors. Psychologists do not consider sexual orientation to be a conscious choice that can be voluntarily changed.

Numerous false stereotypes and unwarranted prejudices exist toward individuals who have bisexual or homosexual orientations. As a result, the process of "coming out," or publicly confirming one's sexual orientation, can be difficult and may cause emotional pain. Lesbian and gay people often feel "different" and

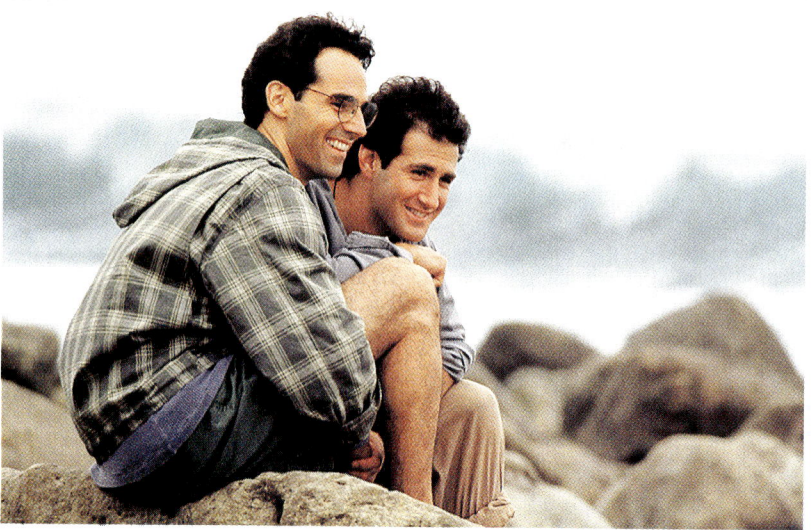

Scientists have not yet explained the origin of sexual orientation, but psychologists do not consider it to be a conscious choice that can be voluntarily changed. (Source: © Tony Stone Images/Bruce Ayres)

alone when they first become aware of same-sex attractions. They may also fear being rejected by family, friends, coworkers, and religious institutions if they do come out.

American society has traditionally discriminated against homosexual and bisexual individuals by declaring sexual acts between same-sex partners illegal, by not recognizing gay marriages as legal, and by denying custody or adoption of children to same-sex partners. After decades of gay rights activism, however, there has been some movement toward reducing the amount of discrimination based on sexual orientation, and an increasing number of gay couples are marrying or maintaining legal partnerships and raising families.

Critical Thinking Question

> Psychologists believe that negative attitudes toward homosexuals as a group do not result from actual experience with lesbians or gay men but rather from stereotypes and prejudices. What can be done to address the prejudice and reduce the acts of violence against homosexuals?

Communicating about Sex

HEALTH SKILLS

For many reasons, communicating about sex is difficult. For some college students, lessons learned as a child, such as "don't talk about sex in mixed company," can create communication gaps between couples. For others, the language available to talk about sex is simply too limiting. For still others, sharing intimate thoughts and desires is psychologically threatening.

The fact is, we communicate about sex whether we know it or not. Our sexuality is communicated through the clothes we wear, the pattern of our speech, and even the way we walk. Our facial expressions and voice tones can communicate sexual attraction, or rejection, even when the subject "sex" is never broached. And we miscommunicate about sex. We may inadvertently send a signal of rejection that we do not really mean. Or we may inadvertently "turn on" someone when our intent is just the opposite.

To avoid the problems that miscommunication brings to a relationship, a couple should first acknowledge the importance of communicating openly about sex. Good communication can result in a more fulfilling relationship for both parties. In contrast, poor communication can result in dissatisfaction and tension and ultimately bring about the breakup of the relationship. Good communication is obviously important for couples who are sexually involved. It is just as important, however, to couples who practice sexual abstinence. **Sexual abstinence** is a behavioral choice, not an indication of the absence of sexuality. Therefore, even though vaginal intercourse is avoided, the couple expresses sexual feelings and sexual behaviors that can range from fondling and kissing to sexual massaging, mutual masturbation, and anal intercourse. Another way that healthy couples who abstain express their sexual feelings is through verbal communications.

sexual orientation A person's enduring attraction to individuals of a particular gender.

heterosexual A person who has a sexual attraction to people of a different sex.

homosexual A person who has a sexual attraction to people of the same sex.

bisexual A person who has a sexual attraction to people of both sexes.

gay A homosexual orientation; a homosexual man or woman.

lesbian A homosexual woman.

sexual abstinence A behavioral choice not to engage in vaginal intercourse.

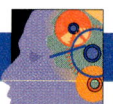

DEVELOPING HEALTH SKILLS

Learning How to Say "No" and "Yes"

The following three steps for saying no represent good advice for the person wanting to either avoid or delay sexual contact. By considering these, you can avoid being caught off guard and not knowing how to handle a situation.

1. Express appreciation for the invitation ("I appreciate your attraction to me."). Perhaps you may also wish to validate the value of the other person ("You are a good person.").
2. Say no in a clear, unequivocal fashion ("I would prefer not to make love, get involved in a dating relationship," and so forth).
3. Offer an alternative, if applicable ("I would like to have lunch sometime.").

Saying no can be difficult, particularly when sexual play has already started. Saying no should effectively bring sexual activity to a halt.

Saying yes can be more complex than saying no because rather than limiting alternatives, saying yes creates even more alternatives. Yes to what? For how long? Often people allow yes to be communicated through nonverbal means. Lovers often assume that they know what their partners want and need. Such assumption amounts to mind reading. Of course, it is not possible to literally read another person's mind, so nonverbal communication is open to misinterpretation.

Source: Based on Robert Crooks and Carla Baur, *Our Sexuality*, 5th ed., (Menlo Park, CA: Benjamin Cummings, 1993), p. 236

Nonverbal communication is a very powerful means of telling a sexual partner about desires, needs, and feelings. Facial expressions such as smiles or frowns clearly communicate pleasure or displeasure. Posture, such as sitting with legs and arms crossed and leaning away from a person, can signal that it is time to stop sexual advances. At the same time, posture that is open, such as two people facing each other with open arms and leaning toward each other, may be seen as an invitation to "go ahead." Sounds such as pleasure moaning also serve to communicate a go-ahead; no sound or sounds of frustration can signal at least one partner's wish to stop.

When nonverbal language and verbal language conflict, an individual sends a mixed message. For example, when one sexual partner says no but his or her nonverbal responses signal pleasure and encouragement, the other sexual partner has a problem deciding what to do. Does he or she continue sexual activity and honor the nonverbal signals, or stop and honor the verbal signals? How well do you communicate? Read the Developing Health Skills box to learn more.

Love: The Basis of Intimate Relationships

"How do I love thee? Let me count the ways," wrote Elizabeth Barrett Browning to her husband, Robert, nearly 150 years ago. Indeed, there are numerous ways to love a person. Now as then, love plays a major role in establishing a lifestyle as well as in the selection of a sexual partner. Read about the current trends in romance in the Cultural View box.

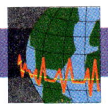

CULTURAL VIEW

Closing the Romance Gap

Is romance in the air? It's definitely evident in current popular culture. Moviegoers have been gobbling up film versions of Jane Austen's genteel stories of love lost and won like so many chocolate bon-bons. *Romeo and Juliet* is back. *The English Patient*, a tale of forbidden love, plays on audiences' heartstrings. But when you ask people how romantic they are, and how romantic others are, a different picture emerges.

Romance may have become a bit of a one-way street. Women are as romantic as ever, but men seem to be less romantic than in the past. Both genders are more likely now than in 1977 to say women are more romantic than men. Sixty-six percent of women did in 1995, up 17 percentage points, and 49 percent of men, compared with 40 percent in 1977. And the percent of men and women who say men are the more romantic gender dwindled, although the shares were never very large.

In addition, fewer men perceive themselves as romantic. Fifty-four percent of men say "they tend to be romantic," compared with 61 percent in 1977. The share of women who say they are romantic was stable between 1977 and 1995, at about 65 percent.

Although the 1990s man may seem to be less like Romeo and more like characters in the TV sitcom *Men Behaving Badly*, there's cause for hope. Men and women agree on the kinds of things that are romantic. At the top of the list are sending or receiving long-stemmed roses (half of both men and women), going somewhere special for the weekend (43 percent of men and 46 percent of women), and going out to a candlelight dinner (about 40 percent of both).

So guys, turn off the TV and get going. Valentine's Day is here, and you clearly know what to do. From what women say, these love's labors won't be lost.

Source: Reprinted from "Closing the Romance Gap," *American Demographics*, February 1997, p. 25, with permission. © 1997 Cowles Business Media, Ithaca, NY 14851

Psychologist Robert Sternberg has identified three components of love:

1. **Intimacy** (the emotional component of love characterized by a desire to be close, to interact at the intellectual level, to share feelings, and to acknowledge each other's desires)
2. **Passion** (the motivational component of love characterized by a desire to give and receive sexual pleasure and to achieve sexual gratification)
3. **Commitment** (the cognitive component of love characterized by a desire to maintain a highly valued relationship, even when self-sacrifice is required to do so)

Figure 16.3, the Triangles of Love, identifies the seven types of relationship that result from the different combinations of these three components. The term *consummate love* is used for the very special relationships in which all three components of love—commitment, intimacy, and passion—are present. This complete love is the goal of many relationships, but it is difficult to achieve and may be even more difficult to maintain.

Romantic love involves intimacy and passion but no commitment. An example is the form of love experienced in a summer affair. It may be very romantic for the duration of the relationship, but it ends when the summer is over.

Fatuous love is exemplified by commitment and passion but no intimacy. Intimacy takes time to develop. Fatuous love usually develops very quickly, as in the case when two people meet, one week later are engaged, and two weeks later are married. Relationships based on this type of love usually do not work out.

intimacy The emotional component of love characterized by a desire to be close, to interact at the intellectual level, to share feelings, and to acknowledge each other's desires.

passion The motivational component of love characterized by a desire to give and to receive sexual pleasure and to achieve sexual gratification.

commitment The cognitive component of love characterized by a desire to maintain a highly valued relationship, even when self-sacrifice is required to do so.

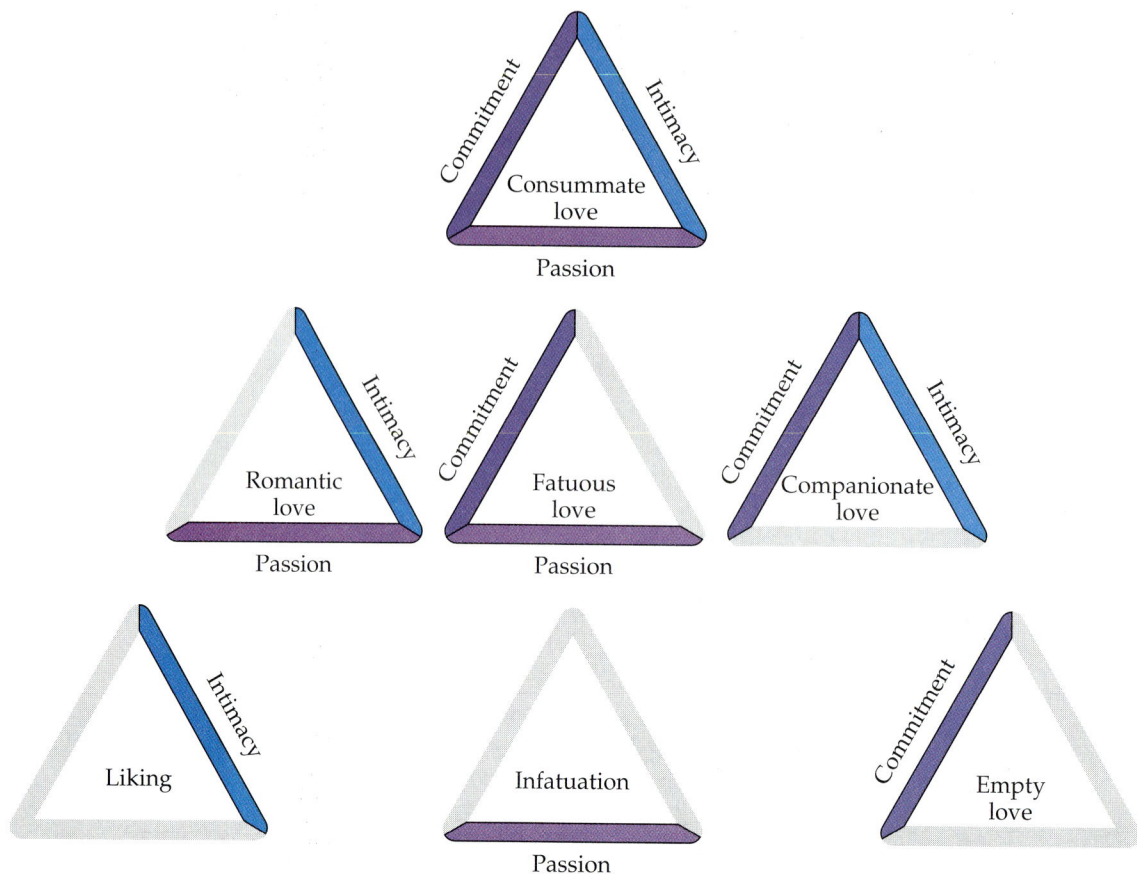

Figure 16.3 The Triangles of Love. *The three components of love are intimacy, passion, and commitment. There are seven types of relationships that result from different combinations of these components.*

Companionate love involves commitment and intimacy but no passion. The long-term friendship and the marriage in which physical attraction has died down are illustrations of this kind of love.

Liking involves only intimacy and refers to a relationship in which communication is possible. Friendship is apparent, there is warmth and closeness, but nothing more. Good friends like each other.

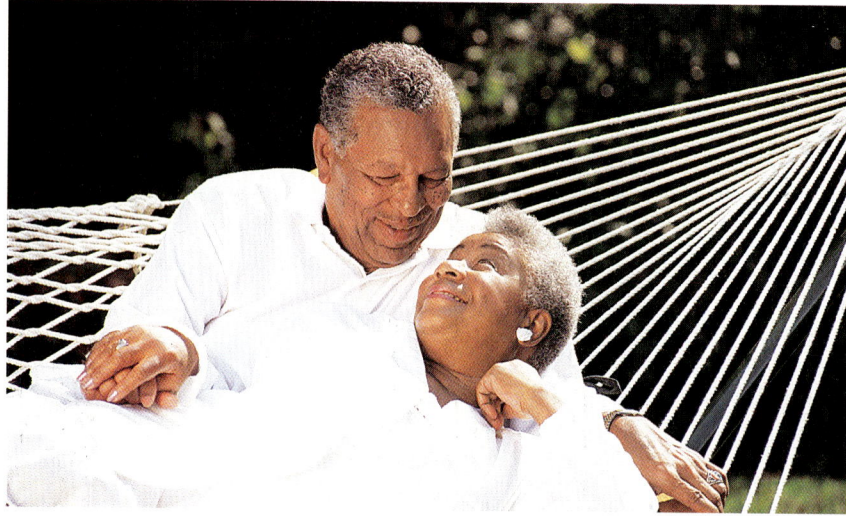

Commitment, along with intimacy and passion, are the three components of love. Commitment involves maintaining a highly valued relationship. (Source: Stock, Boston)

HERE'S LOOKING AT YOU

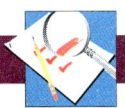

Are You Ready for a Mature Sexual Relationship?

There is no checklist that can determine when a person is ready to have a mature sexual relationship, but having certain personal characteristics can be an indication of readiness. How many of the following personal characteristics do you have?

- Physical maturity
- Patience and understanding
- Knowledge about sexuality and the sexual response
- Empathy and ability to be vulnerable
- Commitment to preventing unintended pregnancies and sexually transmitted diseases
- Ability to handle responsibility for positive consequences
- Ability to handle responsibility for potential negative consequences
- You honestly approve of the sexual behavior

There are also characteristics that can indicate readiness from a couples' perspective. How many of the following characteristics do you and your partner share?

- You trust and admire each other
- You have a relationship that is committed, mutually kind, and understanding
- You have talked about sexual behaviors before they occur
- You have experimented with and found pleasure in nonpenetrative behaviors
- You are motivated in the relationship for pleasure and intimacy
- You are in a safe and comfortable setting for a sexual relationship

Source: Adapted from National Commission on Adolescent Sexual Health, "Readiness for Mature Sexual Relationships—Facing the Facts: Sexual Health for America's Adolescents," 1995. Reprinted by permission of SIECUS, 130 W.42nd Street, New York, NY 10036–7802

Infatuation involves only passion. This kind of love arrives very quickly and can be gone just as fast. You meet a person at a party and are sexually aroused. You go out together, have sex together and then the affair is over. Sometimes infatuation does not even involve an interpersonal relationship. A person can be infatuated with someone without having the nerve to speak to him or her.

Empty love involves only commitment. This kind of love may be seen in a long-term marriage in which the passion is gone and intimacy is only a memory. Habit replaces desire.

A healthy relationship exists when two individuals love each other with the same type of love and within an atmosphere of equality. An unhealthy relationship exists when two people don't "match," yet remain together. Add sex to the formula, and the complexity of relationships becomes greater. A healthy relationship may or may not involve sexual intercourse. When two sexual partners love each other, sexual intercourse may be an appropriate expression of that love. For religious, moral, and other reasons, such as wanting to avoid a pregnancy or an STD, two people who love each other may choose to delay sexual intercourse. To see if you are ready for a mature sexual relationship, see the Here's Looking at You box.

Sexual Relationships

Once the decision is made to have sexual intercourse, it is important to understand biological and psychological sex drives and responses. The sex drive, the practice of giving and receiving sexual pleasure, and physiological sexual response cycles are common to everyone, regardless of sexual orientation or practice.

Sex Drive

The **sex drive** is the biological urge or appetite for sexual activity. It usually arises in the mind and produces feelings of restlessness and an openness to sexual stimuli. The primary biological function of the sex drive is its contribution to human reproduction and continuation of the species. **Libido,** another term for the sex drive, changes according to a number of factors. The hormone testosterone, for example, affects the sex drive in both males and females. When levels of testosterone are relatively low, the drive for sexual activity is likewise low. As the level of testosterone rises, so does the sex drive. Other factors affecting the sex drive are sexual images, memories, and fantasies.

The sex drive is usually satisfied through physical stimulation. This can be achieved through sexual intercourse and/or **masturbation** (self-stimulation). Most studies on sexual behavior report that more than 90 percent of men and 60 percent of women have masturbated. No evidence supports the common notion that masturbation causes any psychological or physical harm. There is reason to believe that it provides a safe and private outlet for sexual desires.

The sex drive serves much more than a biological purpose. It contributes to the development of interpersonal relationships as well. Specifically, it contributes to the initial attraction of one person to another and to the ultimate intimacy of a relationship by providing pleasure and fulfillment. Initial attraction is very important in our culture. Think about how much you deliberate about what to wear before you go out. Couples play out extensive scripts to make a positive impression on each other, including a positive sexual impression. According to a recent study, physical appearance is a far more significant factor for college men in selecting a partner for a sexual or long-term relationship than it is for women. Interpersonal warmth and personality characteristics rated higher for college women. The sex drive is not the only motivating factor that causes people to become interested in each other or to cement that interest. The elements of caring, trust, and affection also need to be considered.

Sexual Pleasuring

Physical stimulation, particularly of certain **erogenous zones** (those areas of the body especially susceptible to sexual arousal, such as the penis, vagina, and nipples), produces an elevated level of sexual excitement and pleasure. Sexual pleasure can be the result of interaction between two individuals, or it can be accomplished through masturbation. Sexual fantasy can also be very effective in stimulating a pleasurable response. One study of college men and women found that the most common purpose of students' fantasies during intercourse was to facilitate sexual arousal.

Foreplay is a term often used for sexual pleasuring. This can be as simple as touching or hugging. Kissing represents a more intimate form of sexual pleasuring. Manually stimulating each other's genitals represents even more intimate sexual pleasuring, sometimes referred to as **outercourse.** Because of the threat of sexually transmitted diseases and unwanted pregnancy, many couples are choosing this as an alternative to intercourse.

The term **intercourse** literally means "running between." Other formal terms for intercourse include *copulation* (coupling or joining) and *coitus* (a coming together). Perhaps the most common term for sexual intercourse is *making love.*

HealthLinks
Alan Guttmacher Institute
http://www.agi-usa.org
A direct link with one of the top research institutes in the country dedicated to sexual behavior and human reproduction.

sex drive The biological urge or appetite for sexual activity; also called libido.

libido The biological urge or appetite for sexual activity; also called sex drive.

masturbation Sexual self-stimulation.

erogenous zones Those areas of the body especially susceptible to sexual arousal such as the penis, vagina, and nipples.

foreplay Sexual pleasuring.

outercourse Mutual masturbation; when two people manually stimulate one another's genitals to achieve sexual pleasure.

intercourse Sexual behavior involving penetration, usually of the penis of a man into the vagina of a woman; a description of a variety of sexual behaviors, including anal, vaginal, and oral stimulation and/or penetration.

vasocongestion The pooling of blood in tissues during sexual excitement; also called tumescence.

myotonia Muscle tension in response to sexual stimulation.

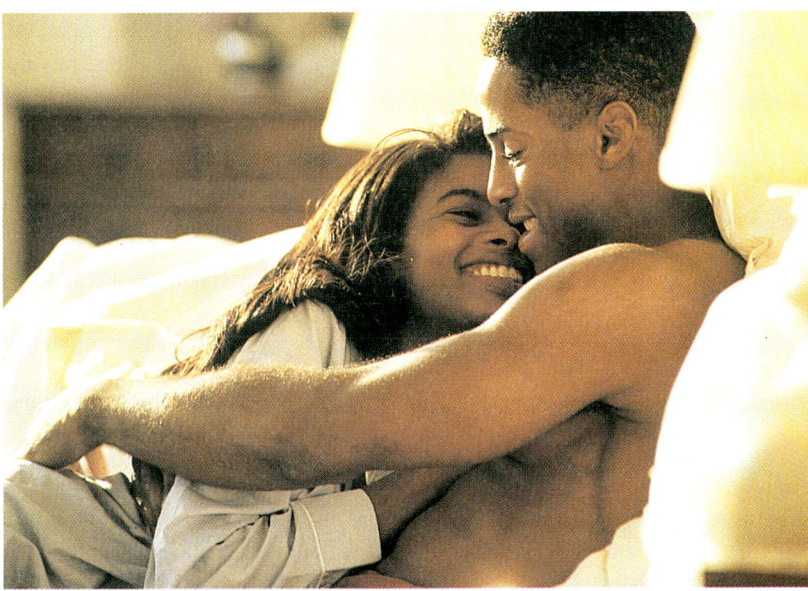

Physical stimulation can produce an elevated level of sexual excitement and pleasure. It can be as simple as hugging or more physically involved as stimulating certain erogenous zones. (Source: © Tony Stone Images)

Intercourse is traditionally defined in terms of heterosexual relations. When a man and a woman have sexual intercourse, the penis enters the vagina. *Intercourse* is also a term used to define widely sexual activity between members of the same sex, for example, anal intercourse. Intercourse serves several functions, including achieving and giving physical gratification, expressing love, communicating, and reproducing.

The Body's Sexual Response

What happens to the body before, during, and after sexual activity? The human sexual response is highly individualized. If asked, each person is likely to describe different physical and emotional responses. However, common physiological changes take place in both men and women.

Physiological Changes

The two major processes that play a role in how the body responds to sexual stimulation are vasocongestion and myotonia. **Vasocongestion** refers to the pooling of blood in tissues that takes place during sexual excitement. Under normal circumstances, the inflow of blood through the arteries is balanced by an outflow through the veins. During sexual arousal, however, the flow of blood into the veins is increased by dilation of the arteries. This increase in blood results in engorgement of certain areas of the body, including the penis, testicles, clitoris, labia minora, and nipples.

Myotonia refers to muscle tension, a normal response to sexual stimulation. Some of these motions are voluntary, such as muscle flexing; others are involuntary, such as muscle spasms during orgasm.

Vasocongestion and myotonia each build up during sexual excitement and release afterwards. Havelock Ellis, the British pioneer in writing about sexual behavior around the turn of the century, first explained the sexual response in two stages, tumescence (the buildup) and detumescence (the release). Today's health professionals who study sexual behavior have replaced Ellis's terminology with more descriptive words.

Critical Thinking Question

> The *Healthy People 2000* objectives include the following: "Increase to at least 85 percent the proportion of people aged 10 to 18 who have discussed human sexuality, including correct anatomical names, sexual abuse, and values surrounding sexuality, with their parents and/or have received information through another parentally endorsed source, such as youth, school, or religious program." Is it possible to know the extent to which this age group is involved in such "sex education"? At what age do you think sex education should begin? Who should be the primary sex educator? What role do schools, religious institutions, parents, and peers serve with respect to sex education?

Masters and Johnson Four-Stage Model

In the 1960s, sex therapists William Masters and Virginia Johnson proposed their four-stage model of sexual response after studying hundreds of individuals during sexual activity. These stages are excitement, plateau, orgasm, and resolution. The stages may vary tremendously in length and intensity, and considerable variety in both may be expected even within individuals. The order of the stages, however, remains the same (see Figure 16.4).

Excitement is the period of time when the body initially responds to sexual stimulation. In the man, the first evidence of excitement is erection of the penis.

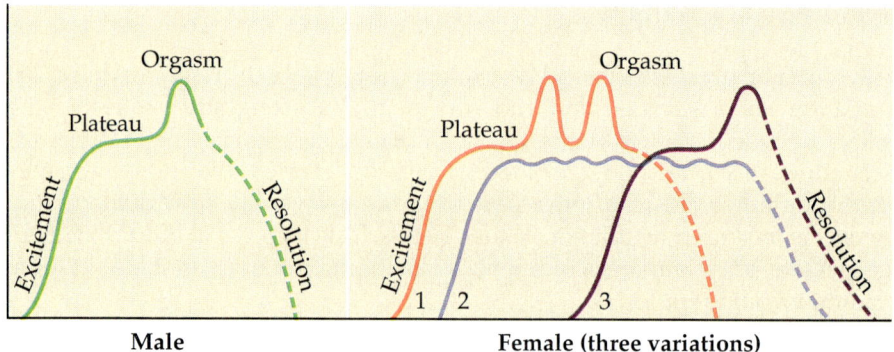

Figure 16.4 The Four Stages of Response. *Masters and Johnson's four-stage model of sexual response includes excitement, plateau, orgasm, and resolution.*

In the woman, the first signs include vaginal lubrication and often nipple and clitoral erection. In both sexes, the heart rate increases, as does the rate of breathing. The excitement stage can last less than a minute or as long as several hours.

The **plateau** phase is the stage of sexual stimulation just prior to orgasm. The word *plateau* connotes a leveling off, but as a sexual response, it may be a period of increasing and decreasing sexual stimulation. The plateau phase varies in length from a very brief, undetectable period of seconds to a very lengthy period of an hour or more.

During the plateau phase, muscle tension remains evident and may increase, deep breathing continues, and the heart rate remains elevated. The clitoris often retracts during this phase of sexual excitement. This normal occurrence should not be misread as a sign of loss of sexual desire. In both sexes, a sex flush, a reddening of the skin due to surface circulation of blood, may spread, causing the sexually stimulated person to feel hot to the touch. The term *hot* has come to mean sexually stimulated.

The **orgasm** is perhaps the least understood phase of the sexual response cycle because each person experiences it in a different way. Scientists have been much more successful in learning what an orgasm is not than in learning what it is. For example, scientific study has shown that Sigmund Freud's theory about orgasm and masturbation is incorrect. He believed that there is a difference between orgasm reached during intercourse (mature orgasm) and that reached through masturbation (immature orgasm).

Physiologically, an orgasm is a reflex action usually elicited by tactile stimulation. It is the shortest phase of the sexual response cycle and typically lasts just a few seconds. Just prior to orgasm, the sexually stimulated person usually experiences a sensation of inevitability, a no-turning-back-now response. A tremendous buildup is followed by a rush, an explosion of feeling or a sense of euphoria. Following the orgasm, a great sense of relief from the tension that was building up is experienced.

In men, an orgasm is accompanied by ejaculation of semen. The semen is a milky fluid containing sperm from the testicles, sugars, bicarbonate buffers, and coagulators. These are all necessary to ensure that sperm have a chance to reach an unfertilized egg. In women, the orgasm is accompanied by quick rhythmic contractions of the uterus and vagina. In both men and women, orgasm does not necessarily happen in every sexual encounter.

Resolution follows orgasm, and the physiological responses reverse. Vasocongestion and myotonia subside. A sense of gratification is felt, and relaxation overcomes the body. Some individuals experience exhaustion and sleep. Women may experience multiple orgasms before completing the resolution phase. This is an uncommon occurrence among men.

Psychological Component

Although the Masters and Johnson model is the most accepted representation of the physiological response to sexual stimulation, in the late 1970s, sex therapist Helen Singer-Kaplan added an important psychological component: desire. (Her model identifies three stages of sexual response: desire, excitement, and orgasm.) By including desire as a part of the sexual experience, Singer-Kaplan expanded the study of sexual intercourse to include the motivations of a person to seek sexual activity or to become available for the sex act.

All sexologists today agree that there is considerable variation between and within the sexes concerning sexual response. Although the ability to respond to sexual stimulation is similar, the rate of response appears to be different in men and women. Women tend to respond more slowly than men, but, as noted earlier, once stimulated, they are more capable of reaching multiple orgasms than are

excitement The period during which the body initially responds to sexual stimulation; includes erection of the penis in men and vaginal lubrication and clitoral erection in women.

plateau The stage of sexual stimulation just prior to orgasm consisting of increasing and decreasing sexual stimulation.

orgasm The climax phase of sexual excitement.

resolution The stage of sexual response following orgasm in which physiological responses reverse and a sense of relaxation overcomes the body.

men. Most men experience a recovery period, or a **refractory period**, after orgasm. This period can last from a few minutes to a few hours and even longer in older men. During the refractory period, no amount of stimulation can bring on another orgasm. There are other differences in sexual response between the sexes, but as more and more is learned, the similarities discovered far outnumber the differences.

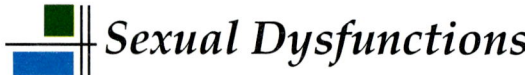

Sexual Dysfunctions

Unfortunately, not everyone can respond normally to sexual stimulation. Collectively, the disorders that interfere with the ability to enjoy a healthy sexual experience are called **sexual dysfunctions.** They may be very mild and create only slight discomfort, or they may be so severe as to completely prevent a person from participating in sexual activities.

Some sexual dysfunctions have an *organic* cause and are due to structural problems or result from a disease involving the sexual organs. Others are the result of medications that interfere with normal sexual functioning. More commonly, sexual dysfunctions result from psychological causes, such as traumatic sexual experiences or simple ignorance about sexual practice.

Inhibited sexual desire is a sexual dysfunction that affects both men and women. The *Diagnostic and Statistical Manual of Mental Disorders IV Revised* defines this dysfunction as "persistent or recurrent deficient (or absent) sexual fantasies and desire for sexual activity." It is difficult to define this problem because there is no normal level of desire. One criterion is how often a person's desire for sex matches his or her partner's. Frequent mismatches may lead to frustrations, misunderstandings, and communication problems. Severe desire problems may result from incorrect sex education (for example, believing that the genitals are dirty and should be avoided) or sexual trauma such as rape. Less severe problems result from temporary situations such as the birth of a baby or simple fatigue.

It is important to note that sexual problems may arise when the goal of sexual behavior is orgasm or mutual orgasm. It is not dysfunctional if one or both partners do not experience an orgasm during each sexual encounter. In fact, the expectation of orgasm can become a form of performance anxiety and actually lead to dysfunction.

Although the "I-have-a-headache" syndrome is a common means of communicating a disinterest in sex, it does not necessarily represent a sexual dysfunction. Each individual's desire for sex varies greatly. Only when the lack of desire persists and threatens the relationship can it be considered dysfunctional.

At the opposite end of the spectrum are people who are addicted to sex. As with all other addictions, sex addiction is an attempt to fill a vacuum resulting from inadequacies and/or insecurities. For these individuals, sex is a consuming passion and overwhelming need that must be satisfied, even if it means risking their jobs, their families, or other relationships. Men and women who are addicted to sex usually have low self-esteem. After a sexual encounter, a sex addict is typically overcome with feelings of worthlessness, anxiety, agitation, guilt, depression, or shame and is driven to have sex once again.

Male Problems

Among the many male sexual dysfunctions, two types appear more often than others: premature ejaculation and erectile impotence.

---

refractory period The recovery period experienced by most men after orgasm; during this period a man does not respond to sexual stimulation.

sexual dysfunctions Disorders that interfere with the ability to enjoy a healthy sexual experience.

inhibited sexual desire Persistent or recurrent deficient (or absent) sexual fantasies and desire for sexual activity.

premature ejaculation Persistent or recurrent ejaculation occurring after minimal sexual stimulation or before, on, or shortly after penetration and before the person wishes it.

impotence Persistent or recurrent inability to attain erection or to maintain it until completion of the sexual activity.

HEALTHWISE CONSUMER

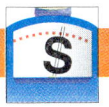

New Treatments for Impotence

"I feel like I'm thirty years old," says one sixty-three-year-old man, who suffered from impotence after an operation for prostate cancer. His fountain of youth comes in the form of a pill that he takes one hour before sex, which gives him the stimulation he needs to get an erection.

There are so many options on the market today that experts who specialize in sexual behavior are talking about a new sexual revolution that could turn the estimated 20 million U.S. men who suffer from impotence into "virile teenagers" again. In the 1960s, sex researchers believed that nearly all impotence was psychological. Today, urologists (specialists in the genitourinary tract in males and urinary tract in females) believe the causes are most often physiological. As one urologist says: "Really, it's all hydraulics."

Treatments available today include:

- A drug taken twenty minutes to an hour before sex works in response to physical stimulation to cause an erection. Success rates for an erection range from 60 percent with few side effects to 80 percent with headaches and diarrhea.
- A suppository inserted into the top of the penis and applied five to ten minutes before sex can cause an erection. It is not recommended for use with a pregnant partner.
- An injection in the base of the penis twenty minutes before sex can cause an erection. It is effective in more than 50 percent of cases, but some of the injection therapies may be painful and cannot be used every day.
- A pump placed around a sheathed penis just before sex causes an erection until the elastic ring at the base of the penis is taken off. While it is clumsy and sometimes makes ejaculation difficult, the pump has few physical side effects.
- Surgery that repairs arteries to boost the blood supply to the penis can restore the ability to have a normal erection. This procedure is effective only when the impotence problem is caused by a simple vascular injury.
- A penile implant, which is either malleable or inflatable and contains a pump and reservoir of saline solution, can cause an erection that lasts until the implant is unbent or drained. It can destroy erectile tissue.

Medical interventions will still not solve all problems. For example, taking an impotence drug or injection to solve marital difficulties may not do the job. There are reports that an injection that works well in the doctor's office will not work at home when there are underlying marital problems. It might be better, says one sex therapist, for couples to learn how to accept each other's changing bodies. But one patient who had his prostate removed says, "If women can get face-lifts, why shouldn't men do this?"

Rapid or **premature ejaculation** is considered the most prevalent sexual dysfunction in men. Rapid ejaculation is defined mainly in terms of the man's sexual partner. Ejaculation is considered too rapid only if the sexual partner is unable to achieve orgasm because of the premature ejaculation and subsequent loss of interest on the part of the man.

There is no clearly defined time limit defining what rapid ejaculation is. It might be ten seconds in one relationship and ten minutes in another. Sex therapist Singer-Kaplan defines it in terms of control. This suggests that therapy for rapid ejaculation should focus on developing a sense of control rather than on an extension of time. It is impossible to determine just how many men experience rapid ejaculation, but the number is probably quite large given the fact that young healthy men tend to experience it naturally.

Another common sexual dysfunction in men is an erectile dysfunction, called **impotence.** This is the inability to achieve and maintain an erection long enough to participate in sexual intercourse. Occasional erectile problems are very common and with an understanding partner present little or no difficulty for the relationship. Erectile problems may be of psychological and/or physical origin. They may result from fear of failure or fear of the inability to perform sexually. They may also result from diseases such as hypertension, diabetes, and prostate cancer. Erectile problems can also be traced to substance abuse. When erectile problems occur in a chronic manner, over a long period of time, or repeatedly to the extent that the relationship is hurt, therapy is recommended.

Female Problems

Just as with men, many sexual dysfunctions occur among women. Two major ones are lack of orgasm and penetration problems.

The failure to reach orgasm by women is called **female orgasmic disorder.** It is attributed to a number of factors, including psychological inhibition and the fear of losing control. It may also result from limited sexual experience. For example, an inexperienced woman might not reach orgasm because her partner has had a premature ejaculation. Failure to experience orgasm during intercourse alone is not a sexual dysfunction. Repeated failure to the point of creating relationship problems, however, does suggest the need for some form of therapy. Better communication between sexual partners is often the only change needed.

A second and far more serious set of problems relates to penetration of the penis into the vagina. Vaginismus and dyspareunia are examples of two penetration-related conditions that cause serious interference with healthy sexual expression. **Vaginismus** is the involuntary constriction of the vagina. When this occurs, intercourse is impossible. Vaginismus usually has psychological origins, such as negative ideas about sex. Women who have been raped sometimes develop vaginismus. This condition requires therapy but is treatable.

Dyspareunia is a term that refers to painful intercourse. Pain and discomfort can be felt if lubrication is insufficient or if a disease is present. Lubrication problems that produce painful intercourse can sometimes be treated simply by extending the period of foreplay to allow adequate sexual excitement to occur. If adequate lubrication remains a problem, topical lubricants can be purchased at a pharmacy. Painful intercourse caused by diseases such as yeast infections or by allergic reactions to douches or birth control methods such as foam are relieved as soon as the disease causing the problem is cured or the source of allergic reaction is eliminated. In some cases, dyspareunia persists and requires more extensive therapy.

Therapeutic Interventions

Treatment of sexual dysfunctions involves medical, educational, and/or psychological interventions. A medical evaluation is necessary in many sexual dysfunctions in order to diagnose possible organic causes of the problem. A physician looks for structural problems and for diseases that may contribute to the sexual dysfunction. Drug treatments are available for both male and female sexual problems (see the Healthwise Consumer box).

Therapy may involve basic sex education, including instruction in methods of sexual technique and expression. Although sex is seen as a natural process that requires no instruction, evidence is clear that some knowledge of how the body responds to sexual stimulation can be beneficial.

Another form of therapy involves learning more about how to communicate sexual feelings. **Sensate focus** is a therapeutic technique in which a couple is taught the nonverbal communication of touching. It is used in treating couples

female orgasmic disorder Persistent or recurrent delay in, or absence of, orgasm in a female following a normal sexual excitement phase.

vaginismus Recurrent or persistent involuntary spasm of the musculature of the outer third of the vagina that interferes with sexual intercourse.

dyspareunia Painful intercourse.

sensate focus A therapeutic technique in which a couple is taught the nonverbal communication of touching in order to help alleviate difficulty having sexual intercourse or performance anxiety.

who have difficulty having sexual intercourse or who experience performance anxiety.

The most complex problems related to sexual dysfunction require psychotherapy. For example, victims of rape or incest or individuals who have developed aversions to their genitalia may require extensive therapy.

To function well sexually, an individual must be able to abandon himself or herself to the erotic experience. A healthy sexual response is one that is unencumbered by guilt and anxiety.

Key Concepts

1. Sexuality is the embodiment of a collection of qualities that make up a person's sexual attitudes and behaviors and his or her sexual relationships with others.
2. Attitudes of a specific individual toward sexuality vary over time. Major sexual life-cycle changes include puberty, marriage, pregnancy, child rearing, menopause, and postmenopause.
3. Sexual orientation refers to the focus of a person's sexual interest—people of the opposite sex, the same sex, or both.
4. Good communication can result in a more fulfilling sexual relationship.
5. When nonverbal language and verbal language conflict, an individual is sending mixed messages.
6. Three components of love are intimacy (the emotional component), passion (the motivational component), and commitment (the cognitive component).
7. The sex drive, or libido, is the biological urge or appetite for sexual activity. It usually arises in the mind and produces feelings of restlessness and an openness to sexual stimuli.
8. Masters and Johnson's four-stage model of sexual response includes excitement, plateau, orgasm, and resolution.
9. Sexual dysfunctions can have an organic cause, due to structural problems or a disease, or a psychological basis, due to traumatic sexual experiences.
10. Treatment of sexual dysfunction involves medical, educational, and/or psychological interventions.

Review Questions

1. Define the term *sexuality* by drawing a comparison between it and the concept of "personality."
2. Differentiate between gender identity and sex role relative to sexuality.
3. Provide evidence of behavioral variance across cultures.
4. Explain the function of androgens and estrogens relative to sexual development and secondary sex characteristics.
5. Explain the similarities and differences between the heterosexual, homosexual, and bisexual sexual orientations.
6. Explain the importance of communication between two sexual partners and give an example of how verbal and nonverbal communication may conflict.
7. List seven types of love according to Sternberg and explain the role of intimacy, passion, and commitment in each type.
8. Describe the difference between masturbation, outercourse, and intercourse.
9. Diagram and explain Masters and Johnson's four-stage model of human sexual response.
10. Identify two sexual dysfunctions common to men and two sexual dysfunc-

tions common to women, and describe the symptoms and possible origin of each.

Selected Bibliography

Boston Women's Health Book Collective. *The New Our Bodies, Ourselves.* New York: Simon and Schuster, 1992.

Irvin, J.M. *Sexuality Education Across Cultures: Working with Differences.* San Francisco: Jossey-Bass, 1995.

Kaplan, H.S. *The Illustrated Manual of Sex Therapy,* 2nd ed. New York: Brunner/Mazel, 1987.

Laumann, E.O., Gagnon, J.H., Michael, R.T., and S. Michaels. *The Social Organization of Sexuality: Sexual Practices in the United States.* Chicago: The University of Chicago Press, 1994.

Masters, W., and V. Johnson. *Human Sexual Response.* Boston: Little, Brown, 1996.

Rathus, S.A., Nevid, J.S., and L. Fichner-Rathus. *Human Sexuality in a World of Diversity,* 2nd ed. Boston: Allyn and Bacon, 1996.

Rossi, A.S. *Sexuality Across the Life Course.* Chicago: The University of Chicago Press, 1994.

Sears, J.T., ed. *Sexuality and the Curriculum: The Politics and Practices of Sexuality Education.* New York: Teachers College Press, 1992.

Smith, T.W. *The Demography of Sexual Behavior.* Menlo Park, CA: The Henry J. Kaiser Family Foundation, 1994.

HealthLinks: Web sites for Developing Healthy Relationships

You can access better health as it relates to this chapter by checking out some of the following sites on the Internet. These and sites identified within the chapter can be accessed directly when you visit the *HealthStyles* Web Site located on the Allyn and Bacon home page at **http://www.abacon.com.**

Planned Parenthood
http://www.ppfa.org/ppfa/index.html
An online source for sexual and reproductive health information.

Go Ask Alice
www.columbia.edu/cu/healthwise/alice.html
An interactive question and answer line out of the Columbia University Health Services. "Alice" is available to answer questions each week about any health-related issues, including relationships, nutrition and diet, exercise, drugs, sex, alcohol, and stress.

Health Hotlines: Developing Healthy Relationships

American Association for Marriage and Family Therapy (AAMFT)
(202) 452-0109
1133 15th St. NW
Suite 300
Washington, DC 20005

Impotence Information Center
(800) 843-4315
P.O. Box 9
Minneapolis, MN 55440

Sex Education and Information Council of the United States
(212) 819-9770
130 W. 42nd Street
New York, NY 10036

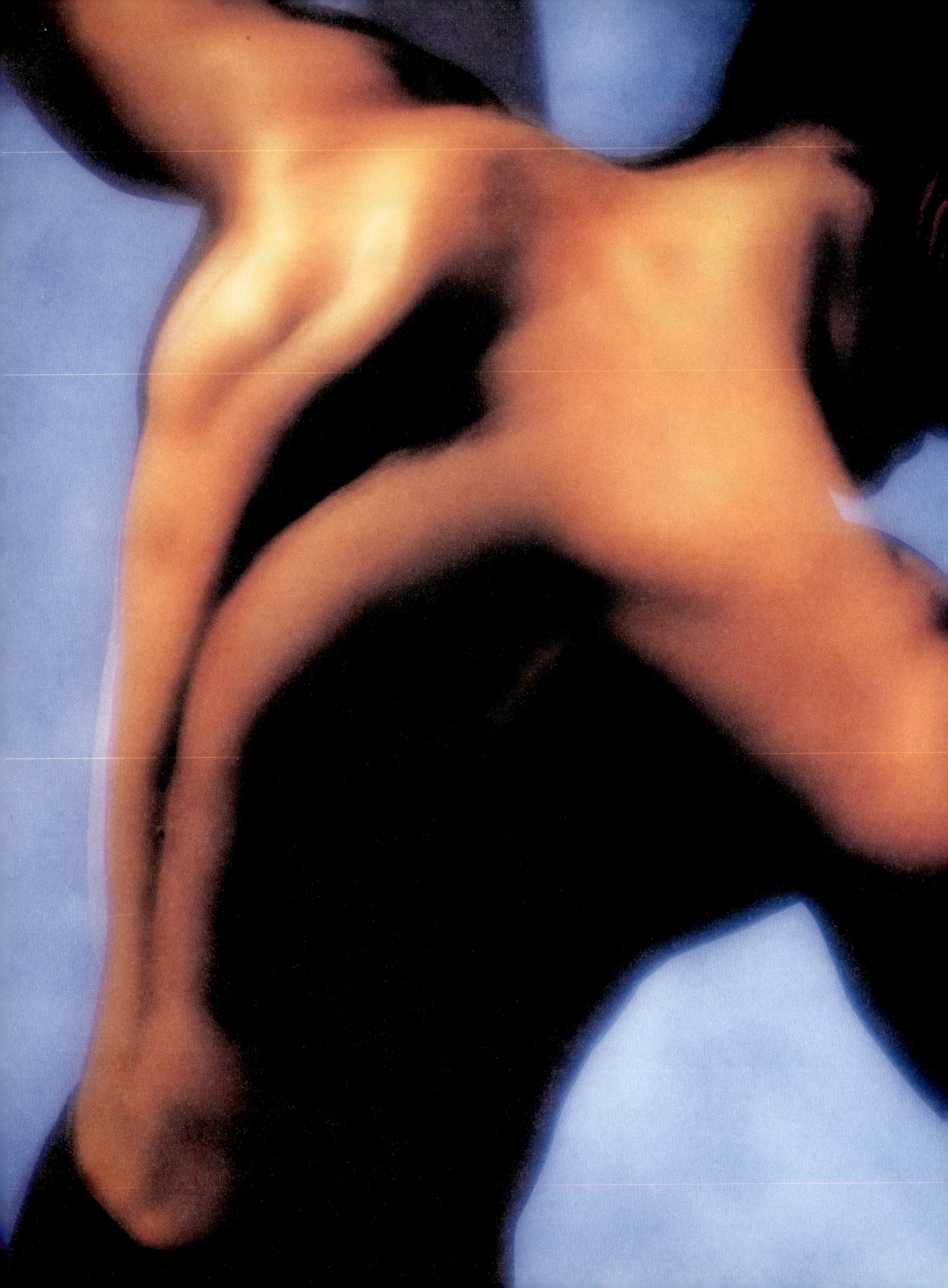

Your Sexual Body

A Primer on Reproductive Anatomy and Physiology

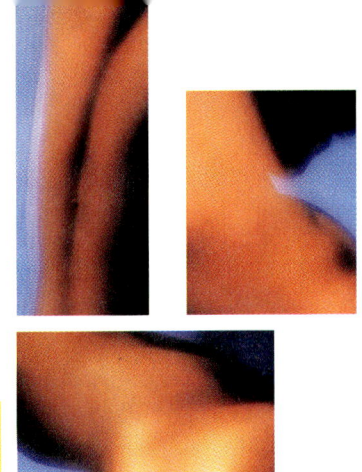

Maintaining a healthy life involves making many decisions that relate to diet, exercise, sleep, smoking, and other health styles. Such health-related decisions generally do not require a full understanding of human anatomy and physiology. For example, you do not need to know the cell structure of skin to know that ultraviolet rays from the sun can cause damage and may result in cancer.

Decisions related to sex and sexuality, however, do require an understanding of human anatomy and physiology. When you want to avoid pregnancy or sexually transmitted infections, it pays to understand the reproductive system. Likewise, when you want to have a baby, it is important to know the mechanics of the reproductive system in order to improve your chances of becoming pregnant.

This special primer examines sex and sexuality from an anatomical and physiological perspective so that you can better understand the biological functions of the male and female reproductive systems. The *reproductive system* is a collective term for the tissue and organs responsible for the production of egg or sperm cells and the secretion of sex hormones. The structures of the reproductive systems of the male and female are also designed to facilitate fertilization of an egg and gestation and delivery of a baby.

In this primer, the male reproductive anatomy and physiology are described first, then female anatomy and physiology, followed by a brief introduction to the menstrual cycle.

Reproductive Anatomy and Physiology of the Male

One of the primary male reproductive functions is to produce sex cells called *sperm*. They are visible only with a microscope yet contain the genetic information necessary for reproduction. The male reproductive system is designed to facilitate the movement of sperm from the sites of production (the testicle) and storage (the epididymis and vas deferens) into the vagina of a female to allow possible union of sperm and egg. Sperm are deposited through a process called *ejaculation*, the expulsion of the semen, including sperm, that usually takes place at the peak of sexual excitement, or *orgasm*.

A second function of the male reproductive system is to produce *androgens*, a family of masculinizing hormones. Androgens account for the development of primary male characteristics, including the sex organs, as well as secondary sex characteristics, such as facial hair, deep voice, and muscular build. *Testosterone* is the major androgen produced.

A third male reproductive function relates to sexual response. The external surfaces of the male genitalia have nerve endings responsive to touch and are thus important during sexual interaction. The external organs of the male include the scrotum and the penis. The internal organs include the testes, epididymis, vas deferens, seminal vesicle, prostate gland, and Cowper's gland.

External Organs of the Male Reproductive System

The *scrotum* is a muscular sac located between the penis and the rectum (see Figure 1). It forms a pouch for holding the testicles. The word *scrotum* comes from the Latin word meaning "bag," an appropriate description of this structure. The *testicles*, oval-shaped organs, reside inside the scrotum. Sperm are produced in the testicles at a temperature that is three to five degrees below normal body temperature. The muscle of the scrotum, the *cremaster muscle*, serves as a temperature regulator, and plays a critical role in fertility. When the temperature of the testi-

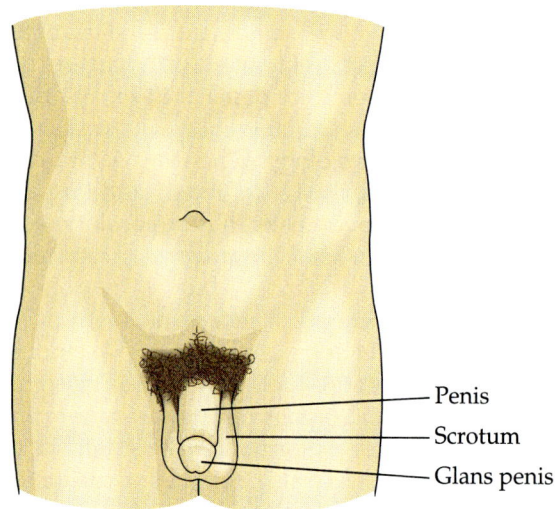

Figure 1 External Male Reproductive Anatomy.

cles is perceived to be too high, the muscle relaxes, allowing the testicles to hang away from the body, thus lowering their temperature. When the temperature of the testicles is perceived to be too low, the muscle contracts, pulling the testicles up close to the body to provide warmth. It is not uncommon for fertility problems to arise from factors such as tight-fitting underwear, excessive time spent in hot tubs, or continual long-distance driving. In each case, the work of the scrotum is compromised, leading to reduced production of sperm. The cremaster muscle may also respond to emotional stress. Thus, some fertility problems may result from continuous contraction of the cremaster muscle due to stress and tension.

The male organ responsible for the transportation of sperm to a female is the *penis*. The size of the penis varies from man to man and also varies during the stages of sexual excitement. The size of a penis is not associated with virility or fertility.

The penis is an extremely sensitive and responsive organ that becomes hard and erect during sexual excitement. This process is called *erection* and is necessary for insertion of the penis into a woman's vagina in order to deposit sperm. In an unexcited state, the penis is a limp, tubular organ. In an excited state, the penis is firm, elongated, and capable of penetrating the vagina. The penis is made up of three cylinders of tissue that, upon sexual excitement, fill with blood, thus making the penis erect. After excitement subsides, each cylinder of tissue releases the blood, and the penis returns to a normal, flaccid state. Running through the penis is the *urethra*, the outlet of the bladder allowing elimination of urine. Actually, the release of semen and the release of urine take place through the same opening of the penis.

At the tip of the penis is the head, or *glans penis*, a highly sensitive area particularly responsive to tactile stimulation. The head is covered with a *prepuce*, a layer of tissue that is sometimes removed in a surgical procedure called *circumcision*. The prepuce is also called the foreskin. Some evidence suggests that circumcision may be an effective means of promoting good hygiene and avoiding not only infection but also perhaps some cancers. It is also done for religious reasons. In total, about 60 percent of U.S. males are circumcised.

Internal Organs of the Male Reproductive System

The organs of a man's body responsible for the production of both sperm and male hormones are the *testes*. During fetal development, the testes usually descend through the inguinal canal and into the scrotum, where they will reside. This migration of the testes from within the abdominal cavity to a location outside the abdominal cavity is necessary to produce the lower temperature needed for the production of viable sperm. Failure of testicles to descend is called *cryptorchidism*. The problem of undescended testicles usually corrects itself during the first few months of a baby's life. It may also be corrected surgically later.

Inside each oval-shaped testicle are numerous *seminiferous tubules* where sperm develop. Surrounding the seminiferous tubules are the *interstitial cells*, the site of hormone production. Although the interstitial cells are not the only place where male sex hormones are produced, they are by far the most important source of these hormones, particularly testosterone.

Through the process of *meiosis*, or reduction division, the cells lining the interior walls of the seminiferous tubules divide and develop into immature *spermatids* that will eventually break away to form sperm. This process of sperm production takes approximately seventy days and continues nonstop from puberty through adulthood.

A normal sperm is microscopic and shaped like a tadpole (see Figure 2). The head contains the genetic material necessary for union with an egg, while the tail

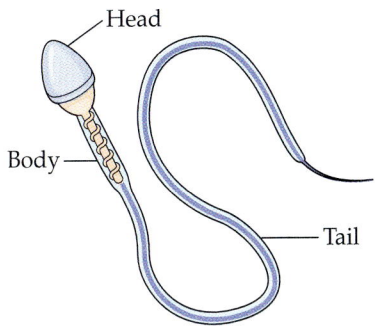

Figure 2 A Single Sperm.

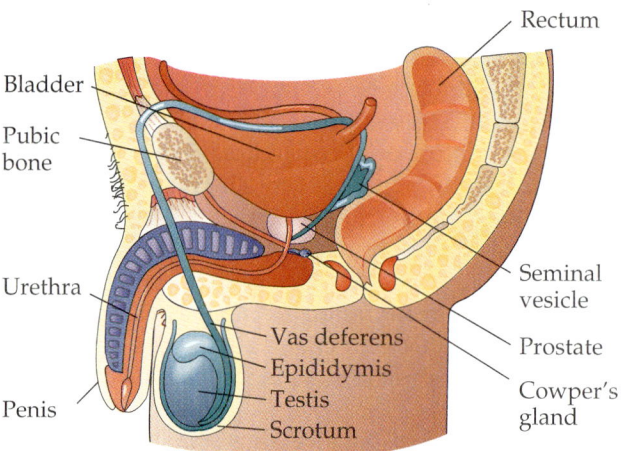

Figure 3 Internal Male Reproductive Anatomy.

is responsible for moving the sperm once it is deposited at the cervical opening to the uterus of a woman. Covering the head are enzymes necessary to penetrate the wall of an egg cell should the sperm come in contact with one.

Sperm produced in the seminiferous tubules migrate to the *epididymis*, where they reside for the two to four weeks it takes to reach maturity. The epididymis is a coiled organ that functions to move sperm from the testicle to the vas deferens for eventual ejaculation (see Figure 3). The epididymis also plays a major role in the ability of the sperm to move once they have been ejaculated. In the epididymis the sperm are surrounded by a nourishing fluid that contains proteins necessary for sperm mobility. The time spent in the epididymis is critical to fertility because immature sperm, or sperm that have not been exposed to proteins necessary for the activity of the tail, do not function effectively once deposited, and therefore may not find the egg cell.

The tube that connects the epididymis to the penis is the *vas deferens*, sometimes called the ejaculatory duct (see Figure 4). This tube is lined with smooth

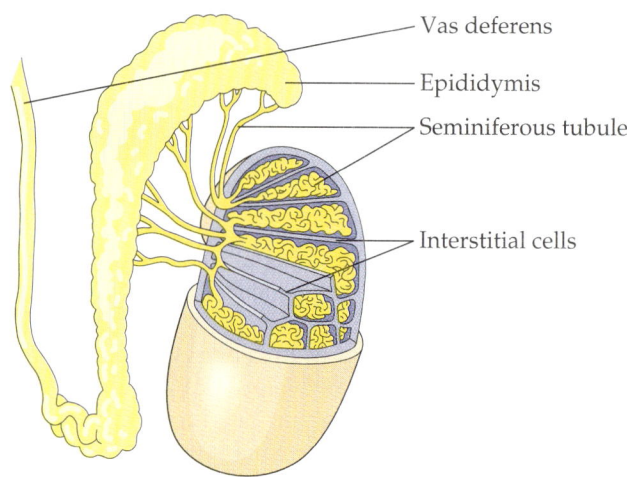

Figure 4 Cross-Section of the Testicle.

muscle. During ejaculation, the muscle contracts rapidly, moving semen and sperm through the penis and out. *Semen* is the fluid that carries sperm during ejaculation. Between 200 million and 400 million sperm are contained in the semen of each ejaculation. Semen is produced in a variety of locations, including the epididymis, the seminal vesicle, and the prostate gland. The *seminal vesicle* produces about 60 percent of semen. This secretory gland was once thought to be the storage site of sperm, thus the name seminal vesicle, but now is known as a source of fluid. It secretes water, fructose sugar to be used for energy by the sperm, and coagulators to assure the thickening of semen once it is deposited. The thick semen allows sperm to maintain contact with the opening to the uterus from the vagina, thus increasing the chances of successful union of sperm and egg.

The vas deferens passes through the *prostate gland*, where approximately 20 percent of semen is produced. The prostate gland contributes bicarbonate buffers necessary for maintaining a basic environment needed for sperm viability and more coagulators. Located near the shaft of the penis are the *Cowper's glands*, two small, pea-like glands that secrete bicarbonate buffers and mucus for lubrication. Secretions from the Cowper's glands occur early in sexual excitement. They counter the acid environment of the pineal portion of the urethra, thus preparing it for ejaculation.

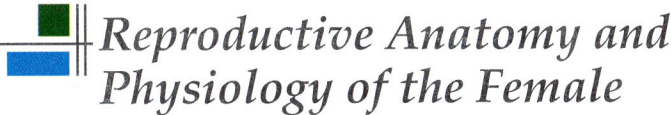

Reproductive Anatomy and Physiology of the Female

The female reproductive system is designed to carry out several functions, including the production of egg cells, the production of hormones, and the gestation and delivery of a baby.

The primary reproductive function of the *ovaries* is to produce egg cells, called *ova*. One ovum (sometimes two or more) is produced in the ovary approximately every month of a woman's fertile period, which lasts from the onset of menstruation until menopause. The egg is produced in response to hormonal signals, which arise from the ovary and from the pituitary gland in the brain. The production of the hormones estrogen and progesterone is an especially important function of the ovaries. These hormones account for many female characteristics as well as contribute to the success of pregnancy.

The structure of the female provides for reception of sperm. The *vagina* is a tubular opening leading to the cervix, where sperm must be deposited if pregnancy is to occur. The *fallopian tubes* provide a place for fertilization and the *uterus* provides a location for fetal development as well as the musculature necessary to expel a full-term baby. Finally, like the male, the female genitalia play a primary role in sexual responsiveness.

The external organs of the female include the mons veneris, labia majora, labia minora, clitoris, and breasts. The internal organs include the ovaries, fallopian tubes, uterus, cervix, and vagina.

External Organs of the Female Reproductive System

Collectively, most of the external reproductive organs of the female are referred to as the *vulva*. The vulva includes the mons veneris, labia, clitoris, and hymen (see Figure 5). The breasts, although not a part of the vulva, may be considered external reproductive organs.

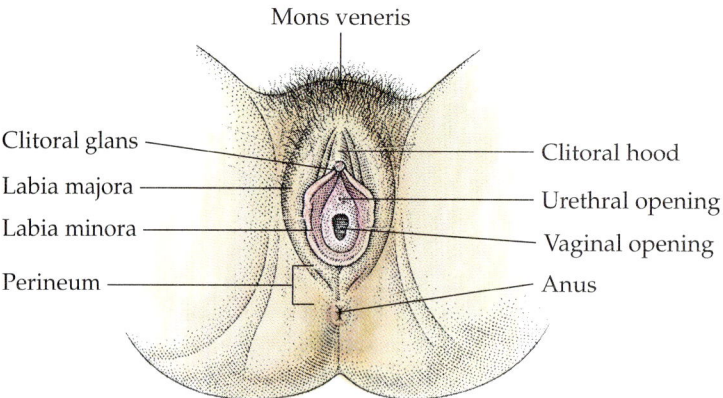

Figure 5 External Female Reproductive Anatomy

The *mons veneris* is a layer of tissue covered with pubic hair located above and forward of the remainder of the vulva. The *labia majora* are the large outer folds of tissue extending from the mons veneris and surrounding the opening of the vagina and urethra. The external sides of these folds of tissue are covered with hair and are pigmented, while the internal sides of the folds are smooth and contain numerous sweat glands. During sexual arousal, the blood flowing into the pelvic area causes the labia majora to swell in size and separate to some degree. The sweat glands serve to lubricate the area, thus facilitating sexual intercourse.

Inside the labia majora (or outer lips) are the labia minora (or inner lips). The *labia minora* are a smaller, thinner set of skin folds that also respond to sexual stimulation, secrete lubrication, and become engorged with blood during sexual excitement.

At the point where the labia minora join, a hood is formed that covers the *clitoris*, a sensitive organ that is responsive to tactile stimulation. The clitoris apparently has no function other than female sexual gratification. It is composed of erectile tissue and upon sexual excitement becomes engorged with blood. The head of the clitoris, the *glans clitoris*, is a highly sensitive portion of the organ.

In some women, the entrance to the vagina is covered with a partial covering called the *hymen*. This tissue serves no apparent function, but has become the focus of many myths, particularly those related to virginity. Because the structure of the hymen varies widely, it is not a means of determining whether a woman has had sexual intercourse.

Although not actually part of the genitalia, the breasts are considered a part of female external sexual anatomy (see Figure 6). The breasts are modified sweat glands that develop during puberty. They are composed of fat cells, glandular tissue, and some fibrous tissue. Combined, these tissues perform an important function—nourishing the newborn. They are mammary, or milk-producing, glands and supply total nourishment to an infant.

The size and shape of breasts vary widely. Breast size is not related to fertility or even the ability to breast-feed. The breasts function sexually in two ways. Some women find pleasure from the stimulation of the breasts, particularly the nipple and the *areola*, the pigmented area surrounding the nipple. Also, because the nipple is erectile tissue, upon sexual excitement, it engorges with blood and becomes erect.

Internal Organs of the Female Reproductive System

The *ovary* is the primary sex gland that produces eggs and sex hormones including estrogen, progesterone, and androgens (see Figure 7). At birth, a baby girl pos-

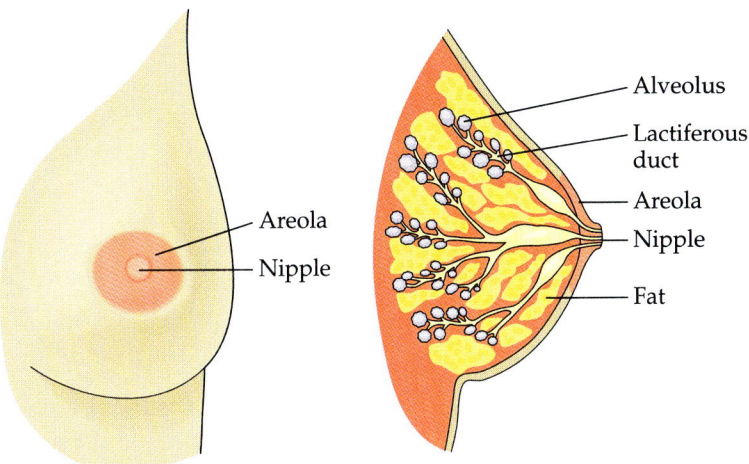

Figure 6 Frontal View and Cross-Section of the Female Breast.

sesses all the potential egg cells, called *follicles*, necessary for her to remain fertile throughout a normal period of fertility. These cells, however, remain in an immature state until they receive hormonal signals from the blood, causing the follicles to begin the maturation process. Many follicles will begin the maturation process each month, but only one (on rare occasions two or more) will become fully mature as an egg and be released into the abdominal cavity to begin the migration to join the sperm. The release of an egg from the ovary is called *ovulation*.

The *fallopian tubes* are small tubes extending from the uterus into the abdominal cavity. Named for Gabriele Fallopius, the tubes provide passageways for an egg to move from the abdominal cavity to the uterus. Finger-like structures called *fimbriae* fan out from one end of each fallopian tube, in search of a released egg. The released egg is then carried down the fallopian tube where fertilization

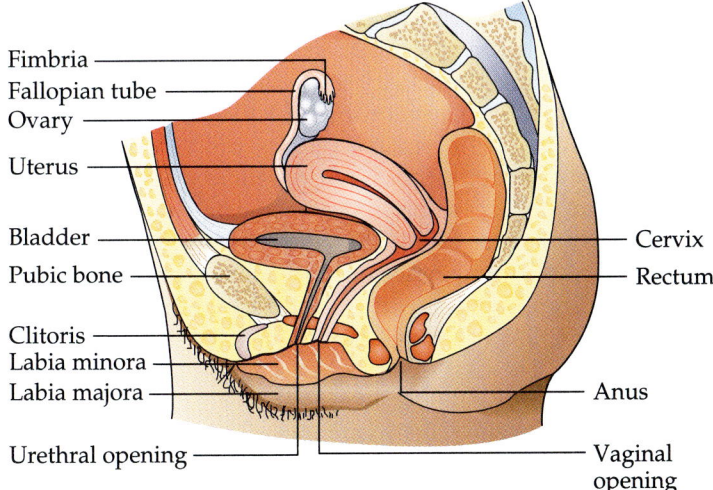

Figure 7 Internal Female Reproductive Anatomy. *(Source: From* Fundamentals of Anatomy and Physiology, *4th ed., by Frederic H. Martini, p. 1055, © 1988. Reprinted by permission of Prentice-Hall, Inc., Upper Saddle River, NJ)*

can take place with sperm that have found their way through the uterus and up the other end of the fallopian tube. The union of sperm and egg takes place in the tube, but implantation and growth of the embryo occurs in the uterus.

The *uterus,* also called the womb, is a muscular organ shaped like a pear. It is composed of three layers. The *perimetrium* is the outer thin covering of connective tissue that serves to contain the uterus. The *myometrium* is a thick middle layer of smooth muscle tissue. This layer is important in that it becomes the muscle that expels a baby at the time of birth. It also provides assistance with menstrual flow by contracting (sometimes cramping). The inner layer, the *endometrium,* is the mucus membrane where the fertilized egg implants and grows. It provides the nourishment and environment for fetal development.

At the opening of the uterus is the *cervix.* The actual opening is called the *cervical os* and is filled with a plug of mucus that changes characteristics according to the hormonal signals of the body. Sometimes this mucus plug is hostile to sperm. At other times, particularly around the time of ovulation, it is not hostile and in fact serves to aid in the transport of sperm into the uterus and eventually up the fallopian tube.

Finally, the vagina is a thin-walled muscular tube that receives the penis during sexual intercourse. This passageway expands at the time of birth to allow movement of a baby from the uterus out of the body.

The Menstrual Cycle

The process of preparing the female body for pregnancy occurs in a cyclic manner beginning at *menarche,* the first sign of menstrual flow, and ending with *menopause,* when fertility and regular menstruation cease. Approximately every month, in response to hormonal signals, the uterus develops the capability of supporting a pregnancy. If pregnancy occurs, the uterus provides a location for fetal development over a nine-month period of gestation. If pregnancy does not occur, the uterus discharges the tissue and fluid built up in preparation for sustaining a pregnancy and begins again the process of preparing for a possible pregnancy. This discharge of tissue and fluid is called *menstruation.*

Although the average menstrual monthly cycle takes about twenty-eight days, it varies greatly from woman to woman. It is just as common for a woman to have regular periods of twenty-three, twenty-five, or twenty-six days, as it is for a woman to have regular periods of thirty-two or thirty-three days. Some women seldom have what are considered regular periods beginning at a predictable time. Irregular periods, in which menstrual flow begins at unpredictable times, are seldom a health problem. Because of the difficulty of predicting the time of ovulation, however, this could become a fertility problem for women attempting to get pregnant or attempting to avoid pregnancy. An important health practice for women is to keep a calendar record of the day when menstrual flow begins. This record provides critical information and should be shared with the physician conducting an annual gynecologic examination.

The easiest way to understand the menstrual cycle is to number the days from the beginning of menstrual flow (day one). Given a twenty-eight-day cycle, several phases can be identified. The first five to seven days are considered the *menstrual phase.* It is the time of menstrual flow. During this phase, the tissue and fluid from the last month's preparation for pregnancy are sloughed off and passed out of the body. It is during this phase as well that the process of developing a new group of follicles for potential ovulation begins. Menstruation is triggered by a drop in the level of both estrogen and progesterone (see Figure 8).

After menstrual flow is well under way, *follicle stimulating hormone* (FSH) is secreted into the blood by the pituitary gland, thus stimulating the ovary to begin the process of preparing egg cells for possible ovulation. This follicular growth takes several days and falls approximately between days six and thirteen in the menstrual cycle. It is influenced by the presence of estrogen levels that rise in response to FSH. This phase of the menstrual cycle is referred to as the *follicular phase.*

The end of the follicular phase is signaled by a sharp rise of another pituitary hormone, *luteinizing hormone* (LH). The rise in the concentration of LH, sometimes called a spike, causes one (and sometimes more) of the follicles to burst and release its contents, including one egg cell, into the abdominal cavity. The release of the egg from the ovary is called *ovulation.* In theory, the ovulated egg floats freely in the abdominal cavity. Actually, the finger-like structures at the end of the fallopian tube quickly locate the egg cell and start it on a path down the fallopian tube toward the uterus. It is at this time (around mid-cycle, or day fourteen) that a woman who has sexual intercourse is most apt to become pregnant.

After ovulation, the level of luteinizing hormone remains higher than at other times during the cycle. This causes the tissue that was once the follicle containing an egg cell to alter slightly and begin secreting higher levels of progesterone. This altered secretory tissue is called the *corpus luteum,* a term meaning yellow body. The hormone progesterone is critical to the maintenance of pregnancy, and in fact the name *progesterone* means "for pregnancy." The level of progesterone remains high for several days following ovulation. This phase of the menstrual cycle is called the *luteal phase* because it is dominated by luteiniz-

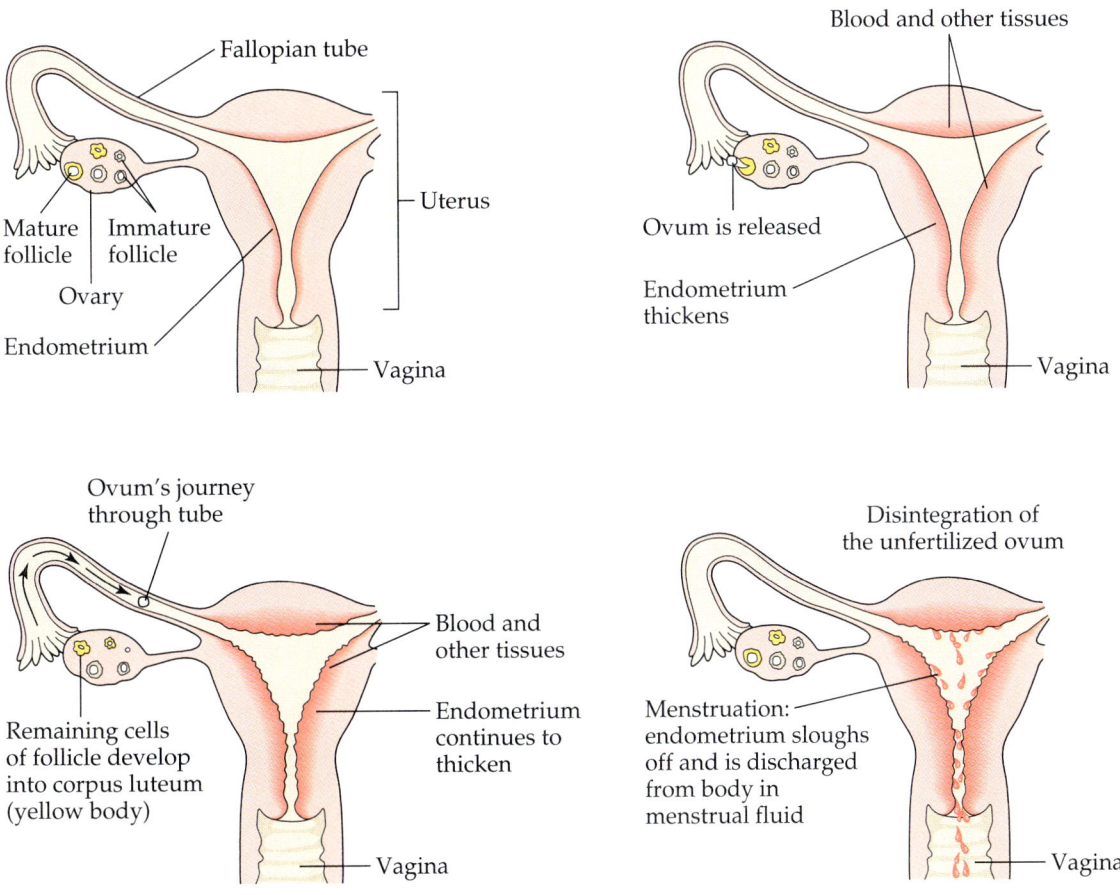

Figure 8 **The Menstrual Cycle.**

ing hormone. The luteal phase usually lasts about fourteen days, even in women who have irregular periods. If pregnancy occurs, signals from the embryonic tissue maintain the level of progesterone and thus delay the onset of menstruation in favor of fetal development. If pregnancy does not occur, however, the level of luteinizing hormone drops, leading to a drop in the level of progesterone, bringing about a breakdown of the endometrium of the uterus. The luteal phase ends with the beginning of menstruation, day one of the next cycle.

■ Test Yourself

Use the following terms to fill in the blanks below.

breasts	follicular phase	ovulation
cervical os	implantation	testosterone
Cowper's gland	labia majora	seminal vesicle
cremaster muscle	ejaculation	luteal phase
epididymis	menstruation	uterus
erection	mons veneris	vas deferens
fallopian tube	myometrium	

1. _____ is the expulsion of semen, including sperm, that usually takes place at a peak of sexual excitement.
2. A powerful masculinizing hormone produced in the testicle is _____.
3. As the penis engorges with blood, it becomes hard and erect, a process known as _____.
4. The _____ serves as a temperature regulator for the testicle, a critical role in fertility.
5. The _____ is a coiled organ that functions to move sperm from the testicle to the vas deferens and provides proteins that affect sperm motility.
6. Another name for the ejaculatory duct is the _____.
7. Once thought to be a storage place for sperm, the _____ is actually a secretory gland that produces a portion of the semen.
8. The _____ secretes a substance that prepares the penis for the passage of sperm.
9. A layer of tissue covered with pubic hair located above and forward of the remainder of the vulva is the _____.
10. The _____ are the large outer folds of tissue extending from the mons pubis and surrounding the opening of the vagina and urethra.
11. Modified sweat glands that develop from puberty into adolescence are _____.
12. Fertilization normally occurs in the _____.
13. _____ refers to the release of the egg from the ovary.
14. The muscular layer of the uterus that may cramp during menstruation is the _____.
15. Normally filled with mucus, the _____ provides a passageway for sperm to reach the uterus and eventually the fallopian tubes.
16. Also called the womb, the _____ is a muscular organ shaped like a pear.

17. The sloughing of built-up uterine tissue is ――――――.
18. The second phase of the menstrual cycle during which estrogen is the dominant hormone is the ――――――.
19. The final phase of the menstrual cycle during which progesterone is the dominant hormone is the ――――――.
20. ―――――― is the burrowing of the embryonic tissue into the wall of the uterus.

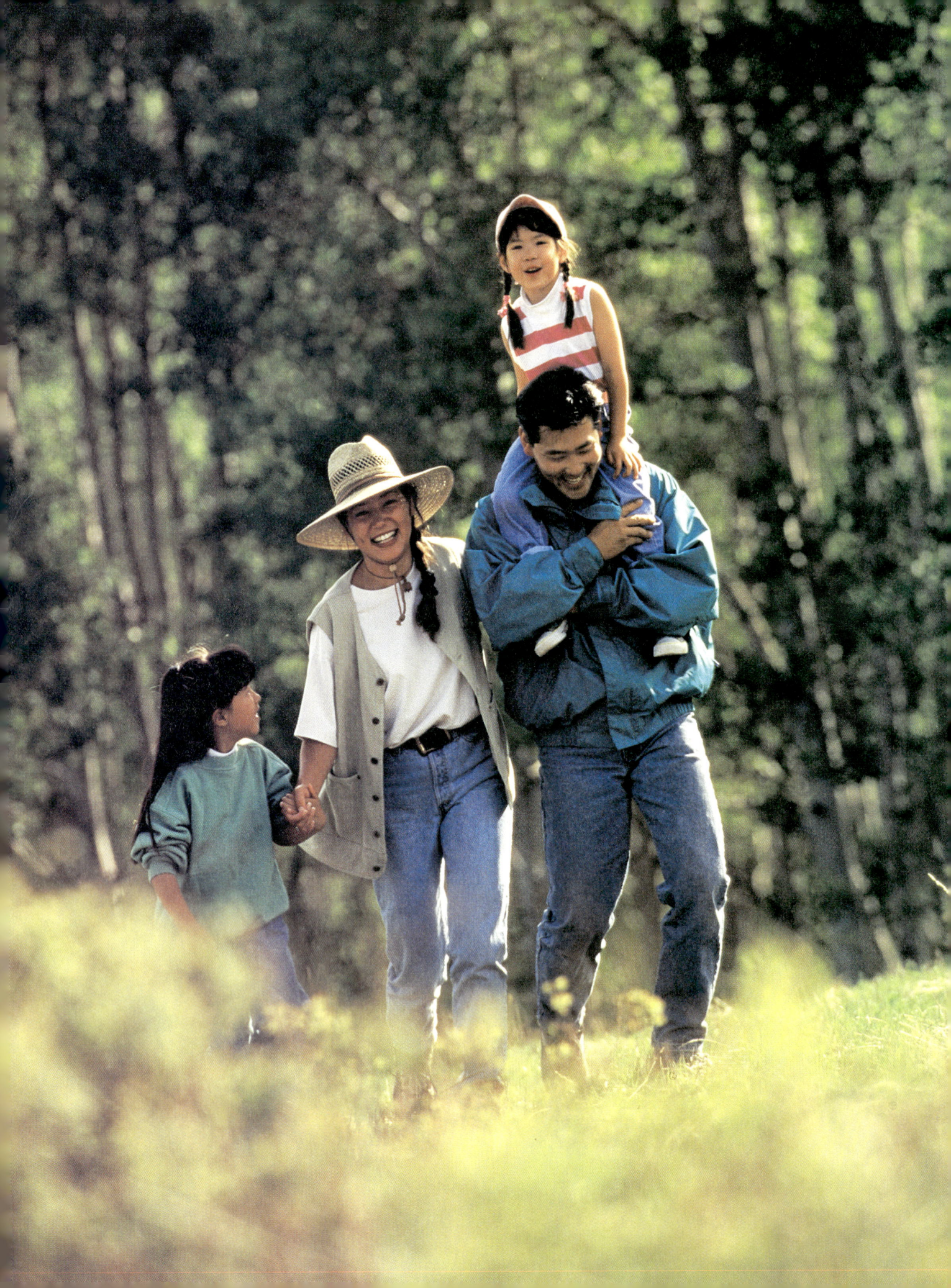

Chapter 17

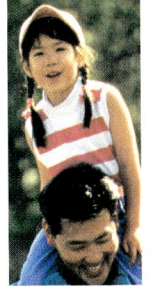
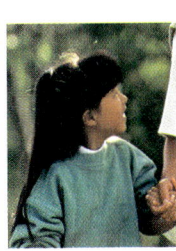
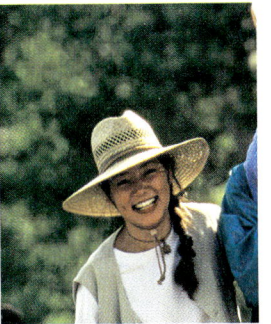

Planning a Family

Objectives

When you finish reading this chapter, you will be able to:

1. Differentiate between family structures, including the nuclear family, the extended family, and the dual-career family and consider the place of traditional marriage in each family structure.
2. Cite conditions that a couple should consider when choosing whether to have children.
3. Identify several factors believed to be associated with infertility as well as medical and social efforts to address such factors.
4. Explain the concepts of and give support for preconception care and prenatal care as important health factors of a pregnancy.
5. Identify two means of studying fetal cells in order to test for the presence or absence of genetic abnormalities.
6. Describe fetal development, beginning with conception and carrying through each trimester to birth.
7. Understand the process of labor and delivery, including the three stages of labor.
8. Understand the place of birth control in overall family planning and identify several methods of birth control that men and women choose.
9. Understand the abortion controversy, including the political importance of this practice, along with characteristics of women who have abortions and why they do so.
10. Recognize that family planning is most effective when based on high-quality information.

What Is Your HealthStyle?

After Indira and Arjun had been married three years, they decided it was time to think seriously about having a family. They had talked about it before they were married, and both agreed that they wanted two children, but until now they were busy settling into married life and furthering their careers.

Indira checked with her family physician to make sure she was in good health, and she began to watch what she ate and drank. Arjun did the same. After all, the consequences could be considerable. Indira and Arjun were lucky. Within four months of deciding it was time to have a family, Indira was happy, healthy, and pregnant.

Louise and Sam form quite a contrast. They, too, had been married for three years, but raising a family was far from what they wanted, at least for now. They were careless about using contraceptives, however, and Louise became pregnant. At first, she didn't know she was pregnant, even after she missed one period. But some other signs, including slightly swollen breasts, told her something was happening. Her physician confirmed that she was six weeks pregnant. Over the course of those six weeks, Louise had had a glass or two of wine several times a week and occasionally shared marijuana with Sam. There was still time to change her health behaviors for the rest of her pregnancy, but she had already compromised at least the first important weeks of gestation.

In Your Opinion

If you look at them without knowing their case histories, Indira and Arjun and Louise and Sam appear to be typical young married couples in the throes of raising a family. Both women are pregnant, one by decision, the other by default. Both wives have discussed the pregnancy with a physician, one in preparation of the event, the other weeks afterwards.

- What were the decisions that Indira and Arjun made that could affect their baby?
- What actions did Louise and Sam take that ignored the implications of having a baby?
- What health skills did Indira and Arjun possess that helped them in this situation?
- How would you handle the decision to have a baby?

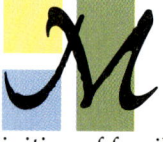

Much has been written about the demise of the American family, but the truth is that, as an institution, it is alive and for the most part well. From a statistical standpoint, the Census Bureau reports that 70 percent of the nation's 99 million households meet its definition of families—people bound by blood, adoption, or marriage.

A family can be defined in numerous ways. The immediate or **nuclear family** consists of parents and/or guardians and their children. It is best understood as those individuals living under the same roof and can include homosexual and lesbian couples. The **extended family** includes those who are connected by blood, marriage, or adoption but who live in another location. It consists of parents, grandparents, aunts, uncles, cousins, and other relatives.

The Beginnings of a Family

The concepts of nuclear and extended family go back to our earliest ancestors, who lived in small bands. The family then, as now, provided a structure for some of the most basic needs in life: psychological, physical, and economic security; sexual satisfaction; and procreation. It also fulfilled several social functions, particularly social support for its members.

In the 1950s, the concept of family was represented—in the movies, on television, by artists, and to some extent in reality—as a working father or breadwinner, a housewife who did not work outside the home, plus two children. This so-called traditional concept of family, although remaining firmly planted in the minds of the public, hardly represents the reality of today.

The family at the turn of the century is noticeably different in many respects. Couples are getting married—and having children—at an older age. And more couples are choosing not to have children at all. (You can read more about one of these trends in the Cultural View box.)

At the same time, there are more **dual-career families.** For economic reasons and personal satisfaction, women are increasingly working outside the home. Today, more than 50 percent of all married women work outside the home, versus 12 percent in 1940. This has had an effect on the structure of the family. Studies show that working women tend to have fewer children than do women who have no work experience outside the home.

Critical Thinking Question

> Politicians are quick to blame many of the social and health problems that face our nation on the breakdown of the family. What argument might support this contention? How might you argue against such a claim? When might a single-parent structure be healthier than a traditional family structure?

Dual-career families demand more of every member of the family. Unless a family assertively works at balancing the expectations of both home and work, problems can develop. For example, consider the woman who is employed full-time outside the home and at the same time is expected (perhaps for reasons of tradition only) to serve as a housekeeper, cook, and head of the family laundry service. Without the help of other family members, the demands of what amounts to two full-time jobs can result in excessive stress and burnout.

Another variation of the nuclear family is the **single-parent family,** which usually consists of a mother and child or children. Only about 10 percent of U.S. single-parent families are headed by a father. Increasingly, single women are choosing to have children or to adopt them so that they can have a family, too. Single men are also adopting children. Because single parents must handle all family roles, they are particularly susceptible to the same stresses and burnout

nuclear family The immediate family; parents and/or guardians and their children, usually living together.

extended family Family members connected by blood, marriage, or adoption, who live in a location outside of one home.

dual-career families Families in which both parents pursue their careers.

single-parent family A family in which only one parent lives in the home and takes care of the children.

CULTURAL VIEW

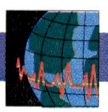

Married, No Kids

The number of married couples without children is rising thanks to empty-nest baby-boom households and baby busters who are finally tying the knot. In 1995, there were 28.6 million married-couple households in the United States without children under age 18 living at home according to the Census Bureau's Current Population Survey. That doesn't necessarily mean there are only two people in the household, though. *American Demographics* estimates that 4.7 million of those married-couple families have adult children over age 18 living at home. The remaining 24 million married-couple families are either truly childless, or are older couples whose children have moved out of the house.

The number of married couples without kids increased 3 percent between 1990 and 1995, slower than the 6 percent increase for all households. However, the number of married couples without children under 18 should grow faster than average into the next century. Between 1995 and 2010, married couples without children under 18 in the home may increase 29 percent, to 36.9 million, according to our projections. The total number of households could increase 16 percent, to 114.7 million, while married couples with children under 13 at home may actually decrease 10 percent, to 22.7 million.

Having adult children at home may not take such a big bite from household spending. Married couples whose oldest child is over age 18, whether living at home or not, have the highest annual expenditures of all married couples, according to the 1995 Consumer Expenditure Survey. This is partly because couples with adult children have an average of 2.7 earners, compared with 1.7 for all married couples.

Married couples without children at home have the lowest expenditures among married couples. But since there are fewer people in their households, they have greater discretionary spending. Child free married couples spend more than average on a number of things, including cash contributions and airline tickets.

—Berna Miller

Source: Reprinted from Berna Miller, "Married, No Kids," *American Demographics,* April 1997, pp. 28–29, with permission. © 1997 Cowles Business Media, Ithaca, NY 14851

---

that occur in dual-career households when the burden of family responsibilities is not shared.

Another lifestyle that is close to but not actually marriage is couples living together. What was once disapproved-of behavior is now practiced by half the population under age forty at some point in their lives. It is estimated that by 2005, half the population under age fifty will be living together without being married. While living together may seem to take the place of marriage, for many it just puts off the wedding date: More than half of all marriages today follow a period of cohabitation. See Figure 17.1 for a look at how family styles have changed over the years.

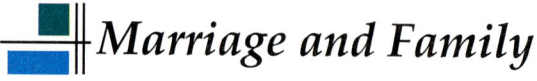

Marriage and Family

Marriage is one of the strongest social and cultural traditions, and most people eventually get married. Statistically, about half of all marriages end in divorce, but most divorced people find new partners and marry again. Specifically, five of six men and three of four women remarry after divorce. Second marriages account for one third of all marriages today. Marriage counselors report that couples are working harder to hold their marriages together and that an increasing number of them are turning to premarital counseling. What couples

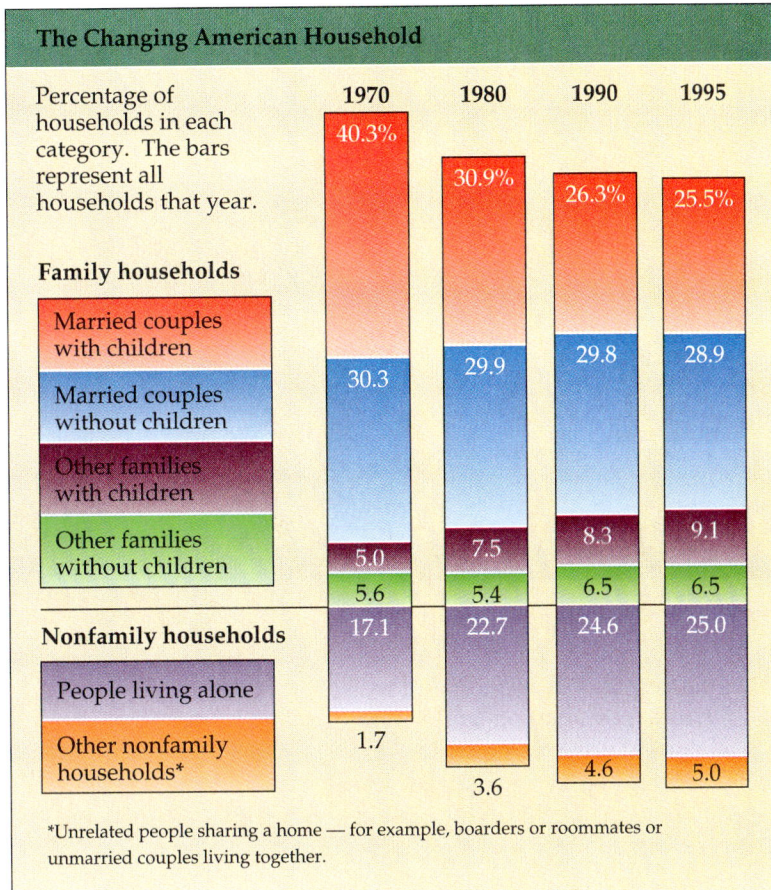

Figure 17.1 The Changing American Household. (Source: Census Bureau)

are looking for, and willing to work on developing, are commitment, bonding, and intimacy.

Marriage is the process of formalizing an interpersonal relationship and establishing a new family core. This makes marriage sound mechanistic, but in fact, it involves elements of romance and psychological and sexual fulfillment

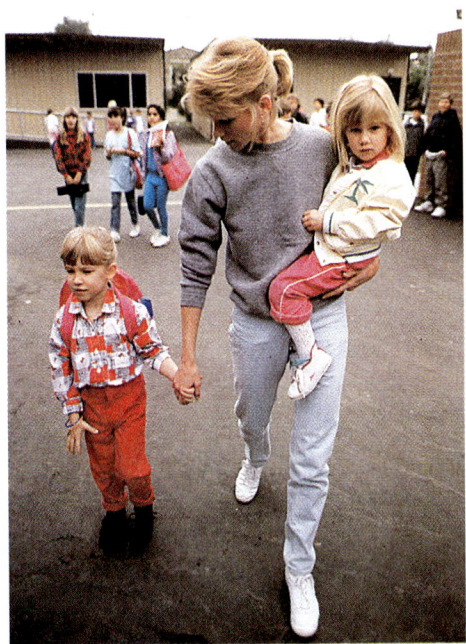

Single parenthood is often the result of divorce; but single women are also choosing to have children or to adopt them to have a family. (Source: Photo Researchers, Inc./© Spencer Grant)

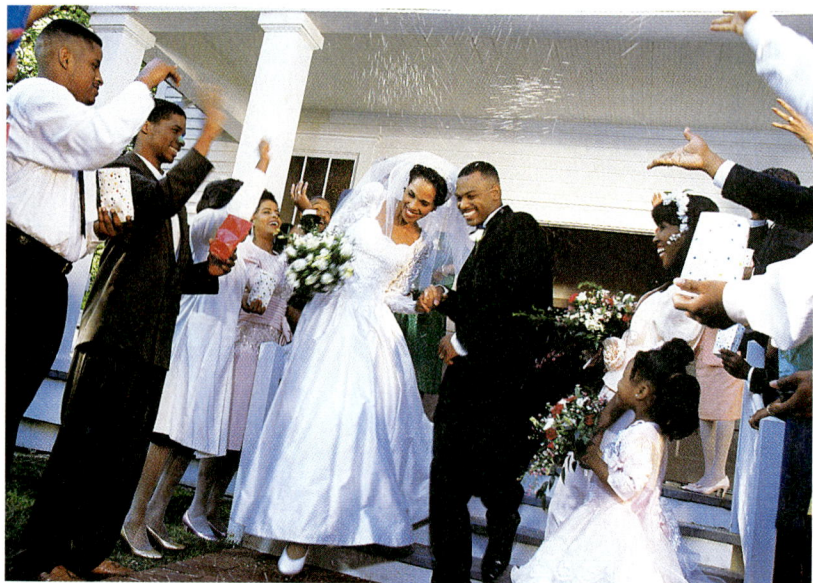

Marriage remains one of our strongest social and cultural traditions. Most people eventually get married. (Source: © Tony Stone Images/Kuluzny/Thatcher)

and offers emotional support and security for both parties. A spouse can be a lifelong friend, a companion, and a buffer against loneliness.

A current controversy exists concerning whether homosexual and lesbian marriages should be recognized. In several cities, these relationships are legitimized. Read about this in the Cultural View box.

HEALTH SKILLS

Deciding to Have Children

Even though premarital sexual activity is common today, one reason why couples marry is to raise a family. Some couples want children right away; others want to wait a period of time to settle into the new relationship. Having children is a serious decision, and not all couples choose this option. No matter how long after marriage a couple actually begins to raise a family, there are certain conditions to consider.

1. *Both sexual partners should want to have a child.* Unwanted children can cause irreparable damage to the marital relationship. More important are the health and safety of such children. Studies document that unwanted children are subjected to higher levels of abuse and neglect than are wanted children. Although some pregnancies result from contraceptive method failures, most unwanted pregnancies result from poor planning and poor decision making on the part of the parents. The obvious way to avoid unwanted pregnancy is through the proper use of effective contraceptive techniques.
2. *Both sexual partners should be physically and psychologically healthy enough to have children and mature enough to accept the responsibility of childrearing.* Raising a family involves a lifelong commitment by both parents. There are periods of extensive nurturing of the very young, support during the sometimes difficult years of adolescence, and guidance in gaining independence in the late teens and early twenties. The demands placed on a family by children in some cases extend well into the adult years.
3. *Both sexual partners should be able to provide the economic support that the child will need to be healthy and properly nourished.* Financial requirements of the young child range from adequate nutrition and quality medical care to day care. During the adolescent years, there are financial demands for social

CULTURAL VIEW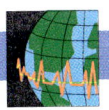

Domestic Partnership

When workers in Washington, D.C. were asked to define their families, they came up with 129 combinations, including living alone, living with a spouse, living in a nuclear family, living with minor children only, living with unrelated children, and living with a same-sex partner.

The changing demographics of the American household are prompting people to reexamine a basic question: What is a family?

Catching Up with Reality?

In cities across the nation, gay and lesbian groups are seeking to expand the traditional definition of a family to include couples of the same sex. The motivation is largely economic: homosexual couples want to get the same share of health and other fringe benefits that married couples get. These benefits can comprise more than 30 percent of a worker's compensation package.

Scores of employers, cities, states, or counties in the United States have granted domestic partnership recognition to unmarried couples, including both heterosexual and homosexual pairs. For the supporters of such ordinances, the law is simply catching up with reality. Matt Coles, a San Francisco lawyer who was present at the creation of the family diversity movement, pointed out, "This movement is not about changing society, because society has already changed. Large numbers of people already live in nontraditional households. History always teaches us that, sooner or later, government has to acknowledge where people are taking society."

Others disagree and see the family as the cornerstone of civilization and defined as people related by blood, marriage, or adoption.

Insurance and Legal Issues

Cities such as San Francisco, Seattle, and Berkeley, which already recognize unmarried relationships, have discovered that they face the worst resistance from insurers. The unspoken fear of some insurers is that they have to pay the catastrophic costs for the treatment of gay partners who have HIV/AIDS. Insurers also worry that a stampede of people will try to create sham partnerships to take advantage of the health benefits. But experience has shown that only a small percentage of employees—the majority of whom are heterosexual—sign up for the domestic partnership plan. In West Hollywood, which created a plan in 1989, just five partners signed up in the first two years of the program.

Berkeley was charged an extra 2 percent fee by a California health maintenance organization (HMO) after it launched a partnership plan in 1985. Three years later, the extra fee was dropped because additional health care costs did not materialize.

Establishing a domestic partnership is a serious step, and to qualify requires proof of a close and committed personal relationship. However, it is not legally the same as a marriage in several ways. Unless there is a will, a domestic partner does not have inheritance rights. Partners do not have a right to each other's pay or property. They cannot share Social Security benefits, immigration rights, veteran's benefits, or even frequent flier miles. They also have no divorce protection, although that matter is likely to be decided in the courts, as couples sue over division of property.

---

activities, clothing, and other day-to-day living expenses. Support for the older child can include expenses of college or job training.

What are the wrong reasons for wanting a child? One often identified by parents is that they thought that having a child would provide stability to their marriage. The presence of a child can seldom do this. In fact, a child often provides just the opposite, interruption, interference, and demands. A second wrong reason is "because I need someone to love me." This response is often heard from pregnant teenagers who feel lonely and out of touch and believe that having a baby will solve their problems. Again, this seldom proves to be the case.

Issues of Infertility

Not everyone who wants to become pregnant can easily do so. Each year about 3 million U.S. couples want to have a baby but cannot successfully conceive one. These couples are said to be infertile.

Infertility is generally defined as the inability of a couple to conceive after one year of intercourse without contraception. Infertility has many causes, including pelvic infections resulting from sexually transmitted diseases, hormonal disturbances in women, and low sperm count in men. Stress, too much exercise, poor nutrition, smoking, and exposure to other environmental hazards can cause bodily changes that impair fertility. Knowing these problems, it is possible to prevent many of the causes of infertility.

Age is also a factor: the older the woman, the higher the incidence of infertility. This is particularly important for women who want to establish their careers before having children. Infertility is a problem for about 2 percent of teenage women, about 10 percent of women in their twenties, and about 14 percent of women thirty to thirty-four. Then it begins to increase steeply to 25 percent of women in their late thirties and 27 percent of women in their forties.

Perhaps the most common way for infertile couples to have children is adoption. But there are other options for women who want to have a birth experience or couples who want some genetic link to a child. One technique used for more than 100 years is **artificial insemination,** in which a woman is artificially impregnated by sperm from an unknown donor or by sperm collected from her partner. Artificial insemination from a sperm bank is also being used today by some single women and lesbian couples who want to have children.

Medical and surgical interventions developed over the last thirty years are successful for 85 percent of infertile couples seeking treatment by inducing ovulation in women and otherwise promoting fertility in both men and women. These interventions include hormones used to stimulate ovulation and surgery to repair damage to the ovaries, fallopian tubes, and testes. Hormone stimulation can cause multiple births, and in 1997, an Iowa woman who had received hormones gave birth to septuplets.

For those still unable to conceive, the breakthrough event took place in 1978 with the birth of Louise Brown, the world's first test tube baby. In the process called **in vitro fertilization** (literally, "fertilization in a glass"), sperm and egg from the mother and father are combined in a glass container, and a fertilized embryo is implanted into the woman. Variations on this process include using a donor egg (not from the mother) or donor sperm (not from the father). These processes are controversial and costly and result in relatively few live births.

One of the most controversial developments is surrogate motherhood, which is when a woman contracts with a couple either to be artificially inseminated with the man's sperm or to have a fertilized embryo implanted in her uterus. The surrogate mother, who typically receives $10,000, carries the pregnancy to term, delivers the child, and gives it to the couple for adoption. This is usually done anonymously—that is, the surrogate mother does not meet the adopting couple. Surrogate motherhood raises many ethical questions, including what to do if the surrogate mother does not give up the baby or, conversely, what to do if the baby is born with defects and the couple does not accept the baby.

HealthLinks
Association of Reproductive Health Professionals
www.arhp.org
ARHP provides numerous resources on reproductive health, including policy updates, newsletters, clinical advances, and patient education information.

HEALTH SKILLS

Preconception Care

The decision to have a baby is a very serious one, and it can have far-reaching implications for the health of the child, the mother, and, in many ways, the family. Good health and a general state of well-being may reduce many of the risks of pregnancy and in fact may even facilitate conception. To help ensure a healthy pregnancy, one that results in a healthy baby and a healthy mother, care should begin before **conception.** Such health care is referred to as **preconception care.**

Preconception care includes a careful evaluation of a potential mother's health status and health behavior as well as environmental factors that may negatively affect the pregnancy. Based on the outcome of such an evaluation, the mother-to-be can take positive steps to eliminate risk factors that may adversely affect her pregnancy. This is important because a large percentage of the pregnancies in the United States are not planned—that is, the mother does not even begin to think she is pregnant until there are telltale signs. By this point, the fertilized egg is developing very rapidly and the risks for harm to developing tissues are far greater than during the rest of pregnancy.

Preconception care has three basic components that, in part, overlap:

1. Risk assessment
2. Health promotion
3. Interventions

A risk assessment includes considering basic factors such as a woman's age, weight, and dietary habits. A woman who is underweight or overweight or who is a vegetarian might seek nutritional counseling to ensure that she is receiving the nutrients needed to sustain a healthy pregnancy. Other risk factors relate to adverse health behaviors, such as smoking, drinking, and taking drugs. As part of her preconception care, a woman may choose to stop smoking. By doing so, she reduces the risk for low birthweight related to tobacco use. Also, she may ask her husband to stop smoking, thus further decreasing the risks to her pregnancy related to passive smoking.

A risk assessment can also identify certain medical conditions that might need special attention during pregnancy. Through preconception care, a woman can learn whether she is at risk for getting rubella, or German measles, which may cause severe birth defects if contracted during pregnancy. If so, she can be immunized against the disease and thus protect her child if she does become pregnant. Not all infectious diseases can be prevented by a vaccine, but once identified, many can be treated before a woman becomes pregnant.

Preconception is the ideal time for genetic counseling in families that have a history of genetic disease or a significant occupational or environmental exposure to toxic agents or when maternal age is a factor. Genetic counseling helps couples better understand their risks and provides the opportunity for genetic testing if necessary. It could also be a determining factor in a couple's decision to adopt children.

Health promotion during the preconception stage includes practicing healthy behaviors, such as proper nutrition and exercise and not smoking or drinking. It also involves counseling about family planning and spacing of pregnancies. During this stage, a couple should begin investigating resources in the community for good prenatal care so the woman can make appropriate arrangements once she knows she is pregnant. It also makes sense to know about your reproductive physiology. See the Your Sexual Body section of this textbook.

The third step of preconception care includes a range of interventions that can be taken to promote a healthy pregnancy. Examples of interventions are getting appropriate immunizations, treating diseases, and getting to the right weight. By taking these three steps, women are in a better position to make informed decisions concerning their pregnancies and their future families.

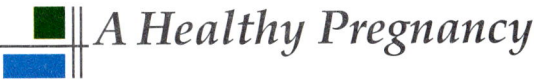
A Healthy Pregnancy

When does life begin? This question prompts some of our culture's hottest debates. Some people believe that life begins at birth. Others believe that life

infertility The inability of a couple to conceive after one year of intercourse without contraception.

artificial insemination Introduction of semen into the vagina by artificial means, using a syringe.

in vitro fertilization A procedure in which the sperm and egg from a man and a woman are combined in a glass container and a fertilized embryo is implanted into the woman.

conception The union of sperm and egg.

preconception care Health-promoting action taken prior to conception for the purpose of reducing health risks to mother and child.

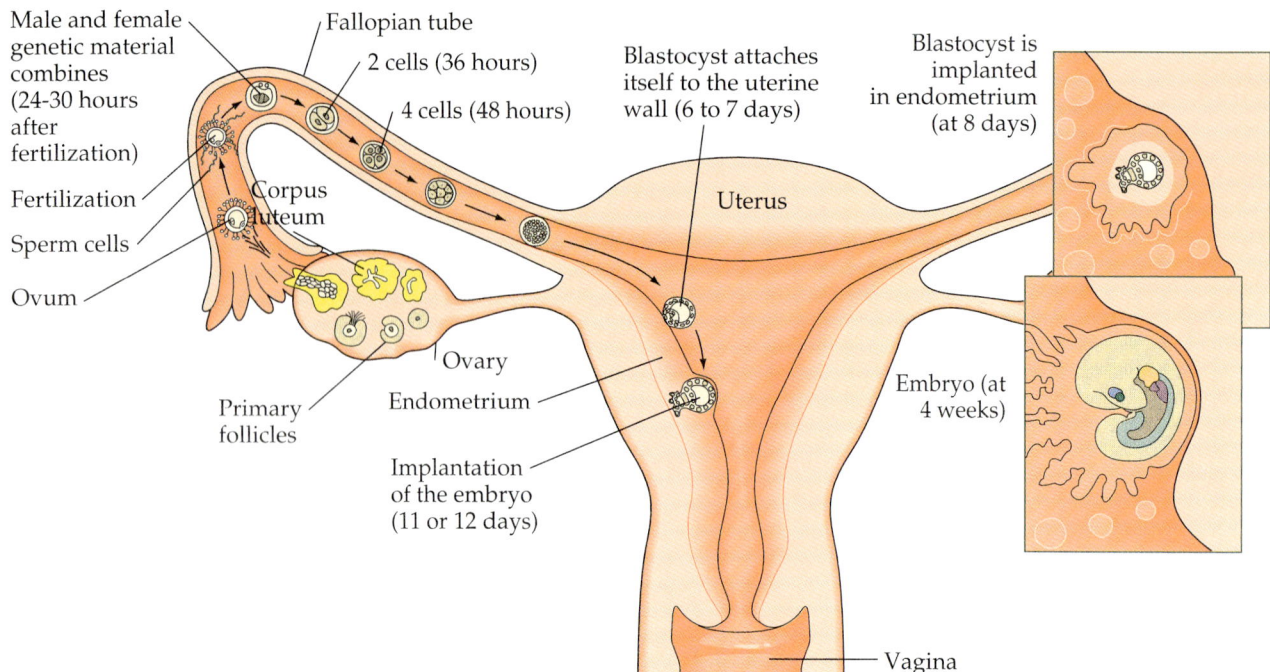

Figure 17.2 The Process of Conception. *Conception takes place in the fallopian tube. A few days later, the embryo is implanted in the wall of the uterus. (Source: Rebecca J. Donatelle and Lorraine G. Davis,* Access to Health, *5th ed., p. 200 (Figure 8.8). Copyright © 1998 by Allyn & Bacon. Reprinted by permission of Allyn & Bacon)*

begins when the fetal heartbeat is heard. Still others believe that it begins at the moment of conception. Although we cannot settle the "life" question, we can establish the point at which pregnancy begins. Pregnancy technically begins at the moment of conception. Conception is that point when sperm and egg unite. It takes place in the fallopian tube, and a few days later, the new embryo implants in the uterine wall, where it will develop into the fetus. The uterus expands to provide a home for the fetus to grow and serves as a muscular means of expelling the baby at birth (see Figure 17.2).

Early signs of pregnancy include **amenorrhea,** or missed menstrual period, along with breast changes such as fullness and tenderness. Sometimes these symptoms are coupled with nausea (morning sickness) and increased urinary frequency. Because each of these symptoms also occurs in nonpregnant women, they should be considered an indication only that a pregnancy is possible, not that it is probable.

Pregnancy can be accurately detected soon after conception by the presence of a hormone, **human chorionic gonadotropin (HCG),** which is secreted into the urine from placental cells. The **placenta** is a structure that develops from the wall of the uterus and serves as an organ of interchange between the mother and the fetus. Pregnancy tests are available at college health services, family planning clinics, and physicians' offices. Many of the tests sold in drug stores have an effectiveness rate high enough to indicate, along with the signs described above, that pregnancy is probable. If you are using an over-the-counter test, positive signs of pregnancy should be confirmed by a physician.

The Importance of Prenatal Care

While the groundwork for a healthy pregnancy and birth begins before conception, it is also important that care is taken during the pregnancy. Health care during pregnancy is called **prenatal care,** or care before birth. Good health care during this period can increase the chances of a healthy pregnancy and delivery.

During pregnancy, smoking, drinking, drug use, and exposure to sexually transmitted diseases are critical health threats to the fetus. Smoking during pregnancy is associated with higher infant mortality and **low birthweight babies.** Studies show that women who smoke a pack or more of cigarettes a day during pregnancy have about a 50 percent greater risk for having a spontaneous abortion or stillbirth than do nonsmoking women. Babies born to women who smoke during pregnancy are born weighing, on average, six ounces less than babies of nonsmoking women. Passive smoking, when nonsmokers inhale tobacco smoke, can also affect a pregnant woman and her fetus (see Chapter 8).

Alcohol is a particularly powerful drug during pregnancy. Alcohol consumed by a pregnant woman travels through the fetal bloodstream in the same concentration as in the mother's. However, the tiny, developing system of the fetus is not as well equipped to handle this alcohol load. For example, the undeveloped fetal liver burns up alcohol at less than half the rate of an adult liver. This means that alcohol remains in the fetal system longer than in the adult system. Heavy, and sometimes light, drinking by a pregnant woman may result in fetal alcohol syndrome, which can cause irreversible mental and physical impairment. Research indicates that no amount of drinking can be considered safe during pregnancy (see Chapter 9).

Babies born to mothers who are drug users are at risk not only of being addicted to drugs themselves but also of being born with significant health problems, including mental retardation, low birthweight, and a tendency toward premature death. Widespread drug use among pregnant women has led to nationwide concern about **crack babies,** babies born addicted to crack cocaine, and babies born already infected with the human immunodeficiency virus (HIV). New drugs for treating AIDS are proving effective in reducing the number of babies born with HIV infection.

Certain medications taken during pregnancy can also harm the fetus. The drug **thalidomide,** taken as a sedative during the early 1960s even though it was not approved for use in the United States, caused severe deformities in developing fetuses' extremities. Thousands of children were born without hands, arms, and/or legs. (Based on studies that show thalidomide's ability to regulate the immune system, it is being used again in the United States to treat certain cancers, AIDS, and some autoimmune diseases; its use, however, is very strictly controlled for women of childbearing age.) More recently, the drug Accutane, used to treat severe acne, was found to cause fetal malformations.

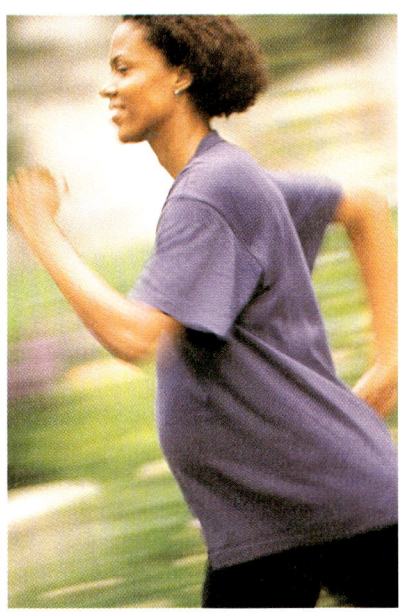

An important component of prenatal care is exercise. Being physically fit can help prepare a woman for the physical work involved in the delivery of a baby. (Source: © Tony Stone Images/ Penny Gentieu)

amenorrhea An abnormal absence or suppression of menstruation.

human chorionic gonadotropin (HCG) A hormone secreted from placental cells; a pregnancy test looks for the presence of this hormone.

placenta The structure that develops from the wall of the uterus and serves as an organ of interchange between the mother and the fetus.

prenatal care Health-promoting action taken after conception and before birth for the purpose of reducing health risks to mother and child; medical care during pregnancy.

low birthweight babies Babies born weighing less than 2,500 grams, or five pounds eight ounces.

crack babies Babies born addicted to crack cocaine.

thalidomide A drug taken as a sedative in the early 1960s and subsequently found to cause severe deformities in the extremities of developing fetuses.

How seriously are these risks viewed by pregnant women? Unfortunately, not seriously enough. For example, of women aged eighteen to forty-four who had given birth to a child recently and who were smoking before they learned they were pregnant, nearly one third reported that they continued to smoke during the pregnancy.

Good prenatal care includes careful monitoring by a physician or certified nurse-midwife, proper diet, and appropriate exercise. The recommended weight gain during pregnancy is twenty-five to thirty-five pounds for an infant weight between six and a half and nine pounds, according to an Institute of Medicine report—considerably more than the fifteen pounds recommended by many physicians in the 1950s and the twenty to twenty-five pounds recommended in 1970.

Gone are the days when pregnant women were confined to home. Today, they are seen jogging, playing tennis, and taking aerobics classes. While most pregnant women should not start a highly strenuous exercise program, most physicians agree that healthy women can continue an exercise program through most of the pregnancy. Exercise helps prepare women for the physical work involved in delivering a baby and can result in an easier delivery. It also helps the mother's body return to normal after the baby is born.

Diagnostic procedures that can be performed during pregnancy to test the health of the fetus are another component of prenatal care.

Testing the Health of the Fetus

The first picture in the baby book used to be the one taken at the hospital within twenty-four hours of delivery. Increasingly, this is being replaced by the **sonogram,** a diagnostic tool that allows the physician indirectly to see the developing fetus and its individual organ systems. The sonogram is useful in determining fetal age, position, and size as well as in detecting certain abnormalities. This information can help a physician determine if the fetus is developing on schedule.

A growing number of other diagnostic procedures help physicians evaluate the health of the fetus. A test of the mother's blood, taken between the thirteenth and twentieth weeks of pregnancy, can detect levels of alpha-fetoprotein (AFP), a substance produced by the fetus's kidneys. High levels of AFP could indicate a neural tube defect, which could result in conditions such as spina bifida; low levels could be a sign of Down syndrome. The AFP blood test is a screening procedure. If a pregnant woman has a questionable level of AFP in her blood, she should speak with her physician about having further diagnostic tests.

Amniocentesis provides physicians with a reliable way to study fetal cells to test for the presence or absence of certain genetic conditions, such as Down syndrome. In this procedure, a needle is inserted through the uterus and into the amniotic fluid that surrounds the fetus. Fluid that contains cells shed by the fetus is drawn out. The test is performed between the fifteenth and eighteenth weeks of pregnancy, when a sufficient number of fetal cells are available for study. It takes an additional two to three weeks to culture the cells and get results from the study. If the test results show a birth defect, the mother can consider whether to continue with the pregnancy or terminate it.

As helpful as amniocentesis is, a woman is into her twentieth week of pregnancy—midway through it—before she gets the results of the test. This time lag has been reduced in recent years with a technique called **chorionic villus sampling (CVS).** The chorionic villi, hairlike projections on a membrane surrounding the interior of the uterus, contain the same information found in the amniotic fluid. The advantage of CVS is that it can be performed earlier in pregnancy—between the ninth and twelfth weeks—and results are available in six to twenty-four hours.

Both amniocentesis and CVS involve some risk to the mother and fetus, including miscarriage (spontaneous abortion) and infection. CVS is also linked to

---

sonogram A diagnostic tool that allows the physician indirectly to see the developing fetus and its individual organ systems.

amniocentesis Means of testing amniotic fluid to indicate the presence or absence of certain genetic conditions, such as Down syndrome, in a fetus.

chorionic villus sampling (CVS) A technique in which the chorionic villi, hairlike projections on a membrane surrounding the interior of the uterus, are tested to determine the presence or absence of certain genetic conditions.

missing or underdeveloped fingers or toes, which are rare abnormalities. These tests should not be done unless a legitimate reason exists. CVS carries slightly more risk for the fetus than amniocentesis and does not detect as many defects.

Critical Thinking Question

Among the kind of information revealed by amniocentesis and chorionic villus sampling tests is the sex of the fetus. Do you think determining the sex of a fetus alone is a legitimate reason for having amniocentesis or CVS? Why might some people oppose the use of these tests for the purposes of sex determination?

Growth by Trimesters

Pregnancy is divided into trimesters of thirteen weeks each. Most of the organs and much of the development of the fetus take shape during the first trimester. Sex, for example, is determined genetically at conception, but it takes about three months before physical differences between males and females can be observed. The head, meanwhile, is disproportionately large (it accounts for nearly half of the fetus's size) because of the developing brain. The effects of drug use and

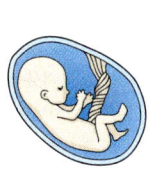
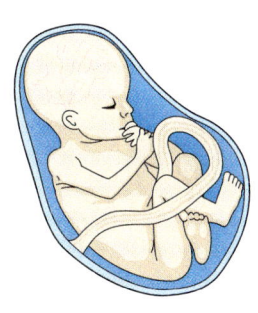
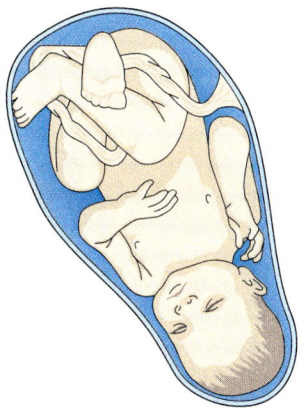

First trimester completed   Second trimester completed   Third trimester completed

Figure 17.3 The Nine Months of Pregnancy. *(a) First trimester completed. After 8 weeks as an embryo, the baby is now called a fetus. Fingers and toes have soft nails. Mouth has 20 buds that will become baby teeth. A special instrument can pick up the baby's heartbeat at 10 to 12 weeks. By the end of month 3, the fetus is 4 inches long and weighs a little over 1 ounce. (b) Second trimester completed. Skin is red and wrinkled and covered with fine, soft hair. The fetus is usually too small and its lungs not ready for life outside its mother. If born now, the fetus might survive with intensive care. Eyelids begin to part and the eyes open. Finger and toe prints can be seen. By the end of month 6, the fetus is 11 to 14 inches long and weighs 1 to 1½ pounds. (c) Third trimester completed. At 38 to 40 weeks, the baby is full term. Lungs are mature and ready to function on their own. During the final month, the baby gains about ½ pound a week. The baby usually drops into a head-down position and rests lower in the mother's abdomen. By the end of month 9, the baby weighs 6 to 9 pounds and is 19 to 21 inches long.*

infectious diseases on the fetus are particularly damaging during this trimester when so much development is going on. By the end of three months, the fetus is approximately four inches long and weighs one ounce.

During the second trimester, the fetus grows to about one foot long and one to one and a half pounds. Its eyes are open, but the lungs and intestinal canal are not yet completely developed. During this time, the mother begins to feel its movements, a sensation called **quickening.** The fetal heartbeat becomes audible through a stethoscope. The mother's breasts grow, and the initial signs of pregnancy, such as morning sickness and frequent urination, usually subside.

The third trimester is a time of growth and fine-tuning for the fetus. Fingernails are already grown and sometimes even need cutting. Some babies are born with scratch marks from their nails. More crucial to life, however, are the respiratory and digestive systems, which are the last systems to be fully developed. The last trimester is a period of great weight gain and growth. A full-term baby, born thirty-nine weeks after conception, weighs six to nine pounds and is about twenty inches long. The mother becomes somewhat uncomfortable with the weight gain associated with carrying a full-term baby, particularly with the crowding of her internal organs. She feels pressure on her bladder. She also feels the fetus kicking and hiccuping. Between two and four weeks before birth, the baby "drops," or positions itself to be delivered through the vaginal canal (see Figure 17.3).

Preparing for Childbirth

Until the 1960s, preparation for childbirth was limited to making regular visits to the physician, getting ready for a quick departure to the hospital, and creating a list of telephone numbers to call when the sex of the baby was determined. During childbirth itself, the father was traditionally banished to a waiting room, where he paced the floor and waited for the announcement from the delivery room. Meanwhile, in the delivery room, the mother most often was put to

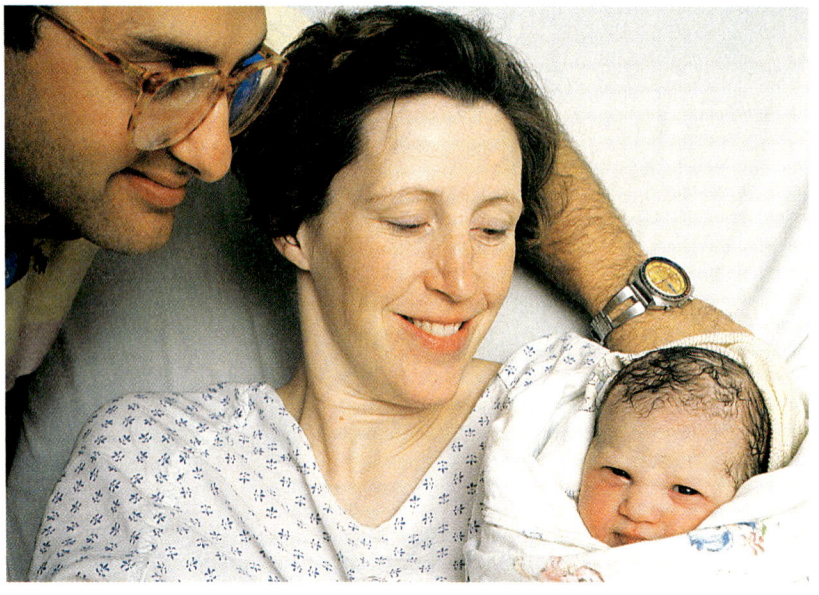

The first family portrait reflects the special bond that exists between parents and children. (Source: © Tony Stone Images/ Penny Gentieu)

"sleep" with anesthesia, shaved, and given an enema and a variety of drugs but very little information about what was actually happening to her and her baby. Having a baby was treated like an illness.

Things have changed, in great part as a result of the women's movement. Many women are choosing **natural childbirth,** and instead of relieving pain with drugs, they rely on a system of breathing and relaxation techniques, based on the principles of Fernand Lamaze, a French obstetrician. In cases in which mothers receive pain medication, the effects are localized and the mothers are awake during the birth. Fathers are also more involved and are usually present at the time of delivery. They give support to the mother and sometimes assist the physician.

An increasing number of women are choosing to have their babies delivered by **nurse-midwives** either in the hospital or in freestanding birthing centers, which are located outside hospitals. These centers, which are usually home-like settings and staffed by certified nurse-midwives, offer a lower-technology alternative to a hospital delivery. Doctors are available as consultants in case a complication arises.

Studies show that birthing centers are as safe as hospital deliveries and cost about half as much money. A key factor in the birthing centers' good record is that they appear to serve very low-risk populations. Their patients tend to be women who are well-nourished, middle-class, educated, married, and over age eighteen. In addition, they did not smoke, drink, or take other drugs during pregnancy.

First-Stage Labor

During the first stage of **labor,** the **cervix,** the opening to the uterus, gradually **effaces,** or thins, and **dilates,** or opens. (Effacement can take place as much as three weeks in advance of labor.) Dilation of the cervix is necessary to allow eventual passage of the baby through the birth canal. It is brought about by a series of contractions of the uterus, which are usually rhythmic in nature. The contractions of the uterus in the early part of the first stage of labor feel like a tightening of the lower abdomen. These contractions are spaced several minutes (perhaps twenty minutes) apart and are generally not uncomfortable. As the first stage of labor progresses, however, the tightening of the uterus during the contraction becomes more and more severe and the contraction brings about a feeling of increasing pressure. At some point during the first stage of labor, the amniotic fluid is released. This fluid is a substance that surrounds and protects the fetus throughout the development process. The release of the amniotic fluid is sometimes referred to as the breaking of waters (see Figure 17.4).

Dilation and effacement of the cervix usually occur within a few hours. In some cases, especially in first births, the process may take much longer, perhaps days or weeks. In the case of second and third births, the process may take only a few minutes. When the cervix is dilated two to three inches (five to six centimeters), the intensity of labor increases and the resting time between contractions is decreased as the body secretes a hormone that brings on the hard contractions needed to expel the baby. The first stage of labor is considered complete when the cervix is completely effaced and dilated to ten centimeters and the baby's head can be seen. This is called **crowning.**

Second-Stage Labor

During the second stage of labor, the baby is actually born. The second stage of labor is usually much shorter than the first stage. It should never be allowed to last longer than one to two hours. Longer second-stage labor can be hazardous to the mother and child (see Figure 17.5).

quickening Fetal movements felt by the mother.

natural childbirth Delivery of a baby "naturally," without the aid of drugs.

nurse-midwife Registered nurse who has completed advanced training in gynecology and obstetrics.

labor The process of childbirth from the initial contractions of the uterus to the delivery of the baby and the placenta.

cervix The opening of the uterus into the vagina.

effacement The thinning of the cervix during the process of childbirth.

dilation Opening of the cervix either for examination or for delivery of a baby.

crowning The point of labor at which the cervix is completely effaced and dilated to ten centimeters and the baby's head can be seen.

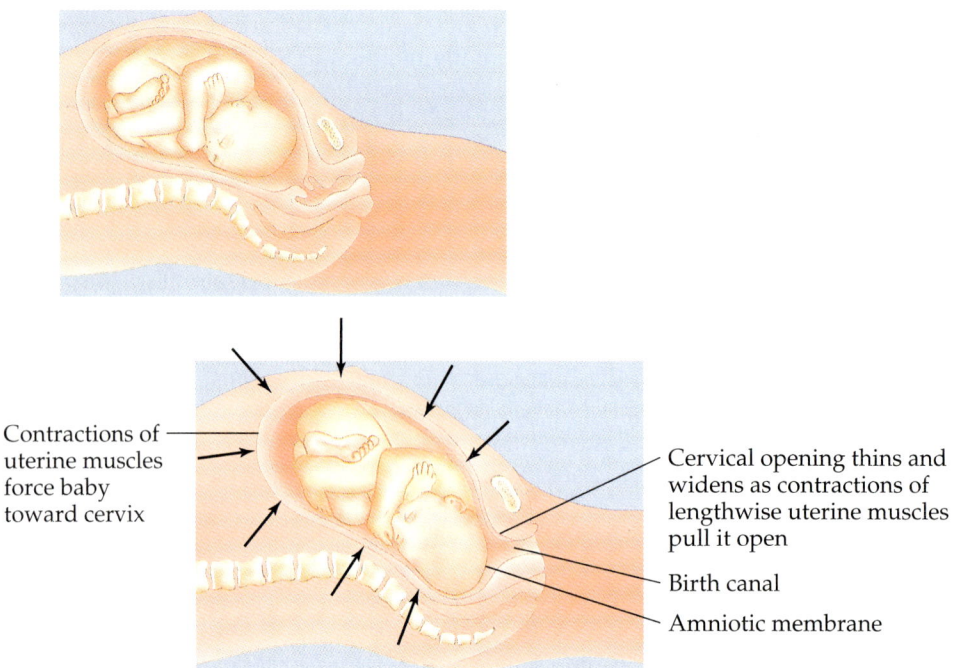

Figure 17.4 First Stage of Labor. *(Source: Rebecca J. Donatelle and Lorraine G. Davis,* Access to Health, *5th ed., p. 205 (Figure 8.10). Copyright © 1998 by Allyn & Bacon. Reprinted by permission of Allyn & Bacon)*

Several positions may be used for the delivery of the baby, including squatting or sitting, but the most common position for delivery in the United States is with the mother lying on her back with her legs apart placed in stirrups, to provide the physician with easy access to the baby when birth takes place.

In the second stage of labor, the uterine contractions increase in frequency and intensity. At the same time, the mother uses her abdominal muscles to help push the baby out. The baby's head is normally the first part of the body to move

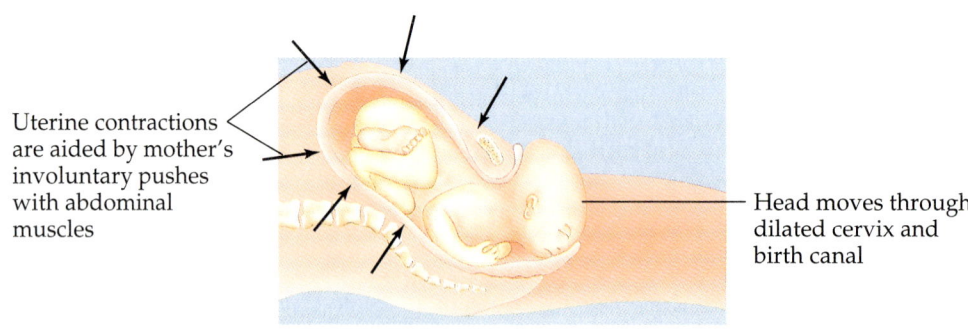

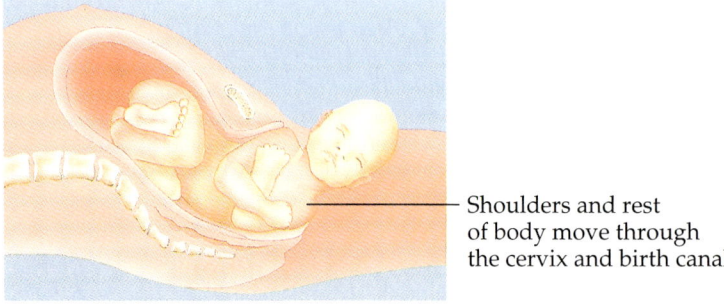

Figure 17.5 Second Stage of Labor. *(Source: Rebecca J. Donatelle and Lorraine G. Davis,* Access to Health, *5th ed., p. 205 (Figure 8.10). Copyright © 1998 by Allyn & Bacon. Reprinted by permission of Allyn & Bacon)*

through the cervix and out the birth canal. The physician may make a small incision from the vagina toward the anus called an **episiotomy** to ensure easier passage of the baby's head through the birth canal and to prevent tearing of the tissue. This procedure may cause discomfort to the mother during the recovery period due to the stitches needed to repair the incision. Some health professionals do not consider it necessary to do an episiotomy routinely believing that relaxation, pushing, manually stretching the area, and patience by the physician can eliminate much of the need for one.

In some cases, the physician may recommend delivering the baby by **cesarean section** (C-section), that is, removal of the baby through an incision in the abdominal wall rather than through the birth canal. Cesarean sections are done in approximately 25 percent of births in the United States. Physicians recommend cesarean sections for a number of reasons: The birth canal may be too small to accommodate delivery; the labor, for a variety of reasons, may not be progressing correctly; the position of the baby may be feet or bottom first, known as **breech presentation**; fetal distress may be evident; or natural delivery may be otherwise perceived as too risky.

The lives of many mothers and infants have been saved through the use of cesarean sections. But this method of delivery is controversial because it may be chosen too often. The procedure is also more expensive than natural delivery and requires that the mother and child stay in the hospital longer. By some estimates, perhaps one third of all cesarean sections are unnecessary. Some physicians are believed to perform them due to fear of a malpractice suit if they wait until a baby is ready to be born naturally. Women who are over age thirty and/or who have private health insurance are more likely to have cesarean section deliveries than are younger women and those who have no health insurance or who are receiving public health benefits such as Medicaid.

Until recently, it was widely held that once a woman had had a cesarean section delivery, she had to have one for all subsequent deliveries. Now physicians believe that some women who have had a cesarean section can have a vaginal delivery in future pregnancies. Today, about one in four women who have had a previous cesarean birth deliver a subsequent child vaginally.

Third-Stage Labor

In the final stage of labor, the placenta separates from the uterine wall and is expelled. This is done naturally through a continuation of uterine contractions. The placenta is examined by the physician to determine if it is intact. The placenta must be completely removed from the woman or complications in recovery from childbirth can result. These complications include bleeding and infection (see Figure 17.6).

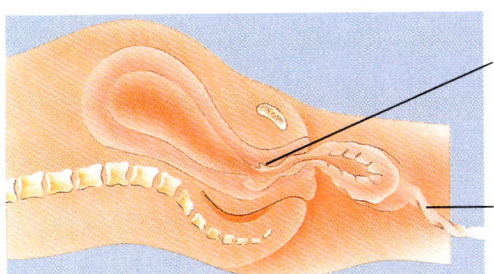

■ **Figure 17.6 Third Stage of Labor.** (Source: Rebecca J. Donatelle and Lorraine G. Davis, Access to Health, 5th ed., p. 205 (Figure 8.10). Copyright © 1998 by Allyn & Bacon. Reprinted by permission of Allyn & Bacon)

episiotomy The small incision made between the opening of the vagina and the anus to ensure easier passage of the baby's head through the birth canal and to prevent tearing of the tissue.

cesarean section Removal of the baby through an incision in the abdominal wall rather than through the birth canal.

breech presentation Positioning of the baby's feet or bottom first in the birth canal.

This ends the long process of having a baby. The process began before conception, as plans were made about the timing of the pregnancy. Ahead lie years of parenting and decisions about future pregnancies.

Family Planning

Pregnancy does not occur with each sexual encounter, but it can happen often enough that **family planning** becomes an important aspect of family life. Family planning is the process of establishing the preferred number and spacing of children in one's family and choosing the means by which this is achieved. The concept of family planning emphasizes the importance of both family and planning. It acknowledges that few events can be more treasured than the discovery of an intended pregnancy. Even though 1997 data indicate that one quarter of all births were unintended—that is, they were either mistimed or not wanted—few events are more potentially damaging to a family than the discovery of an unintended pregnancy. Table 17.1 shows who has babies who are mistimed (a child or children are desired but not at this time) or unwanted (no child or children are desired).

Family planning is usually carried out through the application of one or more **birth control** methods or devices. Birth control is hardly a new idea. Many cultures have provided instruction on pregnancy prevention, including such recommendations as eating the genitalia of an animal prior to intercourse, squatting and attempting to sneeze following intercourse, and covering the penis prior to intercourse with a skin membrane of an animal (the first condom).

The Comstock Law of 1873, named after Anthony Comstock, then secretary of the New York Society for the Suppression of Vice, made it illegal to disseminate contraceptive information through the U.S. mail because such information was considered obscene. Many states passed "little Comstock laws," some of which banned the use of contraceptives. Birth control pioneer Margaret Sanger had to flee to Europe to avoid prosecution after she opened her birth control clinic

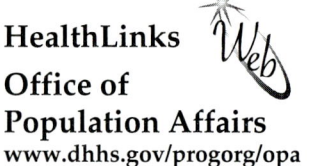

**HealthLinks
Office of
Population Affairs**
www.dhhs.gov/progorg/opa

The OPA provides resources and policy advice on population, family planning, reproductive health, and adolescent pregnancy issues.

TABLE 17.1 Who Has Unintended Babies

	Ever had an unintended birth	Percentage of these births mistimed	Percentage of these births unwanted
All women	24.4%	80.4%	19.6%
By age			
Under age 20	6.1	83.4	16.5
Ages 20–24	22.5	84.7	15.3
Ages 25–29	28.5	73.6	26.4
Ages 30–44	38.1	56.8	43.2
By marital status			
Never married	14.2	78.4	21.6
Currently married	34.2	82.6	17.4
Formerly married	47.0	67.5	32.5

Source: National Center for Health Statistics, 1997

in 1916 in Brooklyn, where women could get diaphragms that she had shipped from abroad.

The social acceptance of birth control grew during the mid-twentieth century. In 1962, the birth control pill was approved for marketing in the United States; in 1965, the Supreme Court declared laws prohibiting the sale and use of contraceptives to be unconstitutional, calling them a violation of the right to privacy. Condoms are now sold openly in drug stores and on college campuses and are given away free in some high schools and other public settings. Women purchase nearly 50 percent of condoms sold for use by males. Condoms are now available for women.

There are several reasons why birth control is so acceptable today:

- The development and availability of a variety of effective and safe methods of birth control
- The changing role of women and their entry into the work force so that family planning is more critical
- An increase in the rate of sexual activity among both the unmarried and the married populations

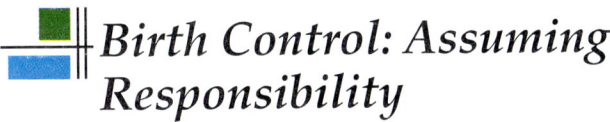

Birth Control: Assuming Responsibility

Each time a couple has sexual intercourse, the woman is at risk for getting pregnant. Thus, abstinence is the only totally effective birth control method known. A fact of life, however, is that most adults are sexually active.

For some women, birth control provides the means to choose the number and spacing of children. Others have significant health reasons for using birth control. Teenage mothers, for example, face an increased risk for having low birthweight babies. Older mothers, meanwhile, face a higher risk for having children who have Down syndrome. In some situations, pregnancy might be harmful to the mother, particularly if she has other health problems, such as cancer or heart disease.

The Range of Birth Control Choices

When choosing from the wide range of birth control methods, it is important to become well informed about the various options. This can be done by visiting with a physician, college health professional, or birth control counselor who will review the various options and the advantages and disadvantages of each and discuss how each might or might not fit within your lifestyle. It is unwise to choose a birth control method based on incomplete information or information from an unreliable source. The following section discusses some of the options available today. Before you make a decision about birth control, however, you should seek more information.

A term that has become synonymous with birth control is *contraception*. **Contraception** is the intentional prevention of conception, the union of sperm and egg. Modern science has produced several means of contraception. Non-technological methods also exist, but they are relatively ineffective in preventing pregnancy.

family planning A process of establishing the preferred number and spacing of children in one's family and choosing the means by which this is achieved.

birth control Prevention of pregnancy for the purpose of family planning.

contraception The intentional prevention of conception.

Critical Thinking Question

The *Healthy People 2000* objectives include the following: "Increase to at least 90 percent the proportion of sexually active, unmarried people aged 15–24 who use contraception, especially combined methods of contraception that both effectively prevent pregnancy and provide barrier protection against disease." Baseline data suggest that at the time of first intercourse, only 63 percent of women in this age category use contraception and dramatically fewer use a combination of methods. If the prevention of unintended pregnancy is a simple matter of applying existing technology, why the reluctance on the part of this age group to apply such technology? Could it be that they have misconceptions about contraceptive methods? Or is it because they deny the possibility an unintended pregnancy? What do you think?

The **rhythm method** relies on knowing when a woman ovulates (releases an egg) and then calculating when her fertile and infertile periods are. To use the rhythm method, a woman needs to calculate by calendar when she ovulates and to take her temperature regularly. Ovulation is often represented by a slight increase in temperature. Once the monthly anticipated day of ovulation is determined, abstinence from intercourse is necessary for the rhythm method to be effective. However, women often ovulate at unexpected times during the month, and even if all procedures are followed correctly, it is not uncommon for women who rely on the rhythm method of birth control to become pregnant. It has a failure rate of 24 percent. This means that 24 out of 100 women practicing the rhythm method for one year become pregnant.

Another nontechnological method is **withdrawal,** in which the man withdraws his penis from the vagina before ejaculating so that sperm are not deposited at or near the birth canal. The failure rate for withdrawal is high, and it is considered to be ineffective in preventing pregnancy. The main reason for the failure of this method of birth control is that during intercourse, sperm are present even when ejaculation has not taken place. Withdrawal, therefore, does not ensure that sperm are not placed in a position to bring about pregnancy.

With the introduction of the **birth control pill** in the 1960s, a dramatic increase in the effectiveness of contraceptives took place. The pill consists of chemicals that are similar to hormones normally produced in a woman's body. When taken regularly for a full monthly series, this drug keeps the ovaries from releasing eggs. No egg, no conception. The pill has a 1 percent failure rate with "perfect" use and a 6 percent failure rate with average use—which includes forgetting to take it on schedule. See Table 17.2 for failure rates of all contraceptives.

The pill is available in a variety of doses and is prescribed by a physician. It must be taken exactly as prescribed or may not be effective. There were many problems associated with the pill in the 1960s and 1970s, including stroke among women who smoked, but with significant changes in the pill over the years based on extensive research, it is now viewed as a relatively risk-free method of birth control. This is not to say that there are no risks. Risks are always present, but compared with the risks of carrying a baby to term, the pill is very safe. Some

---

rhythm method The method of contraception that relies on knowing when a woman ovulates and then calculating when her fertile and infertile periods occur.

withdrawal The method of contraception in which the man withdraws his penis from the vagina before ejaculation.

birth control pill A pill, consisting of chemicals similar to hormones normally produced in a woman's body, that prevents pregnancy.

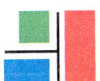

TABLE 17.2 Birth Control: How Often Does It Fail?

Method	Average use	Perfect use
No method (chance)	85.0	85.0
Spermicides	30.0	6.0
Withdrawal	24.0	4.0
Periodic abstinence	19.0	9.0
Cervical cap	9.0* 26.0**	6.0
Diaphragm	18.0	6.0
Condom	16.0	3.0
Pill	6.0	0.1
Intrauterine device	4.0	0.6
Tubal ligation	0.5	0.4
Depo-Provera	0.4	0.3
Vasectomy	0.2	0.1
Norplant	0.05	0.09

Figures are the estimated percentage of women experiencing an unintended pregnancy in the first year of use.
*For women who have never given birth
**For women who have had two or more children
Source: Reproduced with the permission of The Alan Guttmacher Institute from The Alan Guttmacher Institute, "Contraceptive Use," *Facts in Brief*, New York and Washington, 1998

people believe that there would be fewer unintended pregnancies if the pill were available without a prescription (see the Healthwise Consumer box).

An injectable birth control drug, Depo-Provera, was approved for use in the United States in 1992 and made available in 1993. It provides three months of birth control with just one "shot" and has a very high level of effectiveness. As with the pill, it must be prescribed by a physician. Side effects of Depo-Provera include weight gain, some reports of depression or mood disorders, and irregular menstruating cycles and excessive bleeding between cycles.

Another contraceptive that became available in the United States in the early 1990s is Norplant, a surgically implanted hormone-releasing device. Once implanted, it protects against pregnancy for up to five years. Its success rate is extremely high. Fertility returns once the implant is removed or it has run its full course. This device provides all of the advantages of the birth control pill without the disadvantage of having to remember to take a pill every day at a prescribed time, and it is longer-lasting than the injectable drug. The most common physical side effect of Norplant is menstrual irregularity, but that decreases after the first year of use.

Depo-Provera and Norplant also carry social side effects. Initially, there was concern that something as easy to do to prevent getting pregnant would discourage condom use, which is necessary to prevent STDs. But a study carried out among teenage, inner-city mothers who had just given birth at the University of Pennsylvania Hospital compared women on Norplant with those on the pill and found that Norplant did not change condom use behavior. Researchers found that 40 percent of those on Norplant said they had used a condom the last time

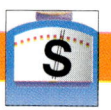

HEALTHWISE CONSUMER

Should Birth Control Pills Be Sold Over the Counter?

Yes There's no scientific reason why the Pill should be available only by prescription. This is a simple product, and people should have cheap, easy access to it. Evidence indicates that the more available birth control is, the less likely people are to have abortions and unintended pregnancies.

Of course, there are risks with all drugs. But fewer people die from the Pill than from aspirin. You don't need a doctor to tell you whether you have one of the two big risk factors for the Pill: You know whether you're over 35 or smoke. All you need is a warning on the label. As with any other over-the-counter drug, the package could instruct the consumer to see a doctor if she experiences any problems.

Right now we're not doing well in instructing women on how to take the Pill. Doctors aren't the most appropriate people to do this because the time they spend with patients is expensive and brief. The fine-print inserts that come with oral contraceptives are written for lawyers, not consumers. We need simple instructions, plainly written. There also could be an in-store videotape to provide information and a toll-free number to call with questions.

Those who oppose an over-the-counter Pill argue that the cost might go up with free market competition and television advertising. Well, certainly the present price is totally out of line with reality. This is an old product, it's been around for 30 years, and still it costs $20 a packet. It is a rip-off to sell something for a hundred times its manufacturing cost.

I'm pretty sure that if the Pill were sold without a prescription, some generic manufacturer would offer it for a reasonable price.

Malcolm Potts, professor of planning at the University of California at Berkeley, first advocated selling birth control pills without prescription in 1975.

No If everyone in America had access to primary care, we'd have less trouble with the idea of the Pill going over the counter. But for now, birth control is a poor woman's ticket to health care. The family planning clinic visit is her annual exam, when she gets a Pap smear, blood pressure check, and general health information.

The Swedes experimented with selling birth control pills over the counter, and it wasn't successful. Women used the Pill incorrectly, and many got pregnant.

Women need face-to-face discussion about how to use the Pill. They need to be told that if they take certain antibiotics or vomit frequently, birth control pills are less effective. They need to understand that you can't take fewer pills just because you're having sex less often. It's also a crucial time to tell women they've got to do something additional—use condoms—to protect themselves from HIV.

Women going on the Pill also need to be able to discuss their concerns with a health-care provider. For instance, according to recent studies, it appears that if you take the Pill for five years or more before you get pregnant, you slightly increase your risk of breast cancer at a young age. That's a legitimate worry that needs to be discussed.

Then there's the cost issue. For women who pay for the Pill out of pocket now, an over-the-counter version could be good, because the price might drop. But for women whose insurers or for whom federal subsidies pay for prescription birth control pills, this would be unmitigatedly bad. They'd be forced to pay for over-the-counter pills themselves, and many simply couldn't.

Cindy Pearson is program director of the National Women's Health Network, which opposes over-the-counter birth control pills.
Source: "Should Birth Control Pills Be Sold Over the Counter?" *Health,* March–April 1995, p. 20. Reprinted by permission of Time Inc. Health

they had intercourse, and 46 percent of a similar group taking the pill said they had used a condom. The difference is not statistically significant.

Another concern is that injectibles will be used coercively—for example, women could be required to have a contraceptive shot or implant as a condition of being paroled or of getting welfare. A California court required a woman con-

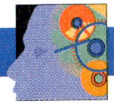

DEVELOPING HEALTH SKILLS

Correct Use of a Male Condom

For condoms to provide maximum protection, they must be used *consistently* and *correctly*. *Consistent* use means using a condom from start to finish every time you have sex. *Correct* use means to:

1. Use a new latex condom for each act of intercourse—whether vaginal, anal, or oral.
2. Be careful when opening the condom. Do not use your teeth, fingernails, or other sharp object to open the condom wrapper because you might tear the condom inside.

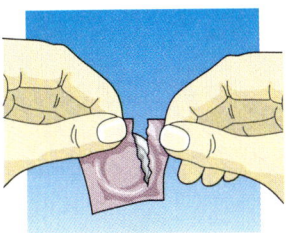

3. Put the condom on after the penis is erect and before any sexual contact.

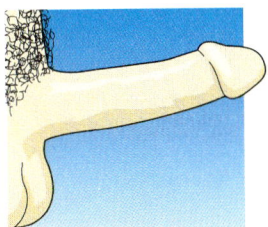

4. Hold the tip of the condom and unroll the condom all the way down the erect penis—the rolled rim should be on the outside. Leave space at the tip of the condom for semen, but make sure that no air is trapped in the condom's tip.

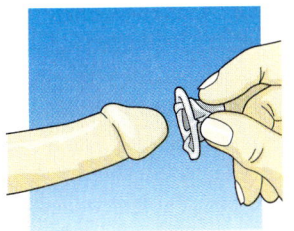
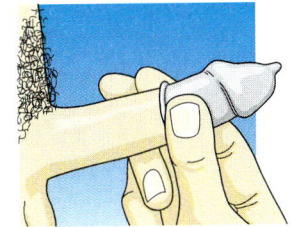

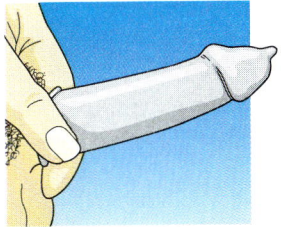

5. If additional lubrication is needed, lubricate the outside of the condom if it is not prelubricated. Use only water-based lubricants. You can purchase a lubricant at any pharmacy. Your pharmacist can tell you which lubricants are water-based. Oil-based lubricants, such as petroleum jelly, cold cream, hand lotion, cooking oil, or baby oil, weaken the condom. It is recommended that a spermicide be used in conjunction with the condom. This not only serves as a lubricant, but also enhances the condom's effectiveness in preventing unwanted pregnancy and disease.
6. Withdraw from your partner while the penis is still erect. Hold the condom firmly to keep it from slipping off.

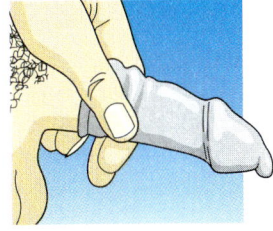

7. Throw the used condom away in the trash.

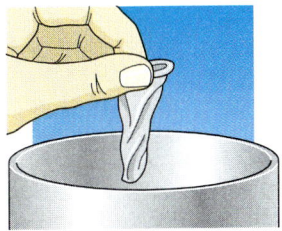

8. Never reuse a condom.
9. If the condom breaks during sex, withdraw from your partner and put on a new condom.

Source: Centers for Disease Control and Prevention

DEVELOPING HEALTH SKILLS

Correct Use of a Female Condom

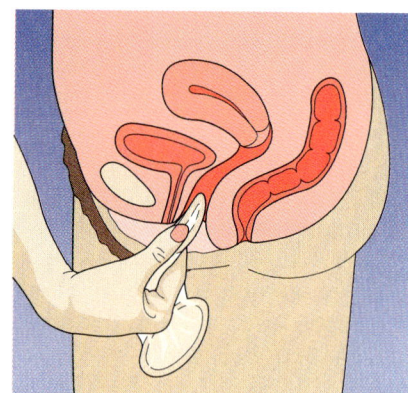

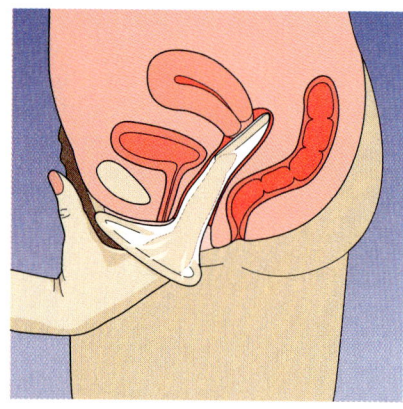
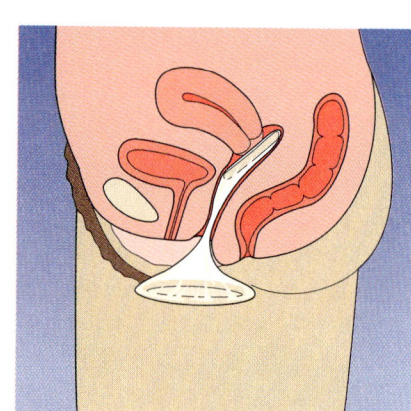

1. Inner ring is squeezed for insertion
2. Sheath is inserted, similarly to a tampon
3. Inner ring is pushed up as far as it can go with index finger
4. Condom in place

- Make sure the condom is in place and that your partner goes into the condom.
- Use enough lubricant.
- Use a new condom for each sex act.
- Throw the condom into a trash receptacle. Do not flush condoms down the toilet They are not biodegradable.

Source: Courtesy of The Female Health Company

victed of child abuse to use Norplant on being paroled. The case was ruled moot when she violated her parole by using drugs, but it illustrates the point.

There are several **barrier methods** of contraception that physically separate the sperm from the egg. The **male condom** is a thin rubber sheath for the penis that collects semen ejaculated during intercourse. This inexpensive method of birth control also protects against most sexually transmitted diseases (see Chapter 15). The condom, when used in conjunction with a spermicide, is considered a highly effective method of birth control (see the Developing Health Skills box). Failure of the condom can occur when a man does not hold the condom when withdrawing his penis. It is highly unusual for a condom to be manufactured with a defect.

Barrier methods for women include the **female condom** and the **diaphragm.** The female condom prevents sperm from reaching the cervix (see the Developing Health Skills box). It lines the inside of the vagina and keeps a barrier between the cervix and the penis, like the male condom. It also provides protection against some sexually transmitted diseases. The female condom is relatively new and has been sold in drugstores only since 1994. Its availability gives many women a greater sense of control in the prevention of pregnancy and STDs. Thanks to the female condom, they no longer have to depend on a man's actions for protection. This birth control device, however, is not widely used due to its awkward design. The effectiveness of the female condom remains somewhat unclear, although it is considered nearly as effective as the male condom.

The diaphragm is a soft rubber cup that covers the entrance to the uterus and holds **spermicide,** an acidic substance that kills sperm.

All barrier methods of birth control have added advantages of helping to prevent STDs. None is considered risk-free, however.

Spermicides include creams, foams, vaginal suppositories, and vaginal film. They form a chemical barrier that either kills sperm or makes them inactive and thus unable to pass through the cervix to the egg. Spermicides are available without a prescription and present no known risk to general health. They are less effective, however, than other contraceptive methods, but when they are used with a condom, their effectiveness can be increased significantly.

Contraimplantation refers to preventing implantation of the fertilized egg. The **intrauterine device (IUD)** is a small plastic object inserted by a physician into a woman's uterus. Some IUDs release copper or a hormone. It is not fully understood why the IUD prevents implantation, but it changes the lining of the uterus in some way that prevents implantation and thus prevents pregnancy. One IUD, the Dalkon Shield, was taken off the market in the 1980s because it was associated with internal scarring, infertility, and, in some instances, death. As a result, the availability of all IUDs has fallen, and most companies have stopped producing them.

Sterilization is a form of birth control in which steps are taken to permanently end fertility. Sterilization, sometimes called voluntary surgical contraception, is by far the most popular method of birth control among married men and women. The most common forms of sterilization are vasectomy for men and tubal ligation for women (see Table 17.3).

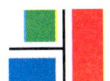

TABLE 17.3   Chosen Methods of Contraception

Method	Percentage of users
Tubal ligation	27.7%
Pill	26.9
Male condom	20.4
Vasectomy	10.9
Withdrawal	3.0
Depo-Provera	3.0
Periodic abstinence	2.3
Diaphragm	1.9
Other methods	1.8
Norplant	1.3
Intrauterine device	0.8
Total	100.0

NOTE: Use of the female condom is too new to be reflected in these figures.
Source: Reproduced with the permission of The Alan Guttmacher Institute from The Alan Guttmacher Institute, *Facts in Brief,* New York and Washington, 1998

barrier methods Methods of contraception that physically separate the sperm from the egg; include condoms and diaphragms.

male condom A thin rubber sheath for the penis that collects semen ejaculated during sexual intercourse; acts to prevent pregnancy and sexually transmitted diseases.

female condom Lines the inside of the vagina and covers the cervix; acts to prevent pregnancy and sexually transmitted diseases.

diaphragm A soft rubber cup that covers the entrance to the uterus.

spermicide An acidic substance that kills sperm.

contraimplantation Preventing implantation of the fertilized egg.

intrauterine device (IUD) A small plastic birth control device that is inserted into the uterus by a physician.

sterilization A form of birth control in which steps are taken to permanently end fertility.

Vasectomy involves surgically cutting and tying the vas deferens of the man, thus preventing the passage of sperm. The vas deferens carries sperm from the testicles to the penis. Vasectomy does not interfere with normal sexual activity or the amount of semen ejaculated, but it does mean that no sperm are present in semen.

Tubal ligation is a surgical procedure in which the fallopian tubes are cut and tied in order to prevent the passage of the egg and the subsequent union of sperm and egg. Both procedures are considered permanent, although reconnecting the tubes or the vas deferens has been done with limited success.

Critical Thinking Question

The *Healthy People 2000* objectives include the following: "Increase to at least 95 percent the proportion of females aged 15–44 at risk of unintended pregnancy who use contraception." The current usage rate is around 90 percent. On the surface, these data suggest a healthy trend. The use of contraception appears to be widely accepted. Yet, unintended pregnancies continue to occur. Why, given the available and accessible methods of birth control, do you think unintended pregnancies continue?

Emergency Contraception

Occasionally an "emergency" form of birth control is needed. The **"morning-after pill"** is the nickname of the emergency approach to contraception. It provides a backup if, for example, a condom breaks, a diaphragm becomes dislodged, or a woman forgets to take the pill. The morning-after pill is also used in cases of unplanned and unprotected sexual intercourse or unwanted sexual intercourse, such as occurs with rape or incest. A specific number of estrogen/progesterone birth control pills are taken within the first seventy-two hours following unprotected intercourse. This form of contraception, which can cause nausea and vomiting for a day or two, can prevent implantation. It is 75 percent effective in preventing pregnancy.

While most gynecologists know about the pills, they seldom prescribe them because they wait for women to ask. And most women do not know enough about them to ask for them. A recent survey conducted by Louis Harris & Associates found that 60 percent of women polled said they had heard about emergency contraceptives, but only 20 percent knew that the pills were effective for up to three days after intercourse.

Another factor related to the use of the morning-after pill is that some druggists refuse to fill prescriptions for it because it conflicts with their personal beliefs about when life begins. While recognizing pharmacists' rights of refusal, the American Pharmaceutical Association says that right must not override a patient's right to treatment.

HEALTH SKILLS

Deciding about Birth Control

There are pros and cons relating to safety, efficacy, and convenience associated with each form of birth control. Who is responsible for weighing the pros and cons? Who is responsible for birth control or for making the decisions about birth control? The best decisions are those made when both sexual partners are involved. And the best decisions are made long before beginning sexual activity. The decision of which form of birth control to use, if any, is a highly personal one. Several criteria should be considered.

SAFETY No one should consciously place his or her own health at risk in order to practice a form of birth control. The package inserts for the birth control pill identify specific conditions that indicate when the pill should not be used—for example, if a woman has diabetes or is over age forty and smokes. For safety reasons, women who choose to use the pill should be honest with their physicians about their medical histories and honest with themselves concerning their current health.

EFFECTIVENESS Many methods of birth control are more effective theoretically than they are actually. The condom, for example, is theoretically 97 percent effective. Yet, because of improper use, its actual effectiveness is closer to only 84 percent. All contraceptive and contraimplantation methods have been studied enough to yield both theoretical and actual effectiveness rates. When choosing a birth control method, couples should find out the risk of pregnancy and take that risk into consideration. There is no perfect birth control method except total abstinence.

ACCEPTABILITY This represents the extent to which the birth control method fits within an individual's values and lifestyle. Acceptability is measured in a number of ways, including availability, ease of use, reversibility, and impact on sex drive. Each of these considerations influences how acceptable a form of birth control is to an individual. For example, sterilization is more likely to be an acceptable form of birth control for someone who has decided to have no more children than for someone who has not made up his or her mind about this.

Because the choice of a contraceptive is a highly personal decision, it's important that the choice be made carefully and only after considering the range of complete information. The Here's Looking at You box provides a test for checking a contraception's appropriateness.

The Abortion Controversy*

Abortion is one of the most controversial topics in modern U.S. society. An **abortion** is the termination of pregnancy. Some abortions take place spontaneously in the form of a miscarriage. In fact, it is estimated that 33 percent of all pregnancies end in a **miscarriage**, or spontaneous abortion. The controversy arises over **elective abortions**, those that are medically induced for the purpose of ending unintended pregnancies.

According to the Alan Guttmacher Institute (AGI), more than 50 percent of pregnancies among U.S. women are unintended and half of these are terminated by abortion. The rest are carried to term. Each year, 3 out of every 100 women of reproductive age have an abortion; 47 percent of them have had at least one previous abortion and 55 percent have had a previous birth. At current rates, an estimated 43 percent of women will have had at least one abortion by the time they are forty-five years old. In addition:

- The majority of women getting abortions are young: 55 percent are under twenty-five, 33 percent are aged between twenty and twenty-four, and 22 percent are teenagers.

*Portions of "The Abortion Controversy" are reproduced with the permission of The Alan Guttmacher Institute from The Alan Guttmacher Institute, "Induced Abortion," *Facts in Brief*, New York and Washington, 1997

vasectomy Surgically cutting and tying the vas deferens of the man, thus preventing the passage of sperm.

tubal ligation A surgical procedure in which the fallopian tubes are cut and tied in order to prevent the passage of the egg and the subsequent union of sperm and egg.

morning-after pill A form of hormonal contraception used within the first seventy-two hours after unprotected sexual intercourse; generally considered an emergency method of birth control that prevents implantation.

abortion The termination of pregnancy.

miscarriage Spontaneous abortion.

elective abortions Abortions that are medically induced.

HERE'S LOOKING AT YOU

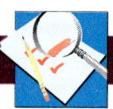

What Is Your Contraceptive Confidence?

What method of birth control are you considering using? _____

Have you had problems using this method before?   Yes   No

How long did you use this method? _____

Answer yes or no to the following questions:

Am I afraid of using this method?

Would I really rather not use this method?

Will I have trouble remembering to use this method?

Have I ever become pregnant while using this method?

Will I have trouble using this method correctly?

Do I still have unanswered questions about this method?

Does this method make menstrual periods longer or more painful?

Does this method cost more than I can afford?

Could this method cause me to have serious complications?

Am I opposed to this method because of any religious beliefs?

Is my partner opposed to this method?

Am I using this method without my partner's knowledge?

Will using this method embarrass my partner?

Will using this method embarrass me?

Will I enjoy intercourse less because of this method?

If this method interrupts lovemaking, will I avoid using it?

Has a nurse or doctor ever told me NOT to use this method?

Is there anything about my personality that could lead me to use this method incorrectly?

Am I at any risk of being exposed to HIV (the AIDS virus) or other sexually transmitted infections?

Total number of yes answers: _____

Most individuals will have a few yes answers. Yes answers mean that potential problems may lie in store. If you have more than a few yes responses, you may want to talk to your physician, counselor, partner, or friend. Talking it over can help you to decide whether to use this method or how to use it so it will really be effective for you. In general, the more yes answers you have, the less likely you are to use this method consistently and correctly.

Source: Hatcher, R.A., et al. *Contraceptive Technology: 1991, 1992.* Manchester, NH: Irvington, 1992

- Most women (66 percent) who have an abortion intend to have children in the future.
- Women who report no religious affiliation are about four times as likely as women who report some affiliation to have an abortion. However, Catholic women are 29 percent more likely than Protestants to have an abortion and are about as likely as all women nationally to do so.
- While white women obtain 61 percent of all abortions, their abortion rate is well below that of minority group women. Black women are nearly three times as likely as white women to have an abortion, and Hispanic women are roughly two times as likely.
- Most abortions are obtained by never-married women.
- Women give three major reasons for choosing abortion: three quarters say that having a baby would interfere with work, school, or other responsibilities; about two thirds say that they cannot afford a child; and one half say

vacuum aspiration   A method of abortion performed in the first trimester that involves dilation of the cervix and removal of the contents of the uterus by suction.

they do not want to be a single parent or are having problems with their husbands or partners.
- About fifteen thousand women have abortions each year because they became pregnant after rape or incest.

It is impossible to know the exact number of abortions that occur, but AGI estimates that in 1994, 1.4 million abortions took place, down from 1.5 million in 1992. There are several possible reasons for this drop in the abortion rate:

- Changes in attitudes about having an abortion
- Reduced access to abortion services
- Fewer unintended pregnancies
- More women are becoming less fertile as the nation's population ages

Abortion became legal in 1973 with the *Roe v. Wade* Supreme Court decision. From that time through 1994, more than 31 million women in the United States have chosen to have an abortion rather than carry an unwanted child. The abortion rate prior to *Roe v. Wade* is not known because most abortions took place illegally and were unreported, but it is assumed that many women risked their lives having abortions in unclean places, performed by ill-trained persons using unsafe and sometimes ineffective techniques. Today, abortions take place in special clinics or in hospitals.

Ninety percent of elective abortions are performed during the first trimester of pregnancy. At this time, the fetus is very small, ranging in size from microscopic to approximately three inches long. Abortion is extremely safe during the first three months of pregnancy. In fact, at this stage, abortion presents fewer physical health risks than are present when carrying a pregnancy to term.

First-trimester surgical abortion methods are **vacuum aspiration** or suction curettage. Both techniques, which are performed by a physician under local anesthesia and on an outpatient basis, involve dilation of the cervix (it is gradually opened) and insertion of a small tube into the uterus. The contents of the uterus are removed by a machine that forms a suction.

A controversial early abortion procedure is RU-486, a pill that is taken after implantation to induce miscarriage. (This is in contrast to the morning-after pill, which prevents implantation.) The drug, a synthetic steroid called mifepristone, makes it difficult for the fertilized egg to adhere to the uterus's lining. It triggers

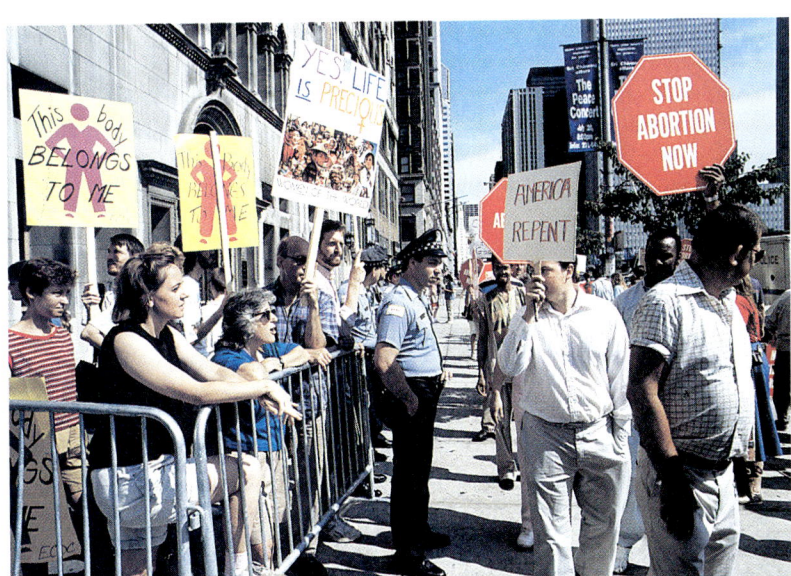

The two sides of the abortion issue make their position clear. Pro-choice advocates believe that a woman has the right to choose whether or not she wishes to continue a pregnancy, and pro-life advocates believe that the developing fetus has the right to live and needs someone to advocate for those rights. (Source: © Tony Stone Images/Robert Kusel)

uterine contractions and the result is an abortion. RU-486 is also called a medical abortion and is strongly opposed by foes of abortion.

Unlike a surgical abortion, RU-486 is effective in producing abortions in the very early weeks of pregnancy—usually in the first forty-nine days, but it can be used safely up to the sixty-third day. Also unlike a surgical abortion, which is a one-step procedure, RU-486 requires three visits to a physician or clinic over fifteen days to administer and monitor the drug. Side effects include bleeding, cramping, nausea, and vomiting.

Developed in France, RU-486 received conditional approval for use in the United States in 1996, which means that the Food and Drug Administration has ruled it safe and effective. As of 1998, it is not yet produced here. It is effective in 95.4 percent of cases.

Abortions that are performed in the second trimester are more complicated (because the fetus is much larger) and slightly more risky. About 10 percent of abortions are done in this period. The methods used for second-trimester abortion are dilation and evacuation, and induction. In the **dilation and evacuation** method, the cervix is dilated, and suction is used to remove the contents of the uterus much as in the first trimester. **Induction** involves artificially inducing labor, usually through the administration of a drug, prostaglandin. Prostaglandin is the same substance that causes uterine contractions during labor. Induction often involves a limited hospital stay. Fewer than 3 percent of women having an abortion in the United States choose the induction method.

Late-term abortions are probably the most controversial of all, even though only 1 percent of abortions are performed after more than twenty weeks of pregnancy. The procedure used is called intact dilation and extraction and the fetus is vaginally delivered. Women seek late-term abortions because they face grave health risks or their fetuses have fatal abnormalities.

Regardless of the stage of development of pregnancy, when a woman chooses to seek an abortion, counseling is offered. What to do about an unwanted pregnancy may be an easy decision for some women, but for others, there may be many factors that make abortion seem wrong.

The two sides of the abortion issue are politically represented by pro-choice and pro-life points of view. **Pro-choice** advocates support the idea that a woman has the right to choose whether or not she wishes to continue a pregnancy. **Pro-life** advocates, on the other hand, believe that a pregnant woman must carry the pregnancy to term because the developing fetus is a human being and has a right to live. Both factions agree that an abortion represents a failure to control conception, whether intentional or unintentional.

The health risks of abortion remain widely debated. There is growing evidence, however, that abortion does not represent a major risk, either psychologically or physically. The risk for abortion complications is minimal, and fewer than 1 percent of all abortion patients experience a major complication such as serious pelvic infection, hemorrhage requiring a blood transfusion, or unintended major surgery. The psychological complications from abortion are much more difficult to measure, but with proper counseling and follow-up, such complications are normally kept to a minimum.

dilation and evacuation A method of abortion performed in the second trimester in which the cervix is dilated and medical instruments are used to remove the contents of the uterus.

induction The method of abortion in which labor is artificially induced.

pro-choice A political position that supports the idea that a woman has the right to choose whether or not she wishes to continue a pregnancy.

pro-life A political position that supports the idea that a pregnant woman must carry the pregnancy to term because the developing fetus is a human being and has a right to live.

A Final Word on Planning a Family

Decisions relating to family planning are among the most important that you will make. This is because they affect not only your health but also the health of others in your family. With many of these decisions, you are likely to face controversies that are publicly debated. Information that you might need to make family planning decisions is constantly changing as new research is reported and other new developments take place. Your decisions should be based on the best available information.

Key Concepts

1. The nuclear family consists of parents and their children, typically living under the same roof. Members of an extended family are connected by blood, marriage, or adoption but live in different locations.
2. Half of all marriages end in divorce, but most divorced people find new partners and marry again.
3. The early signs of pregnancy include amenorrhea, or a missed menstrual period, along with fullness and tenderness of the breasts.
4. Smoking during pregnancy is associated with higher infant mortality and babies having lower birthweights.
5. Good prenatal care includes careful monitoring by a physician or certified nurse-midwife, proper diet, and appropriate exercise.
6. During the first stage of labor, the cervix gradually opens or dilates to allow eventual passage of the baby through the birth canal. During the second stage of labor, the baby is born. In the final stage of labor, the placenta separates from the uterine wall and is expelled.
7. Contraception is the intentional prevention of the union of sperm and egg. Contraimplantation methods prevent implantation of the fertilized egg in the uterine wall.
8. An abortion is the termination of pregnancy. Ninety percent of elective abortions are performed during the first trimester of pregnancy.
9. Pro-choice advocates support the idea that a woman has the right to choose whether or not she wishes to continue a pregnancy. Pro-life advocates believe that a pregnant woman must carry the baby to term because the developing fetus is a human being and has a right to live.
10. Effective family planning requires extensive and objective information.

Review Questions

1. Describe different family structures, including the nuclear family and the extended family. How have the dual-career family and the single-parent family changed our view of what constitutes a family?
2. List three conditions that a couple should consider when choosing whether or not to have children.
3. Define infertility and identify several medical and social interventions designed to correct infertility.
4. Differentiate between preconception care and prenatal care and establish a case for the importance of each.
5. Differentiate between amniocentesis and chorionic villus sampling. What is each test designed to do?
6. Divide a normal pregnancy into three trimesters. Identify significant developmental landmarks that should, under normal conditions, be complete during each trimester.
7. Explain the major events that take place during each of the three stages of labor.
8. List several methods of birth control that men and women choose and identify the advantages and disadvantages of each.

9. Differentiate between the pro-choice and pro-life positions on the abortion issue. What are the health implications of each proposed practice?
10. Describe the importance of high quality information to the process of planning a family.

Selected Bibliography

Facts in Brief. New York: The Alan Guttmacher Institute, 1997. The series includes "Contraceptive Use," "Induced Abortion," and "The Limitations of U.S. Statistics on Abortion."

Hatcher, R.A., et al. *Contraceptive Technology: 1991–1992.* Manchester, NH: Irvington, 1992.

Journal of Marriage and Family (published monthly).

Medical Aspects of Human Sexuality (published monthly).

HealthLinks: Web Sites Related to Reproductive Sciences

You can access better health as it relates to this chapter by checking out some of the following sites on the Internet. These and sites identified within the chapter can be accessed directly when you visit the *HealthStyles* Web Site located on the Allyn and Bacon home page at **http://www.abacon.com.**

American Society of Reproductive Medicine
www.asrm.com
The ASRM is a voluntary nonprofit organization devoted to advancing knowledge and expertise in reproductive medicine and biology. The site provides the latest information on reproductive care, state infertility laws, and current clinical trials.

American College of Obstetricians and Gynecologists
www.acog.org
A link into the nation's leading group of professionals providing health care for women. The site provides women with the latest information on women's health issues.

ASPO/Lamaze Association
www.lamaze-childbirth.com/index.htm
Lamaze International promotes natural childbearing experiences for women and families through education, advocacy, and reform.

LaLeche League International
www.lalecheleague.com
Web site for the organization dedicated to providing education, information, and support to women who want to breast feed. Information includes updates on local support groups and other help.

Health Hotlines: Planning a Family

Association of Women's Health, Obstetric, and Neonatal Nurses
(800) 673-8499
700 I Street NW, Suite 600
Washington, DC 20005

Be Healthy: Positive Pregnancy and Parenting Fitness
(800) 433-5523
RR1 Box 172
Glenview Road
Waitsfield, VT 05673

International Childbirth Education Association
(800) 624-4934
P.O. Box 20048
Minneapolis, MN 55420-0048

National Adoption Center
(800) 862-3678
1500 Walnut Street, Suite 701
Philadelphia, PA 19102

Planned Parenthood Federation of America
(800) 829-7732 (National Office)
(800) 230-7526 (for nearest local office)
810 Seventh Avenue
New York, NY 10019

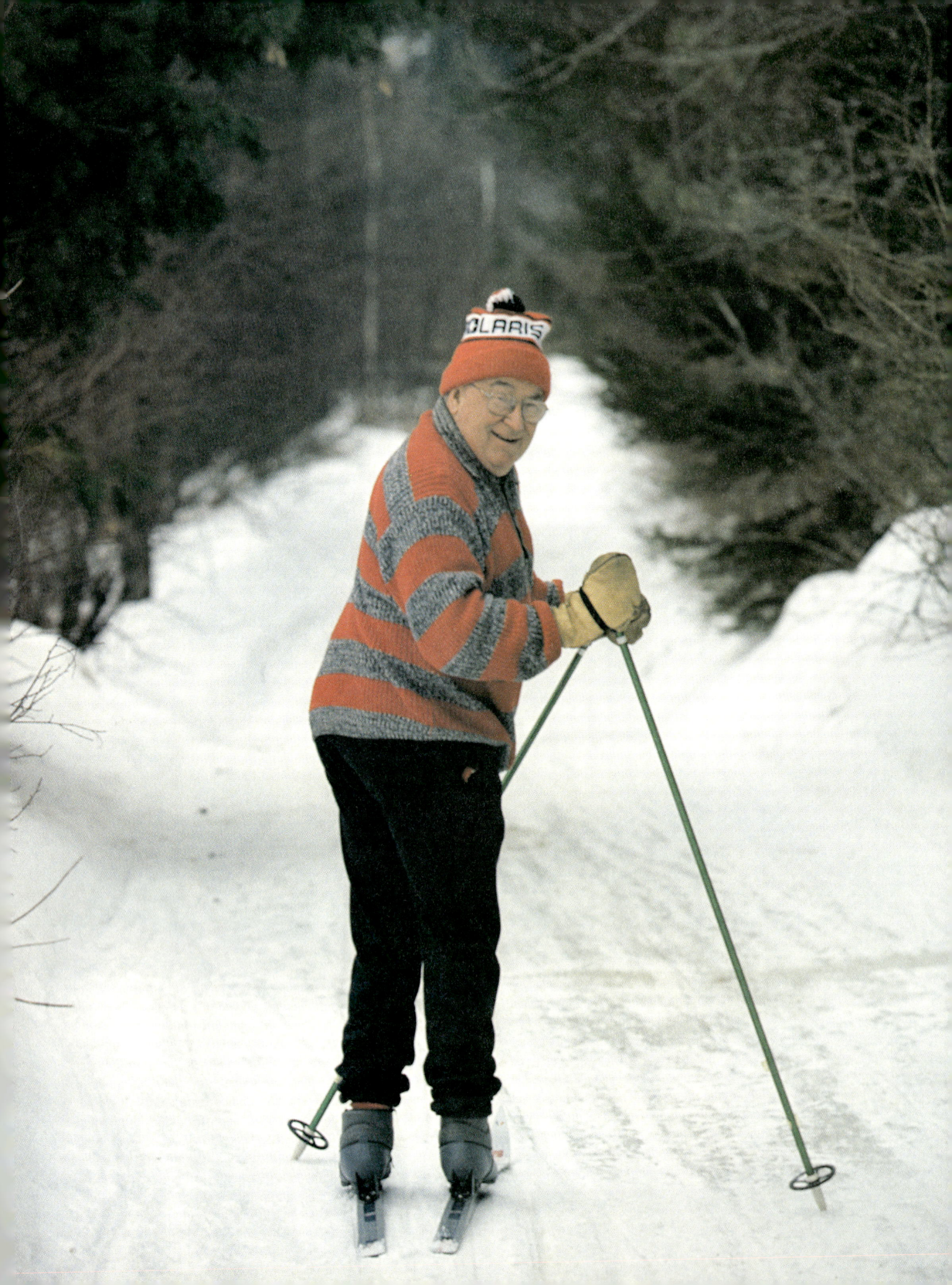

Chapter 18

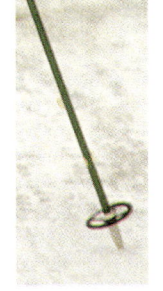
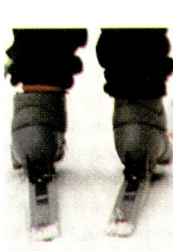
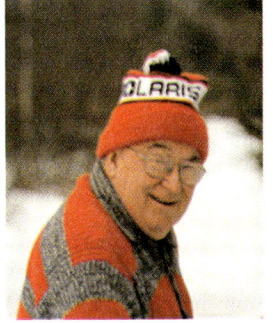

Aging

Growing Older, Keeping Healthy

Objectives

When you finish reading this chapter, you will be able to:

1. Differentiate between chronological, functional, and psychological methods of measuring age.
2. Describe the "typical" elderly person according to gender, marital status, living arrangements, and health status.
3. Recognize some of the misconceptions about aging, including the misconception that older people are not sexually active.
4. Recognize the great variety in how people age—the different styles of aging.
5. Describe how aging influences health status.
6. Understand what happens to the bones, the senses, and the brain during the aging process.
7. Recognize Alzheimer's disease and become familiar with some of the myths surrounding this cause of dementia.
8. Test your knowledge concerning aging and the brain.
9. Understand how to prevent some of the major health concerns of aging including depression, medicine abuse, and falls.
10. Recognize the importance of regular physical activity and nutritious diet as key elements of healthy aging.

What Is Your HealthStyle?

Sam McNeil had owned an auto repair shop for thirty-five years. When he started having an increasing number of aches, pains, and other physical ailments, he decided it was time to retire. He sold his business, and although he talked a lot about his retirement, he made no plans for what he would do with his time.

Even though his upcoming retirement was his choice, Sam grew depressed over it. He would miss the daily interactions with the people in his shop and the customers, and he would miss the work. Sam wasn't sure what he'd do with all his time—helping his wife with chores around the house or, more realistically, getting in her way wasn't filling him with excitement. Sam had a lot of skills that would be highly valued if he volunteered on community projects—from repairing machinery to balancing a budget—but he thought of himself as too old and too tired to get involved.

Charles Hill, in contrast, was looking forward to his retirement from teaching high school social studies. He had served the school well for more than thirty years and had guided thousands of students, including one who had followed in his footsteps and was teaching in his department. Charles felt that he had been a good mentor to many of his students.

But now it was time to move on and pursue new activities—activities he did not have time for when he had classes to teach and other school responsibilities. He was interested in doing some work with an environmental group and had talked about volunteering at a local historical museum. But first on his agenda was a three-month trip around the country with his wife.

In Your Opinion

Older age just may live up to your expectations. If you expect the worst, you may get it, just as Sam did. If you expect it to be an enhanced time of your life, that too is possible. At least it was for Charles.

- How would you rate your parents' and grandparents' approaches to aging?
- Do they take the Charles Hill approach or the Sam McNeil approach? What factors influence their approaches?
- What health skills might Charles Hill possess that affect his positive attitude about his approaching retirement?
- Make a list of activities that you want to be doing when you are sixty-five years old. How might the list change when you are seventy-five years old? *Will* it change?

When you think of yourself as "old," what age do you have in mind? For a twenty-one-year-old college student, being thirty can seem old because it carries an image of responsibilities far beyond what is expected of students—for example, having a full-time job or being a parent or a homeowner. Over the span of a lifetime, however, being thirty is not really very old because a person born today can expect to live for seventy-six years—up considerably from a century ago, when life expectancy was only about forty-seven years.

Given these statistics, what age do you now have in mind when you think of yourself as old? What do you expect the quality of your life to be when you are sixty-five years old? What about when you are eighty-five years old? These questions are often raised but seldom given serious consideration until the later years of life become a reality for you or your parents.

Although some elderly people are sickly or otherwise lead impaired lives, most people over age sixty-five are active and involved members of the community. They lead productive lives, have paid or volunteer jobs, take classes, get advanced degrees, and have sexual experiences. Growing older for these people is a testament to good health due to their genetic makeup, their health styles, and advances in medicine.

Whether you like it or not, you—a college student—show signs of aging. Some of them are visible—maybe a few gray hairs, "smile" wrinkles around your mouth, or a thickening around your waist. Inside your body, other signs of aging are taking place, such as hormonal changes.

Fortunately, none of these changes is life threatening, so rather than fret about getting older, think of yourself as fortunate to be living in an age and environment in which healthy aging is natural.

Growing Older

If you think of aging as a numbers game, it starts at age sixty-five. The Census Bureau defines people aged sixty-five to seventy-four as elderly, people seventy-five to eighty-four as aged, and people eighty-five and more as very old. The very old are the fastest growing age group in the United States, and demographers estimate that by 2050, there will be 18 million Americans over age eighty-five versus 4 million in 1997.

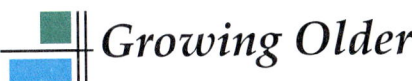

Critical Thinking Question

> The *Healthy People 2000* objectives include the following: "Increase years of healthy life among people aged sixty-five and older to at least 14 more years." Currently, a sixty-five-year-old can expect nearly twelve more years of healthy life. Interestingly, this figure has not changed in the last ten years. Why do you think no change has occurred? Given the enormous gains in medical science in the past ten years, what might account for the stability of these data?

Gerontologists, specialists who study the social, biological, behavioral, and psychological aspects of aging, see enormous differences among people of these various age groups. Some of the so-called young-old—people in their sixties—might be in nursing homes, whereas some of the old-old—eighty-five and older—are still living independently. The reasons for the differences are a continuous source of study.

Several biological theories have surfaced concerning why and how people age:

- The wear and tear theory contends that simply as a consequence of living for many years, the effects of disease and damage over time produce aging.

gerontologists Specialists who study the social, biological, behavioral, and psychological aspects of aging.

- The free radicals theory suggests that foreign elements in the blood build up over time in the body and produce aging.
- The biological clock theory assumes a relationship between time and biological decline.

Several sociological and psychological theories have been proposed as well. The bottom line is that gerontologists are not in agreement as to what causes aging. They do agree, however, that aging is an inevitable element of living and is a process influenced by lifestyle decisions. Aging can be healthy or less healthy, depending on factors within the control of the individual.

Measuring Age

There are three common measures of age. **Chronological age,** represented in the number of years since birth, provides markers to differentiate life stages. It is also used as a qualifier for certain privileges. For example, an eighteen-year-old is old enough to vote, join the armed forces, and serve on jury duty. Privileges for people age sixty-five years and older include Social Security payments and reduced "senior citizen rates" for buses and movie tickets. Even people in their fifties are offered senior rates in some places.

From a health standpoint, chronological age may be misleading, especially in older adults. **Functional age** is a better way to represent the physiological capacity of the body. An eighty-five-year-old tennis player, for example, may have a functional age of fifty-five in terms of cardiopulmonary output.

People who feel old before their time use **psychological age** to measure their years. By saying, "I am old," they may be looking for an excuse to retire from work, be dependent, or become inactive. On turning age fifty a shoe salesman who was in good health said he now "felt" old. He began taking naps in the middle of the afternoon and soon took early retirement because he found work too strenuous for "an old man like myself."

Who Are the Elderly?

In spite of wide variations in aging, it is possible to draw a picture of the typical older American using demographic statistics.

GENDER Older women far outnumber older men. There are more than double the number of women than men aged sixty-five and older.

MARITAL STATUS Because of these differences between genders, about 75 percent of the men age sixty-five and older are married, but only 35 percent of the women are still married. These differences increase over the years, so that women are more likely to spend their final years alone.

LIVING ARRANGEMENTS Most elderly live independently in their own homes, an apartment, or, increasingly, in a retirement community. Fewer than 5 percent of those age sixty-five and older live in nursing homes. Again, there are vast differences among the elderly: of those aged sixty-five to seventy-four, less than 1 percent live in nursing homes, compared with 22 percent of those aged eighty-five or older. At some point in their lives, 43 percent of the elderly enter a nursing home at least once (see Table 18.1).

HEALTH STATUS The noninstitutionalized elderly—the 95 percent who are not in nursing homes—view themselves as relatively healthy. Overall, 68 percent rate their health as excellent, 21 percent as fair, and only 11 percent as poor. Nevertheless, of this group, one in five needs help from another person in at least one activity of daily living, such as dressing, bathing, walking, or shopping.

chronological age A number representing the number of years since birth.

functional age A number representing the ability to function; a tool for comparing actual age with ability to function.

psychological age A number representing a perceived age (how old you feel).

ageism The term used to describe prejudice and discrimination against the elderly based on misconceptions regarding age.

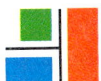

TABLE 18.1 Living Arrangements of the World's Elderly

	China	Japan	Sweden	U.S.
People over age 65	6%	11%	18%	13%
Living in group/nursing home	1	5	10	5
Living with adult children	66	67	4	5
Living alone or with spouse	33	28	86	90

Misconceptions about Aging

Some very real changes occur as you age. But we also have many misconceptions about what actually takes place in old age based on misinformation, biases, and stereotypes. **Ageism** is the term used to describe prejudice and discrimination against the elderly based on these misconceptions.

What is the source of these stereotypes? You start learning them early in life from examples in children's books. Researchers at the University of Maryland's Center on Aging analyzed more than 650 books in the Montgomery County Public Library and found that three words—old, little, and ancient—accounted for 80 percent of the adjectives used to describe elderly people. Elementary school textbooks compound this negative image. They present the elderly as useless and helpless. Such thinking becomes reinforced throughout life, so that even some elderly view themselves as not contributing to society. See the Cultural View box on how positively the Japanese think about the elderly.

Consider the following misconceptions and the factual responses to them:

What some people believe	What actually happens
All old people are alike.	More variability exists among the elderly than in any other segment of the population.
Old people are senile.	Short-term memory loss does take place in older age, but it does not impair intellectual judgment or clarity of thinking. True senility is a disease state that affects only a small percentage of the elderly.
Older people can't learn.	Except for those who have neurological problems, the elderly can assimilate as much overall knowledge as younger people. However, it may take an older person slightly more time to absorb new knowledge.
The elderly are useless.	More than 10 percent of those aged sixty-five and older continue to work. Volunteering is also increasing among the elderly through programs such as the Retired Senior Volunteer Program and Foster Grandparent Program.
Older people aren't interested in sex.	Sexual activity does decrease in older age, but it is mostly because of a lack of a partner rather than a lack of interest.

HealthLinks
Administration on Aging
www.aoa.dhhs.gov/

A link to the Health and Human Services agency dedicated to addressing the health needs of the elderly.

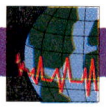

CULTURAL VIEW

Respect for the Elderly in Japan

In Japan, gray is beautiful. Most older Japanese make no attempt to hide gray hair and wrinkles because there the elderly have traditionally been treated with great respect. It is quite proper to ask older Japanese their age and to congratulate them on it. In the United States such a remark would be considered rude.

Families celebrate the coming of old age by treating the "honorable elder" to a special 61st birthday party. An annual national holiday, Respect for Elders Day, is set aside to encourage younger people to understand the needs of the elderly, and older people to improve and enrich their own lives.

Deeply Rooted in Culture

Respect for the elderly is deeply rooted in Japanese culture. The ancient Confucian concept of filial piety held that children should remain devoted to their parents no matter how despotic or disagreeable they were. This tradition has been questioned by modern Japanese. Now the ideal is that the elderly earn affection and respect from the family by demonstrating fairness, wisdom, and helpfulness.

In Japan, nearly all relationships are defined according to a delicately graded hierarchy. It is difficult for Westerners to imagine that Japanese relationships could be truly affectionate, based as they are on authority and responsibility on the one hand and

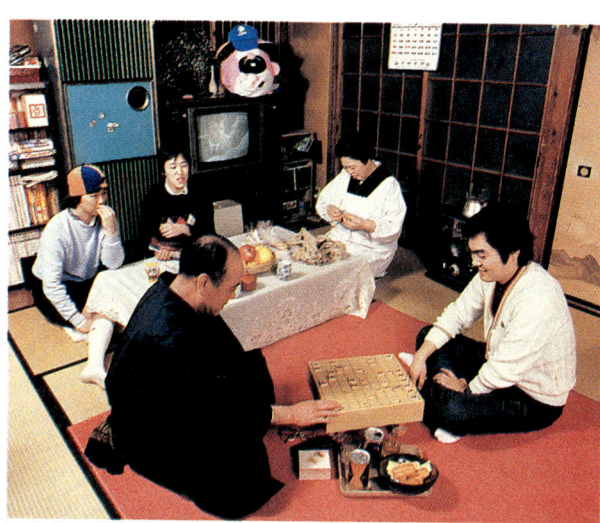

Traditionally, most older Japanese have lived with their children and grandchildren. Times are changing, however, many adult children do not have the room to care for their elderly parents. (Source: © Tony Stone Images/Paul Chesley)

Psychology of Aging

Why do some people in their seventies feel good in spite of a series of ailments while the fifty-year-old shoe salesman sees himself as weak and tired in the absence of any signs of ill health? There are several theories about how people age differently. These are called styles of aging. We discuss three of them here and give an overview of the psychological tasks of aging.

CONTINUITY STYLE OF AGING Some people do not change very much as they grow older. There is a continuity in how they lead their lives. If they were very rigid as young adults, they remain rigid as older people. If they were flexible as young adults, they remain flexible when they are older. Healthy young adults are usually healthy in older age, and people who experienced health problems as young adults usually experience health problems in their old age. This approach to aging suggests that your behavior today clearly influences your behavior in later life.

ACTIVITY STYLE OF AGING Remaining active is the key to a healthy and long life for some people. Based on the premise that you are as old as you feel,

deferential subservience on the other. But the Japanese see no conflict.

The Japanese language both reflects and defines these deferential relationships. There are three forms of speech, each complete with its own vocabulary, grammar, and syntax. Elders and social superiors are addressed in the honorific form of speech, the middle form is for equals, and the plain or blunt form is reserved for younger persons or social inferiors.

Japan, like other Asian societies, has prided itself on respect for the old. Ancestor worship was the foundation of Japanese religions, and it logically followed that respect and duty toward living parents and grandparents were the second most important things in life.

Families have customarily shown respect for the elderly by using the honorific form of speech, giving the aged the best seats, catering to their tastes in food, serving them first, allowing them to go through doors first, bowing and letting them use the family bath first. Traditionally, most older Japanese have lived with their children and grandchildren, providing valued services in the household.

A Change in Traditions

These customs survive most strongly in rural areas and among families that have traditional occupations and among households where there are middle-aged or older people. However, many of these practices of respect have declined among young people living in the cities.

Rapid urbanization and industrialization in Japan have disrupted ancient family patterns. Families living in tiny urban apartments have no room to care for elderly parents. An expected 40 percent increase in social security and other taxes—needed to provide services to Japan's exploding elderly population—will strain each family's ability to care for its own aged.

Japan has a tradition of forced retirement at age fifty-five. It also has the highest life expectancy in the world. This leaves many people with decades left to live in which they cannot support themselves. In the twenty-first century, respect for the elderly may have to be redefined. Perhaps the retirement age will be raised, perhaps more social programs and pension plans will help the aged in ways that have traditionally been the province of families.

Shinji Takada, sixty-five, a fisherman, cared for his mother until her death at age ninety-two. His own children have long since left for Tokyo and Osaka, where they have no room for him when he is older. "These are modern times, and I cannot expect one of them to return to the family home when I become very old," he said. "Just as jobs no longer pass from father to son, so family responsibilities no longer pass from generation to generation."

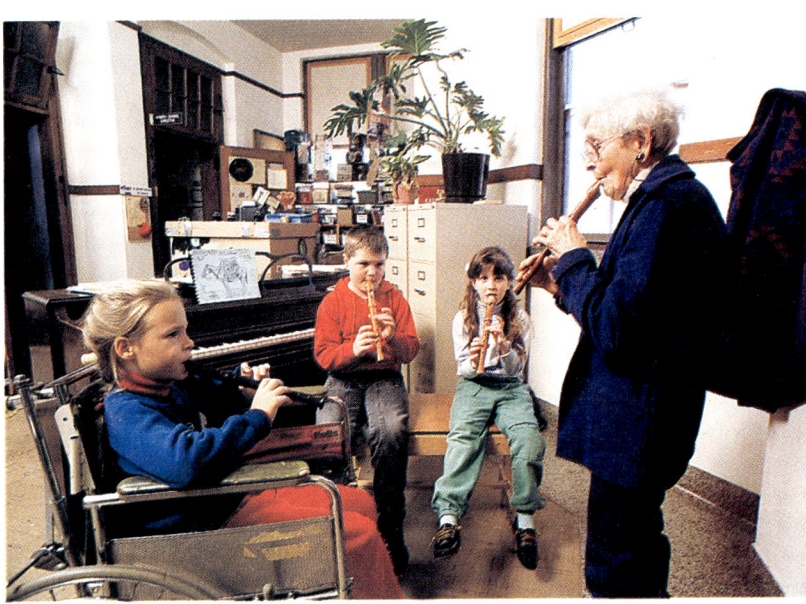

Some elderly thrive on being around the younger generation, whether as grandparents or great-grandparents, or as volunteers with the Foster Grandparent Program. (Source: © Tony Stone Images/Paul Meredith)

many older people use walking, playing tennis or golf, and participating in hobbies and civic activities as ways to stay "young" and involved. However, this could cause problems for some individuals, particularly elderly people who take on too many activities or too strenuous a load.

DISENGAGEMENT STYLE OF AGING In contrast to staying active, some people withdraw from society as they age. They reduce their commitments to the community and let the younger generation take over. This style of aging enables older people to have more time to be reflective. The disengagement style can backfire, however, if the older person disengages too early or is pushed out before he or she is ready to go. Such events may be a blow to one's self-esteem.

PSYCHOLOGICAL TASKS OF AGING According to Erik Erikson's model of aging, every developmental stage of life involves tasks that need to be completed before one moves on successfully to the next stage. An individual's sense of worth is closely associated with how well these tasks are accomplished. During early childhood, some of these tasks involve developing trust, autonomy, and initiative. Tasks of early and middle adulthood include learning how to make commitments to others and developing a sense of **generativity,** or concern for family and society (see Table 18.2).

Erikson's eighth and last stage of maturity involves the task of developing a sense of personal integrity strong enough to withstand physical disintegration. People who achieve this can look back on their lives with warm feelings of accomplishment. Those who do not may feel despair, especially if they believe that it is too late to make amends.

One ninety-year-old woman who leads an active life sees her aging as a blessing and a privilege. "To see your children and grandchildren become adults is a joy, but to watch your great-grandchildren grow up is the ultimate happiness." She feels fulfilled with what she has done over her lifetime and has successfully mastered Erikson's final stage in life.

Critical Thinking Question

There are many styles of aging. According to the disengagement theory, as individuals age, they are simultaneously released by society from social roles and withdraw psychological energy from social ties and activities. Retirement, for example, represents society's permission to disengage. Ideal aging occurs when the elderly person and society disengage from each other at the same time. Dysfunction occurs when one party disengages before the other is ready for it. What is your opinion of this theory of aging? Is it an effort to justify existing conditions, or is it a clear explanation of "the way things are"? Why do you think mutual disengagement is important?

Caring for an Elderly Parent

What will happen to your parents as they age, and how involved will you be in their later-in-life decisions? A Gallup poll conducted for *Health* magazine of adults age eighteen and older who had at least one living parent shows that most

generativity A concern for family and society.

people are devoted to their families and are prepared to help their parents age gracefully (see Table 18.3).

Perhaps one of the most difficult things for adult children to do is to ask their parents the "what-if" question—what if they get old and need help? While most people have not made plans for this possibility—in some cases, eventuality—with their parents, they have at least broached the topic:

- 36 percent have talked but made no plans
- 14 percent have worked together to prepare legal documents for finances, housing, and medical care
- 12 percent have discussed plans for finances, housing, and medical care but have not done so in a legal form
- 37 percent have not discussed this topic with their parents
- 1 percent didn't know

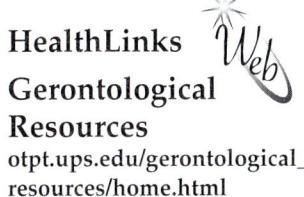

HealthLinks Gerontological Resources

otpt.ups.edu/gerontological_resources/home.html

Part of a larger site, this site is dedicated to meeting the educational needs of the elderly and their caregivers, particularly in the areas of occupational and physical therapies.

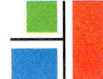

TABLE 18.2 Erikson's Life Cycle of Developmental Tasks

Stage	Aproximate age	Important event	Description
1. Basic trust versus basic mistrust	Birth to 12–18 months	Feeding	The infant must form a first loving, trusting relationship with the caregiver or develop a sense of mistrust.
2. Autonomy versus shame/doubt	18 months to 3 years	Toilet training	The child's energies are directed toward the development of physical skills, including walking and controlling the sphincter. The child learns control but may develop shame and doubt if not handled well.
3. Initiative versus guilt	3 to 6 years	Independence	The child continues to become more assertive and to take more initiative but may be too forceful, which can lead to guilt feelings.
4. Industry versus inferiority	6 to 12 years	School	The child must deal with demands to learn new skills or risk a sense of inferiority, failure, and incompetence.
5. Identity versus role confusion	Adolescence	Peer relationships	The teenager must achieve a sense of identity in occupation, gender roles, politics, and religion.
6. Intimacy versus isolation	Young adulthood	Love relationships	The young adult must develop intimate relationships or suffer feelings of isolation.
7. Generativity versus stagnation	Middle adulthood	Parenting and work	Each adult must find some way to satisfy and support the next generation.
8. Ego integrity versus despair	Late adulthood	Reflection on and acceptance of one's life	The culmination is a sense of acceptance of oneself as one is and a sense of fulfillment.

Source: Lester A. Lefton, *Psychology*, 6th ed., pp. 374, 390. Copyright © 1996 by Allyn & Bacon. Reprinted by permission of Allyn & Bacon

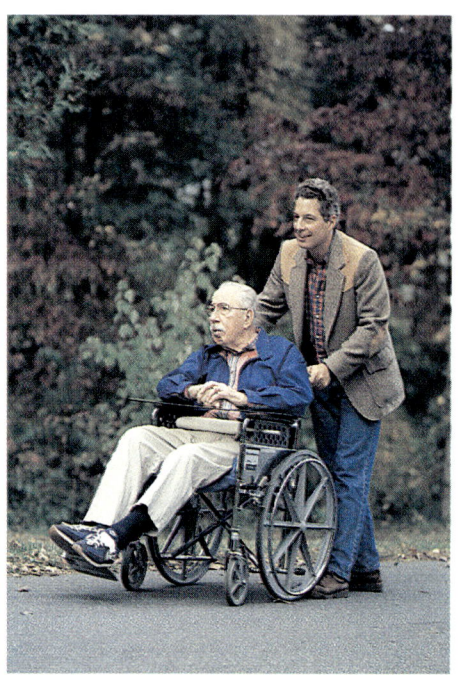

As parents age, a reversal of roles often takes place—adult children help with the care of their elderly parents. How involved do you think you will be in the care of your parents when they get older? (Source: © Tony Stone Images/David Young-Wolff)

Interestingly, responses to the Gallup poll differed by age. People in the eighteen-to-twenty-nine age group were less likely to have talked to their parents about "what-if" than older children, but they were much more likely to say they might ask a parent to move in with them than did those age fifty and older. How would you respond to the questions in Table 18.3?

TABLE 18.3 Children and Their Aging Parents

Question	Yes	No	Don't know
Do you think it's an adult child's responsibility to care for his or her parents as they grow older?	85%	6%	9%
Is it still the child's responsibility to care for his or her parents even if the parents and child have never gotten along well?	66	20	14
Would you consider placing your parents in a nursing home if they were too sick to care for themselves?	52	39	9
Would you consider asking your parents to move in with you if they could no longer live alone?	85	12	3
Do you think your parents should use up their savings to pay for their long-term care, even if that means there will be nothing left for you to inherit?	84	13	3

Source: Condensed from "Tough Choices for American Families: A *Health*/Gallup Poll," *Health*, October 1993, pp. 44–45. Reprinted with permission from *Health*, © 1993

Aging Body and Mind: Changes that Occur over Time

The one constant in the three viewpoints mentioned in the Psychology of Aging section is that changes occur with age. Some changes occur rapidly, such as when a child becomes taller or in puberty when breasts enlarge and pubic hair and other secondary sex characteristics appear. Other changes are not visible and develop only over a long period of time, such as a buildup of plaque in the arteries. Intellectual changes, too, develop slowly. Slight deficits in memory or thought processes are often not noted immediately by the older person himself or herself or even by family and friends. It may take years before the cumulative effect is realized.

Health Status

Are older people sicker than younger people? Such a question is like asking whether a glass is half full or half empty. The answer: It depends.

Surveys consistently show that the majority of elderly people say that their health is good or excellent even though they suffer from more illnesses than do younger people. Clearly, older people have more chronic conditions. The wear and tear of daily life—year after year, decade after decade—does take its toll. Although chronic and degenerative diseases are not usually the cause of death or disability in early adulthood or middle life, for many older people these threats become a reality. More people over age sixty-five die of heart disease than of any other cause. The second leading cause of death in this age group is cancer.

Older people also have more illnesses related to their weakened immune systems. Aging immune systems may become less adept at recognizing invaders. They may also become less resistant to infection. A common viral infection such as influenza can be life threatening for the elderly. An aging immune system sometimes mistakes the body's own cells for invaders, causing autoimmune diseases. Research suggests that arthritis might be an autoimmune disease.

With age comes a reduction in energy. This does not mean that it is time to take naps in the afternoon and retire, as the shoe salesman did. Nor does it have much effect on normal functioning. But it is a sign to slow down a bit. What is behind this loss of steam? Research on the heart and lungs illustrates some of the causes.

The heart of an older person, for example, might pump at the same pace as it did when he or she was younger, but now it pumps less efficiently and less powerfully. This means that in carrying out normal activities, an older person's vital organs receive less blood flow than do those of a younger person having the same heart rate. During exercise, the differences are even greater, and a seventy-year-old circulates far less blood per minute than does a thirty-year-old participating in the same activity.

The lungs are among the most resistant organs to change due to aging—provided they are cared for. Even so, a natural reduction occurs in the maximum amount of air exchange as a person gets older. This is in part due to the reduced effectiveness of the bronchial tubes' lining, which helps filter the air in the lungs.

Telltale Signs

One of the most visible signs of aging is a loss of the fatty and connective tissues that provide skin tone. The result is wrinkles. For many people, wrinkling begins in the early twenties and is usually first seen on the forehead. By age thirty, it is common to find "crow's feet" beside the eyes. In the forties and fifties, more pronounced aging lines develop, including radial and vertical mouth lines, baggy eyes, and jowls. Excess exposure to sunlight may contribute to a more rapid wrinkling of the skin than would otherwise be the case.

The cosmetic industry caters to people concerned with wrinkles, offering creams, mud packs, and other products to rejuvenate skin. These products offer temporary fixes—for example, adding moisture to the skin makes eyes look less baggy—but they do not make you free of wrinkles. The face-lift option promises a wrinkle-free result, but this, too, is not long lasting, and women (and increasingly men) are having multiple face lifts during their lifetimes.

Changes in hair provide another indication of aging. Although some people are prematurely gray at age twenty-one, graying of hair usually begins in the late thirties and forties. The balding process is almost entirely determined by genetics and is seen mostly in males. If your father or grandfather lost his hair as a young man, you are very likely to lose your hair at approximately the same age. Women, too, can have a genetic predisposition to thinning hair. This can develop in the forties but is more prominent in the seventies and eighties.

There are numerous solutions to graying and balding, including dyes, hair transplants, and hair growth drugs and creams. As with all prescription and over-the-counter drugs, these should be taken only in consultation with a physician.

A change in weight occurs with age, perhaps not as it shows on the scale but certainly as it shows in the mirror and in how clothes fit. For example, the body of a typical twenty-year-old female is about 17 to 20 percent fat. Over the years, the female body becomes proportionally more fat, and by age sixty, fat accounts for about 40 percent of body weight.

Aging muscles undergo change as well. Older muscles undergo a loss of contractility and flexibility and become susceptible to strains, pulls, and cramps. As people get older they also shrink in height as a result of muscle weakening, decreased space between the bones of the spine, and **osteoporosis.** It is not uncommon for a person to be two to three inches shorter in old age than in young adulthood.

Critical Thinking Question

> The *Healthy People 2000* objectives include the following: "Reduce to no more than 90 per 1,000 people the proportion of all people aged sixty-five and older who have difficulty in performing two or more personal care activities, thereby preserving independence." Baseline data for this objective were 111 per 1,000 for people sixty-five years and older and 371 per 1,000 for people eighty-five years and older. To what extent do you think independence is a matter of physical fitness? How might the definition of *fitness* differ for the adolescent, the middle-aged adult, and someone over eighty-five years of age?

Bone Density

In young people, living bone constantly renews itself and bones become harder and stronger. However, bones reach a peak mass—their maximum density and strength—around age thirty-five. After that, bone mass begins to diminish. This is particularly harmful to women.

osteoporosis A disorder in which bone density decreases, making the bones more likely to break.

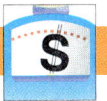

HEALTHWISE CONSUMER

Eye Care

You can help your elderly relatives prevent vision loss by discussing the following advice with them. Even though it was written for senior citizens, some of these tips make sense for younger people, too, such as protecting your eyes against sun damage.

- *Get regular eye examinations.* Have a complete examination every two to four years between ages forty and sixty-five and every one to two years after age sixty-five. If you have a family history of eye disease, such as glaucoma or macular degeneration, or a chronic condition that can affect your eyes, such as diabetes, you may need annual examinations. A complete eye examination typically includes a thorough history, eye function tests, and an examination of the appearance of your eyes.
- *Control chronic health conditions.* By treating chronic medical conditions such as diabetes or high blood pressure, you minimize the risk of developing associated vision problems.
- *Recognize symptoms.* Get immediate care if you have these symptoms: sudden loss of vision in one eye, sudden hazy or blurred vision, flashes of light or black spots, or halos or rainbows around lights. They may signal a serious medical problem such as acute glaucoma or a stroke.
- *Protect your eyes against sun damage.* Wear sunglasses that block 90 to 100 percent of UVA and UVB light. When buying sunglasses, read product information carefully to determine the amount of protection provided. For greater protection, choose a wrap-around style. Dark glasses that don't block UV light may actually cause more damage than wearing no sunglasses; they dilate your pupil, allowing more light in without blocking the damaging rays. In addition to sunglasses, wear a brimmed hat. Fifty percent of sunlight comes from directly overhead and can get by most sunglasses.
- *Eat a variety of foods.* A deficiency of certain nutrients may increase your risk of some eye diseases. However, the American Academy of Ophthalmology recommends getting adequate nutrients by eating a variety of foods rather than by taking supplements.
- *Make the most of the vision you have.* Be sure to always use good lighting, such as a gooseneck lamp, that directs illumination onto your reading or work area. You need more light as you grow older whether you have vision problems or not. If your vision becomes impaired, take advantage of the variety of low-vision aids available. Devices include everything from magnifiers to items such as large-size clocks and game boards

Source: Adapted from "Vision and Your Eyes: Managing Common Problems," in the October 1995 *Medical Essay: Supplement to Mayo Clinic Health Letter*, with permission of Mayo Foundation for Medical Education and Research, Rochester, Minnesota 55905

Thinning bones, a condition called osteoporosis, affects one in two women and one in three men over age seventy-five. It develops less frequently in men in part because they have heavier bones than women to begin with. It is believed that estrogen, a female hormone secreted during the childbearing years, helps ensure a strong skeleton. After menopause, women are at significantly increased risk for osteoporosis. As a result, many women are prescribed estrogen replacement therapy (called hormone replacement therapy, or HRT). HRT can significantly increase bone density and reduce the odds of bone fracture—as well as the risk of heart disease and stroke—but it can also increase the risk of breast cancer for some women. The benefits and risks of HRT should be discussed with a doctor.

The dangers of thinning bones are multiple. Although you do not die of thin bones, this condition can significantly affect your quality of life. For a person who has osteoporosis, a simple stumble or fall can lead to a crippling fracture or compression of the vertebrae, which can result in severe back pain as well as a disfiguring stooped appearance.

Heredity plays a role in osteoporosis: It is more prevalent among fair-skinned people, and a woman is more likely to develop this condition if her mother or grandmother had it. Other risk factors are cigarette smoking and heavy alcohol consumption because they can impair calcium absorption. The best time to prevent osteoporosis is during young adulthood. Having a good diet with adequate amounts of calcium, doing weight-bearing exercise (walking, playing tennis), and not smoking can help keep bones thicker (see Chapter 7).

The Senses

Almost everyone's visual capacity declines with age. As people age, their eyes take longer to adjust to changes in light or to see darker colors, for example. Another difficulty that begins in the late thirties but becomes very pronounced by age sixty—affecting nearly 100 percent of the elderly—is **presbyopia,** which involves difficulty in reading materials at close range. Presbyopia (*presby* means elders) is easily corrected with glasses or contact lenses.

Another eye condition common among older people is **cataracts,** a clouding of the lens. About half of Americans between ages sixty-five and seventy-four—70 percent of those older than age seventy-five—have cataracts, and removal of cataracts is the number one surgical procedure performed on people aged sixty-five and older. See the Healthwise Consumer box for tips on good eye care for the elderly.

Hearing loss is also common among older people, particularly with high-frequency sounds such as *s, z, t, f,* and *g*. Most college students can hear people talk in a whispered voice, but many older people need the sound to be about ten decibels louder. It is believed that some of this hearing loss is preventable. Years of bombardment by noises can result in permanent hearing deficits in later years (see Chapter 20). Another cause of hearing loss is the buildup of fatty deposits in the ears as a result of diet. This is similar to the buildup of plaque in the arteries.

Sexual Activity

Lovers at age seventy? Not only is it possible, it is happening to people who might be just like one of your grandparents—physically and mentally active, lonely, and "looking around." Both science and common sense suggest that people become less satisfied with sex and have more trouble responding sexually during later life. Yet a recent study from the Mayo Clinic suggests that we should reconsider the role of aging in sexual satisfaction.

It is true that older men are more likely to have reduced sex drive and problems with erections and that older women are likely to experience vaginal dryness or a decline in sexual responsiveness. Nonetheless, the Mayo researchers found that more of their older research subjects were satisfied than dissatisfied.

According to gerontologist Robert N. Butler, "The romance of many older people can be very tender, very sensitive. It may have intercourse. It may not." A study carried out by researchers at San Francisco State University of men and women aged 80 to 102 living in retirement homes found that the most common sexual activity was touching and caressing without intercourse, as reported by 72 percent of the men and 40 percent of the women. Sexual intercourse was third: 63 percent of the men and 30 percent of the women reported doing it. Based on this study, living in a retirement home does not preclude sex, and for 42 percent of the respondents, it actually increased their chances.

As for ability, for 90 percent of women over age sixty, sex is reported to be as good as or better than when they were younger. Although many men think that

presbyopia A difficulty in reading materials at close range; common in older persons.

cataracts Clouding of the lens of the eye.

neurotransmitters Chemicals that facilitate the passage of impulses in the brain.

neurons The basic cells of the nervous system.

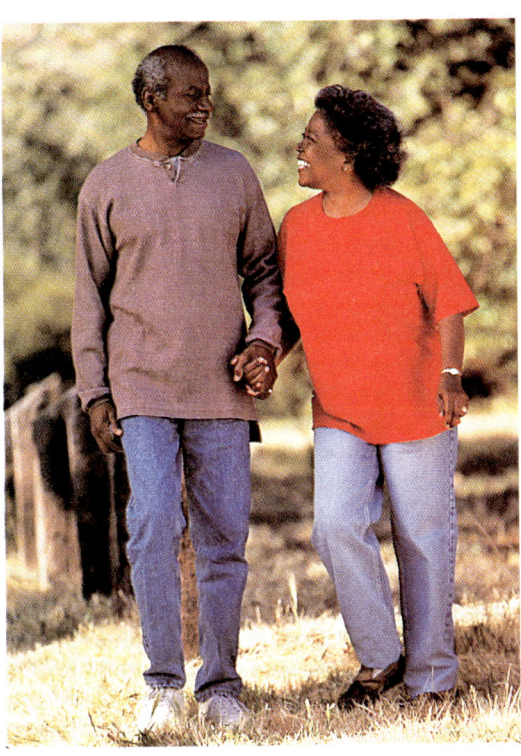

Contrary to popular belief, sexual interest is alive and well for senior citizens. For many people, living in a retirement home actually increases their chances of meeting someone. (Source: FPG International/© Ken Chernus)

by the time they reach age sixty, they will be too old to have an erection, the truth is that impotence is due to factors that can happen at any age and not to the aging process alone. Overall, studies consistently show that sexual activity is possible into the eighties and nineties.

Mental Ability

One of the greatest fears about getting old is the decline of mental faculties. The good news is that research shows that age alone does not necessarily cause a loss of brain function or reasoning ability. According to the National Institute on Aging, disease—not age in itself—may underlie many or even most cases of mental decline in the elderly.

People of all ages can learn new things. Older people, however, may not learn as rapidly as they did when they were younger. Older people also are not as quick to recall things from their long-term memory. This is a normal function of information retrieval, not memory loss. In effect, the older you are, the more information you have to sort through in your memory. Moreover, intelligence does not decline with age. Studies show that when intelligence tests are given to the same people over a period of many years, their scores remain the same.

Short-term memory is a different issue. It is a complex process that involves the release of chemicals called **neurotransmitters,** which facilitate the passage of impulses in the brain. The aging brain produces smaller amounts of neurotransmitters, and unless steps are taken to keep brain **neurons** stimulated, short-term memory slows down considerably in older people. Studies show that mental

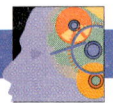

DEVELOPING HEALTH SKILLS

Exercising Your Memory

Mnemonics, the art of improving short-term recall and ferreting out stored facts, depends on strong visual images and meaningful associations. It's a system for cross-indexing stored information in arresting ways. These methods take only a little time to master. They work because they seize the attention and demand concentration. The more outrageous the connections you set up, the better.

Use "loci" (Latin for "places"). Take a string of facts to be remembered: for instance, points you want to cover in a talk. Match each one to a specific site you can visualize easily—your living room, perhaps, or your street. If you're giving a talk on substance abuse, make a tour of the living room, stationing your introductory remarks on drug cartels on the table left of the fireplace. On the mantel, store what you're planning to say about government policy. To the right of the fireplace, in the bookcase, situate drug education—and so forth, around the room. When you give your talk, make another mental tour of the room and "pick up" your notes. You can adapt the same loci to something more innocuous, like a grocery list: pasta on the table, tomato sauce on the mantel, salad greens in the bookcase.

Make up rhymes. Nobody ever forgets the useful "*I* before *E*, except after *C*." But to remember home chores, make up your own rhymes: "Skitty, skat, let in the cat," for instance. The cornier the better.

Compose mental pictures, particularly when you're trying to remember a name: Helen Decker, say, might conjure up a vision of Helen of Troy on shipboard.

Repeat or rehearse new facts. "How do you do, Helen," you say when introduced at a party. A few minutes later you say to yourself, "That's Helen Decker." And a minute or so after that. "Can I get you anything to drink, Helen?" You probably won't forget Helen's name.

Make up acronyms or sentences. "Maple" could help an out-of-towner in New York City

---

exercise, much like physical exercise, can help keep you alert even late in life. Examples of mental exercises are provided in the Developing Health Skills box. The Here's Looking at You box tests your knowledge about aging and the brain.

Memory problems in the elderly can also be caused by poor nutrition, depression, **hypoglycemia** (low blood sugar), and adverse reactions to medication. In most cases, these problems are reversible with appropriate and timely treatment of the underlying condition. Alzheimer's disease and other forms of **dementia** are not treatable.

Living with Alzheimer's Disease

Most people forget someone's name, a telephone number, or where they put the car keys. This is normal forgetfulness. **Alzheimer's disease** is not normal forgetfulness. It is a serious progressive and irreversible disease that affects the cerebral cortex and produces dementia in middle to late life. This disease affects about 5 percent of people over age sixty-five and 20 percent of the over-eighty population; it accounts for about half of the dementia cases in the United States. Alzheimer's disease starts with an inability to find the right word but progresses to misusing words, asking the same question over and over again, writing many reminder notes, wearing the same clothes every day, not paying bills, and not taking medicine. Personality changes include abusive behavior, disorientation, paranoia, depression, and other cognitive and behavioral deterioration.

At some point, people living with Alzheimer's disease cannot write or speak coherently, do not understand when people speak to them, and may not recog-

hypoglycemia Low blood sugar.

dementia A disorder characterized by the general and often slow decline of mental abilities.

Alzheimer's disease A degenerative disorder that causes dementia in middle to late life.

incontinent Unable to control one's bowels or release of urine.

remember the order of Madison, Park, and Lexington Avenues. "The postman at Sutter's Mill was bushed from pining for California" could help a visitor remember the order of five San Francisco streets, Post, Sutter, Bush, Pine, and California.

Chunk or regroup clusters of data to give them a pattern. Telephone numbers are already partially grouped, but you can give them further meaning. Helen's three-number exchange, 744, is easy to remember, but you won't forget the rest of the number either, 4591, when you reflect that she looks to be 45, almost halfway to 91.

Write things down. Writing notes and making lists will often fix things in your mind. You may not even have to refer to your notes or lists.

Structure your life. Even the hook for the house keys by the back door is a mnemonic device: you'll always look there first. Similarly, keep your checkbook in the drawer of your desk, or park your reading glasses on the night table.

Ease your mind. If you feel you are forgetting too much, consider the following:

- Give yourself time. The sky won't fall in if you forget a name or a number, and if you employ a few delaying tactics (don't rush right up to the friend whose name you've forgotten), the missing data may surface. If they don't, don't make a big fuss over it. Just admit you've forgotten.
- Don't expect too much. If you're nervous about forgetting, you usually do.
- Play games. Crossword puzzles, Scrabble, and card games are all good exercises for improving memory.
- Improve your mind. Going to lectures, taking classes, and joining groups will introduce new stimuli and keep your neurons transmitting.

Source: "Exercising Your Memory," reprinted with permission from the *University of California at Berkeley Wellness Letter*, October 1988. © Health Letter Associates, 1988. To order a one year subscription, call 800/829-9170

---

nize themselves in a mirror. In time, they cannot feed themselves or even chew and swallow. They become bedridden and **incontinent** and eventually lose consciousness and die. On average, the course of the disease may last seven to nine years, but it can last as long as twenty years.

Alzheimer's disease is not new. It was first identified in 1907 by a German neurologist, Alois Alzheimer. There are two major reasons why there seems to be an upsurge in the incidence of the disease today. One is that people are living longer—long enough to have the symptoms appear. The second is that autopsy studies reveal that Alzheimer's disease is far more prevalent than physicians had previously thought.

Autopsies show that people who have Alzheimer's disease often have tangles in their brain tissue and abnormally high amounts of some brain chemicals and deficiencies in others. One chemical that is deficient in Alzheimer's patients is acetylcholine, which is necessary for the transmission of messages from one part of the brain to another. Whereas the brains of older people who do not have Alzheimer's disease have less acetylcholine than the brains of younger people, those who have Alzheimer's disease have as much as a 90 percent loss of acetylcholine. Scientists do not know what causes this chemical abnormality, but taking acetylcholine supplements does not change the course of the disease.

Theories concerning the cause of Alzheimer's disease are numerous. Possible causes include a slow virus, a malfunction of the immune system, and a genetic abnormality. None has been proven or rejected. For example, a person who has several close family members whose symptoms of the disease appeared before age sixty-five has a much higher risk for developing Alzheimer's disease than do

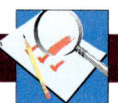

HERE'S LOOKING AT YOU

What's on Your Mind? A Quiz on Aging

What changes to the brain do you think occur as people age? There's a great variation in emotional, intellectual, and physical changes that occur among the elderly. It's probably safe to say that what we know about changes to the brain as we age is far less than what we don't know. Complete the following statements and questions to see just how much *you* know.

1. *"You can't teach an old dog new tricks" is a saying*
   a. that recent scientific experiments have shown is true for older people.
   b. that only applies to dogs, cats, and other non-human species.
   c. that is outdated and scientifically incorrect.
2. *How does aging affect intelligence?*
   a. Brains in older people don't work as fast, but knowledge based on experience grows in later life.
   b. Older people are really more intelligent because they have been using their brains for so many years.
   c. Older people don't learn as much as they did when they were younger.
3. *Creativity in old age is*
   a. enhanced by experience.
   b. a lost art.
   c. difficult because of changes in the brain.
4. *Depression is a problem for many older people. The condition is*
   a. acceptable, given their age and illnesses.
   b. just a normal part of growing older and can't be reversed.
   c. frequently treatable once its cause is pinpointed.
5. *Psychotherapy, or "talk" therapy, for people over age 65 is*
   a. a waste of time. People that age don't have much time left.
   b. a good idea. At age 65, people continue to live a long time, making it even more important that they seek help for mental health problems.
   c. a waste of effort. Older people are so set in their ways that there really isn't much point in trying to deal with their mental health problems.
6. *Nerve cells in the adult brain gradually die over the years. What is the result?*
   a. It means that memory loss in old age is inevitable.
   b. Not much, because people continue to learn as they grow older.
   c. Over time—and with a proper diet, physical exercise, and mental stimulation—the brain replenishes the nerve cells it loses.
7. *Which of the following has been shown to cause Alzheimer's disease in some patients?*
   a. alcohol or drug abuse.
   b. aluminum deposits in the brain.
   c. a genetic defect in some families.
   d. lack of education.
8. *Most typically, memory loss in older people is caused by*
   a. Alzheimer's disease.
   b. too many things to remember.
   c. a variety of factors, such as overmedication or illness.
9. *Which of the following is true?*
   a. Alzheimer's disease can be cured if diagnosed early enough.
   b. Alzheimer's disease can be treated to slow the progress of the disease.
   c. There is no known cure for Alzheimer's disease.
10. *What is the best method for conclusively diagnosing Alzheimer's disease?*
    a. the Myers-Briggs personality test.
    b. a diagnostic blood test.
    c. psychiatric evaluation.
    d. tissue analysis after death.
11. *True or false? Solving puzzles and other "mental gymnastics" can keep the aging brain healthy.*
    a. False. Mental exercises won't keep your brain sharp in later life.
    b. True. Intellectual and creative pursuits help adults avoid dementing diseases.
    c. Neither. The value of mental exercise for brain fitness has yet to be demonstrated.
12. *Personality changes in later life are*
    a. rare in healthy people. People stay pretty much the same throughout life.
    b. normal because experience makes people

very different than they were as children and young adults.
c. inevitable because people become cranky and difficult as they age.

13. *Dreading death is a preoccupation among*
    a. older adults who, as they grow yet older, see friends dying.
    b. many healthy adults in middle age who are struggling with "midlife crisis."
    c. both of the above.

14. *True or false? Older people worry too much.*
    a. False. Worry is not really a characteristic of old age.
    b. True. People become much more anxious as they age.

15. *A "tip-of-the-tongue" (TOT) experience—when you know a word or name but just can't seem to retrieve it from your memory—*
    a. is always a sign of Alzheimer's disease in an older person.
    b. is usually a temporary glitch.
    c. means that once you have forgotten a name or word, you will never remember it again quickly.

16. *Sexual problems in older adults*
    a. are a normal part of aging. Women lose interest in sex after menopause and men are often impotent.
    b. are mostly caused by emotional or mental health problems.
    c. are caused by changes in brain function that affect parts of the brain associated with sexual satisfaction.

17. *A stroke is a sudden disruption in the flow of blood to the brain. The likelihood of a stroke can be reduced*
    a. by quitting smoking, adopting sensible eating habits—low-cholesterol and low-fat diets—and controlling high blood pressure.
    b. by keeping under control and not allowing a bad temper to explode.
    c. somewhat. Research shows that the death rate from stroke has fallen only slightly despite preventive measures.

18. *Many older people complain that they don't sleep as well as they used to. Their sleep may be troubled because*
    a. they take more medications.
    b. they are anxious about retirement and other major life changes.
    c. they have a variety of medical problems, such as arthritis or cardiovascular disease, that are common with age.
    d. all of the above.

Answers

1. **c** Older adults can and do learn new skills relatively easily. In fact, in properly designed programs, older individuals can benefit from training as much as, and sometimes more than, younger people.

2. **a** Good news: Experience-based intelligence remains stable or improves slightly well into late adulthood. In many jobs, the expertise of older workers allows them to be among the safest and most productive employees. The speed and efficiency of processing information can decline, however, with increasing age. Recent scientific experiments show that, with practice, older adults can reverse some of these effects.

3. **a** Picasso painted until his death in his nineties and Grandma Moses kept painting until she died at age 101. In addition, many not-so-famous older adults take on second or third careers, try new hobbies, or begin closer interpersonal relationships after age 65.

4. **c** Depression can be treated successfully and should be taken seriously because it is a major risk factor for suicide. It is not a normal part of aging, although many older adults suffer from it. Adverse drug reactions, illness, certain life events, and other factors can cause older people to become depressed.

5. **b** Psychotherapy ("talk" therapy) has proven successful for older people, and its benefits can last for many years. At age 65, people continue to live an average of 16.8 years. Those over age 85 represent the fastest-growing age group.

6. **b** It is true that nerve cell loss begins by about age two and progresses throughout life. But normal nerve cell loss is not believed to have a significant effect on overall performance because people continue to learn as they age. Excessive nerve loss associated with illness can cause problems.

7. **c** Studies indicate that a small but important percentage of Alzheimer's disease patients come from families in which the disease occurs more often than in the general population. This suggests that genetic factors play an important

role in those families. Scientists have not yet been able to establish how much of a role genetics plays in the vast majority of families, however, and they have yet to identify other factors causing the disease.

8. **c** Memory loss in older people can have many causes and can often be treated. While Alzheimer's disease or other dementing disorders can cause memory loss, other factors can include depression, reactions to some drugs, and head injury.

9. **c** There is no known cure for Alzheimer's disease, but much can be done to treat the symptoms of the disease that cause suffering and discomfort. Several medical or social interventions can be used, including drug therapy for depression and simplifying the patient's environment.

10. **d** A diagnosis of Alzheimer's disease can be confirmed by autopsy only after death. In the living patient, the diagnosis is strongly suggested only after all other possible causes of dementia are systematically ruled out.

11. **c** Neither. Scientists have not proven that "mental gymnastics" can keep an aging human brain healthy that otherwise might have begun to decline, but they have found that there might be some benefit to "exercising" the brain. Laboratory research shows that animals in stimulating environments can release chemicals in their brains related to keeping nerve cells healthy and active.

12. **a** When an older person shows significant personality or behavior changes, it is usually a signal that something else is wrong. For example, a new, growing hostility in relationships with others can mask serious, hidden depression.

13. **b** A dread of death is not typical for healthy older adults. When it occurs in older people, it is usually related to depression or a struggle with terminal illness. In healthy adults, a fear of death is actually more common in middle age.

14. **a** False. For the vast majority of older adults, worry is not a problem. One recent study of people in their nineties found that over 70 percent report that they are in good spirits, never feel lonely, and are free from worry.

15. **b** TOTs are often just temporary mental glitches, although word-finding problems may be slightly more frequent among older adults. Scientists are studying TOTs to see how the brain stores and retrieves information, hoping to explain a range of language and memory problems, such as those that occur after a stroke. In some cases, however, word-finding problems can be a sign of Alzheimer's disease. Older adults should be monitored closely to see if word finding becomes a serious difficulty.

16. **b** Emotional state plays a greater role than normal aging changes in causing sexual problems in older adults. Depression can significantly interfere with sexual interest, motivation, and fantasy life in one's later years. It is one of the most common causes of impotence in older men and is treatable.

17. **a** These approaches have been so successful that the death rate from stroke has fallen as much as 50 percent since 1970. The decline also has been due to more advanced diagnostic tests and treatments.

18. **d** Although the quality of sleep can change as people age, most older people spend the same amount of time sleeping as they did when they were younger. Good sleep habits, including exercising, avoiding alcohol and caffeine, and going to sleep at the same time every night, can help with troubled sleep.

Source: National Institute on Aging

others. However, not even such a high-risk person will necessarily get the disease.

Without a known cause or treatment, Alzheimer's patients and their families are left to cope with the disease at home and in nursing homes. About two thirds of people who have Alzheimer's disease are cared for at home, and more than 50 percent of all nursing home patients have either Alzheimer's disease or a related condition. Caring for someone who has Alzheimer's disease can involve feeding, dressing, bathing, handling incontinence, watching to make sure the patient is not doing something unsafe, and dealing with his or her wanderings at all hours of the night. It is no wonder that these caretakers talk about the thirty-six-hour day.

Preventable Health Problems

Your grandmother seems confused. When you call her on the phone, she isn't always sure who you are. You worry whether it is Alzheimer's disease, but you might do better to have someone check her medication. One of the serious misdiagnoses among the elderly may be misinterpreting confusion due to **overmedication** as a symptom of a disease.

Many of the health risks that the elderly face are preventable. Key among these are depression and other mental states, overmedication, and falls.

Sadness in Old Age

Depression is the most common psychological disorder among older people. It can be triggered by two very common situations for an elderly person: the loss of a loved one or the onset of a disease. Perhaps the elderly are right to be depressed and to feel lonely and abandoned. How do you think you would act if your spouse died after fifty-five years of being together? How would you cope with living alone again—and at age seventy-five? How would you respond to the onset of and increasing disability caused by not one or two but four and even six different medical conditions?

Other causes of depression in the elderly can be conditions that are treatable, including thyroid abnormalities, nutritional deficiencies, and infections. In general, the mental health needs of the elderly are not being met, in part because the elderly themselves think that it is natural to be depressed when you are old. Insomnia, for example, is one of the signs of depression, but it is also a fairly common complaint among the elderly. Research shows that aging reduces the amount of sleep a person can expect to get at any one time, and by age seventy-five, some people may find that they are waking up several times each night.

Suicidal thoughts often accompany depression for people of all ages, but the elderly have the highest suicide rate of any age group. The elderly also receive only 2 to 4 percent of inpatient and outpatient mental health services, which suggests a large gap between the amount of care they may need and what they actually receive. Depression can be successfully treated in most older people with psychotherapy, antidepressants, or a combination of the two.

Medication Abuse

In some respects, the senior citizen drug scene is similar to what you might expect among teenagers and young adults—misuse, accidental abuse, and sharing of drugs. The difference is that for senior citizens the drugs of choice are most often prescriptions: 86 percent of the elderly have one or more chronic conditions, many of which require drug treatment. Consider the following conversation in a retirement community as an example:

Charles: I couldn't sleep last night. I had such chest pains. I bet it was indigestion from that big dinner we had.

overmedication Consuming a high dose of medication, or combination of medications, resulting in symptoms (side effects) that compromise accurate medical care.

depression A mental disorder marked by sadness, anxiety, fatigue, underactivity, sleeplessness, and reduced ability to function and relate to others.

Louisa: What you need is my heart medicine. Remember I used to have chest pains, too, but thank goodness not since my doctor gave me something that really works. Here, take some of mine. I promise you'll feel better.

Unrealistic, you think? Have you ever shared a medication with a friend? Perhaps for menstrual cramps, or a migraine, or weight loss. Sharing medications is no less common among the elderly. Unfortunately for Charles, if he takes Louisa's "miracle" drug, he might end up in the hospital either with an adverse drug reaction or as a heart attack patient if in fact he was having early signs of an attack and did not seek appropriate treatment for the real cause of his chest pain.

Older people are particularly sensitive to the effects of medicine and suffer reactions including confusion, decreased coordination, mental deterioration, and tremors. Even so, numerous studies show that the elderly lack knowledge about appropriate drug use. It is estimated that about 60 percent of the elderly do not comply correctly with medication directions. They might decrease the proper dosage to stretch the prescription out or take a larger dose thinking that if a little is good, more might be better. Either situation could result in an adverse reaction. Drug misuse is not limited to prescription drugs. It is common for older people to misuse over-the-counter drugs as well. And because many older individuals take several medications, problems related to drug interactions are common.

Each year, more than a quarter of a million older adults are hospitalized because of adverse reactions to drugs, thirty-two thousand have hip fractures caused by drug-induced falls, and more than one hundred sixty thousand suffer mental impairment caused or worsened by drugs.

Although the following advice is important to people of all ages, it is particularly important for the elderly:

- Before leaving the physician's office or the pharmacy, make sure the instructions for taking your elderly relative's medicine are clear to you and your relative or another family member or friend.
- Make sure to notify your relative's physician of any symptoms that he or she develops after starting a new drug. They may be caused by the drug.
- Ask your relative's primary care physician or pharmacist to coordinate all drug use—both prescription and over-the-counter.

Falls

The elderly are at particularly high risk for unintentional injuries. Fall-related injuries send almost 8 percent of people over age seventy to the emergency room each year. Some 40 percent of people hospitalized for fall-related injuries do not go home, but are discharged directly into nursing homes.

Hip fractures are by far the most dangerous fractures associated with falls among the elderly. Because osteoporosis is a primary cause of fractures in this age group, women are affected more than men. By age ninety, it is estimated that one in three women will have sustained a hip fracture. In addition to the pain and medical expense involved, hip fractures can seriously limit independent living on a temporary and sometimes permanent basis. Self-esteem and self-confidence can be lessened with repetitive falls, which can lead to diminished activity and increased dependency.

Although some falls have a single, obvious cause, researchers believe that most falls are due to a combination of factors:

- Mental changes such as confusion, dementia, or mini-strokes
- Cardiovascular or circulatory problems, especially an inability to adjust blood pressure to sudden changes in posture, which can cause fainting

- Antianxiety drugs, antidepressants, and other sedating medications
- Effects of diseases, such as the pain of arthritis or the tremors of **Parkinson's disease**
- Muscular weakness and overall decline in physical vigor
- Changes in vision, hearing, reflexes, and coordination
- Environmental hazards

As many as 40 to 50 percent of all falls are caused by potentially avoidable environmental factors. Most of the elderly fall at home, where simple environmental corrective measures can be easily introduced. These measures include improved lighting, repairing or replacing worn carpeting, tying electrical cords to the wall so they don't trail on the floor, installing stairway banisters, and wearing rubber-soled corrective footwear. Additional preventive measures include exercise and strength and balance training—proven means of reducing the risk of falls. With carefully adjusted home environments and with increased physical skill comes reduced risk, resulting in less fear of falling and less social decline associated with falls.

Promoting Healthy Aging

The quality of life in old age is influenced to a great extent by health style choices made in younger years. A lifelong exercise program, for example, can help prolong and prevent the onset of osteoporosis and thus improve the quality of life for an eighty-year-old woman. And a decision made in his early thirties to stop smoking is appreciated almost daily by a healthy and active seventy-five-year-old man.

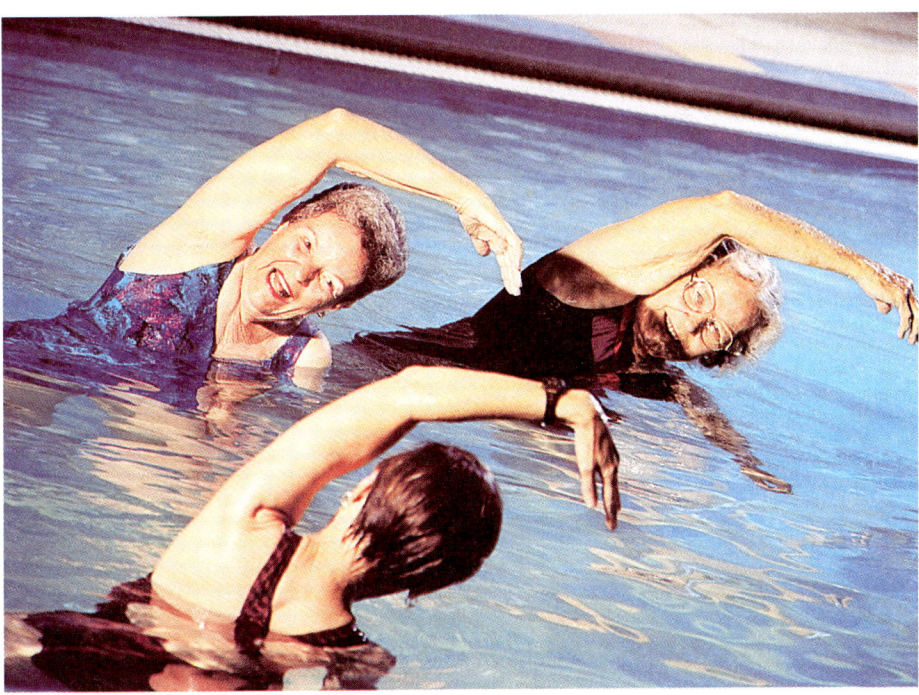

Maintaining an active lifestyle, which includes regular exercise, is a key component to healthy living throughout the lifespan and can be particularly beneficial in later adulthood. (Source: © Tony Stone Images/Zigy Kaluzny)

Parkinson's disease A serious illness marked by progressive loss of normal muscle function; over time, the muscles become stiff, causing shaky movements.

Critical Thinking Question

> The perception of time changes as we age. From the perspective of a four-year-old, two years represents half a lifetime. The same two years, however, are viewed as only a brief period in life by an eighty-year-old. How can younger generations learn the value of time? Would such a value influence their health-related decisions? How might the development of health skills influence an appreciation of time?

For those who put off exercising, good nutrition, and other healthy lifestyles when they were younger, there is still time for a second chance. In fact, gerontologists say that no single group can benefit more from exercise than the elderly. And it does not have to be an elaborate exercise plan. Researchers report that simply walking four hours a week can decrease the risk for future hospitalization for heart disease. Another moderate exercise, T'ai chi (which is discussed in Chapter 4 as a way to reduce stress), probably improves balance, reduces the risk for falls, and may increase strength. According to the Centers for Disease Control and Prevention, regular physical activity by older people may also reduce risks for chronic disease by maintaining normal body weight, blood pressure, glucose tolerance, and lipoprotein lipid levels.

Surveys suggest that today's elderly are more active than before, based on the fact that they have become healthier and more functional in daily life. Researchers at Duke University's Center for Demographic Studies, which periodically samples 20,000 Americans over age sixty-five, found a 15 percent decrease between 1982 and 1994 in what it calls "chronic disability rates" as measured by ability to perform daily activities such as feeding or dressing oneself.

As a result of findings such as these, health education and fitness programs for senior citizens are cropping up across the country, and participation in athletic events for older people is increasing. Each year, more than one hundred thousand people between the ages of fifty-five and ninety-nine participate in U.S. National Senior Sports Organization (USNSSO) competitions in more than seventy cities. Most senior sports enthusiasts are not lifelong athletes, and at least half of the senior competitors had not done their sport until they were in their fifties, according to USNSSO.

Because so many Americans expect to live a long life, the idea of age sixty-five as the gateway to old age seems old-fashioned. Although it might be the point of retirement from the workplace for some people, it can be the starting point for adult education classes, health promotion, community involvement, and what one psychiatrist calls a "psychic aliveness."

Key Concepts

1. The Census Bureau defines people aged sixty-five to seventy-four as elderly, people seventy-five to eighty-four as aged, and people eighty-five and more as very old.
2. There are more than double the number of women than men aged sixty-five and older.

3. Ageism is the term used to describe prejudice and discrimination against the elderly based on misconceptions and stereotypes.
4. The majority of elderly people say that their health is good or excellent even though they suffer from more illnesses than do younger people.
5. One of the most visible signs of aging is a loss of the fatty and connective tissues that provide skin tone. The result is wrinkles.
6. Memory loss due to poor nutrition, depression, hypoglycemia (low blood sugar), and adverse reactions to medication is both preventable and reversible.
7. Alzheimer's disease is a progressive and irreversible disease. It may be caused by a slow virus, a malfunction of the immune system, or a genetic abnormality, but none of these theories has been proven.
8. Each year, more than a quarter of a million older adults are hospitalized because of adverse reactions to drugs.
9. Hip fractures are by far the most dangerous fractures associated with falls among the elderly.
10. According to the Centers for Disease Control and Prevention, regular physical activity by older people may reduce risks for chronic disease by maintaining normal body weight, blood pressure, glucose tolerance, and lipoprotein lipid levels.

Review Questions

1. Describe three methods of measuring age: chronological, functional, and psychological.
2. List characteristics of elderly persons in the United States using gender, marital status, living arrangements, and health status as categories.
3. State five misconceptions about aging often held by the general public. Correct those misconceptions with factual information.
4. Name three styles of aging and give an example of how each is reflected in behavior.
5. Compare the normal health status of an aging person with that of a young adult and a middle-aged person.
6. Identify the primary health concerns related to the bones, the senses, and the brain during the aging process.
7. Describe the symptoms of Alzheimer's disease.
8. Identify ten misconceptions concerning Alzheimer's disease.
9. List actions that can be taken to prevent depression, medicine abuse, and falls among the elderly.
10. Make a list of reasons why regular physical activity and a nutritious diet are important for healthy aging.

Selected Bibliography

Aging Research and Training News (published 22 times a year).
Health after 50: The Johns Hopkins Medical Letter (published monthly).
Truth about Aging: Guidelines for Accurate Communications. Washington, DC: American Association of Retired Persons, 1986.

HealthLinks: Web Sites for Healthy Aging

You can access better health as it relates to this chapter by checking out some of the following sites on the Internet. These and sites identified within the chapter can be accessed directly when you visit the *HealthStyles* Web Site located on the Allyn and Bacon home page at **http://www.abacon.com.**

American Association of Retired Persons
www.aarp.org
The nation's leading organization for people 50 and older, providing information and education, advocacy, and community services offered by a network of local chapters and experienced volunteers throughout the country. Explore back issues of *Modern Maturity* magazine and the monthly *AARP Bulletin,* and examine the latest information on tax and policy changes.

National Institute on Aging
www.nih.gov/nia/
The National Institute on Aging (NIA) is one of the National Institutes of Health. The NIA promotes healthy aging by conducting and supporting biomedical, social, and behavioral research and public education. The site includes recent announcements of significant findings from NIA-supported research, upcoming events, and employment opportunities. In addition, you will find publications on health and aging topics for health professionals and the public.

Health Hotlines: Aging: Growing Older, Keeping Healthy

Alzheimer's Association
(800) 272-3900
919 North Michigan Avenue, Suite 1000
Chicago, IL 60611-1676

American Association of Retired Persons
(800) 424-2277
601 E Street NW
Washington, DC 20049

Eldercare Locator
(800) 677-1116
National Association of Area Agencies on Aging
1112 16th Street NW, Suite 100
Washington, DC 20036

National Council on Aging
(800) 424 9046
409 Third Street SW, 2nd Floor
Washington, DC 20024

National Institute on Aging Information Center
(800) 222-2225
P O. Box 8057
Gaithersburg, MD 20898-8057

Older Women's League
(800) 825-3695
666 11th Street NW, Suite 700
Washington, DC 20001

Chapter 19

Death and Dying

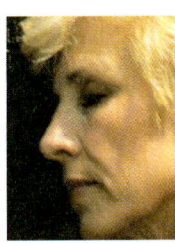
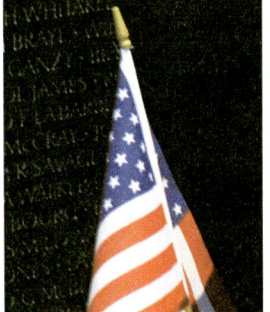

Objectives

When you finish reading this chapter, you will be able to:

1. Recognize death as it is biologically, legally, and religiously understood.
2. Understand different forms of euthanasia and the controversy surrounding this end-of-life decision.
3. Differentiate between the understanding of death by children, by adolescents, and by adults.
4. Differentiate death from the process of dying and know the meaning of the living–dying interval.
5. Recognize five stages of dying according to Elizabeth Kübler-Ross.
6. Understand the function of a hospice and its goal to provide comfort for dying patients.
7. Recognize the tasks that survivors must undertake in the event of a loved one's death.
8. Recognize the importance of documents such as a will, a durable power of attorney for health care, and a uniform donor card.
9. Recognize the three stages of grieving—impact, recoil, and recovery.
10. Understand death and loss as inevitable elements of life and that grief can lead to an inspiration or recommitment to life.

What Is Your HealthStyle?

George was a junior in high school when he was diagnosed with bone cancer and his left leg was removed above the knee. He was fitted with a prosthesis and got along well with his life. Unfortunately, when he was a junior in college, his cancer returned and spread to other parts of his body. This time, his condition was terminal, and George was having difficulty coping with this fact. He sank into a depression and gave up hope. In his final weeks of life, he refused help, including an appropriate level of pain medication. He could have made many decisions concerning his medical care, his funeral, and his personal belongings, but George steadfastly refused to discuss these issues.

Several weeks before he died, George could no longer handle the pain and he was admitted to the hospital. He was placed on a life support system that involved numerous tubes being inserted into his body—although his family had no idea whether this accorded with his wishes. Despite visiting often, his parents and sisters were not in the hospital when he died.

Krista's fatal illness was leukemia. Like George, she thought she had beaten a childhood disease, but soon after she entered college, the symptoms began to reappear, beginning with weight loss and extreme fatigue. She managed to complete her freshman year, but by summer, she was fading rapidly.

With support from her parents and brother, Krista chose to enter a hospice care program to enable her to lead as high-quality a life as possible in her final weeks and to die at home. With proper pain medication, Krista remained alert and involved. She read books, listened to music, and kept in touch with the people most important to her. Her hospice team helped her not only with pain management but also with planning her own funeral. Krista wanted her roommate to recite a poem they both loved. She and her brother spent long hours talking about her impending death and gaining strength from each other. As she neared death, Krista was at home, where her surroundings were familiar and she could be at peace with herself.

In Your Opinion

George and Krista dealt with dying in different ways. George thought he was being brave by "fighting" death; Krista "fought" in another way.

- What could George have done to make his last weeks more manageable for himself and his family?
- Do you think he gave up by going to the hospital?
- What health skills do you think Krista had that helped her through this time?
- How would you compare the quality of the last few days of George's and Krista's lives?
- Which would you choose for yourself, and why?

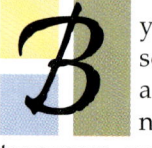

By this time in your life, you have probably known at least one person who has died. For most college students, this usually means a grandparent or another elderly relative. Death, however, does not happen only to those who have led full lives. Children, teenagers, young adults, and your middle-aged parents can also die of diseases and accidents.

The Hollywood image of dying is one of romantic suffering. When death finally takes place at the end of the film, everyone is ready for it. When he was thirty-eight years old, the Welsh poet Dylan Thomas wrote:

Do not go gentle into that good night,
Old age should burn and rave at close of day;
Rage, rage against the dying of the light....*

Although Thomas was to die two years later, he wasn't yet ready to face death.

Contrast this to the ninety-four-year-old man who broke his hip and had a hip replacement because, as he said, "he didn't want to spend the rest of his life in bed." At ninety-nine, however, he said that he "heard the angels sing" and wanted no more medical interventions. He was ready for death, which came a year later.

A basic fact of life is that it will end in death. This is true for all living species because no person or living thing lives forever. People die. Pets die. Plants die. In spite of the inevitability of death, few people want to talk about it. So great is the ability to deny mortality that more than two thirds of all Americans do not have a living will, which stipulates which medical treatments are and are not to be used in the terminal days of life.

This reluctance to face something so inevitable appears to be universal. As Woody Allen said, "I'm not afraid of dying. I just don't want to be there when it happens." Or as W. C. Fields wanted for his own epitaph, "On the whole, I'd rather be in Philadelphia." (This epitaph was not used. His tombstone contains only his vital statistics.)

Humor is one of the many positive ways to talk about death. This is why at wakes and other memorial gatherings people often talk about funny things that happened to the person who died. Such humorous accounts are shared out of love and respect and can help give meaning to death.

College students face the issue of death more often than you think. By age eighteen, one in twenty students has lost a parent. Suicide, AIDS, cancer, and automobile accidents have also taken the lives of classmates. To help students better understand the concepts of death and dying, colleges have instituted courses and other studies on the topic. The study of death and the psychological and social problems associated with it is called **thanatology**. In Greek mythology, Thanatos was death personified.

The Meaning of Death

Death is a certainty, but defining it is not simple. Depending on who you are and what your relationship is to the dying person, death can take on different meanings. For a friend, death can mean the tremendous loss of a close personal companion. For a relative, death can mean not only a crushing personal loss but also dealing with legal requirements such as a will. For a physician, death can mean following a set of criteria to determine when—or whether—death has actually occurred. The meaning of death changes as the point of view changes.

---

*Source: "Do Not Go Gentle into That Good Night" by Dylan Thomas, from *The Poems of Dylan Thomas*. Copyright © 1952 by Dylan Thomas. Reprinted by permission of New Directions Publishing Corp. and David Highman Associates

thanatology The study of death and the psychological and social problems associated with it.

Critical Thinking Question

> Out of nearly 320 objectives in *Healthy People 2000*, only 26 are tracked using mortality data. In other words, cause of death is critical to only 26 objectives. There are no death-with-dignity objectives that examine such issues as the number of people attached to life support systems who do not want life support. Among the health objectives for the nation, should more or less emphasis be placed on the prevention of death? Why might death with dignity be a public health issue?

The Biological Perspective

From a biological perspective, death is a natural event that happens to all living things. Animals and plants are created, live, and, with age, wither and die. When a once-living creature is dead, it no longer breathes, moves, or perceives the world around it. It no longer experiences sensations such as heat, cold, pain, or happiness.

A biological definition of death may address the irreversible loss of all body functions. According to the traditional biological definition, death takes place when spontaneous cardiac or respiratory activity ceases—that is, when heartbeat and breathing stop.

Medical advances have made this definition obsolete because with the help of a respirator, or breathing machine, a person can "live" indefinitely. Breathing is controlled by the brain, so if a person no longer has brain activity, then he or she is called **brain dead.**

In 1968, the Harvard Medical School Ad Hoc Committee to Examine the Definition of Brain Death developed criteria that base death on cessation of brain activity rather than on functioning of the heart and lungs. The Harvard criteria call for confirming—and reconfirming twenty-four hours later—total unresponsiveness in the patient, including a flat reading on an **electroencephalogram (EEG),** which measures brain activity. After such reconfirmation, family and hospital staff are notified and death may be declared. At that point, the respirator is removed and the artificial breathing ceases. The criteria have been adopted by several states and have been the basis of numerous court decisions.

To date, no consensus exists on the biological definition of death, and it remains one of the great ethical controversies facing the nation.

Critical Thinking Question

> The study of death and dying has always been controversial. The prevention of death has been a primary goal of public health. Untimely death, such as that of a child, is often viewed as the ultimate loss. At the same time, the death penalty is an option in nearly forty states and is a part of federal law. Likewise, death can be a goal during war. In other words, some forms of death are socially acceptable—others are not. To what extent is the social acceptability of death a matter of culture? Of nurture? Of nature?

The Legal Perspective

The difference between the biological and legal perspectives on death is a bit fuzzy because they both hinge on the same question, "When does death take place?" Medical and technological advances have significantly clouded the legal perspective on death by allowing persons to remain technically alive, despite biological or religious beliefs that they are dead. An estimated 5,000 to 10,000 Americans in a persistent vegetative state are kept alive with machinery that helps them breathe, eat, and remove bodily wastes. A person in a vegetative state is completely unresponsive and has no awareness of his or her environment. But is this living? Physicians, lawyers, judges, ethicists, and family members have debated the issue, but the legalities of the right to die are still unclear. Families have sought the answer to this question in state courts, and the case of Nancy Cruzan went to the U.S. Supreme Court.

In 1983, when she was twenty-five years old, Nancy Cruzan was in a serious automobile accident. Her car went off the road and rolled over several times. She was tossed into a watery ditch, face down. Her heart stopped. It was at least fourteen and possibly twenty minutes before paramedics were able to restart her heart and lungs. After four minutes without oxygen, the brain begins to deteriorate. By the time they initiated life support, the paramedics could not undo the damage to her brain.

Nancy survived but never regained consciousness and remained in a vegetative state. She lay awake, but not aware, for many years in a Missouri nursing home. Convinced that she would not have wanted to be kept alive under such circumstances, her parents requested that her feeding tube be removed. They argued that her constitutional right to privacy included her right to die. The Supreme Court heard the case in 1990 and ruled against it based on the fact that more evidence was needed of Nancy Cruzan's desires not to be kept alive under such circumstances. The Cruzan family was subsequently able to reconstruct discussions with Nancy before her accident that confirmed her desires not to stay alive on mechanical devices. The feeding tube was removed and she died soon after.

The Religious Perspective

From a religious perspective, death may be considered the irreversible loss of the soul from the body—a necessary event in the passing of the soul from its existence on earth to an existence elsewhere. An afterlife, or heaven, is part of the religious perspective on death.

Some religions describe afterlife in concrete terms. Other religions have an ambiguous image of an afterlife state but nonetheless hold a firm belief that there is something more after death. The confidence that an afterlife exists greatly influences the personal and social behavior of the living.

The death of a person is often celebrated through a religious service, a funeral. Funerals provide a means of showing respect for the deceased. They also provide a means of celebrating the person's life by allowing kind words and fond memories to take center stage. Following a religious funeral, a religious burial is conducted in accordance with tradition and ritual handed down by generations. For more on the religious perspective on death, read the Cultural View box.

Euthanasia

Due to complex medical technology advances, not only the moment of death but also the manner of dying have increasingly become a matter of choice. And, as with other choices, the morality and legality of end-of-life decisions are hotly

brain dead A state that occurs when there is no longer brain activity.

electroencephalogram (EEG) A device that measures brain activity.

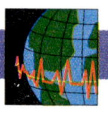

CULTURAL VIEW

Religious Traditions about Death

What happens to human beings after death? Every religion has an answer to this important question. And while the answers are different, they all have this in common: The belief that there is some kind of life after death. It may be the Christian belief of death and resurrection or the Buddhist belief in the rebirth of the soul to another person.

The hope that life in some way goes on seems to be an almost instinctive response among people since human history began. Just as there are enduring beliefs about the afterlife, there are funeral rites in every culture that mark the transition between the two phases of existence.

Paying Respect

Until modern times, funerals in all known societies were religious rites. In the Western world, there is a small but growing trend toward secular rites. This trend emphasizes the universal human need to respond to the disruption caused by death, even among those who are not religious. Funerals are a means of showing respect for the dead, while at the same time providing an occasion for mourners to express their grief and find comfort from friends and family members.

The mourning period after death is well defined in several religions. It is set aside as a special time to express grief, so that the survivors can gradually disentangle themselves from the deceased and eventually continue with their lives unencumbered by unresolved relationships.

Thousands of years before the development of modern psychology, Judaism defined four phases of mourning that are very similar to the cycle of bereavement and the modern insights about the benefits of expressing grief rather than the repressing it. At the end of the mourning period, Jews are expected to get back to business as usual, and Jewish tradition chides anyone who mourns beyond the prescribed period.

Burial Traditions

While Jews bury their dead as soon as possible, in a plain shroud and wooden coffin to level distinction of wealth at the time of the funeral, Christian burials in the United States have become expensive and elaborate, leading to a barrage of criticism.

The common practice of a wake, where the face is made up and the body is embalmed and viewed in a comfortable-looking coffin, is regarded as reinforcing the denial of death, because the corpse is made to appear as if it is only sleeping.

---

passive euthanasia Indirect action taken to bring about death, such as withholding something needed by a dying person to sustain life.

active euthanasia Direct action taken to bring about death, such as taking a dying person off life supports.

physician-assisted suicide A form of active euthanasia in which the patient is allowed to bring about his or her own death by self-administering a lethal drug provided by the physician.

debated. Contributing to the debate have been the activities of Michigan physician Jack Kevorkian, sometimes called "Dr. Death" due to his persistence in assisting patients with suicide despite legal restrictions to the contrary. As of 1997, Kevorkian has acknowledged assisting more than sixty patients who had chronic and painful conditions to terminate their lives with a lethal injection device. His actions have made the issue of euthanasia one of national interest.

The term *euthanasia* has a Greek origin meaning "good death." It refers to ending a person's life when that person's life quality has declined so that death presents a better option than continuing to live. Cancer patients, for example, may be unable to relieve the intense pain resulting from their terminal disease. Rather than continuing to live in pain, they often consider euthanasia as a positive choice.

Euthanasia can be either passive or active. In both cases, the goal is bringing about death with dignity. **Passive euthanasia,** the more common of the two, involves withholding something needed to maintain life, such as not putting a dying person on a respirator. **Active euthanasia** occurs when action is taken to bring about death—for example, when a dying person wants to be taken off life supports. **Physician-assisted suicide,** the type of euthanasia practiced by Dr. Kevorkian, is a form of active euthanasia in which the patient is allowed to bring

In the United States, burial is most common but cremation is gaining acceptance despite prescriptions against it in the Jewish and Christian faiths. Hindus and Buddhists normally dispose of their dead through cremation. In the Hindu religion, all the relatives of a dead person are looked on as ritually impure and the mourners are secluded from the rest of the world for ten days after the funeral. Daily ceremonies are performed to give the naked soul of the dead person a new spiritual body with which it may pass on to the next life. The soul is reborn after death to live in another body and continue an endless round of birth, death, and rebirth. There are some differences between Buddhist and Hindu beliefs about the transmigration of the soul, but essentially, both religions believe in rebirth.

Unlike Buddhists and Hindus, Muslims bury their dead. They believe in the promise of a paradise where they will be rewarded for faithfulness to Allah and for any suffering they endured in this life.

Among Native American Plains Indians, the most common forms of burial were scaffold and tree burials. In a traditional tree burial the body remained there until it decomposed. Burial grounds were usually avoided by Indians because they feared that the grounds were haunted by spirits of the deceased. At the time of the burial, close relatives would come to linger near the corpse, preparing food for the spirit's journey to the hereafter, which was described as a duplicate of the living world. The hereafter was the place where spirits were reunited with their dead relatives. To show their grief, mourners would often cut their hair short, gash their arms and legs, and blacken their faces. It was also customary for relatives of the dead to give away their belongings to the needy.

Modern Plains Indians, such as the Indians of the Lakota tribe, combine elements of Christian burial with ancient Indian customs. Although the tree or platform burials are no longer allowed, Indians still follow the custom of giving away the deceased's belongings either at the time of death or one year later. Indians still gather one year after the death of a loved one to honor the deceased and release his or her spirit to the hereafter.

Today in the United States and Western Europe, the elaborate apparel of mourning common in the nineteenth century, such as black buntings draped over buildings, arm bands, and widows' weeds (black clothing), have disappeared. This is seen by some as a sign that death has become taboo in our culture and that mourning is considered morbid. Without such outward signs, traditionalists worry that the bereaved will be left to suffer alone, aggravating their sense of loss. Traditions, however, are strongly rooted; those discussed here, and others, are likely to continue in some fashion.

about his or her own death through a lethal injection or other means provided by the physician.

In 1997, the Supreme Court unanimously ruled that there is no constitutional right to die with the aid of a physician. The ruling allows patients to have artificial life supports disconnected, but upholds state laws in Washington and New York that make it a crime for physicians to give lethal drugs to dying patients who want to more quickly end their lives. According to the Court's decision, "When a patient refuses life-sustaining medical treatment, he dies from an underlying fatal disease or pathology, but if a patient ingests lethal medication prescribed by a physician, he is killed by that medication."

The Supreme Court ruling leaves the responsibility of banning or legalizing physician-assisted suicides to each state. In 1994, Oregon became the first state to make it legal for doctors to help terminally ill patients die. There was a ballot initiative in 1997 to repeal the law, which was overwhelmingly defeated: 60 percent voted to keep the death with dignity law. Other states are likely to take some action on this issue.

A recent nationwide poll found that 51 percent of Americans think it should be legal for a physician to help a terminally ill patient commit suicide. And in Kevorkian's home state of Michigan, 56 percent of physicians surveyed recently

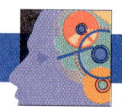

DEVELOPING HEALTH SKILLS

At Issue: Should Doctors Be Allowed to Help Terminally Ill Patients Commit Suicide?

Yes It would be a great comfort to people who face terminal illness to know they could get help to die if their suffering became unbearable. All pain cannot be controlled, and it's arrogant for anybody to say that it can. Quality-of-life decisions are the sole right of the individual.

It's nonsense to say that death shouldn't be part of a doctor's job—it already is. We all die. Death is a part of medicine. One of a doctor's jobs is to write death certificates. So this idea of the doctor as superhealer is a load of nonsense. The fact is that it's not so easy to commit suicide on your own. It's very hard for decent citizens to get deadly drugs. Even if they do, there's the fear that the drugs won't work. There are hundreds of dying people who couldn't lift their hand to their mouth with a cup of coffee, let alone a cup of drugs. They need assistance.

Of course, people who are depressed or who feel they are a weight on their families should be counseled and helped to live. But you have to separate those instances from people who are dying, whose bodies are giving up on them. If you think there is a cure around the corner for your malady, then please wait for it. That is your choice. But sometimes a person realizes that her life is coming to an end, as in the case of my wife, whose doctor said, "There is nothing else we can do."

We're not talking about cases in which a depressed person will come to a doctor and ask to be killed. Under the law the Hemlock Society is trying to get passed, the doctor must say no to depressed people. A candidate for assisted suicide has to be irreversibly, terminally, hopelessly ill and judged to be so by two doctors.

Derek Humphrey is the founder of the Hemlock Society and author of Final Exit, *a book advising terminally ill people on how to commit suicide.*

No If it's a question of someone's wanting the right to die, I say jump off a building. But as soon as you bring in somebody else to help you, it changes the equation. Suicide is legally available to people in this country. Just don't ask a doctor to help you do it. That would violate the traditions of medicine and raise doubts about the role of the physician.

One of my worries is that people will be manipulated by a doctor's suggesting suicide. A lot of seriously ill people already feel they're a burden because they're costing their families money. It would be easy for a family to insinuate, "While we love you, Grandmother, and we're willing to spend all our money and not send the kids to college, wouldn't it be better if…?" There is no coercion there, but you build on somebody's guilt. We'd have a whole new class of people considering suicide who hadn't thought about it before.

Then, too, I don't believe that you could successfully regulate this practice. The relationship between the doctor and the patient begins in confidentiality. If they decide together that they don't want anybody to know, there is no way the government can regulate it. The presumption is that physicians would only be helping people commit suicide after everything else had failed to end their suffering. But a lot of people won't want to be that far along. None of the proposed regulations take into account a person who is not suffering now, but who says, "I don't want to suffer in the future. Let me commit suicide now." I can imagine a doctor who would say, "Yes, we're going to make sure that you don't have to suffer at all."

Daniel Callahan is a bioethicist and director of the Hastings Center, a medical ethics think tank in Briarcliff Manor, New York.

Source: "Should Doctors Be Allowed to Help Terminally Ill Patients Commit Suicide?" *Health,* May–June 1993, p. 22. Reprinted by permission of Time Inc. Health

said they support allowing a doctor to help a patient commit suicide. The American Medical Association is against physician-assisted suicide, but has recently promulgated guidelines to help people die with dignity. What is your position on this? See the Developing Health Skills box to gain added insight.

Living Will Declaration

Declaration made ___(enter date)___ ,
I, ___(your name)___ being of sound mind, willfully and voluntarily make known my desires that my dying shall not be artificially prolonged under the circumstances set forth below, and do declare:

If at any time I should have an incurable injury, disease or illness certified to be a terminal condition by two physicians who have personally examined me, one of whom shall be my attending physician, and the physicians have determined that my death will occur whether or not life-sustaining procedures are utilized and where the application of life-sustaining procedures would serve only to artificially prolong the dying process, I direct that such procedures be withheld or withdrawn, and that I be permitted to die naturally with only the administration of medication or the performance of any medical procedure deemed necessary to provide me with comfort care or to alleviate pain.

OTHER DIRECTIONS:

In the absence of my ability to give directions regarding the use of such life-sustaining procedures, it is my intention that this declaration shall be honored by my family and physician(s) as the final expression of my legal right to refuse medical or surgical treatment and accept the consequences from such refusal.

I understand the full import of this declaration and am emotionally and mentally competent to make this declaration.

_____
_____
_____
_____

(Your signature and address)

I believe the declarant to be of sound mind. I did not sign the declarant's signature above for or at the direction of the declarant. I am at least 18 years of age, and am not related to the declarant by blood or marriage, entitled to any portion of the estate of the declarant according to the laws of interstate succession of ___(name state)___ or under any will of declarant or codicil thereto, or directly financially responsible for the declarant's medical care. I am not the declarant's attending physician, an employee of the attending physician or an employee of the health facility in which the declarant is a patient.

_____
_____

(signatures of two witnesses)

Figure 19.1 Living Will. *This signed and witnessed declaration lets physicians and family know your wishes about using life-sustaining procedures.*

A federal law took effect in 1991 that ensured that every adult patient entering a hospital, nursing home, or hospice be told about the right to choose—and refuse—treatment in the event of terminal or incapacitating illness. Since then, patients are asked if they have a **living will** or other written declaration about what happens if they become unable to make decisions about their own medical care (see Figure 19.1). Such a written declaration is called an **advance medical directive.** An advance medical directive allows you to stipulate under what conditions you wish and no longer wish to have medical treatment, including artificial life supports such as respirators or intravenous feeding, in the event that you cannot express these preferences to physicians or relatives. If an individual does not have an advanced medical directive and wants one, the hospital can provide the appropriate form. You can modify the form in any way you choose and add any conditions you like as long as they comply with the laws in your state.

The Patient Self-Determination Act was designed to ease medical decision making and reduce the needless prolonging of death in hopeless cases. It does not change the situation of anyone without an existing advance medical directive. An advance medical directive can be brought about by preparing a living will, or a person may give such decision-making authority to a relative or friend through a **durable power of attorney for health care** document. Traditionally, power of attorney is used to empower someone to handle your finances and make other legal decisions. A durable power of attorney for health care names a representative to speak for you about your health care if you are unable to do so. This representative does not have to be an attorney but rather can be anyone you name. For your own sake, this person should be someone who is aware of your wishes and understands what is and would be important to you if you were in a vegetative state or otherwise unable to make health-related decisions.

It is important to let your family physician and family members know that you have an advance medical directive that you want followed. They should also

living will A will that stipulates which medical treatments are and are not to be used in the final days of life.

advance medical directive A person's written declaration about what should happen if he or she becomes unable to make decisions about his or her own medical care.

durable power of attorney for health care A document that identifies a representative to speak for a person about his or her health care if the person is unable to do so.

be aware of your durable power of attorney for health care. Such documentation should be kept as part of your medical records. A recent study of nearly 5,000 terminally ill patients found that most did not have directives, and of those who did, their physicians knew about it only 25 percent of the time. Medic Alert Foundation, which markets bracelets for people with chronic illnesses, recently began allowing users to keep on file their preferences for end-of-life treatment. A Notice to Health Care Providers card is another way to protect yourself. Make up a card like the one shown in Figure 19.2 and carry it where it can be found, such as with your driver's license.

Critical Thinking Question

Opponents of euthanasia raise the argument that voluntary euthanasia may "slip" into involuntary euthanasia. In other words, there is no way of assuring that a person's choice to end his or her life is "firm" or that a physician is truly acting on the patient's wishes. Therefore, they argue, euthanasia should be illegal. Can you propose a way of assuring that euthanasia remains voluntary and does not "slip" into involuntary action? What would constitute a "slip"?

Death as Seen throughout the Life Cycle

How a person perceives death also relates to how old he or she is. Very young children view death as a departure or sleep-like state that is reversible. They are unable to comprehend the permanence of death and believe that the person who died will eventually wake up and play with them again. Starting at about age five, children begin to understand death but tend to blame it on an external force, such as a "bogeyman." This permits them to believe they can avoid death by outsmarting or running away from the bogeyman. Psychologists believe that by age nine, children comprehend that death is part of the life cycle and that all things eventually die, including themselves.

Figure 19.2 Notice to Health Care Providers. *Fill out and carry a card like this along with your driver's license. It is one way to make sure people know about your health care decisions.*

Notice to Health Care Providers

I, _____ , have appointed:
(your name)

_____
(agent's name)

_____
(address)

Phone: _____ _____
(day) (evening)

as my agent to make health and personal care decisions for me if I am unable to do so. He/she has a copy of my complete health care power of attorney.

_____ _____
(date) (signature)

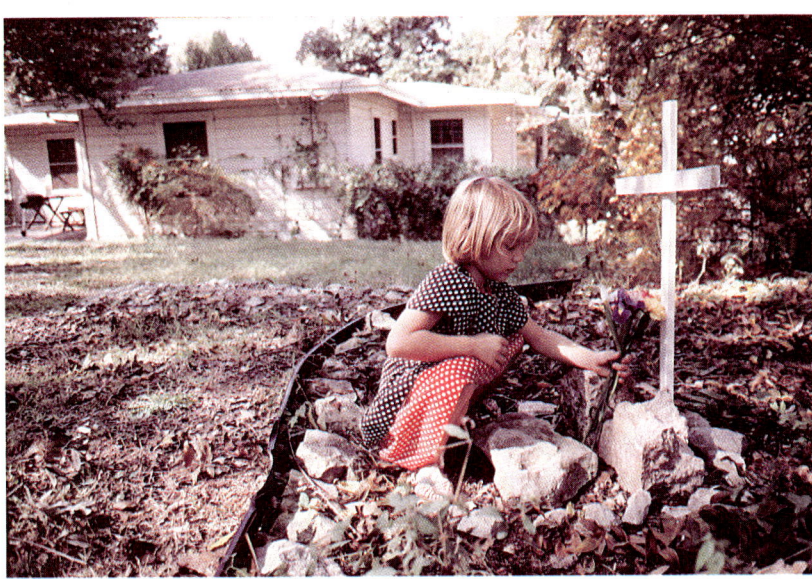

Laying flowers at a pet's backyard grave is a meaningful experience for this youngster. Children begin to understand the concept of death at about age five. (Source: The Image Works/ © John Moore)

Adolescence is a period of intense growth, development, independent expression, and experimentation. Teenagers have a sense of invincibility, which in part contributes to self-destructive behaviors such as smoking, drug abuse, and reckless driving. When a classmate dies, most teenagers are ill prepared to confront that death.

For young adults aged eighteen to twenty-two, understanding death may be a factor of experience. An eighteen-year-old who matures late and is exposed to little or no death among family members or classmates may know about death only from the movies, television, or newspaper stories. Risk-taking behavior for this person may continue with little concern for the so-called frailty of life, and his or her understanding of death is closer to that of an older adolescent—"it couldn't happen to me" or "that is someone else's problem." Another eighteen-year-old may have a completely different attitude about death if he or she has lost a best friend to a drunk driving accident or a relative to a terminal disease. Young adults gradually learn to accept that the longer they live, the more they are exposed to death.

With adulthood comes a more philosophical attitude toward death. In part, this is because most adults have given thought to the age-old question, What is the meaning of life? Although adults recognize the inevitability of their own deaths, they assume that it will happen much later in life—during old age. The death of their own parents seriously confronts them with their own mortality. Interestingly, risk-taking behavior tends to subside as this sense of mortality increases.

The longer a person lives, the more often he or she is confronted with the death of family and friends. A study of attitudes toward death among the elderly showed that about 45 percent of older people are optimistic about life and only 10 percent are actually fearful of dying. The rest repress thoughts about dying, just as younger people do.

As to the quality of life of older people near the end of life, the news is encouraging. Based on findings from the National Institute of Aging's Last Day of Life Study, which involved interviews with close family members of elderly people who had recently died, researchers found that most older people were in excellent health a year before they died; as many as 11 percent felt they were in

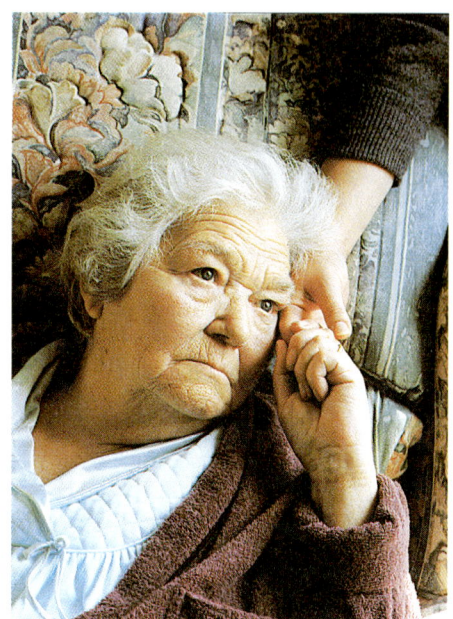

For a small percentage of elders, later adulthood can be a pensive time as they reflect on the past. The support of family and friends is particularly important during these times. (Source: © Tony Stone Images/Ian Shaw)

good health the day before they died. They also were not left alone to die, as many older people fear: 99 percent of the elderly saw various members of their families in the last three days of their lives.

Dying as a Process

Death is a state. Dying, on the other hand, is a process. At what point in life do we begin the process of dying? Some people say that the process of dying begins at birth. This is a way of suggesting that everyone will die at one time or another but it tells very little about the actual process of dying. A more functional understanding of the dying process suggests that dying begins with the diagnosis of a terminal disease or condition and continues until the point of death. The time between the diagnosis and death is called the **living–dying interval.**

A twenty-year-old person who is diagnosed with a brain tumor, for example, may be given two or three years to live. That person's living–dying interval begins when he or she is informed of the tumor and ends with death. On the other hand, a twenty-year-old in a fatal automobile accident has a brief living–dying interval—perhaps lasting only a few hours or even seconds.

It is important to remember that aging is not dying. Aging is the process of growing older; dying is the process leading to death, and it happens to people of all ages.

Stages of Dying

Although everyone would prefer to be healthy and not sick, studies show that more than 80 percent of the people asked say they would want to know if they were dying when they are very ill to enable them to better prepare for their own deaths.

Psychiatrist Elisabeth Kübler-Ross said that the issue is not whether patients should be told they are dying but rather how to tell them this news. For example, a physician can tell a patient that he or she has an incurable disease but still give a window of time for living. A patient might feel hopeful if he or she knew that 60 percent of the people with the same illness live as long as three to five years.

living–dying interval The time between the diagnosis of a terminal condition and death.

denial The stage of dying in which the person does not believe that death is going to happen to him or her.

anger The stage of dying in which the person is angry at almost anything.

bargaining The stage of dying in which the person bargains for more time.

depression The stage of dying in which anger is replaced with a sense of loss.

acceptance The stage of dying in which the person understands that death is inevitable.

hospice A specialized health care program, usually for the last weeks or months of life, emphasizing the management of pain and other symptoms associated with terminal illness, in contrast to treatment.

Hope is crucial for coping with dying. Hope helps sustain the dying person through the days, weeks, or months of suffering. In her classic book, *On Death and Dying*, Kübler-Ross delineated five stages that terminal patients go through in accepting the fact that they are dying. Hope usually persists throughout all these stages.

The first stage is **denial**—"No, it can't be happening to me." One patient is convinced that her mammograms were mixed up with someone else's and that she does not have breast cancer. Another wants to get a better explanation of his problems in the hope that the first physician's diagnosis was wrong. In this period of denial, the patient is still in shock and cannot believe that he or she is going to die.

The second stage is **anger**—anger at almost anything. The patient is angry at the physician for giving him or her the diagnosis or for not having a cure. The patient is angry with relatives and friends because they will live long after he or she is dead. The patient is angry at other patients who aren't as sick or who are responding better to experimental treatments. And the patient is often angry at God for giving him or her such an illness.

At some point, the patient reaches the third stage, **bargaining**, when he or she bargains for a little more time. "Let me live long enough to graduate from college," or, "Give me just a few days without pain." If this "wish" is granted, the patient usually bargains for more time again. One woman wanted only to live long enough to see her eldest son married. She was taught self-hypnosis so that she would be able to be comfortable for several hours—the length of time she needed to attend the wedding. After the wedding, she was both exhilarated and exhausted and said to the physician: "Now don't forget I have another son."

Depression is the fourth stage of accepting death. This sets in when the patient can no longer deny that he or she is dying and can no longer bargain for extra time. The reality is sinking in, and the anger that had been experienced earlier is replaced with sadness and a sense of loss. This is called a preparatory depression—preparatory for the final separation from this world.

The final stage is **acceptance**, when the patient understands that he or she is dying. When patients accept death, it is often a painful time for the survivors, who may misinterpret it as a rejection of their caring efforts. But how could someone ever be ready to die and, at the same time, continue to hold onto meaningful relationships? With acceptance, the struggle is over and, as one patient put it, it is time for "the final rest before the long journey."

Patients who have worked through these stages of the dying process are able to detach themselves slowly and peacefully and more or less come to terms with their fate. It is important to note that these stages are not universally experienced—some people never accept the fact that they are dying. And, when the stages are experienced, they do not necessarily occur in lock-step fashion. Some individuals accept the fact that they are dying long before they bargain for more time.

Hospice: Comfort for the Dying

Because dying is a process and not an event, where do people go when they are dying and what do they do? At the onset of the living–dying interval, most people continue with their regular daily activities—going to school, to work, caring for their children, mowing the lawn. But as the illness progresses, pain increases and physical limitations set in. The three greatest fears of a dying person are fear of pain, fear of loss of control, and fear of isolation and abandonment.

Hospice care is designed to lessen these three major fears and to help the dying person live as fully as possible. Hospice is a specialized health care program emphasizing the management of pain and other symptoms associated with terminal illness. It is palliative, not curative. This means that the goal of hospice

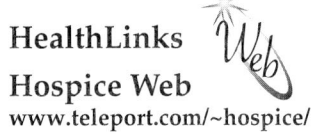

HealthLinks
Hospice Web
www.teleport.com/~hospice/
A link to numerous resources for and information about hospice care, including a link to similar resources and a listing of hospices around the country.

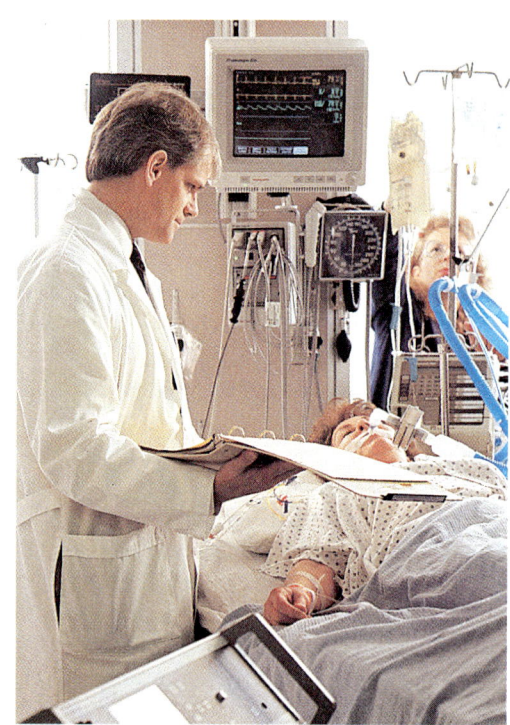

As an alternative to being hooked up to monitors and receiving treatment as they die, many people choose the hospice alternative—palliative care at home surrounded by family and close friends. (Source: © Tony Stone Images/Stewart Cohen)

care is not to correct the terminal condition and thus save the life of the ill person. Rather, the goal is to relieve the pain and suffering associated with the dying process. Hospice care provides support to the family as well as to the patient. In the middle ages, a hospice was a way station for travelers. It comes from the Latin words *hospes*, which means "host" or "guest," and *hospitum*, which means "hospitality."

Most hospice care is received at home, but there are also special inpatient hospice facilities. Typically, a hospice program offers support services to patients and families through a team of professionals, including physicians, registered nurses, therapists, home health aides, social workers, chaplains, and volunteers. This team effort addresses not only physical distress but also any emotional, social, financial, or spiritual problems that may be troubling the patient or family.

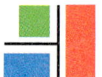 **TABLE 19.1** Who Gets Hospice Care Services

Primary diagnosis	Percent
Cancer	58.6%
Cardiovascular diseases	12.7
Alzheimer's and other degenerative diseases of the central nervous system	6.7
Chronic lung diseases	6.6
Kidney failure	3.2
Infectious diseases	3.1
AIDS	3.1
All other diagnoses	6.0

Source: National Center for Health Statistics

bereaved Survivors of a recently deceased person who experience a sense of loss and grief.

Hospice care is highly personalized, and patients and their families can play an important role. Volunteers are particularly helpful for family members who need to continue with their own lives while assuming the responsibilities of twenty-four-hour home care for their loved ones.

Hospice care is truly end-of-life care. Patients include those in the last stages of diseases such as cancer or other terminal illnesses such as AIDS (see Table 19.1). The average length of care is 50 days—less than two months. A person who leaves hospice care almost always does so by dying, surrounded by family members and in the familiar home setting.

For Survivors: A Time of Decisions and Bereavement

Coping with the death of a loved one does not stop with the death itself. The **bereaved,** or the survivors of the recently deceased person, are left to plan the funeral, handle financial matters, and, above all, work through the grieving process. This is not as simple as it might appear because grieving family mem-

National Kidney Foundation
Please detatch and give this portion
of the card to your family.

This is to inform you that, should the occasion ever arise, I would like to be an organ and tissue donor. Please see that my wishes are carried out by informing the attending medical personnel that I have indicated my wishes to become a donor.
Thank you.

Signature Date

For further information write or call:
National Kidney Foundation
30 East 33rd Street, New York, NY 10016
(800) 622-9010

Uniform Donor Card

of ____________________
(print or type name of donor)

In the hope that I may help others, I hereby make this anatomical gift, if medically acceptable, to take effect upon my death. The words and marks below indicate my wishes.

I give: ☐ any needed organs or parts
☐ only the following organs or parts

specify the organ(s), tissue(s) or part(s)

for the purposes of transplantation, therapy, medical research or education;
☐ my body for anatomical study if needed.

Limitations or special wishes, if any: __________

Figure 19.3 Uniform Donor Card. *By signing a uniform donor card to donate body parts upon death, the gift of life can be a part of death.*

HERE'S LOOKING AT YOU

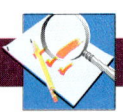

What Do You Know about Organ Donation?

How much do you know about organ donation in the United States? For example, did you know that 83 percent of patients that have had heart transplants live for at least one year after transplantation, and 75 percent live for at least three years? Take the following quiz to see how up-to-date you are on these important issues.

1. How many people in the United States die each year because of the shortage of organs for transplantation?
   a. 200
   b. 800
   c. 1,200
   d. 2,800
2. Which of these is NOT transplanted?
   a. Cornea
   b. Large intestine
   c. Pancreas
   d. Tendon
   e. Lung
3. Which religion opposes organ donation?
   a. Catholicism
   b. Judaism
   c. Greek Orthodox
   d. Islam
   e. Jehovah's Witness
   f. None of the major world religions opposes organ donation
4. How many lives can be saved when one person agrees to donate organs?
   a. 1 or 2
   b. Up to 4
   c. 6 or more
   d. Up to 50
5. True or False: Most organ transplants go to the wealthy.
6. True or False: My doctors will not try as hard to save me if they know my organs will be used to save 6 people if I die.
7. What is the most important thing to do if you want to donate your organs after your death?
   a. Write out a last will and testament
   b. Fill out an organ donor card
   c. Tell your family
   d. Write a living will
8. On average, a new name is added to the national waiting list for organs every:
   a. 2 days
   b. 8 hours
   c. 18 minutes
   d. 45 seconds
9. The first successful human kidney transplant was in:
   a. 1902 (Vienna, Austria)
   b. 1933 (Ukraine, USSR)
   c. 1954 (Boston, Massachusetts)
   d. 1968 (Stanford, California)
10. True or False: Transplanting livers to people that abused their own liver is unethical.

ANSWER:

1. **d.** Despite the fact that nine out of ten people in this country support the concept of organ donation, organs are donated less than one third of the time. Since not enough organs are donated, eight people die each day waiting for organs.
2. **b.** Large intestine
3. **f.** All the major religions permit, allow, and support transplantation and organ donation. For Jehovah's Witnesses, donation is a matter of individual conscience with the provision that all

---

HealthLinks
TransWeb
www.transweb.org/
A site dedicated to organ transplantation and donation.

bers must make important decisions. Some people have written specific directions in their wills about how to dispose of their bodies, what kind of casket to buy, and what hymns to sing at their funerals. Such planning allows family members to proceed as smoothly as possible in following these wishes.

Decisions about the Body

There are several decisions that have to be made right away about the physical remains of a body. One of the first is whether or not you want to donate any organs for medical or research purposes. Many body parts can be transplanted

organs are drained of blood prior to transplantation.
4. c. The lungs can be transplanted individually to two patients, the heart to another patient, the liver to yet another, and the kidneys to two others. The pancreas and small bowel may also be used. In addition, many other patients may have their lives improved by corneal transplants, heart valves, bone and tendon grafts, and skin grafts.
5. **FALSE.** In 1984 the U.S. Congress passed the National Organ Transplant Act that mandated the establishment of a national organ procurement and transplantation network to equitably and fairly distribute organs. The United Network for Organ Sharing (UNOS) was then formed to undertake the responsibility of administering this network. It is illegal in the United States to buy or sell human organs. UNOS expends great effort to ensure that organ allocation is not prejudiced along racial, economic, geographical, gender, or any other basis.
6. **FALSE.** The medical care provided to patients is not affected by whether organ donation is planned or not. Organ donation does not occur until after one is declared dead. In order to preserve organs for transplantation it is absolutely necessary to give the best medical care possible to the patient prior to death.
7. c. The single most important thing to do if you want to donate organs is to tell your family. The next of kin have the responsibility of giving permission for organ donation once death has occurred. If they know your feelings on the matter they will be able carry out your wishes. Organ donor cards are important, but even in states where they legally override the wishes of the next of kin, they often can't be found in time to make a difference. Although a will is important to have for many reasons, wills may be difficult to locate, they are commonly not read for several days following death, and they have to be authenticated before they are acted upon. A Living Will is meant to indicate how you want medical care to be given in the event that you are unable to make decisions. It is for when you are still living but incapacitated, not for when you have died.
8. c. 29,000 new patients are added to the waiting list for organ transplants each year. This is equivalent to 2,400 new patients waiting every month.
9. c. 1954 (Boston, Mass.) Dr. Joseph E. Murray performed a kidney transplant from one woman to her identical twin in 1954. Dr. Murray received the Nobel Prize in Medicine for this accomplishment.
10. **FALSE.** This is an incorrect concept based on both medical principles and general concepts of justice. For example, alcohol use is not always associated with liver disease. Many people consume excessive alcohol for their lifetime without developing liver disease. No one understands who is predisposed to liver disease due to alcohol consumption, but it is clear that some people develop liver failure after consuming four drinks a day. Since liver transplants are life-saving, it is the same as sentencing patients to death if they are denied liver transplantation as an option. Nevertheless, if the primary disease (alcohol dependence) is not in remission, liver transplantation is withheld.

Source: Excerpted from "How Much Do You Know About Organ Donation in the United States?" an online quiz from TransWeb: All About Transportation and Donation (www.transweb.org)

immediately following death and give life to others. These organs and tissues include bone, bone marrow, eye, heart, kidney, liver, lung, pancreas, and skin. By signing a uniform donor card (see Figure 19.3), a person over age eighteen can agree to donate all or part of his or her body upon death. If no plans were made to donate organs prior to the death, family members can make this decision afterwards. Time is crucial in this process because the organs must be removed soon after the death, before they deteriorate. The Here's Looking at You box tests your knowledge about organ donation.

Depending upon the circumstances of death, some families may request an **autopsy,** a surgical postmortem examination of the body to determine cause of

autopsy A surgical examination of the body to determine the cause of death.

death. This information can be useful in learning more about sudden, unexplained deaths, in investigating infectious diseases that may be harmful to the public, and as evidence in legal proceedings and for insurance purposes. An autopsy can include examining tissue; checking for drugs, chemicals, or toxic substances; looking for bacteria and other causes of infection; and performing other tests. Organs can still be donated after an autopsy is performed.

Some people wish to have the body embalmed. **Embalming** is the use of chemicals, internally and externally, to temporarily preserve the body for open casket viewing and/or if the body has to be sent to a distant destination for burial. Embalming is not required in all states. It is often presented to the grief-stricken as needed but may be an unnecessary added expense. Another option that is becoming more acceptable is **cremation,** or having the body burned. Cremated remains can be privately scattered, scattered at sea, scattered by airplane in unpopulated areas, kept by the family in an urn at home, entombed in a niche in a special vault for urns called a **columbarium,** or buried in a cemetery.

In 1965, fewer than 4 percent of the deceased in the United States were cremated; today, more than 20 percent are cremated. An even greater percentage of Americans say they want to be cremated. Forty percent of people surveyed said they would choose cremation for themselves or their loved ones because they want to save money (25 percent) or land (17 percent), it is convenient or simple (13 percent), and they don't want the body in the earth (11 percent). People said they reject the idea of cremation for reasons including not believing in it (36 percent), religious objections (12 percent), and not wanting the body destroyed (3 percent).

Planning a Funeral

At the same time that decisions are being made about what to do with the body, the family must also make funeral plans. The funeral is a ceremony connected with burying or cremating the dead. This is a time-honored ceremony, and anthropologists who have studied different cultures generally agree that all civilizations show some evidence of honoring the dead with a funeral.

A funeral is an important aspect of a death because it provides family and friends the opportunity to celebrate the life of the deceased and to offer support to the bereaved. It also brings a sense of closure to that person's life. A eulogy delivered by a close friend can be a meaningful way to express these feelings. Religious and cultural rituals—an Irish wake, the Jewish seven-day mourning period of *shiva*—also provide opportunities to share grieving.

Most people choose to be buried in a cemetery. Family members can select a wide array of caskets from a simple pine box to an ornate copper or bronze one. Selecting a headstone and the epitaph to go on it is another decision that the family must make. This is usually done months after the burial.

A Time of Bereavement

During this time, the most difficult issue at hand for loved ones of the deceased is dealing with **grief,** the deep sadness caused by a loss. **Bereavement** is the period during which a sense of loss is felt as a result of the death of a loved one. Both grief and bereavement suggest a state of feeling that varies in intensity.

Mourning is another word used to mean expressing grief at someone's death, for example, by wearing black clothes. It is also a period during which the family mourns the dead. The length of time a family mourns and the behaviors they exhibit in this period are usually defined in cultural terms. An example of cultural mourning is an Irish wake to "celebrate" the deceased person's life.

Having a well-written and up-to-date will can ease matters considerably. If you wish to be cremated or buried in a simple pine box, for example, these

---

embalming The use of chemicals, internally and externally, to temporarily preserve the body for open casket viewing and/or transportation.

cremation The burning of a dead body into ashes.

columbarium A special vault for urns containing ashes of cremated bodies.

grief A deep sadness caused by a loss.

bereavement The period during which a sense of loss is felt owing to the death of a loved one.

mourning Expressing grief at someone's death.

impact The stage of bereavement in which loved ones react with shock, disbelief, and denial.

recoil The stage of bereavement in which the bereaved superficially carry on and try to return to normal.

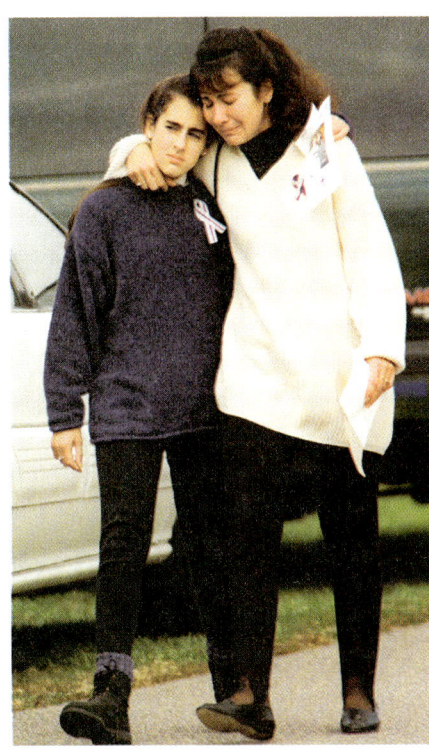

For survivors, there are emotional stages of grieving, starting with the impact of hearing the news to recovery to a more normal life without the person. During the early stages of grieving, family members and friends need support from each other. (Source: The Image Works/Stephen D. Cannerelli)

instructions should be in your will and not left to family members to decide or debate. No matter how much thought and preparation are given to the tasks that follow death, coping with the death of a loved one takes time.

The grieving process is much like the dying process; they both involve stages of gradual adaptation to loss. For the dying person, the loss is permanent. The grievers, however, must adapt to this loss and return to leading their lives much as they did before. In many ways, of course, life will never be the same without the person who died.

Although there are three basic stages of bereavement—impact, recoil, and recovery—in actuality, the stages are not as sharply delineated. People handle these stages quite differently, and they frequently shift back and forth among stages to meet the needs of the moment.

The **impact** of the news of the death of a loved one is usually met with shock, disbelief, and denial, even when the person has been sick and was expected to die. Such reactions may last only a few minutes or may linger for several weeks. This period of shock provides the bereaved with a buffer from reality in order to make an adjustment that is needed—accepting the loss of a loved one and life without him or her.

The second stage of the grieving process is a long period of **recoil,** during which the bereaved find themselves in a vacuum, superficially carrying on and trying to return to normal. One mother, for example, set a place at the table for her teenage son for months after he died of leukemia. There is no longer a "normal" for the bereaved family. New norms have to be established.

During this stage, which can last for as long as a year, grievers feel continued sadness and despair and are usually preoccupied with thoughts about the deceased person. There is great variability at this time, and grievers can become irritable, angry, restless, and depressed. This period is best described as a series of steps forward and backward. Only time appears to increase the steps forward and reduce the number of slides backward. It is important to point out that slid-

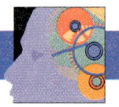

DEVELOPING HEALTH SKILLS

How to Help a Friend

Many people feel uncomfortable and awkward calling or visiting a friend who is grieving. But if you really care for your friend, you can help by the simple act of communicating your feelings of shared grief and concern.

- *Get in touch.* Call, write, or visit and let your friend know your concern.
- *Attend to practical matters.* You might be needed to call people and let them know when the funeral will take place. This kind of help can create a special bond.
- *Encourage others to visit or help.* Call on your network of friends to help out. You might want to schedule some visits so that everyone doesn't come at once in the beginning and then no one comes later on. Ask people to prepare food.
- *Be a good listener.* Your friend might want to talk emotionally about the deceased. But don't force conversation. Be prepared to accept silence. It is better than aimless chatter.
- *Don't tell the bereaved how he or she feels.* Good friends think they are helping with statements such as, "I know you must feel relieved now that your mother is out of pain."
- *Do not probe for details about the death.* If your friend offers information, listen with understanding.
- *Encourage postponing major decisions.* Wait until after the period of intense grief. Whatever can wait should wait. In time, draw your friend into quiet outside activities. Some people do not have the initiative to go out on their own.
- *When your friend returns to activities, treat him or her as a normal person.* Acknowledge your friend's loss, but don't dwell on it.

---

ing backward is not bad, and, in fact, may be necessary in order for the bereaved to deal with many intense feelings.

The third stage usually takes place within twelve to fifteen months after the death when the bereaved person begins **recovery** from the loss and shows signs of returning to a more normal life. This stage does not mean that he or she no longer grieves. Indeed, grief for the deceased person can last for years. Loss of a loved one can be particularly intense at the time of the person's birthday or when the family gets together to celebrate holidays. Overall, the stage of recovery signals an acceptance of the person's death and is characterized by fewer and fewer bouts with despair. Gradually, the bereaved builds a new life. See the Developng Health Skills box about how to help a friend grieve.

Loss as a Creative Force

Facing death, whether a close friend's or your own, is seldom easy. With preparation, however, thanatologists believe that the loss experience of death can be a creative force for the living. They suggest that preparation for death involves attempting to answer several questions. They emphasize that it is not as important to reach answers to the questions as it is to become involved in the process of seeking answers. When facing death, the following questions may be important:

- What do I believe about life and about death?
- Is there purpose in my living? What is life all about?
- Is there more to life than what I have perceived thus far?
- What happens when I die?
- Is death something to be fought off and postponed for as long as possible?

recovery The stage of bereavement in which the bereaved begin to show signs of returning to a more normal life.

- Are there circumstances in which death is something to be welcomed?
- How do I feel when I accept that someday I will die?

The answers to these questions, and the process of seeking answers to them, are influenced by our experiences, what we have learned from those around us, and what we have come to understand about our existence from our cultural and religious heritage. The experience of death can have a positive side. When a loved one dies, the grief that must follow cannot be avoided, but grief can lead to an inspiration or recommitment to life. In this way, loss may actually become a creative and healthy force.

Being healthy does not necessarily mean avoiding pain, loss, and adversity. Certainly, it cannot mean avoiding the experience of death. Healthy people respond to normal human experiences with a positive outlook, constructive mind set, and the determination to make decisions that result in a higher quality of life—even when those experiences have involved death. A commitment to life is a lasting tribute to someone who has died.

Key Concepts

1. A biological definition of death may address the irreversible loss of all bodily functions.
2. A religious definition of death may include the concept of the irreversible loss of the soul from the body.
3. A living will stipulates under what conditions you wish and no longer wish to have medical treatments that will extend your life.
4. A durable power of attorney for health care names a representative to speak for you about your health care if you are unable to do so.
5. Most people say they would want to know if they were dying when they are very ill to enable them to better prepare for their own deaths.
6. The dying person goes through five stages: denial, anger, bargaining, depression, and acceptance.
7. Hope helps maintain the dying person through the days, weeks, or months of suffering.
8. Hospice is a specialized health care program emphasizing the management of pain and other symptoms associated with terminal illness.
9. A funeral provides family and friends with the opportunity to celebrate the life of the deceased and to offer support to the bereaved.
10. The grieving process, much like the dying process, involves stages of gradual adaptation to loss, including impact, recoil, and recovery.

Review Questions

1. Write a definition of death from a biological, legal, and religious perspective.
2. Define *active* and *passive euthanasia*.
3. Explain why the actions of Dr. Jack Kevorkian have prompted a national debate on end-of-life decisions.
4. Differentiate between how children, adolescents, and adults view death.
5. Define the *living–dying interval* and give an example of how this period can be brief or lengthy.
6. Name the five stages of dying according to Elisabeth Kübler-Ross and briefly describe the nature of each stage.

7. Identify the primary goal of hospice care and describe how it provides comfort for dying patients.
8. Identify the significant tasks that survivors must undertake when a loved one dies.
9. Name several important written documents that should be completed by everyone in order to assure that personal end-of-life desires are known by medical providers and family members.
10. Describe the impact, recoil, and recovery stages of grieving and estimate the time involved in negotiating each stage.

Selected Bibliography

Approaching Death: Improving Care at the End of Life. Washington, DC: Institute of Medicine, National Academy Press, 1997.

DeSpelder, L.A., and A.L. Strickland. *The Last Dance: Encountering Death and Dying.* Mountain View, CA: Mayfield, 1992.

Foley, D.J., et al. "Recounts of Elderly Deaths: Endorsements for the Patient-Self-Determination Act". *The Gerontologist* 35, no. 1 (1995): 119–121.

Kübler-Ross, E. *Death: The Final Stage of Growth.* Englewood Cliffs, NJ: Prentice-Hall, 1975.

Lemnin, M.R., and G.E. Dickinson. *Understanding Dying, Death, and Bereavement,* 2nd ed. Fort Worth, TX: Holt, Rinehart, and Winston, 1990.

Neeld, E. *Seven Choices: Taking the Steps to New Life after Losing Someone You Love.* New York: Clarkson N. Potter, 1990.

Shape Your Health Care Future with Health Care Advance Directives. Washington, DC: American Association of Retired Persons and American Bar Association, 1995.

HealthLinks: Web Sites for Dealing with Death

You can access better health as it relates to this chapter by checking out some of the following sites on the Internet. These and sites identified within the chapter can be accessed directly when you visit the *HealthStyles* Web Site located on the Allyn and Bacon home page at **http://www.abacon.com.**

Choice in Dying

www.choices.org

Choice in Dying is a national not-for-profit organization dedicated to helping patients and their families participate in decisions about end-of-life medical care. As the creator of living wills, they provide advance directives, counsel patients and families, train professionals, advocate for improved laws, and offer a range of publications and services, such as the *Right-to-Die Law Digest,* that summarize important developments in the field and describe changes in the law.

Last Acts: Care and Caring at the End of Life

www.lastacts.org

Last Acts call-to-action campaign is designed to raise the nation's awareness of the need to improve care of the dying and to promote the sharing of issues and solutions at the national, state, and local levels. A visit to this site will find an electronic newsletter, the searchable Resource Directory, and general information about the Last Acts Campaign.

Health Hotlines: Death and Dying

Children's Hospice International
(800) 242-4453
2202 Mt. Vernon Avenue, Suite 3C
Alexandria, VA 22301

Choice in Dying, Inc.
(800) 989-9455
200 Varick Street, Number 1001
New York, NY 10014-4810

Grief Recovery Helpline
(800) 445-4808
8306 Wilshire Boulevard, Suite 21A
Beverly Hills, CA 90211

Living Bank
(800) 528-2971
P.O. Box 6725
Houston, TX 77265

National Hospice Organization
(800) 658 8898
1901 North Moore Street, Suite 601
Arlington, VA 22209

United Network for Organ Sharing
(800) 24-DONOR (243-6667)
P.O. Box 13770
Richmond, VA 23225-8770

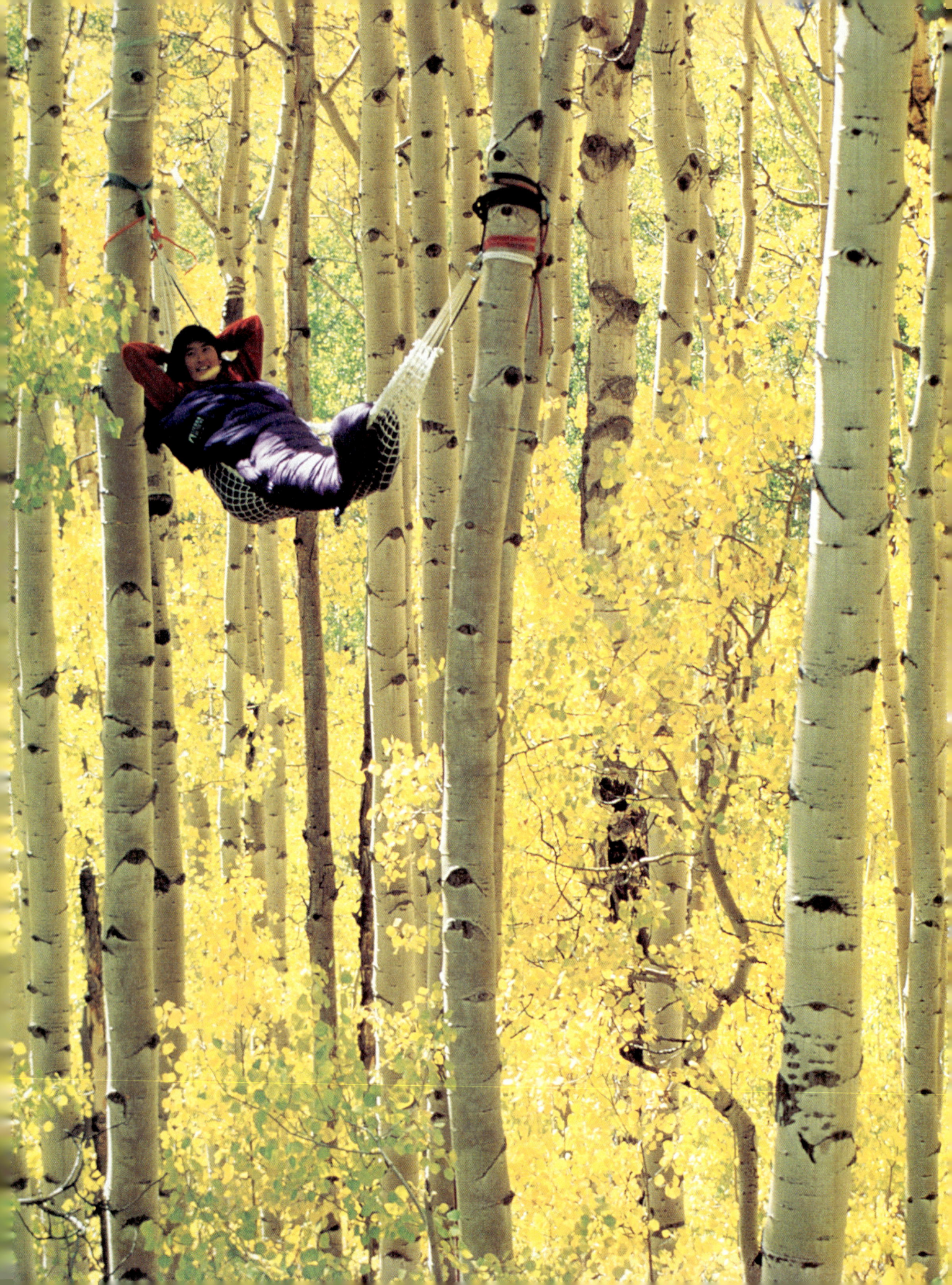

Chapter 20

Living in a Healthy Environment

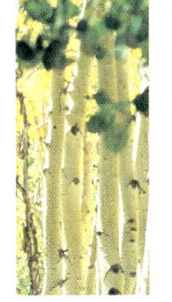
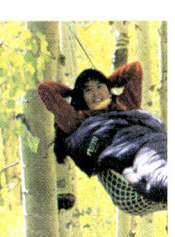
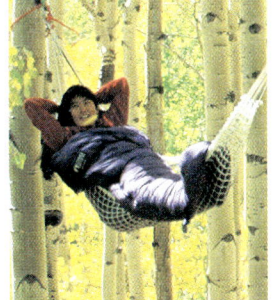

Objectives

When you finish reading this chapter, you will be able to:

1. Differentiate between serious environmental threats and threats that are perceived to be serious but that actually present little risk to the global environment.
2. Recognize the difficulty of measuring environmental health threats.
3. Understand the meanings of carcinogen, teratogen, and mutagen.
4. Describe the health effects of air pollution and list the principal air pollutants along with the primary source of each.
5. List the principal water pollutants and identify the source of each.
6. Understand the health threat of solid waste.
7. Recognize the practices of precycling and recycling and their potential for reducing solid waste.
8. Understand the health hazards of toxic wastes in the environment.
9. Recognize noise as an environmental pollutant.
10. Recognize a range of opinion concerning environmental policy and action.

What Is Your HealthStyle?

Angela wasn't really interested in joining the Outdoor Recreation Club on a ten-mile hike in the woods on Sunday, but her roommate, Lynn, had pressured her into going. Lynn ticked off the reasons for going: It would be fun, it would be a change from being indoors in a stuffy building, they would get some exercise and burn off calories, and there might be some interesting people there.

Angela went along with this and, much to her surprise, enjoyed herself on the trip. The next day, however, she got an upset stomach, which in two days developed into a serious case of diarrhea. At the student health department, Angela got medication to help her condition after finding out that she had gotten sick in what she thought would be a "squeaky clean" environment. She had drunk water from the beautiful stream running through the woods, not knowing that it was polluted with *Giardia*, an infectious agent.

Karim was also on the hike, but in contrast to Angela, he drank water from a plastic bottle that he had in his backpack. When he goes on longer camping trips, he takes along iodine drops, and when he is thirsty, he fills his cup with water from the stream and puts in a few drops of iodine to purify the water. He also adds a pinch of lemonade mix to make it taste better.

Another way the two contrasted was that Angela left trash behind when the group stopped for lunch. She wasn't as careful as she should have been when she unwrapped her sandwich, and without thinking, she left a plastic bag on the ground. Karim followed the rules of the outdoors: The only thing he left behind was his footprints.

In Your Opinion

Although the world around you seems so natural, there are many steps you can take to protect the environment and at the same time protect yourself from it.
- What could Angela have done to prepare better for her hike with the Outdoor Recreation Club?
- What lessons had Karim learned that he followed instinctively?
- When you have been hiking or otherwise spent time outdoors, how have you contributed to keeping the environment sound?
- What health skills contribute to the preservation of the environment?

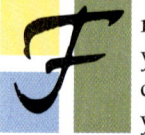

From the air you breathe to the water you drink, the environment that you depend on for life sustenance can cause major health risks. This does not mean that you have to worry about your health each time you go outdoors or drink a glass of water. In fact, there is likely to be a wide difference in perception between what you think is risky and what the scientists think. Even health experts do not agree among themselves about which environmental risks are most harmful to human health. This is in stark contrast to personal lifestyle risks: Health experts universally agree that certain risk factors—particularly smoking cigarettes and eating too much fat—are major contributors to disease and death.

Part of the confusion about environmental health stems from the fact that the science behind assessing environmental risks is still relatively young. Many health specialists believe that the public's concern about chemicals and cancer is out of proportion to the actual risk. This has given birth to the idea of **acceptable risk**. According to this idea, although exposure to a specific chemical or other hazardous material might be capable of causing disease, the likelihood of actually getting sick from it is very small. Other scientists argue against this idea because they believe that there have not been enough studies of the long-term effects of exposure to chemicals and other pollutants to be sure if any level of risk is acceptable.

Critical Thinking Question

Many environmental threats are difficult to quantify. For example, it is difficult to know the impact of air pollution when so many individuals smoke cigarettes. Given our limited ability to measure environmental health, do you think health officials and scientists could be overreacting to environmental health threats? Do you believe there is an acceptable level of risk?

Environmental Health: How Big Is the Problem?

Scientists cannot precisely determine the extent of environmental harm, particularly as it relates to health, for several reasons. First, the impact of pollution on the human body is often subtle and goes unnoticed for long periods of time. Because of this delay, when symptoms do appear, people tend to focus on them and not on their root cause. Furthermore, by the time an environmentally induced disease such as cancer is diagnosed, it is usually too late to correct the problem.

Another reason is that pollutants come from many sources, making a cause-and-effect determination difficult. The compounding effects of **multiple hazards** further complicate the effort to determine the source of the problem accurately.

Finally, people react differently to pollutants and to different exposure levels. Sunbathing over a twenty-year period may cause **melanoma** in one person and nothing much beyond a tan in another. Individual responses are due in part to your genetic composition, exposure to other pollutants, and lifestyle habits, such as cigarette smoking.

Identifying Health Effects

Three terms are becoming familiar to the public as awareness of environmental health hazards increases: *carcinogens, teratogens,* and *mutagens.*

A **carcinogen** is a substance that causes cancer. If the level of exposure is sufficient, the effect of carcinogens on human tissue is generally irreversible. A diagnosis of cancer today may reflect an exposure to a carcinogen many years ago. Similarly, carcinogens added to the environment today may not reveal their damage until many years from now. In addition, substances that are not carcinogenic by themselves may interact with other substances to promote cancer.

HealthLinks
Ecologia
ecologia.nier.org/
Ecologia is a nonprofit organization dedicated to environmental issues of public concern. The site provides policy and technical information about environmental health issues.

acceptable risk A circumstance in which the benefits outweigh the risks; when the likelihood of ill effects is very small.

multiple hazards Simultaneous exposure to more than one health threat.

melanoma A skin cancer that often starts as a mole-like growth and grows in size and changes color; the most serious of the various types of skin cancer.

carcinogen An agent that causes cancer.

Many environmental pollutants are not only carcinogenic but teratogenic and mutagenic as well. A **teratogen** causes birth defects. For example, children born to mothers who have eaten food contaminated by methylmercury frequently develop a disorder resembling cerebral palsy. A **mutagen** causes hereditary changes on the cellular level that may be passed from one generation to another. Although many chemicals are mutagenic in large doses, it is not known whether mutagenic risks exist at the levels at which they currently appear in the environment.

Environmental pollutants have other serious health effects, including damage to the nervous and immune systems, lungs, and kidneys. Exposure to high levels of lead, for example, can result in mental retardation and brain damage. Mercury poisoning also affects the brain as well as the kidneys and bowels.

The Air You Breathe

People have known for centuries that the air we breathe can make us sick. Before the age of sophisticated air-quality monitoring, coal workers took caged birds down into the mines with them. If the birds died, the miners knew that the air they were breathing contained deadly gases that they could not smell. The saying "mad as a hatter" referred to nineteenth-century hat makers who often became irrational—or "mad"—from breathing the fumes from the mercury they used to make felt hats. Today, the automobile is the single most significant cause of air pollution.

Whether the pollutant is invisible, as is mercury, or a cloud of smoke, as is smog resulting from automobile emissions, air pollution can cause serious ill health effects. Environmental scientists are increasingly concerned because, given that high levels of air pollution can cause adverse health effects, it is reasonable to assume that low levels over a long period of time can have negative health effects as well.

Table 20.1 is a listing of major pollutants and the health concerns associated with each. Criteria pollutants are those for which the U.S. Environmental Protection Agency (EPA) sets national standards; there are only six criteria pollutants, but they are discharged in relatively large quantities by a variety of sources. There are thousands of hazardous air pollutants that pose a danger to health, but they are associated with certain, specific sources and usually threaten only people living near large industrial facilities or in heavily polluted urban areas. Hazardous air pollutants are also regulated by the EPA.

Why Dirty Air Is Unhealthy

Toxic gases occur naturally in the environment, and under normal circumstances, the body's excellent filtering system, which includes the nose, mucous membranes, and cilia (small, hair-like projections from cells lining air passages leading to the lungs), assures that we breathe in "safe" air.

Air pollution, however, is not normal. It overtaxes the filtering system of the body. The result is that we breathe in noxious particles and gases. Illnesses related to air pollution include diseases of the lung, throat, bronchial tubes, sinuses, and nose because these organs come in direct contact with the polluted air.

Asthma, for example, is a serious chronic lung disease that is increasing in prevalence, in part due to air pollution. People who have asthma have an allergic overreaction to airborne particulates such as dust. As a result, a flood of antibodies causes lung inflammation, airway restriction, and a life-threatening shortness of breath. More than 14 million Americans suffer from asthma today—up from 7 million in 1982. According to the Centers for Disease Control and Prevention (CDC), about two thirds of asthma sufferers live in areas where at least one fed-

---

teratogen An agent that causes birth defects.

mutagen An agent that causes hereditary changes on the cellular level that may be passed from one generation to another.

air pollution The contamination of air by waste products.

asthma A breathing disorder that causes wheezing, coughing, and difficulty in breathing.

dermatitis A skin disorder in which an area of skin may become red, swollen, hot, and itchy.

benzene A chemical that can cause leukemia in humans.

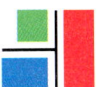

TABLE 20.1 Health Effects of Air Pollutants

Pollutants	Health concerns
Criteria pollutants	
Carbon monoxide	Ability of blood to carry oxygen impaired; cardiovascular nervous and pulmonary systems affected
Lead	Retardation and brain damage, especially in children
Nitrogen dioxide	Respiratory illness and lung damage
Ozone	Respiratory tract problems, such as difficulty breathing and reduced lung function; also, asthma, eye irritation, nasal congestion, reduced resistance to infection, and possibly premature aging of lung tissue
Particulate matter	Eye and throat irritation, bronchitis, lung damage; also impaired visibility
Sulfur dioxide	Respiratory tract problems, permanent harm to lung tissue
Hazardous air pollutants	
Arsenic	Cancer
Asbestos	A variety of lung diseases, particularly lung cancer
Benzene	Leukemia
Beryllium	Primarily lung disease, although also affects liver, spleen, kidneys, and lymph glands
Coke oven emissions	Respiratory cancer
Mercury	Several areas of the brain as well as the kidneys and bowels affected
Vinyl chloride	Lung and liver cancer
Radionuclides	Cancer

Source: U.S. Environmental Protection Agency

eral air quality measure was exceeded. Air pollution inside homes, which are built more tightly and so are not as drafty as in the past, may also play a role because cat dander and dust mites are asthma-triggering substances.

As the pollutants pass from the lungs into blood vessels and throughout the body, other organs are compromised, including the heart. Less life-threatening diseases related to air pollution include allergies, eye irritation, and **dermatitis** (skin reactions).

In some cases, an air pollutant can become even more hazardous when it is breathed along with another pollutant or when the same pollutant emanates from two different sources. *Synergistic effect* is the term used when the simultaneous actions of two separate entities together have a greater total effect than would be expected from the sum of the individual effects. As you read in Chapter 10, this occurs also when two drugs are taken together.

Benzene, a chemical that can cause leukemia in humans, is a good example of this synergistic effect. Benzene is a chemical widely used in the manufacturing of other chemicals and in petroleum refining. It is also contained in cigarette smoke. Although cigarettes emit an insignificant amount of benzene compared to the amount emitted by industry, cigarette smoking is the major source of benzene exposure because smokers directly breathe in this pollutant. Smokers have ten times as much benzene in their breath as do nonsmokers. Passive smoking—tobacco smoke in the environment inhaled by nonsmokers—also raises the risk of benzene exposure.

People who live in the nation's most polluted cities are about 15 percent more likely to die prematurely than are those who live in cities having the clean-

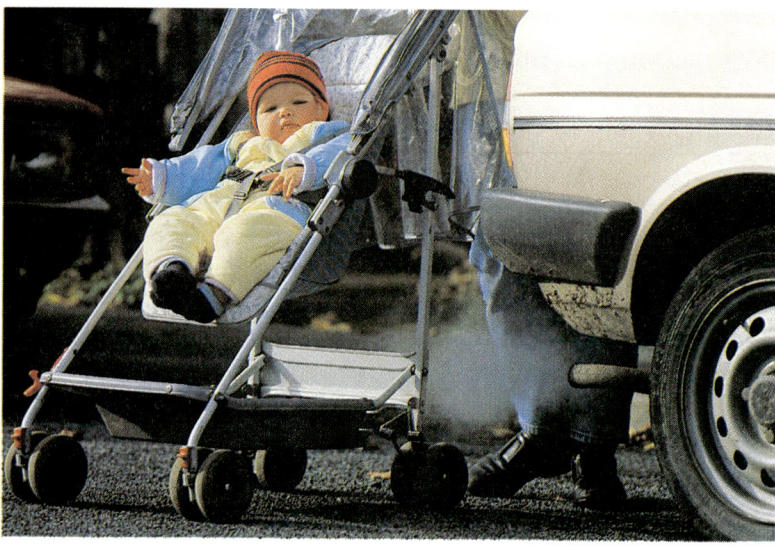

As the world's air quality worsens, the incidence of asthma among children is increasing, in part due to air pollution. (Source: © Tony Stone Images/David Woodfall)

est air. According to calculations made by researchers at the Harvard School of Public Health, people exposed to the dirtiest air run a risk for premature death about one sixth as great as if they had been smoking for twenty-five years. Of the fifteen U.S. cities having the highest air pollution levels, six are in California.

The good news about air quality is that, overall, it is getting better. Ten years ago, the proportion of people living in areas that have not exceeded standards for air pollutants hovered around 50 percent; today, more than 75 percent of Americans live in such areas.

Principal Air Pollutants

Carbon monoxide is a colorless, odorless, poisonous gas produced by the incomplete burning of carbon in fuels. Carbon monoxide is emitted by internal combustion engines, most of which are gas-powered motor vehicles, including automobiles, trucks, and buses. It is by far the most plentiful air pollutant.

Fortunately, this deadly gas usually does not stay in the environment for long. It tends to convert, by natural processes, into harmless carbon dioxide fast enough to prevent any general buildup. However, it can reach dangerous levels in areas having heavy auto traffic and little wind. When breathed, carbon monoxide replaces oxygen in the blood, and, because lack of oxygen affects the brain, one of the first symptoms of carbon monoxide poisoning is impaired perception and thinking. Carbon monoxide poisoning can cause heart failure and loss of consciousness (asphyxiation).

Sulfur oxides are acrid poisonous gases produced when fuel containing sulfur is burned. Electrical utilities and industrial plants, particularly those using coal, are the principal producers of sulfur oxides. Although industry is working to reduce the levels of sulfur oxide emissions, principally by switching to low-sulfur fuels or removing sulfur from fuels entirely, sulfur oxides are still a major pollutant. As the level of sulfur oxides in the air increases, breathing becomes more difficult. Respiratory diseases associated with sulfur oxides include coughs and colds, asthma, bronchitis, and emphysema.

Sulfur oxides combine with moisture in the air to form sulfuric acids. Sulfuric acid dissolves in water droplets in the atmosphere and falls to earth as **acid rain.** This precipitation has a higher level of acid than normal. To illustrate this

---

carbon monoxide   A colorless, odorless, poisonous gas that is produced by the incomplete burning of carbon in fuels.

sulfur oxides   Acrid poisonous gases produced when fuel containing sulfur is burned.

acid rain   Precipitation having a higher than normal level of acid due to the combination of sulfur oxides and moisture in the air.

hydrocarbons   A chemical compound made up of hydrogen and carbon; the major chemical ingredient of many fuels.

smog   A brownish haze that forms when hydrocarbons react with nitric acid in the presence of sunlight.

particulates   A tiny pollutant in the air such as dust, soot, and mold spores.

alveoli   The balloon-like air sacs at the end of the bronchioles of the lung.

lead   A metal found in exhausts, emissions, and paint.

nitrogen oxides   Poisonous gases that are produced when fuel is burned at very high temperatures.

ozone   A poisonous form of oxygen that chemically reacts with a variety of substances.

point, a fog in southern California was measured as having an acidity level equal to a hydrochloric acid solution that is used to clean toilets.

Acid rain can be particularly harmful to trees and aquatic life, especially species that can live only in a narrow range of acidity. Acid rain can also corrode buildings and impair visibility.

Gasoline, which is a mixture of many kinds of **hydrocarbons,** is the major source of hydrocarbon emissions. Hydrocarbon pollution is due in part to gasoline vapors that evaporate from the tank or escape from the tail pipe. Other sources are gasoline stations and industries that use solvents, paint, and dry cleaning fluids.

At the levels usually found in the air, hydrocarbons rarely have an effect on health. In a confined space, however, they can cause asphyxiation. A major problem associated with hydrocarbons is their role in forming smog. **Smog** is a noxious mixture of smoke and fog that develops when hydrocarbons, nitrogen oxides, and other gases are trapped under a layer of warm air.

Particulates are solid particles or liquid droplets so small that they are transported great distances by the winds and can remain in the air for a long time. They range in size from soot to particles too small to detect except under a special microscope. Particulates are produced primarily by coal plants and industrial processes as well as by natural sources, such as forest fires.

The smaller particulates are, the more likely they are to reach the innermost parts of the lungs and clog the **alveoli,** or lung sacs. Diseases associated with particulates include black lung disease, found among coal miners who inhale coal dust, and brown lung disease, found among textile workers who inhale cotton fibers.

Lead enters the air from automobile exhaust and from industries that smelt or process metal. It is absorbed into the body and accumulates in soft tissues and bones, especially affecting the nervous system and kidneys. Children are highly susceptible to lead poisoning from air pollutants and other environmental sources.

Lead-based paints, which were often used in homes built before 1950, are particularly harmful to inner-city children, who tend to live in older houses and who may eat the sweet-tasting paint chips that fall on the floor or are loose on the window sill. Children are more vulnerable than adults to lead poisoning because their body mass is small and their nervous systems are still developing. According to the American Academy of Pediatrics, lead is more dangerous to children than the asbestos found in building materials in older schools.

Lead is also released by automobiles using leaded gasoline and can affect rural as well as urban environments. For example, lead emissions attach to dust and soil and are either breathed in or taken up by plants.

Many efforts to get lead out of the environment have been made over the past thirty years, including banning the manufacture and sale of leaded paint. Although most of the gasoline sold today is lead-free, many gasoline engines and vehicles, including lawn mowers and farm tractors, still use leaded gas.

Nitrogen oxides are poisonous gases produced when fuel is burned at very high temperatures, as in electrical power plants, industrial boilers, and transportation vehicles. At high levels, nitrogen oxides can be fatal. At lower levels, they can irritate the lungs, cause bronchitis and pneumonia, and lower resistance to respiratory infections such as influenza. The principal harm does not come from nitrogen oxides directly but from the photochemical oxidants they form to make ozone and other ingredients of smog.

Ozone is a poisonous form of oxygen and is the principal component of smog. Ozone is not emitted directly into the air but rather is formed by chemical reactions between two other pollutants—hydrocarbons and nitrogen oxides. It irritates the mucous membranes of the respiratory system and can cause coughing, choking, and impaired lung function. It also aggravates chronic respiratory

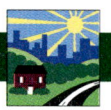

YOUR ENVIRONMENTAL NEIGHBORHOOD

Global Warming and Environmental Effects

Nature and Sources

The earth's climate is fueled by the sun. Most of the sun's energy, called solar radiation, is absorbed by the earth, but some is reflected back into space. A natural layer of atmospheric gases absorbs a portion of this reflected solar radiation, eventually releasing some of it into space, but forcing much of it back to earth. There, it warms the earth's surface, creating what is known as the natural "greenhouse effect," as illustrated in Figure 20.1.

Without the natural greenhouse effect, the earth's average temperature would be much colder and the planet would be covered with ice.

Recent scientific evidence shows that the greenhouse effect is being increased by release of certain gases to the atmosphere that cause the earth's temperature to rise. This is called "global warming." Carbon dioxide (CO_2) accounts for about 85 percent of greenhouse gases released in the United States. CO_2 emissions are largely due to the combustion of fossil fuels in electric power generation. Methane (CH_4) emissions, which result from agricultural activities, landfills, and other sources, are the second largest contributor to greenhouse gases in the United States.

Industrial applications such as foam production, refrigeration, dry cleaning, chemical manufacturing, and semiconductor manufacturing produce other greenhouse gas emissions such as hydrofluorocarbons (HFCs). Smelting of aluminum produces another greenhouse gas called perfluorinated compounds (PFCs). Emissions of nitrogen oxide from automobile exhaust and industrial processes contribute to the formation of ground-level ozone or smog, also a greenhouse gas.

Health and Environmental Effects

Greenhouse gas emissions could cause a 1.8 to 6.3 degree Fahrenheit rise in temperature during the next century, if atmospheric levels are not reduced. Although this change may appear small, it could produce extreme weather events, such as droughts and floods; threaten coastal resources and wetlands by raising sea level; and increase the risk for certain diseases by producing new breeding sites for pests and pathogens. Agricultural regions and woodlands are also susceptible to changes in climate that could result in increased insect populations and plant disease. This degradation of natural ecosystems could lead to reduced biological diversity.

Source: U.S. Environmental Protection Agency, *National Air Quality and Emissions Trend Report*, 1995

diseases such as asthma and bronchitis, which is why people who have these conditions are warned to stay inside during periods of high smog levels. Ozone can also irritate the eye.

Ozone in the air you breathe is not the same as the **ozone layer** in the stratosphere, which filters out ultraviolet rays from the sun and serves as protection against the sun's radiation—and skin cancer. There is much scientific debate about how depleted the ozone layer is, but it is clearly being threatened to a measurable degree. The major contributors to the destruction of the ozone layer are **chlorofluorocarbons (CFCs),** which had been used as aerosol spray propellants and refrigerants and are present in the exhaust of high-flying jet planes. As of 1996, CFCs can no longer be produced in or imported into the United States. Existing stock can be reused and recycled, so CFC prducts are not totally eliminated yet.

Over the past two decades, ozone levels in the United States have fallen to about 5 percent below normal in the summer and 10 percent below normal in the winter. The biggest "hole" in the ozone layer is over the Antarctic, where ozone levels fall to 70 percent below normal.

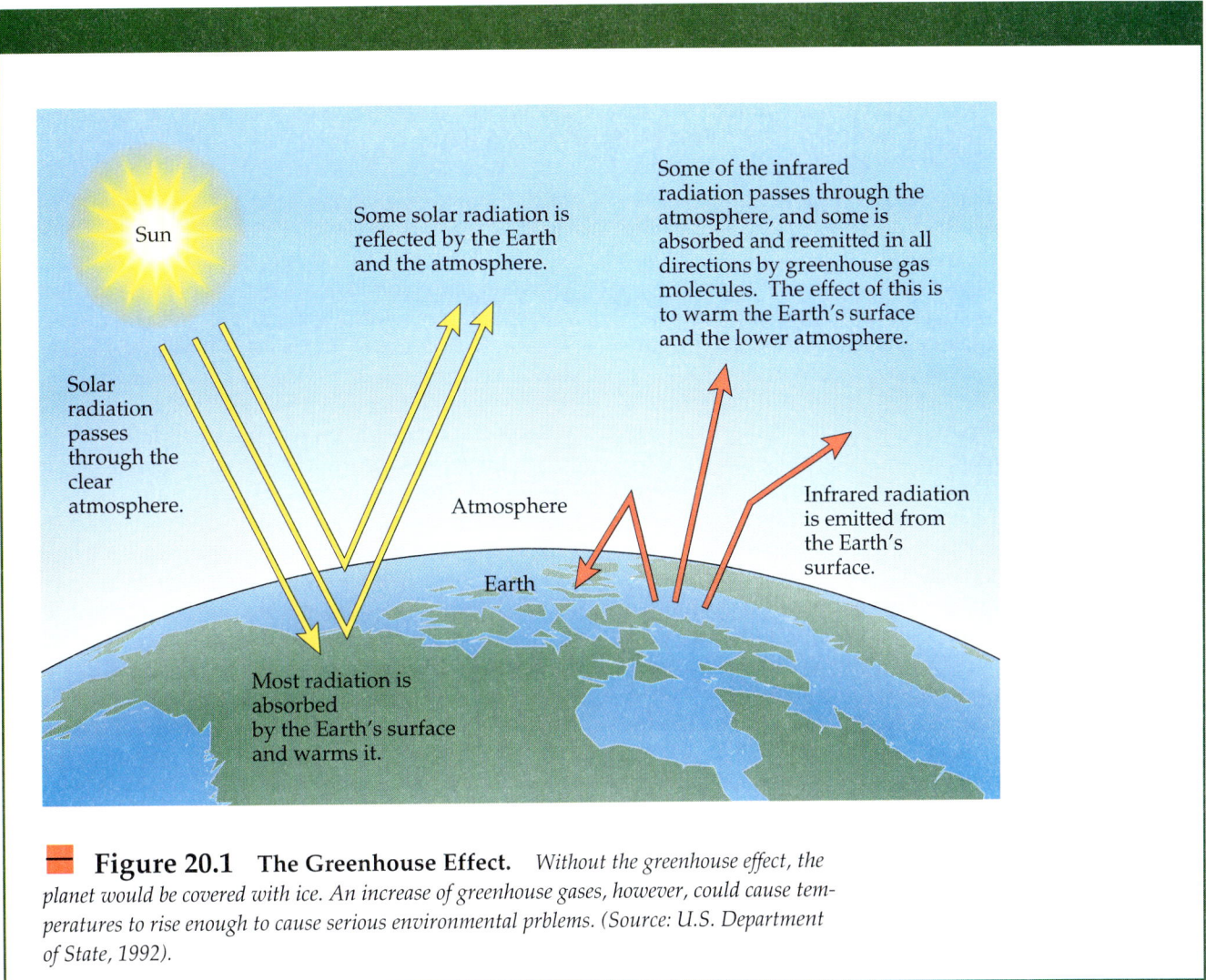

Figure 20.1 The Greenhouse Effect. *Without the greenhouse effect, the planet would be covered with ice. An increase of greenhouse gases, however, could cause temperatures to rise enough to cause serious environmental prblems. (Source: U.S. Department of State, 1992).*

Many of the air pollutants we have discussed combine to cause what is called the greenhouse effect, which some scientists believe can lead to **global warming.** The Your Environmental Neighborhood box explains this phenomenon further and demonstrates what happens in Figure 20.1.

The Automobile: King of Air Pollution

The automobile is a major source of air pollution in most areas of the United States. Although cars are cleaner and more efficient than they were twenty-five years ago, far more automobiles and other vehicles are on the road today. In 1970, there was one car for every 2.5 Americans; today, there is one for every 1.7 Americans.

Not only are more people driving more cars but also they are driving them greater distances. This growth in usage leads to more congestion, which further increases emissions. Improvements in cars, fuels, and the overall transportation system hold the clues for cleaner air in the future. So does the use of "clean" transportation, such as bikes (see the Cultural View box).

ozone layer A region of the stratosphere, which filters out ultraviolet rays from the sun.

chlorofluorocarbons (CFCs) Compounds used as aerosol spray propellants and refrigerants that contribute to the depletion of the ozone layer.

global warming The gradual rise in the average temperature of the earth.

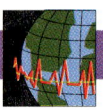

CULTURAL VIEW

The Bicycling City of Groningen, Holland

The myth is that cycling is popular in the Netherlands because the country is so flat. The reality is that biking is widespread because the Dutch toiled to make it that way.

Cycling for recreation and transportation has a long tradition in this small, densely populated country, but cars started making inroads in the 1950s and 1960s. Faced with energy shortages and growing pollution problems in the 1970s, the Dutch looked to their roots for answers.

In 1975, the national government decided to devote at least 10 percent of its surface transportation budget to bicycling. According to Marcia Lowe in her Worldwatch paper "The Bicycle: Vehicle for a Small Planet," the government spent $230 million dollars to build bike routes, parking lots, and other facilities between 1975 and 1985. With 8,370 in miles of bike routes by the mid-1980s in some Dutch cities, bicycles became the mode of transportation used for half of all trips.

Nowhere is this trend more pronounced than in Groningen, an ancient city of about two hundred thousand. Under an ambitious "traffic circulation plan" introduced in 1977, downtown Groningen was divided into four sectors. You can pedal, walk, or take public transportation from one sector to another, but you can't drive. Cars may enter each sector, but to travel between them, drivers must leave the city and use an encircling highway.

The city also encourages commuters to combine bicycling with mass transit by providing parking at train stations. One lot can hold 3,000 bikes—and its capacity needs to be doubled.

The Dutch pay attention to details, too. At traffic lights, stop lines for bikes are in front of those for cars so cyclists aren't overwhelmed with exhaust fumes. Separate traffic lights for bicycles turn green a few seconds earlier than the ones for cars, so that riders can safely cross intersections or turn left. Additionally, bikes can turn right on red, but cars can't.

A giant downtown car parking lot has been turned into a town square. A formerly traffic-snarled thoroughfare is now a bustling open-air market. And, in the ultimate example of no-turning-back policy, Groningen has permitted buildings to be constructed in the middle of the former highways, leaving room for bikes to pass but not cars.

The result of all this is a city that feels like a town. The pace is slower, the scale is smaller. Yet it remains a vibrant and prosperous place to live and work. "It's a phenomenal place," says Andy Clarke of the Bicycle Federation of America, who has been to Groningen twice, including a week-long visit for the International VeloCity Cycling Conference in 1987. "I was pedaling in a group of twenty cyclists. In most cities you would feel like you're part of a mini demonstration. But in Groningen, you just get lost in the crowd."

"It's not a function of geography or heredity," he adds. "It's decisions by people and their elected representatives. Nothing has been done in Groningen that couldn't be done in the United States."

Source: "The Bicycling City of Groningen, Holland," reprinted from the May 1992 issue of *Bicycling Magazine* with permission from Rodale Press, Inc., copyright 1992

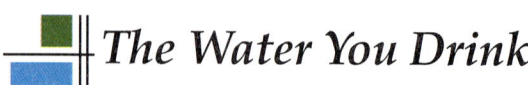

The Water You Drink

When you are thirsty, you turn on the water faucet and expect to get good, clean water to drink. This is true for most people living in the United States, but there are significant pockets of the country where the water supply is contaminated. Toxic chemicals continue to pass through municipal waste water treatment plants, and it is estimated that about one quarter of waterborne illnesses can be attributed to bacteria or viruses from untreated or inadequately disinfected or filtered waste water.

Chemicals are added to the water supply to kill microorganisms, and about 80 percent of U.S. drinking water has chlorine added to it to prevent outbreaks of

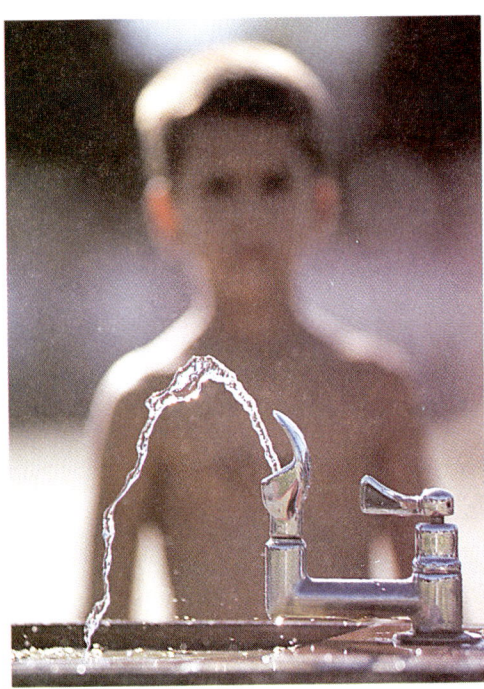

Water continues to be one of our greatest, yet most threatened, natural resources. (Source: The Image Works/© Frank Pedrick)

cholera, typhoid, dysentery, and other waterborne illnesses that were once endemic. A recent cholera outbreak in Latin America, which killed five thousand people and made six hundred thousand very sick, was attributed to inadequate levels of chlorine.

While the number of outbreaks of waterborne illnesses is declining in the United States, large outbreaks do take place. In 1993, for example, four hundred thousand people became ill and about one hundred died in Milwaukee because of a waterborne disease, *Cryptosporidium,* in the water supply. This waterborne parasite, commonly called crypto, is excreted by cattle and other animals. Rainwater washes it into rivers, lakes, and reservoirs, and it gets into the water system. It can also come from overflows from sewage treatment plants. Overall, about nine hundred thousand people a year get sick from the water supply. Chlorine does not kill *Cryptosporidium*.

Drinking Safe Water

While the tap water in most communities is safe, the Milwaukee outbreak illustrates that you never know when something could happen to the water supply where you live. If there is a water emergency in your community, you will be notified about it by news alerts in the papers and on television and radio. The following tips are commonly offered by health departments when there is a water emergency:

- Boil tap water for one minute to kill *Cryptosporidium* and up to ten minutes for other infectious agents.
- If you buy bottled water, remember that some of it comes from aboveground sources (in contrast to underground springs) and could contain the same waterborne diseases as tap water. The safest bottled waters have been distilled or processed by reverse-osmosis.
- If you have an impaired immune system—for instance, if you have AIDS or are on chemotherapy—speak to your physician about your water drinking options.

HEALTH SKILLS

**HealthLinks Web
Environmental Protection Agency**
www.epa.gov

Government agency that oversees all environmental issues. Site provides a wealth of information, as well as links to other environmental and safety resources.

Sources of Water Pollution

There are numerous sources of water pollution, but the major ones are industrial, municipal, and agricultural. The EPA refers to water pollution sources as point and nonpoint sources. **Point source pollutants** enter a body of water at a specific point—for example, at an industrial plant or a sewage facility. **Nonpoint source pollutants** enter a body of water as runoff or seepage.

Discharges from industry can be both point and nonpoint source pollutants. They may be dumped directly into bodies of water and also carried there indirectly by rainfall. For example, when mercury and arsenic particles are released into the air from factories, they often attach themselves to water droplets and return to earth as rain, thereby contaminating a stream or lake—or further contaminating an already polluted one. Accidents such as oil spills also contribute to the problem of water pollution.

Municipal sources of pollution include urban storm water runoff, septic systems leaking, bacteria, and landfill seepage contaminating the water table.

Agricultural sources of pollution include large drainage areas (usually resulting when land is plowed but not yet held in place by vegetation) and runoff of sediment, agricultural nutrients, and pesticides. Nutrients can deplete a body of water's oxygen supply by overstimulating plant and algae growth.

It is estimated that 2.6 billion pounds of pesticides are applied yearly to U.S. crops. In spite of this, crop damage seems to be increasing rather than decreasing because many insects are becoming resistant to the effects of pesticides. The proper use of pesticides is widely debated. For two contrasting opinions, see the Your Developing Health Skills box.

Toxic chemical compounds in use today find their way into both drinking and recreational waters. Organic chemicals, many of which are suspected of causing cancer, are also found in drinking water. For example, **perchloroethylene (PCE)**, a chemical used by the dry cleaning industry, and **trichloroethylene (TCE)**, a chemical used as a degreaser by machine shops, have contaminated large quantities of drinking water because they have leaked into the soil from the waste dumps where they were discarded.

Given all these pollutants, the EPA's 1994 water survey found that nearly 40 percent of surveyed U.S. water bodies are too polluted for fishing, swimming, and other uses. To put this in perspective, looking only at lakes, about 37 percent of surveyed lakes are impaired—the equivalent of six Great Salt Lakes.

Why Dirty Water Is Unhealthy

The Great Lakes basin provides a good illustration of how water becomes unhealthy. According to a Coast Guard study, the Great Lakes are contaminated by more than 400 oil spills and 70 chemical spills every month. In addition, there is concern that the Great Lakes area is overexposed to pesticides and herbicides. Spills in estuaries often make fish unsuitable for eating. When oil in water is ingested by organisms in the food chain, highly destructive pollutants can spread throughout the population.

The main health threat from water pollution, however, comes not from oil spills but from toxic wastes, which can cause cancer, food and chemical poisoning, and even an increase in cardiovascular disease when fertilizers having high sodium levels run off into surface and ground waters. Toxic chemicals move up the food chain from aquatic life to human consumption. Over time, it is anticipated that these contaminants will lead to a variety of problems in humans, including premature births and impaired cognitive and motor development.

As with most pollutants, the effects of water pollution are, for the most part, unknown. But evidence suggests that the cumulative effect of water pollution will result in problems ranging from higher cancer rates to increases in neurological problems.

---

point source pollutant Point source pollutants enter a body of water at a specific point.

nonpoint source pollutant Nonpoint source pollutants enter a body of water as runoff or seepage.

perchloroethylene (PCE) A suspected carcinogen used in dry cleaning.

trichloroethylene (TCE) A suspected carcinogen used as a degreaser in machine shops.

fluoride A trace mineral used to help prevent dental caries.

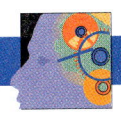

DEVELOPING HEALTH SKILLS

Should Pesticides That Cause Cancer in Animals Be Banned from Our Foods?

In 1958, the Delaney clause was passed requiring that additives causing cancer in animals or humans be eliminated from processed foods. A 1987 court settlement extended the law to include pesticides, in processed as well as some raw foods; recently, the Clinton administration has begun phasing out thirty-seven pesticides. Urged by food processors, Congress is considering legislation that would repeal Delaney.

Yes There is substantial evidence that the incidence of many forms of cancer has increased dramatically over the past thirty years. We're seeing more brain cancer, testicular cancer, breast cancer, and prostate cancer. This is no time to lower our guard.

The Delaney clause is probably the strongest public health statute in the world, and the premise behind it remains sound. We should avoid exposure in the food chain to chemicals that cause cancer in animals. People are quick to say, "Well, it's just lab animals." But the similarities between humans and lab animals are great enough that we should act with caution. After all, we are animals. If something causes tumors in animals, we must assume it will cause cancer in humans, too.

What we understand best about carcinogens is the limited extent of our knowledge. We don't know whether one carcinogen can increase the cancer-causing effects of another.

We should be putting more emphasis on reducing our current use of pesticides. We're now using 2.6 billion pounds annually in the United States. That's a new record. And it's not only the food supply that's affected; these chemicals are polluting the groundwater, lakes, and streams. Less hazardous chemicals and other existing technologies, such as biological controls and crop rotation, could replace many of these pesticides.

Without the Delaney clause, we would be deliberately poisoning our food, then policing the results.

Al Meyerhoff is an attorney with the Natural Resources Defense Council in San Francisco.

No I'm not saying throw caution to the wind. Any group of scientists can come up with a list of carcinogens that do need to be kept out of the food supply. But Delaney does not discriminate between potent carcinogens and those that pose only an insignificant risk. Enormous resources are being spent to address what can amount to zero risk. There are many substances that are not powerful carcinogens and only produce cancer in animals when they're fed very high doses, doses that humans would never ingest.

People don't realize that very often a pesticide may be protecting the crop—and the consumer—from a worse hazard. For example, when a corn crop gets stressed, an insect called a corn borer can get into the ear of corn, carrying the spores that produce aflatoxin, a very powerful natural carcinogen. The synthetic pesticides that are used to control the corn borers are really protecting you against the naturally occurring carcinogen, which is a more serious risk.

Besides, eliminating certain pesticides would most likely increase the cost of produce, so people wouldn't be eating as much of it. And we know that not eating enough fruits and vegetables is a major risk factor for cancer.

We need to compare the risks, make trade-offs. We're not poisoning our food by having a minute quantity of a pesticide in it any more than we're poisoning our water by adding tiny amounts of chlorine to protect us from cholera.

Michael Pariza, a toxicologist, directs the University of Wisconsin's Food Research Institute in Madison.

Source: "Should Pesticides That Cause Cancer in Animals Be Banned from Our Foods?" *Health,* March–April 1996, p. 36. Reprinted by permission of Time Inc. Health

Fluoride in the Water: What Does It Really Do?

Ever since 1945, when the trace mineral **fluoride** was pumped into the water system as a way to harden teeth and prevent cavities, there has been a cloud of controversy over its benefits. It was attacked by people on the right as a communist plot to foul the water system and by those on the left as a government conspiracy to force people to take compulsory medication in their water. Conservatives have objected to the tax costs, and environmentalists say they do not want any additives in anything they eat or drink.

Today, at least 62 percent of the U.S. population drinks water containing fluoride, whether they like it or not. (Fluoride also occurs in the water supply naturally, especially in the South.) In addition, millions of people use fluoride toothpaste daily and consume food and beverages made with fluoridated water.

According to one measure—dental decay—fluoride has been a major public health success. In 1944, more than 90 percent of American children had some form of tooth decay. Today, about 50 percent have never had dental caries.

One burning question is, Can this success be attributed to fluoride in the water? According to the American Dental Association (ADA), the answer is clearly yes. Tooth decay, says the ADA, occurs between 50 and 70 percent less often in fluoridated areas than in nonfluoridated areas. Critics point to surveys that show a drop in tooth decay in children no matter where they live. Although this is true, the National Institute of Dental Research estimates that children who have always lived in fluoridated areas have 18 to 25 percent less decay than their peers living in nonfluoridated areas.

Critical Thinking Question

Despite the noted benefits of fluoridated water, some communities are fighting having fluoride added to their community water supply. How do you feel about this issue? Do the benefits of reduced tooth decay outweigh the unknown risks of fluoride? Does tooth decay represent a compelling threat to public health?

Solid Waste: The Art of Throwing Things Away

America is sometimes called the throw-away society. We have disposable Styrofoam containers for our fast foods, disposable diapers, and convenient trash pickup at our front door. As a result of some of our consumer preferences, **landfills** are bulging to the point of overflow. And in some major cities, solid waste is shipped overland or by barge to other parts of the country simply because there is no longer enough room for the waste. St. Louis ships its trash across the Mississippi River to landfills in Illinois, and many New Jersey towns truck their garbage to Michigan or Ohio, where dumping fees are cheaper than in the East.

In addition, some wastes are dumped illegally. Swimmers along the New York and New Jersey shorelines have come across used syringes and other medical wastes, in spite of stiff penalties for mixing infectious materials with regular trash.

landfills An area where trash and other wastes are deposited and covered with soil.

precycling The practice of choosing products that have the potential for reuse, using packaging that can be used for other purposes, or choosing packaging that has already been recycled.

Solid waste is made up of everything from paper and metal cans to old tires, plastic containers, food, grass and other yard wastes, and motor oil. It is estimated that every person generates about seven pounds of solid waste a day. Most of it—73 percent—goes into landfills, so it is not surprising that our present landfills will soon need to be replaced (see Figure 20.2).

Consider just one product on the trash heap: disposable diapers. They do not degrade—at least not for hundreds of years—so every disposable diaper ever buried is still there, taking up between 1 and 2 percent of all landfill space. Disposables have captured about 85 percent of the diaper market. Each year, about 16 billion more disposable diapers are added to the heap, and on average, each baby uses 4,000 to 5,000 diapers before he or she is toilet trained. (It should be noted that cloth diapers can affect the environment, too. Washing them requires using a lot of hot water, and, as nutrients, phosphates in detergent add to the burden of water pollution.)

Common household waste can contribute to health problems resulting from everything from the creation of breeding grounds for rats, flies, and mosquitoes to the emission of noxious smoke from burning trash. Rainwater seeping through buried wastes percolates down through the soil and contaminates ground water. Other organic wastes, such as garbage and paper products, decompose and can form explosive methane gas. Methane absorbs heat from sunlight and may contribute to global warming.

While solid waste remains a considerable problem, the throw-away rate is dropping—from 3.3 pounds per day per person in 1994 to 3.2 pounds in 1995. A decrease of 0.1 pound might not sound like much, but this means that there were over 1 million fewer tons of waste, according to the EPA.

Critical Thinking Question

The *Healthy People 2000* objectives include the following: "Establish curbside recycling programs that serve at least 50 percent of the U.S. population and continue to increase household hazardous waste collection programs." Baseline data show only 26 percent of the nation has curbside recycling. Is the establishment of an objective such as this adequate stimulus for business development? Given the market for recycled materials such as newspaper and glass, should the development of recycling businesses be left to market economics? How could our government use tax breaks and low-interest business loans to stimulate recycling?

Precycling and Recycling Options

Reducing the amount of solid waste in the environment is dependent on two practices, precycling and recycling. **Precycling** is a concept that refers to eliminating solid waste before it is created. This might be considered primary prevention of solid waste.

Precycling is dependent on wise consumer choice. For example, when given the option of buying fast food that is highly packaged (i.e., Styrofoam boxes placed in plastic coated sacks filled with numerous paper wrappings) or fast food that is only minimally packaged (provided on a simple, recyclable paper

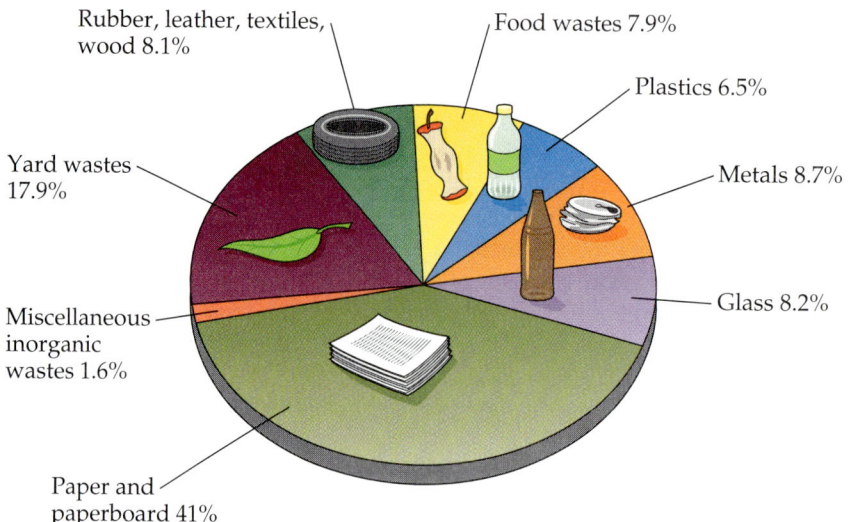

Figure 20.2 What's in Your Garbage. *Every person generates about seven pounds of solid waste a day, and most of it goes into a landfill in your community. Paper and paper products account for most of the solid wastes by weight. (Source: U.S. Environmental Protection Agency)*

plate), a wise and healthy consumer choice would be the latter. The same concept can be applied to grocery shopping, snack buying, and other consumer purchases. Precycling also involves reusing products, using packaging for other purposes, and buying products that are recycled or packaged in containers that can later be recycled locally.

Recycling, a much more familiar concept, refers to the process of collecting and reusing newspapers, plastics, aluminum cans, glass bottles, and many other solid wastes. Recycling can greatly reduce the landfill problem—and save

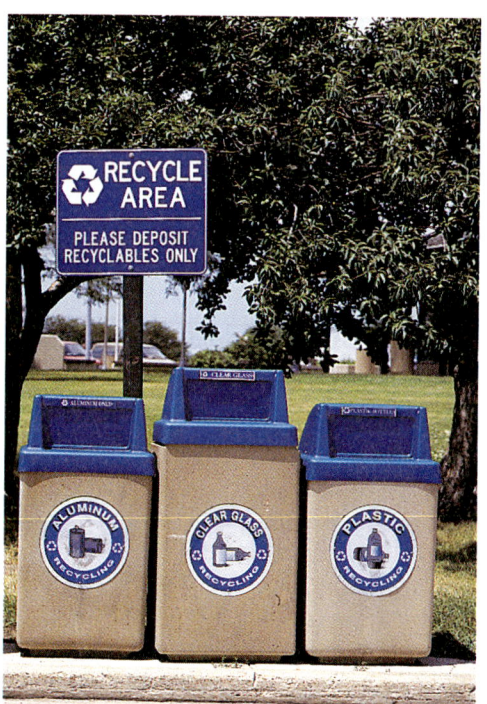

Many communities have convenient places where people can deposit recyclable goods. Recycling aluminum cans, glass bottles, plastics, and newspapers saves money, natural resources, and energy. (Source: The Image Works/© Eastcott/Momatiuk)

recycling The use over and over again of substances such as metal and glass.

HERE'S LOOKING AT YOU

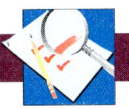

Know Your Recycling

Recycling has been part of the American consciousness long enough for a couple of generations to have ingrained the concepts and philosophy of the movement and adopted the behaviors as part of daily living. Today, a drive through most communities in the country will produce signs of recycling bins and compost piles. But how well informed are you about recycling and with recycling terms? Answer the following questions to check your knowledge, then check your answers.

1. Which of the following are effective in reducing the amount of waste generated from households?
   a. backyard composting
   b. recycling
   c. variable rate trash collection fees
   d. collection of yard waste for composting
   e. all of the above
2. What is cullet?
   a. part of a bird's gizzard
   b. glass sorted and crushed for recycling
   c. a drain pipe for storm water
   d. bundled newspapers
3. What material is most commonly collected by curbside recycling programs? (Hint: It is consistently valuable.)
4. Which one of the following should you not put into your compost bin?
   a. shrub trimmings
   b. grass clippings
   c. coffee grounds
   d. meat scraps
   e. egg shells
5. What is a mobius (as related to recycling)?
6. What recycled material is used in toothpaste? (Clue: It's part of the stannous fluoride ingredient.)
7. This common household recyclable is used to make stuffing for sleeping bags and winter jackets. The stuffing has good insulating qualities. (Clue: It often holds soft drink.)

Answers

1. All of these are effective means of reducing the generation of waste from households. Variable rate trash collection fees, where homeowners pay based on the amount of waste discarded, encourage participation in other waste reduction practices.
2. Cullet is glass which has been sorted and crushed for recycling. The glass should not be broken at home, because then it cannot be sorted and freed from contaminants. Only glass containers should be put out for recycling. Do not recycle light bulbs, drinking glasses, ceramics, baking dishes, window glass, or mirrors. Any metal caps or rings should be removed.
3. Aluminum is collected by 847 of 864 curbside recycling programs in Pennsylvania. The "street price" for aluminum cans in the Mid-Atlantic region of the United States was 27¢–32¢ per pound during the first week of October 1996. (Source: Market Page, Waste Age's Recycling Times)
4. Meat scraps should not be put into a compost bin because they could attract pests or could create odors.
5. A mobius is the chasing arrow recycling symbol.
6. Tin used to make stannous fluoride is made from detinning old steel cans. The body of the can is made from steel but has a tin coating. The resulting tin is very pure and is ideal for use in toothpaste. This is the only domestic source of tin in the United States.
7. PET (polyethylene terephthalate) soft drink bottles are used to make polyethylene fibers for insulation as well as carpets, fabrics, strapping, and engineered resins for the automotive industry.

Source: Adapted from the Pennsylvania Department of Environmental Protection as posted on Web site www.dep.state.pa.us

money, natural resources, and energy. It is estimated that recycling a single press run of the Sunday *New York Times,* for example, would save some seventy-five thousand trees. The Here's Looking at You box tests your general knowledge about recycling.

Currently, about 27 percent of the nation's solid waste is recycled. More than 7,000 communities across the country—from major cities such as Los Angeles to small towns—have curbside pickup of recyclables, and there are nearly 9,000 community drop-off centers. In addition, supermarkets across the country are taking back the empty plastic and paper bags that their customers used to carry home foods and other products. You can do your share to reduce the amount of solid waste in your community by practicing precycling and recycling:

HEALTH SKILLS

- Buy goods having little or no packaging.
- Reuse products, or find alternative uses for products.
- Buy goods in returnable and recyclable containers.
- Establish a recycling center in your home—a place to collect bottles, plastics, newspapers, and cans.
- Learn where you can take items to be recycled.
- Build a compost pile and turn your food wastes, leaves, and grass clippings into fertilizer.
- Find people at your college and in the community who are interested in reducing waste by promoting precycling, promoting recycling, and inventing new uses for old materials.
- Encourage local merchants to sell goods in returnable containers.
- Compare your community with other communities that have successfully addressed solid waste and other environmental problems.

HEALTH SKILLS

Another health skill is to know which products can be recycled or composted and which ones must still be "dumped" in a landfill.

Materials that can be recycled

- Paper (newspapers, corrugated boxes, office papers, mixed papers)
- Plastics (milk, soft drink, and other containers)
- Glass (bottles and jars)
- Aluminum (cans and other aluminum products)
- Steel (appliances and other steel products)
- Wood (e.g., lumber, pallets)

Materials that can be composted

- Leaves, grass, and brush
- Food wastes other than meat, fish, and poultry
- Some organic materials such as paper contaminated with food

Materials that must be deposited in landfills

- Wastes heavily contaminated by food residues, household chemicals, etc.
- Composite materials (plastic-coated paper, furniture, and appliances, other than their metal content)
- Miscellaneous inorganic materials such as street sweepings

Health Hazards from Toxic Waste

The word *waste* indicates that something not wanted is thrown away. When dealing with toxic materials, how that waste is thrown away carries serious health implications. Some **hazardous wastes** are disposed of safely—for example, by burying them in steel containers. But too often, toxic wastes are gotten rid of incorrectly or otherwise leak into the environment, for example, in the form of fumes. In addition, even steel drums rust and corrode over time, so that toxic wastes such as gasoline and other chemicals leak out into the environment.

Chlorinated dioxins, for example, are emitted by some chemical processes and by the high-temperature burning of plastics in incinerators. People are exposed to them in a variety of ways, but the most common way is through air pollution—they are exposed directly by breathing toxic particles or indirectly after the airborne particles fall to earth and are taken up by crops, animals, or fish that are consumed or fall in water that is drunk. As a result, some dioxins accumulate in the body over time and become highly concentrated in human fatty tissue and breast milk.

Toxic chemicals can have both acute (immediate) and chronic (long-term) poisonous effects. Acute reactions are often easy to observe—from watery eyes and irritated skin to unconsciousness and death. It is sometimes years before chronic effects—such as lung disease and neurological symptoms including blurred vision, muscle weakness, and difficulties in balance—become apparent. Even more subtle are the behavioral effects of toxic poisoning: anxiety, depression, and hyperactivity.

Cancer and birth defects due to toxic wastes also develop over a long period of time, so that it is sometimes difficult to trace back to the point of exposure. Love Canal is an example of a toxic waste dump that was associated with a high incidence of miscarriages, stillbirths, urinary and nervous system disorders, and skin disease. More than 20,000 tons of chemicals were buried on the site in upstate New York in the early 1950s, but it took until the late 1970s before the health problems became apparent and people were evacuated.

Landfills are another potential source of toxic waste. One housing development in Savannah, Georgia, was built on a landfill, and when methane gas began escaping from it, residents had to be evacuated.

Another problem associated with toxic wastes is that even when a toxic material is banned, it can harm the environment for decades. Polychlorinated biphenyls (PCBs), which were produced primarily as electrical insulation, have been banned in the United States since 1977. But these chemicals are still found in older appliances, in landfills, and in the fatty tissues of fish and other animals—including the fat and breast milk of people who eat those animals.

Dangers from Noise

If someone was talking, could you tell whether he or she had said the word *beg* or *keg*? Normally, you might be able to, but at a live rock concert, where the noise level is over 110 decibels (where 60 decibels is usually rated as "comfortable"), you might not even know that someone is talking to you.

Noise is something that no one can avoid. This disturbance in the environment has been escalating since the Industrial Revolution. In the 1990s, it is one of the great threats to the quality of life. Noise, unfortunately, is accepted by many as a necessary evil in life. Cars, subways, motorcycles, planes, TVs, video games, Walkman-type personal stereos, power tools, and a multitude of other gadgets have left us in a very noisy world. Sound levels above 85 decibels—roughly equivalent to that produced by a power leaf blower, lawn mower, or food blender—are potentially hazardous. Most Americans live in near-dangerous noise environments, typically experiencing chronic average noise levels of about 70 decibels (see Table 20.2).

hazardous waste Waste that is flammable, explosive, corrosive, or toxic.

toxic chemical A chemical that is poisonous. Exposure can cause bodily reactions ranging from watery eyes to unconsciousness and death.

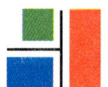

TABLE 20.2   It's a Noisy World: Noise Levels and Human Response

Common sounds	Decibels	Effects
Normal breathing	10	Just audible
Whisper	30	Very quiet
Normal conversation	50–55	Comfortable under 60
Vacuum cleaner	70	Intrusive, interferes with telephone
Garbage disposal	80	Annoying, interferes with conversation; Constant exposure may cause damage
Television	70–90	Very annoying; 85—noise level at which hearing damage begins after eight hours, exposure
Lawn mower	85–90	
Motorcycle at 25 ft.	90	
Snowmobile	105	Regular exposure of more than one minute risks permanent loss over 100 decibels
Power saw, chain saw	110	
Thunderclap, boom box	120	Threshold of sensation is 120 decibels
Stereos (over 120 watts)	110–125	
Jet takeoff	130	Beyond threshold of pain—125 decibels
Shotgun firing	130	

Source: National Institute on Deafness and Other Communication Disorders

Who Is at Risk?

Workers especially vulnerable to hearing loss due to noise levels are firefighters; police officers; construction, airport, and factory workers; musicians; farmers; and truck drivers. There are regulations designed to protect workers from hazardous noise levels, including those mandating the wearing of protective earplugs or earmuffs, but compliance is inconsistent.

Leisure-related threats—those that can occur in your everyday life—include live or recorded high-volume music, some household appliances, woodworking tools, lawn care equipment, and recreational vehicles such as snowmobiles and trail motorbikes. One important feature of noise-induced hearing loss is that it is preventable in all but certain cases of accidental exposure.

Physical Damage Caused by Noise

A sudden loud noise can leave you temporarily deafened, and you may experience a ringing in the ears, but normal hearing usually comes back within a few hours at most. This type of temporary hearing loss is called a **temporary threshold shift (TTS).** An example of a situation that can cause TTS is an explosion.

Over time, repeated exposure to loud noise can result in partial or total hearing loss. This is caused by destruction of the cilia in the **cochlea** (inner ear) and their auditory nerve connections. Any time you are exposed to a loud noise, some of your cilia are destroyed. Prolonged or repeated exposure to noises can cause a total collapse of this sensitive portion of the body.

Noise has other effects on the body, even at levels that do not produce hearing loss. Researchers have found that following a sudden, loud, or unexpected noise, there are bodily changes including increased blood pressure and heart rate. Noise also causes the peripheral vessels in the eyes and brain to dilate, which implicates noise as one of the many possible causes of headaches.

Damage from noise can also occur to the developing ear, and even possibly to the ears of a fetus. Premature babies are exposed to unrelieved noise in neona-

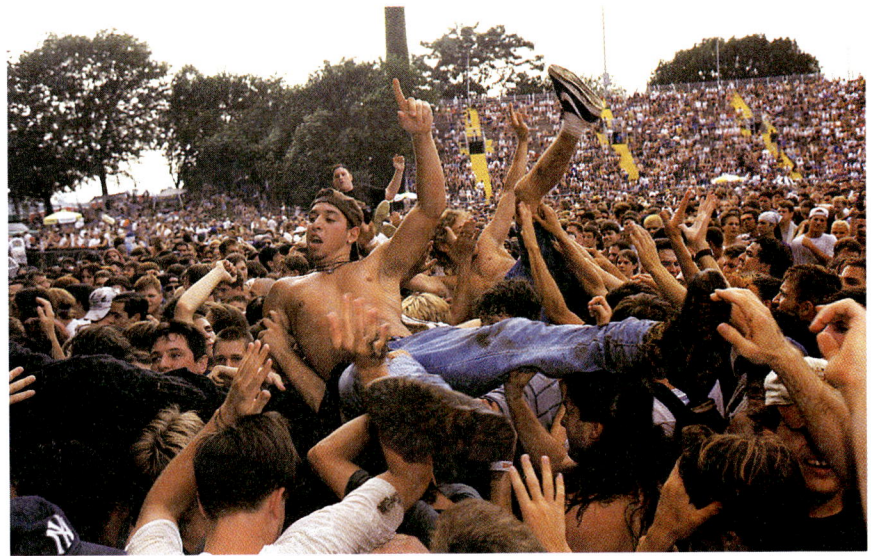

How much is having fun at a rock concert worth to you? Sound levels at rock concerts are in the 110 to 140-decibel range, but anything above 85 decibels is potentially hazardous. (Source: The Image Works/© A. Lichtenstein)

tal intensive care units, where noise levels in incubators can vary from 60 to 80 decibels. A premature baby can spend weeks and sometimes even months living in this environment without any respite from the noise.

Advice from the Wise

In 1989, the U.S. Supreme Court ruled in a six to three decision that no constitutional right exists to play rock music too loudly. The court rejected the argument of a group called Rock Against Racism that New York City's rules for keeping the volume down at Central Park concerts were a violation of the group's freedom of expression. Justice Thurgood Marshall, then eighty years old, was one of the dissenters from the Court's decision. He said: "Judgments that sounds are too loud, noise-like, or discordant can mask disapproval of the music itself." Quoting a music critic, he said, "New music always sounds loud to old ears."

To protect "young" ears, the best advice from the National Institute on Deafness and Other Communication Disorders is to take a break from noise. For those exposed to noise at some chronically high levels, several hours of respite can forestall damage.

Indoor Pollution: Sick Buildings, Sick People

As if there aren't enough dangers resulting from breathing polluted air outside, the air you breathe inside—in your dorm, your home, or your office—can cause adverse health effects. According to an EPA study, people may be exposed to a pollution threat 100 times greater while indoors because that is where they typically spend 80 percent of their time and because the length of exposure multiplies the risk.

The problem in great part stems from the energy crisis of the early 1970s, when building engineers found that they could save on energy bills by better insulating offices, schools, and other institutional buildings and recirculating air within the building. Energy costs fell, but the indoor air became unhealthy as a result of the **tight building syndrome,** and office workers and students began complaining about eye and skin irritation, dry throat, fatigue, dizziness, nausea, and respiratory discomfort, including shortness of breath (see Figure 20.3).

temporary threshold shift (TTS) Temporary hearing loss usually caused by a sudden loud noise.

cochlea The inner ear.

tight building syndrome Characterized by unhealthy indoor air that results from a lack of circulating air or a lack of ventilation.

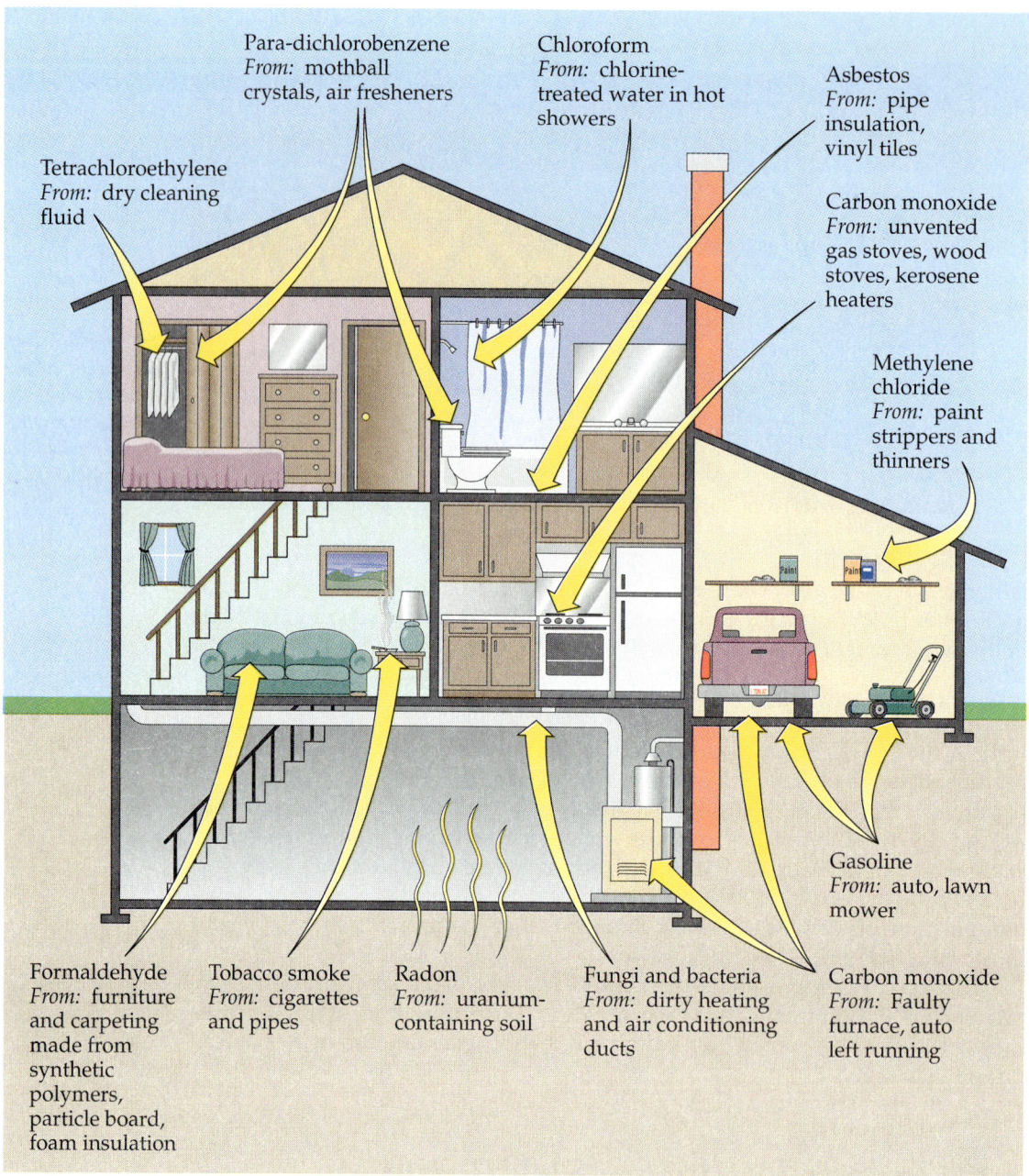

Figure 20.3 Sources of Indoor Air Pollution. *How many of these pollutants might be in your home or dorm? People who are sensitive to outdoor air pollution are also likely to be sensitive to indoor air pollution.*

Meanwhile, in private homes, also in response to the energy crisis, wood and coal stoves began to gain popularity. In some cases, this caused a rise in carbon monoxide and nitrogen dioxide levels inside the house. Such a rise can result in dizziness, slowed reflexes, and respiratory irritation. With heating in the winter and air conditioning in the summer, some homes have little fresh air exchange (see Table 20.3).

In addition, radon—an odorless, colorless, radioactive gas—seeps into millions of homes through basements, openings for utility pipes, floor drains, joints between walls and floors, and cracks in foundations. Some reports indicate that

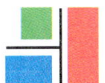

TABLE 20.3 Indoor Air Pollutants

Pollutant	Effects on the body
Asbestos fibers	Fibers widely used in insulation and other building materials that can cause lung disease, including lung cancer
Carbon monoxide	An odorless gas produced by incomplete combustion, such as that occurring in tobacco products, gas stoves, and unvented or improperly functioning heating equipment; interferes with the supply of oxygen to the body's tissues
Formaldehyde	An irritating and probably carcinogenic gas emitted from several types of consumer products, including particle board, plywood, insulation, cigarettes, and fabrics
Nitrogen dioxide	The by-product of high-temperature combustion, such as that occurring in gas stoves, unvented space heaters, and tobacco products; a principal respiratory irritant that may interfere with the body's defense against respiratory infections
Pesticides	Used in approximately 84 percent of U.S. homes; can cause acute toxic reactions after use
Radon	A radioactive gas in the earth's crust that can seep into homes; increases the risk of lung cancer
Tobacco smoke	More than 3,800 chemical compounds, most of which are toxic and 60 of which are known carcinogens; a cause of lung cancer and heart disease
Solvents	Cleaning products that contain some chemicals that can cause birth defects

Source: U.S. Environmental Protection Agency

there is an association between radon in the home and lung cancer; others do not. The EPA and the Department of Energy have identified a number of high-radon areas. If you live in such an area, it is likely that there has been a lot of newspaper coverage on the issue, and you might want to test to see if your home is affected. Call your local EPA office to see if your area is listed. You might want to test even if your area has not yet been studied.

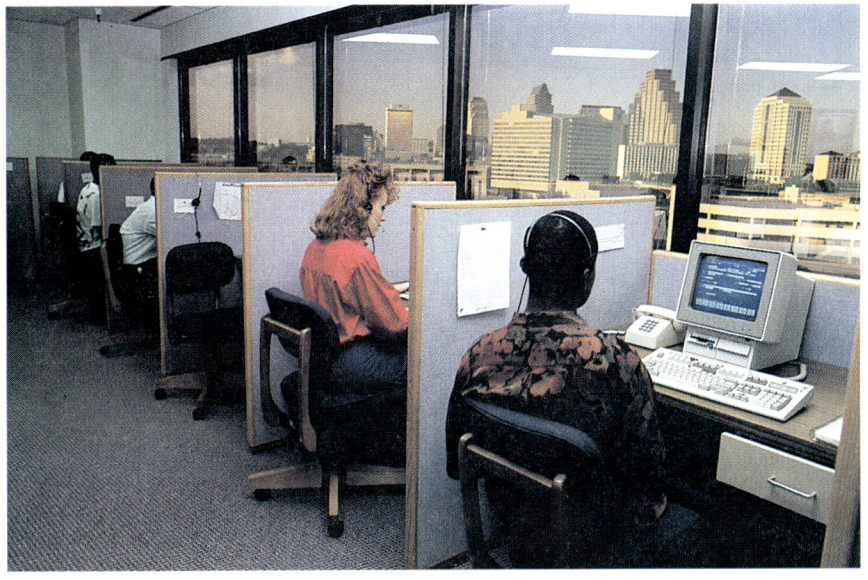

The view may be great, but sealed windows and poor ventilation can result in an unhealthy work environment. Indoor air pollution is invisible and can cause dizziness, nausea, and shortness of breath. (Source: The Image Works/© Daemmrich)

HEALTHWISE CONSUMER

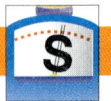

Multiple Chemical Sensitivity

In her late thirties, Karen Stevens began to develop severe reactions to perfumes and building materials while working in an airtight San Francisco office building.

"I had excruciating pain throughout my entire body. My fingers swelled so badly that they looked like purple scars. I could barely hold a pencil. I had cramping, severe pain, and trembling and I sometimes got to the point of crying uncontrollably. I couldn't walk a straight line."

Stevens, a certified public accountant and tax specialist, eventually went on disability. She would like to work at home, but she says she is hypersensitive to her computer.

Stevens is one of thousands of people in the United States suffering from a disorder peculiar to the late twentieth century. They say they are tormented by the chemicals we all encounter in everyday life. Fumes emitted by new carpets, building materials, clothes, cigarettes, and polluted air and water trigger severe reactions in them.

An Illness or a Fantasy?

What is this mysterious ailment? Some call this illness environmental illness, others call it total allergy syndrome, and still others call it multiple chemical sensitivity. There are also those in the medical profession who call it a fantasy.

The American Medical Association and the American Academy of Allergy and Immunology say that psychological problems can cause people to believe that chemicals are making them sick. Other physicians, who call themselves clinical ecologists or specialists in environmental medicine, believe that toxins in the environment are making people ill.

What is clear is that thousands of people are suffering from something. Many people with multiple chemical sensitivity can anchor the onset of their symptoms to times when they were exposed to chronic medium levels of contaminants. In Stevens's case, she says that she was exposed to indoor air pollution. Others became hypersensitive to a variety of substances after an overwhelming chemical exposure, such as a chemical spill on the job. Nearly half of those people said their illness started after a pesticide exposure.

"The world turned into a landmine," said a physician who became incapacitated by the ailment. After a person initially becomes sensitized, very low levels of exposure to chemicals that were easily

Critical Thinking Question

The *Healthy People 2000* objectives include the following: "Increase to at least 40 percent the proportion of homes in which homeowners/occupants have tested for radon concentrations and that have either been found to pose minimal risk or have been modified to reduce risk to health." This is one objective that calls for individual action by occupants of homes. In 1994, only 11 percent of homes had been tested for radon. Have the national objectives overstepped their boundaries by invading the privacy of the home? What compelling public health issues might justify this objective?

indoor pollution The contamination of indoor air by waste products or natural pollutants.

What Are the Risks?

People who are sensitive to outdoor air pollution are also likely to be sensitive to **indoor pollution.** Especially sensitive are infants and young children, pregnant

tolerated previously can set off severe allergic-type reactions. These include respiratory problems, headache, fatigue, flulike symptoms, mental confusion and short-term memory loss, stomach and digestive problems, heart irregularities, skin disorders, muscle and joint pains, irritability, and depression.

Those who are most severely affected have withdrawn from the world. Annabelle Brausieck is one of two dozen people living in Wimberley, Texas, because it is ill suited for agriculture and industry, and thus relatively free of modern pollutants. She sleeps in a porcelain "oasis" structure, in which the walls, ceiling and floors are covered in a nontoxic bathtub-like material. She claims to react to all furniture unless it's made of metal with baked-on enamel. She's also sensitive to draperies, lamp shades, plywood, toiletries, household cleaning products, paper, ink, car exhaust, and more.

The physicians who refuse to accept the existence of multiple chemical sensitivity find it hard to believe that such a wide range of very low-level chemical exposures could cause such a large variety of symptoms in so many organ systems. They also wonder how a person who claims to be sensitized initially by one substance, such as a pesticide, will later be affected by other substances having no obvious chemical relationship to the pesticide. Unlike multiple chemical sensitivity, most of the diseases that physicians are familiar with have a much narrower spectrum of symptoms.

New Clues from Research

New, highly speculative brain research is beginning to suggest ways that airborne chemicals, breathed in through the nose, could affect the brain's olfactory bulb, which ultimately could affect the hypothalamus. Because the hypothalamus is involved in so many body systems, disrupting it could have consequences on many parts of the body.

If multiple chemical sensitivity is eventually recognized as a definite medical illness, the cost to industry and government could be immense. The chemical industry could be faced with costly lawsuits and tens of thousands of workers could claim disability under workers' compensation and social security. Since 1988, the Social Security Administration has listed environmental illness as a disabling condition, but claims for workers' compensation have languished for years.

It took fifty years to begin to understand the subtle effects of lead on the human body. It could take even longer to research an illness based on so many chemical triggers and symptoms. In the meantime, it remains an ailment without an explanation, acceptance, or even an agreed-upon name.

---

women, the elderly, and those who have preexisting chronic illnesses, such as lung or heart disease. Read about people who have multiple chemical sensitivity in the Healthwise Consumer box.

You can do some basic, common-sense things to protect yourself from indoor air pollution at school and at home.

HEALTH SKILLS

- Ventilate your room with fresh outdoor air or recirculated filtered air.
- Remove the source of the irritant (e.g., tobacco smoke).
- Properly use and store cleaning solvents, paints, and pesticides.
- Repair or remove faulty home heaters.
- Follow manufacturer's specifications for room size and fuel when using kerosene heaters.
- Use an air purifier to reduce odors, tobacco smoke, dust, pollen, and some toxic gases, and change the filter regularly.

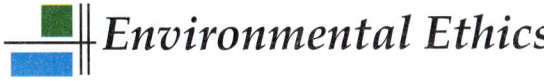

Environmental Ethics

Although environmental awareness is becoming more common in this country, opinions differ greatly on how we should treat the environment. Some people

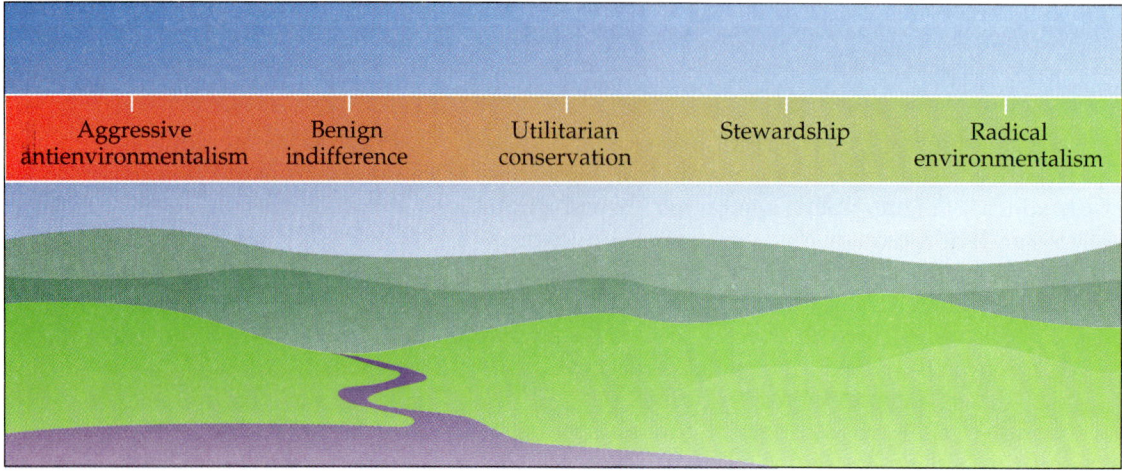

Figure 20.4 Continuum of Environmental Ethics. *Along this continuum, most people subscribe to a practice of stewardship or utilitarian conservation.*

believe that the future of human existence is dependent upon sustaining a healthy environment. Others believe that it is morally appropriate for us to use nature to meet our resource needs without limit. There are others who suggest that our actions today directly influence the health of our children and grandchildren; while others believe that impact is more immediate—that the implications of environmental degradation influence our personal health today. A recent study published in the *Journal of Environmental Education* suggests that there are five different "environmental ethics" which form a continuum, as shown in Figure 20.4. These include:

- *Aggressive antienvironmentalism.* Nature needs to be tamed or controlled to prevent human harm.
- *Benign indifference.* Nature is a useful storehouse of raw materials, so we have unlimited use of natural resources.
- *Utilitarian conservation.* The goods and services found in nature are limited, so we have to exercise caution in their use.
- *Stewardship.* Nature is important to future generations so we have a responsibility to take care of it.
- *Radical environmentalism.* Humans have a moral responsibility to protect all living things, and animals should not suffer needless pain.

The researchers found that most people subscribe to a practice of stewardship and utilitarian conservation and acknowledge the limits of natural resources. They recognize that human beings are dependent on nature for a variety of health-enhancing and life-sustaining benefits and are likely to feel a moral obligation to take care of nonhuman elements of the environment.

It is not necessary to be an environmentalist to feel an obligation to protect the environment and to take appropriate actions. One does not have to participate in a political rally supporting an environmental issue, ride on a Greenpeace ship, or write letters to political leaders to demonstrate personal convictions. Regardless of your philosophical or political position, the day-to-day actions that you take hold the potential of positively or negatively influencing your environment. Perhaps environmental health comes down simply to thinking globally and acting locally.

Key Concepts

1. According to the theory of acceptable risk, although exposure to a specific chemical or other hazardous material might be capable of causing disease, the likelihood of actually getting sick from it is very small.
2. Toxic gases occur naturally in the environment, and under normal circumstances, the body's filtering system ensures that we breathe in safe, filtered air.
3. Air pollution taxes the body's filtering system so that we breathe in noxious particles and gases. The automobile is the most pervasive source of air pollution.
4. The sources of water pollution are numerous, but the major ones are industrial, municipal, and agricultural. The main health threat from water pollution comes not from oil spills but from toxic wastes.
5. Sixty-two percent of the U.S. population drinks water containing fluoride. Fluoride is considered a major health success because it has contributed to a significant decline in dental caries in children.
6. It is estimated that every person generates more than three pounds of solid waste a day. Most of it—73 percent—goes into landfills.
7. Precycling refers to the reduction of household garbage by making environmentally sensitive consumer choices.
8. Recycling newspapers, plastics, aluminum cans, and glass bottles could greatly reduce the landfill problem—and save money, natural resources, and energy.
9. Sound levels above 85 decibels—roughly equivalent to that produced by a power leaf blower, lawn mower, or food blender—are potentially hazardous.
10. People may be exposed to a greater pollution threat from chemicals emitted inside a building than outdoors because that is where they typically spend 80 percent of their time and because the length of exposure multiplies the risk.

Review Questions

1. Differentiate between serious environmental threats and threats that are perceived to be serious but that actually present little risk to the global environment.
2. Cite three reasons why measuring environmental health threats is difficult.
3. Explain the differences between carcinogens, teratogens, and mutagens and give an example of each in the environment.
4. List major pollutants found in the air. Identify a specific disease or health concern associated with each.
5. List major pollutants found in water. Identify a specific disease or health concern associated with each.
6. Differentiate between the practices of precycling and recycling. Explain how each can contribute to the reduction of solid waste.
7. Explain why toxic wastes pose a threat to health and identify an example of the impact of improper disposal of hazardous waste on human health.
8. Describe the physical damage caused by noise.
9. Estimate the cost of environmental cleanup. What would be the benefits of such activity?
10. Identify five points of view concerning the environment and explain how each is represented in an environmentally related action.

Selected Bibliography

Environment (published bimonthly).

EPA Journal. Washington, DC: Environmental Protection Agency, (published bimonthly).

Global Warming & Energy Choices: A Community Action Guide. Washington, DC: Concern, Inc., 1991.

Hall, R.H. *Health and the Global Environment.* Cambridge, UK: Polity Press, 1990.

National Air Quality and Emissions Trend Report. Washington, DC: Environmental Protection Agency, (published annually).

National Water Quality Inventory. Washington, DC: Environmental Protection Agency, (published biennially).

Noise and Hearing Loss (National Institutes of Health Consensus Development Conference Statement). Bethesda, MD: National Institutes of Health, 1990.

One Earth/One Future: Our Changing Global Environment. Washington, DC: National Academy of Science, National Academy Press, 1990.

"Public Health Service Report on Fluoride Benefits and Risks." *Morbidity and Mortality Weekly Report* 40 (1991): 1–8.

The Journal of Environmental Education (published quarterly).

HealthLinks: Web Sites for Living in a Healthy Environment

You can access better health as it relates to this chapter by checking out some of the following sites on the Internet. These and sites identified within the chapter can be accessed directly when you visit the *HealthStyles* Web Site located on the Allyn and Bacon home page at **http://www.abacon.com.**

Keep America Beautiful
www.kab.org

Keep America Beautiful, Inc. KAB is a nonprofit, public education and community improvement organization with local affiliates throughout North America that is committed to preserving the natural beauty, environment, and resources of America and improving waste handling at the community level. This site includes educational material for teachers and students, press releases, a calendar of events, and much more.

National Institute of Environmental Health Sciences
www.niehs.nih.gov

A division of the National Institute of Health, the National Institute of Environmental Health Sciences provides basic research on environment-related diseases. The site includes press releases about scientific discoveries such as the health effects of urban pollution, a monthly journal and supplement that provide the latest in cutting-edge research articles and news of the environment, access to the NIEHS Clearinghouse, and information on employment opportunities.

National Toxicology Program
ntp-server.niehs.nih.gov/

The National Toxicology Program (NTP) coordinates toxicology research and testing activities, provides information about potentially toxic chemicals to regulatory and research agencies and the public, and strengthens the science base in toxicology.

National Center for Environmental Health
www.cdc.gov/nceh/ncehhom.htm
The National Center for Environmental Health collaborates with numerous state and local public and private groups to promote health and quality of life by preventing and controlling disease, birth defects, disability, and death resulting from interactions between people and their environment.

Health Hotlines: Living in a Healthy Environment

Indoor Air Quality Information Clearinghouse
(800) 438-4318
Environmental Protection Agency
P.O. Box 37133
Washington, DC 20013-7133

National Institute of Environmental Health Services
(800) 643-4794
P.O. Box 12233, Mail Drop B2-05
Research Triangle Park, NC 27709

National Lead Information Center
(800) 424-LEAD (424-5323) - Clearinghouse
1019 19th Street NW, Suite 401
Washington, DC 20036-5105

National Pesticide Telecommunications Network
(800) 858-7378
Ag-Chem-Extension
Oregon State University
333 Weniger
Corvallis, OR 97331

Occupational Hearing Service
Dial A Hearing Screen Test
(800) 222-3277 (outside Pennsylvania)
(800) 345-3277 (within Pennsylvania)
P.O. Box 1880
Media, PA 19063

Safe Drinking Water Hotline
(800) 426-4791
Environmental Protection Agency, Mail Stop 4604
401 M Street SW
Washington, DC 20460

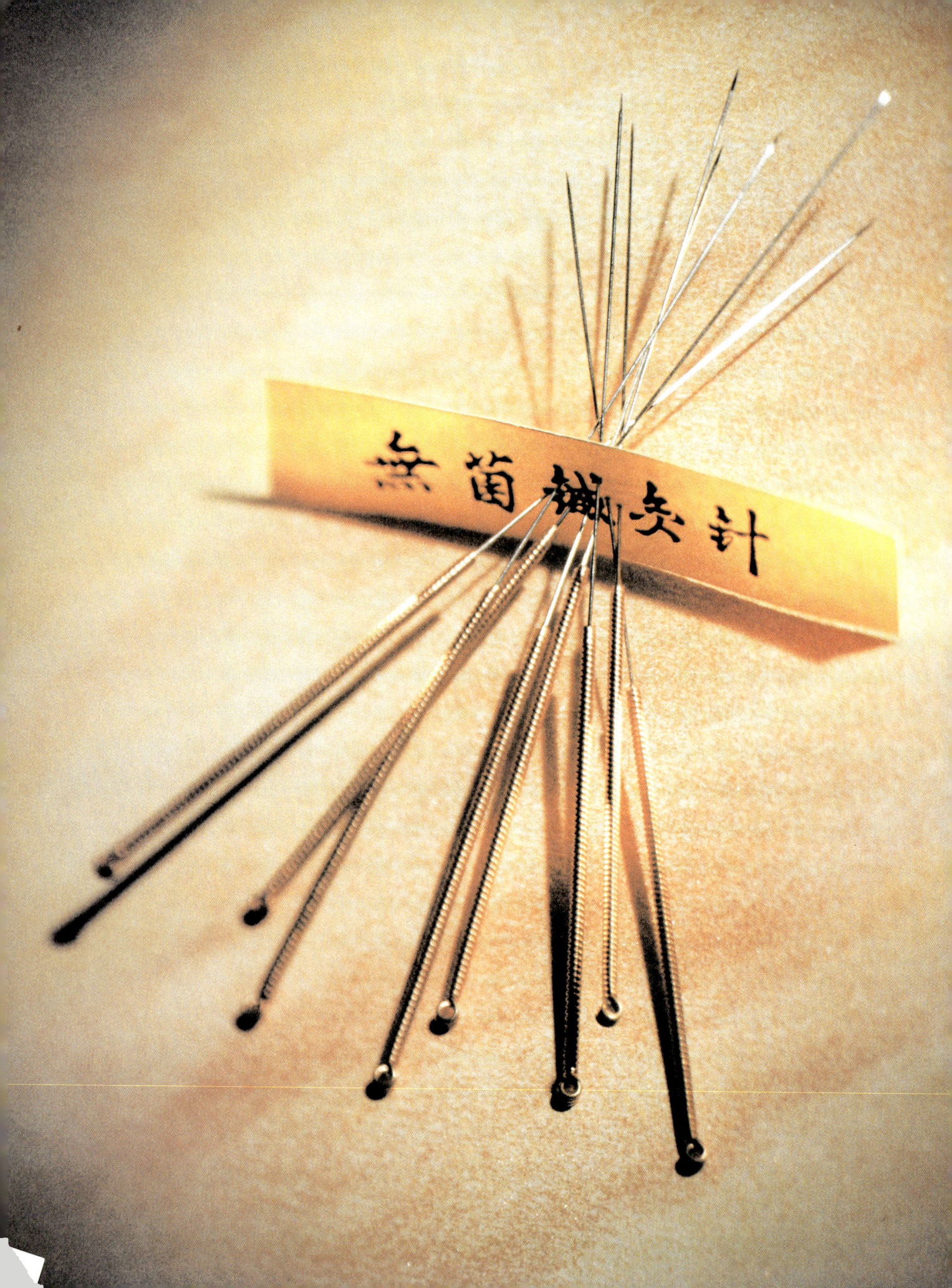

Chapter 21

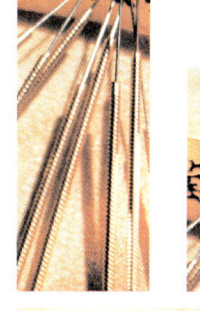
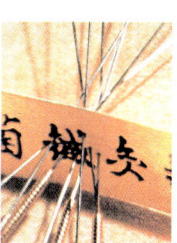
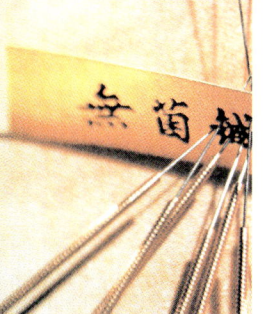

Making Health Care Decisions

Objectives

When you finish reading this chapter, you will be able to:

1. Describe the role of information in consumer decision making.
2. Describe five advertising techniques used to promote health products and services.
3. Recognize quackery and health fraud.
4. State your rights as a consumer of health-related products and services.
5. File a consumer complaint when you are dissatisfied with a product.
6. Make a wise decision by employing several strategies when selecting a physician.
7. Recognize the difference between the insured, the uninsured, and the underinsured.
8. Understand the advantages and disadvantages of traditional indemnity plans, health maintenance organizations, and preferred provider organizations.
9. Differentiate between prescription and over-the-counter drugs and briefly describe how each should be taken.
10. Have access to extensive sources of health information, including hotlines and the Internet.

What Is Your HealthStyle?

While relaxing after classes by reading a fashion magazine, Rani found the perfect solution to her "baggy" body—an amazing, new, miracle tummy reducer for only $49.95. She reviewed the testimonials in the advertisement and liked what she read. She sent off a check that day for a treatment that promised to remove inches from her midsection.

It took some six weeks for the stomach reducer to arrive, and by then, Rani had lost some enthusiasm for it because her friend George had shown her a far cheaper and more effective way to get rid of excess flab. Rani's new stomach reducer sat in the corner and collected dust.

George was also dissatisfied with his flabby midsection and some recent weight gain, and he too decided to do something about it. He went to the college health service and spoke with someone who gave him a nutritionally sound diet to follow. He also began working out at the recreation center three times a week, and on the other days, he took a brisk walk with some friends. George lost ten pounds and looked and felt better than he had before, and all it cost him was time well-spent. In addition, he started helping Rani and has asked her to join the walk-workout group.

In Your Opinion

Rani made a quick and poor health care decision by which she lost money but no weight. George's decision helped him take off the unwanted pounds and also make his body firmer.

- What alarms should have sounded for Rani when she read the tummy reducer ad?
- Have you ever bought or been tempted to buy "miracle" cures? Have they worked for you or your friends?
- Why is George's approach to getting a firmer body likely to work better than Rani's miracle?
- What health skills did George possess that Rani lacked?

Imagine a health care supermarket that has one aisle for insurance products and others for medications, surgery, hospitals, home remedies, and so on. It is not a real place, of course, but such a supermarket does exist in your mind, and each time you need to make a decision concerning your health—which physician to go to, which medication to take, whether to try an alternative therapy—you walk up and down the aisles searching for the right person, place, or product. To do this, you need to be an educated health care consumer. Rani learned how to be a better health care consumer by seeing that good health behaviors could serve her better than buying a so-called health product that wouldn't work.

Americans spend more money on health care than do people of any other country in the world—more than $988.5 billion in 1995—yet there is increasing concern about the quality of care that is delivered. A quick trip to the emergency room for a minor injury that doesn't even require any follow-up visits to a physi-

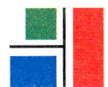

TABLE 21.1 Cost of Health Care in the United States

Year	National health expenditures	Percent of gross domestic product
1970	$73.2 billion	7.1%
1980	247.2	8.9
1985	428.2	10.2
1990	697.5	12.1
1995	988.5	13.6

Source: U.S. Department of Commerce, Health Care Financing Administration

cian can cost more than $200, and a few days in the hospital can run several thousand dollars. The high cost of health care is forcing more people to become involved in these decisions than in the past. Even though most Americans have health insurance and end up directly paying very little for this care, a little bit adds up (see Table 21.1).

Buying Health Care: How Do Consumers Make Decisions?

Whether or not you are aware of it, you make decisions about how to spend your health care dollars virtually every day. Do you go to the physician when you have a cold? There is no treatment for a cold other than symptom relief. Do you buy low-cost generic aspirin or a more expensive brand name, thinking it must be better? Generic drugs can cost between 20 and 85 percent less than their brand name counterparts.

When purchasing any product, you probably look for the best value. In terms of health care, the value is the reasonably priced product or service that will lead to good health and/or the improvement of health status. Sometimes that value is expensive to purchase—as with heart surgery. But sometimes that value can be gained with little or no expense. Sometimes the healthiest and most economical decision is the decision not to purchase a product at all but rather to look for a natural way to improve health. For example, there are times when an aspirin is the appropriate treatment for relief from a stress headache. There are also times when the proper response to a stress headache is simply to relax, perhaps by taking a walk along the beach or through the park. You do not necessarily have to spend a lot of money to be healthy, as Rani found out.

There are plenty of opportunities as a health care consumer to make wise choices—and plenty of opportunities to be the victim of deception or even fraud. To make wise choices and avoid fraud, you need information that is accurate, complete, and unbiased. You also need to understand the nature of advertisements—how health care products and services are presented to the public. Finally, you need to understand the nature of health fraud so you can recognize it when it presents itself.

Decision Making and Accurate Health Information

To make good health care decisions, it is necessary to be actively involved in your own health and to have complete information. What do you know about the drugs you buy, the tests your physician performs, or the diet that promises quick and permanent weight loss? Do you have enough reliable and unbiased infor-

HEALTH SKILLS

HealthLinks

Agency for Health Care Policy and Research
www.ahcpr.gov/consumer/

A reliable link to health information for the public. Provides the latest information on developments in health research, policy changes, and clinical findings.

mation to make reasonable decisions about your health care choices? Unfortunately, many people do not. Figure 21.1 identifies the various ways people participate in their medical care.

Although a lot of accurate information is available, there is also a stream of inaccurate information, and it often is difficult to determine which is which. In part this is because the health field includes many people who claim to be experts. In the field of nutrition, for example, whom do you think you should trust: a registered dietitian who recommends a balanced diet or the owner of a health food store where supplemental vitamins and minerals are sold?

Critical Thinking Question

> The media are filled with information and ads for products making various health claims. Differentiating a true expert from a quack isn't always easy. Do we put too much credence in expertise? Why do you think people are wary of leaving health-related products and services to personal trial and error? What criteria differentiate the true expert from the self-proclaimed expert? What signals alert you to false claims?

In addition to having to sort out who really is an expert, you must also decide what data to trust and how to evaluate risks. Consider the decision to take allergy medicine. Each package contains a **patient package insert,** an information sheet required by the Food and Drug Administration (FDA) which among other

Figure 21.1 Getting Involved. (Source: "How Is Your Doctor Treating You? Getting Information and Getting Involved." Copyright 1995 by Consumers Union of U.S., Yonkers, NY 10703–1057. Reprinted by permission from Consumer Reports, February 1995, p. 88)

Consumer Reports asked its readers ways they got involved in their medical care.	
Here are the percentages who said they had used each tactic:	
Asked physician to explain unclear terms	65%
Asked about any side effects and alternatives to medication	62
Asked about risks involved in tests or surgery	50
Did own research on the condition	48
Asked about alternatives to recommended tests or surgery	44
Asked about other treatments	44
Ascertained the doctor's experience in treating similar cases	43
Questioned doctor's opinions about cause of pain	37
Brought a written record of condition	36
Kept a written record of condition	30
Brought spouse or a friend to an office visit	26
Took notes on what doctor said about the illness	26
Complained that treatment wasn't working properly	25
Sought second opinion about diagnosis or treatment	22
Asked to see medical records	19
Told the doctor the recommended treatment was too painful	18
Told the doctor more information was needed	18
Discussed how treatment costs could be reduced	17

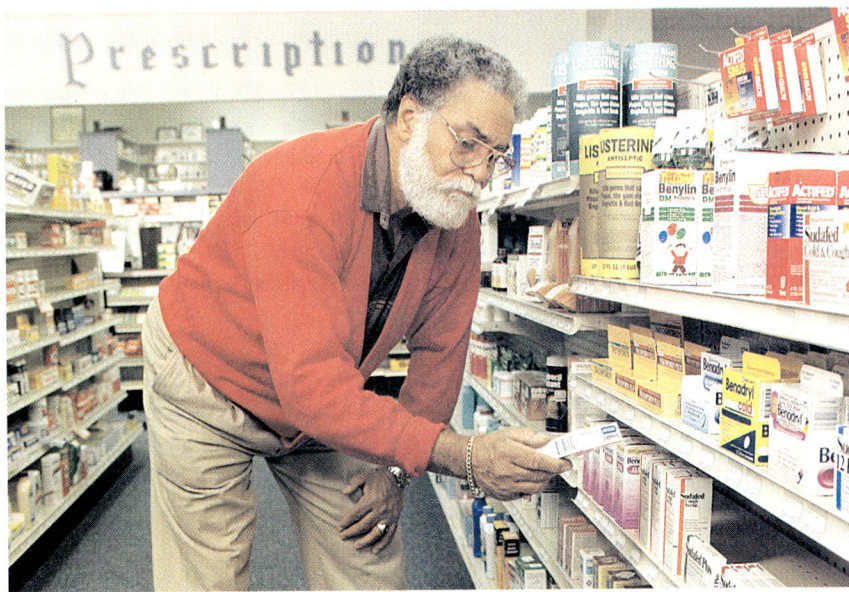

Make good consumer decisions and read about the contraindictions—or side effects—of over-the-counter medications before you buy them. (Source: © Tony Stone Images/Will & Deni McIntyre)

things, warns the consumer of **contraindications,** circumstances that make use of the product inadvisable. The consumer needs to examine the benefits and risks of taking the drug and to decide whether the benefits are worth the risks. You can read about any drug sold in the *Physician's Desk Reference.* Most libraries have this reference book as well as medical dictionaries that define medical terms.

Many good sources for health care information are available, including *Consumer Reports,* the *Harvard Medical School Letter on Health,* the *University of California at Berkeley Wellness Letter,* the *FDA Consumer,* and some medical and health columns in newspapers and magazines. An excellent source of information is the Internet, and a good place to begin searching the Internet is with the Web sites listed within and at the end of each chapter of this textbook. As with any other source of information, however, be critical of what you read on the Internet. The best of the Web sites can still be biased on occasion.

Advertising Health Care

Advertising is the primary way businesses have of informing the public about their products and services. It is also one of the most economical means of selling to the buying public. This is the case with all consumer goods, including health-related products and services. Advertisements of health products and services are seen in magazines, in point-of-purchase displays at the drug store, and on television. An educated consumer uses ads as a means of knowing what health care products are available. At the same time, the wise consumer seldom depends on ads alone as a source of information upon which to base a purchase decision. The reason is that ads, by their very nature, are biased in favor of the product being promoted.

Advertisers attempt to make a product or service as appealing as possible. They do this through several advertising techniques. So-called *scientific studies,* for example, are used in many health-related ads. A common claim might be that "in a doctor-approved research study, brand X relieved headache twice as fast as other brands." Very little data are provided, particularly concerning the research design, study population size, or controls involved in the study. There is nothing

patient package insert An information sheet, required by the FDA, that, among other things, warns the consumer of possible contraindications for use of a drug or medical product.

contraindications Circumstances that make use of a pharmaceutical or medical product inadvisable.

wrong with scientific studies. In fact, good science is how health products and services are designed and developed. But beware of bogus science. And be on guard against ads that quote reputable scientific studies, but present only supportive data. Half-truths can be as effective as outright deception in advertising.

Another technique used by advertisers is the *bandwagon approach.* In this technique, advertisers sell the product by claiming that "everyone is using the product," therefore you must jump on the bandwagon and use it as well. An example of this is seen in ads for exercise equipment when the key selling line is, "over 8,000 of these devices have been sold." Just because a product has been a business success does not mean that it is effective.

Some advertisements rely on *testimonials* to sell their product. The testimonial is usually given by a famous person—or an attractive model—who tells you how the product worked for him or her. Notice the lack of factual data in such ads. After reading the testimonial, the consumer knows little more than that the product exists. The wise consumer does not purchase a product without information on the effectiveness or safety of the product—two components seldom found in testimonial advertisements.

Emotional appeals are used for some products. These are seen in ads that claim that a product is safe or wholesome and are often used for products designed for children, such as cold remedies. A scene showing a sad and obviously ill child being watched over by a loving mother providing a "soothing" medicine is emotionally touching, but like other advertising techniques, provides the consumer with little information.

Finally, some advertisers provide a *comparison to other products* or depend on *price appeal* to sell their products. These approaches are often used with products that are well known to the buying public. Pain relievers, for example, are extremely common, so one way to spur purchase of a particular brand is simply to offer it at a price lower than its competitors'.

Notice that with all the techniques described here the advertiser may bend the truth a little or present half-truths while withholding negative information about the product being advertised. Although there are laws that require truth in advertising, wise consumers view all promotional material with caution. By recognizing the techniques used by advertisers, you as a consumer are better prepared to make wise decisions about health products.

Health Fraud

Some health-related products and services are actually anything but health related. Naive health care consumers in search of the perfect cure for complex health problems seem willing to buy almost anything. In fact, more than 26 percent of Americans surveyed for an FDA poll said that they have used one or more questionable methods of health care to treat medical problems especially prone to quackery.

Quackery—a health claim made for a product or service that cannot be justified by scientifically derived evidence—costs American consumers several billion dollars a year in useless tests and treatments. There are, in addition, serious medical consequences, including getting ill from the use of a product itself or from failure to get the approved, needed therapy when it can be most effective. For example, one quack advertisement noted that 80 percent of women got premenstrual relief by using large doses of vitamin B_6. But the ad neglected to note that the same percentage of women on a placebo thought they got relief, too, or that the doses of vitamin B_6 that were being recommended can cause nerve damage.

The quack, whether selling a product or a service, usually depends on mysticism, sensationalism, and false science. Consider the following lines that are typically found in quack advertisements:

quackery A health claim made for a product or service that cannot be justified by scientifically derived evidence.

DEVELOPING HEALTH SKILLS

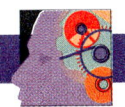

Spotting Health Fraud

Each year, Americans waste billions on bogus treatments that promise to be simple avenues to better health. The problem is so bad that most state attorneys general's offices dedicate tremendous efforts to investigating and prosecuting fraudulent claims. When considering the efficacy of the latest health wonder, ask yourself some simple questions:

- *Does it promise too much too easily?* Unproven remedies are often promoted as cure-alls that will accomplish everything from preventing "aging" to curing impotence.
- *Does it claim immediate or guaranteed results?* Few medical treatments produce immediate benefits for chronic conditions. And even proven therapies can't always guarantee better health.
- *Does it include a secret or exclusive formula?* Legitimate therapies evolve from data collected and reviewed by many scientists.
- *Are testimonials the only proof it works?* Unproven remedies are typically endorsed by "satisfied customers." These people may be paid for their comments or lulled by the power of suggestion into the belief they were "cured."
- *Does it offer a money-back guarantee?* A guarantee is an effective ploy to get you to buy a product. But don't expect anyone to respond to your refund request.

If you question a medical treatment, discuss it with your physician or other health care professional, or write: National Council Against Health Fraud, P.O. Box 1276, Loma Linda, CA 92354.

Source: Adapted from "Health Tips: Spotting Health Fraud," p. 3, in the March 1996 *Mayo Clinic Health Letter*, with permission of Mayo Foundation for Medical Education and Research, Rochester, Minnesota 55905

- "An amazing breakthrough in medical technology..."
- "Our studies prove that ..."
- "Researchers have uncovered the secret that revolutionizes ..."

These words may sound great, especially to the unwary person who is facing a life-threatening illness. Cancer and arthritis are prone to quackery treatments because many patients who have these conditions become desperate for "cures." Also, both diseases tend to go into remission on their own, which allows the quack to claim success (see the Developing Health Skills box).

It is estimated that half of all patients in legitimate cancer therapy also try unproven treatments. Especially popular among cancer patients is metabolic therapy, which includes large doses of vitamins and minerals, a special diet, and detoxification with enemas. Other vulnerable targets for quackery products are people seeking quick weight loss, larger breasts, hair restoration, and removal of wrinkles. If products sound too good to be true, they probably are.

Your Rights as a Health Care Consumer

As a consumer of health care products and services, you have certain rights, including your entitlement to just and fair treatment. You also have certain responsibilities.

You have a right to information. It is your responsibility to ask for it. You can expect to get a certain amount of information from your health care provider. When asked, a pharmacist, for example, will provide basic information about a drug and under what conditions to take it. Sometimes you have to ask for more information, such as how a drug interacts with another prescription drug you take. You may also have to ask for an explanation. One of the keys to making

HealthLinks
Coalition for Consumer Health and Safety
www.healthandsafety.org/

The Coalition for Consumer Health and Safety is a partnership of consumer, health, and insurer groups working together to promote consumer health and safety.

informed decisions about your health care is to avoid being intimidated by your health care providers.

You have a right to safety. It is your responsibility to exercise caution. This may seem obvious, but products that are sold have been tested in the laboratory and gained approval by oversight agencies. This does not mean that you can use a product incorrectly and still expect to have no adverse health effects. You must be careful to use products as directed and to inform your health care professional of all conditions and situations that may affect effective treatment.

You have the right to choose any product you want. It is your responsibility to choose wisely. If given a prescription for a brand name drug, you can ask for a generic version of the same drug. When selecting a physician, you need not be intimidated by the system and accept just anyone. You can ask questions, even interview potential physicians in an effort to feel comfortable and to trust this most important health care professional. Even in a managed care setting such as a health maintenance organization (HMO), you can have a choice of primary care physicians. Read about HMOs on page 572 of this chapter.

You have a right to issue a complaint if you feel that a product or service has not helped you or has been misrepresented. It is your responsibility to do so. Finally, if you feel that you have been deceived as a consumer, there is an action you can take: You can file a complaint.

HEALTH SKILLS

Filing a Consumer Complaint

Reputable companies and manufacturers want their customers to be satisfied. They go to great expense to assure this through customer relations offices that handle complaints. Reputable companies welcome the chance to replace a defective product or refund money for a service that did not fulfill expectations. Many complaints, therefore, can be handled by simply returning the product to the point of purchase or by pointing out your dissatisfaction with the service.

Sometimes, however, companies may not respond to a simple complaint. In such cases you may want to take a more assertive approach by filing a written complaint, first with the company, then with an appropriate local, state, or federal regulatory agency. When preparing a written complaint, first collect all of the information and documentation that you need to make your complaint as clear as possible.

A written complaint can be a simple business letter. Be sure that your letter is addressed to someone who is in a position to respond to your complaint (for example, the customer relations office or the president of the company). Clearly explain the problem that you have with the product or the nature of your dissatisfaction with the service. Describe what you believe to be a fair settlement (for example, a refund of the purchase price, replacement of the product, or credit). Attach all documentation needed to support your claim. In the case of a pharmaceutical product, for example, this might include the receipt for purchase, the patient package insert, and the remaining drugs. If possible, return to where you purchased the product or service and ask to meet with the appropriate person. Deliver your written complaint in person along with a calm explanation of how you would like the situation resolved. An alternative is to send the complaint to the company by registered mail; this provides documentation that the complaint was received.

If you are dissatisfied with the response to your complaint, submit your letter to the Better Business Bureau in your area. You can find the address in the phone book. Depending on the nature and/or severity of your concern, you may also want to issue your complaint to the Consumer Product Safety Commission, a federal office that establishes standards for consumer goods and takes dangerous products off the market, or the Federal Trade Commission, which regulates unfair and deceptive advertising.

Critical Thinking Question

The *Healthy People 2000* objectives include the following: "Increase to at least 75 percent the proportion of the total number of adverse event reports voluntarily sent directly to the Food and Drug Administration that are regarded as serious." A serious adverse event is one that is life threatening and that "requires intervention to prevent permanent damage as well as death, hospitalization, disability, and congenital anomaly." The objective was nearly reached in 1994, when 72 percent of adverse event reports sent voluntarily were serious. Must a consumer experience a life-threatening situation before the FDA is informed? What do you think is the purpose of this objective?

How to Choose Health Care Providers

Suppose you move to a new community and need to find a primary care physician. Who would you choose, and how would you go about making that decision? Similarly, if you had to go to a hospital, either for an emergency or for elective surgery, which one would you choose and why would you make that decision?

The Right Physicians for You

To begin with, there are numerous kinds of medical physicians from whom to choose. Very few physicians graduate from medical school and begin to practice medicine without additional training. Primary care physicians are most often trained in family practice (and are family practitioners) or in internal medicine (and are internists). Pediatricians provide primary care for children, and obstetrician/gynecologists often provide primary care for women. In general, the type of physician you see is usually not as important as the individual physician. For example, a woman can get her primary care from a family practice physician, an internist, or a gynecologist.

In most cases, your primary care physician recommends a specialist for you when you need to see one. Table 21.2 provides examples of some health care professionals and their areas of specialization. It includes some specialists who are not physicians.

There are many kinds of licensed health care practitioners who are not medical doctors (MDs). Psychologists (who provide clinical therapy, counseling, and other mental health care), chiropractors (who provide spine and joint manipulation, often to relieve pain), and podiatrists (who treat foot diseases and ailments) fall into this category. There are also so-called alternative health care practitioners, including acupuncturists, herbalists, and massage therapists. In some cases, an acupuncturist is also a medical doctor. You can read more about this in the Cultural View box.

Naturopaths use a variety of alternative treatments, depending on a patient's individual needs. These methods can include diet; acupuncture; herbal medicine; water therapy; therapeutic exercise; spinal and soft-tissue manipulation;

TABLE 21.2 Health Professionals

Allergist	A specialist who diagnoses and treats allergies	*Nuclear medicine specialist*	A specialist who uses radioactive substances to diagnose and treat various disorders
Anesthesiologist	A specialist who administers drugs during surgical procedures to reduce pain or induce unconsciousnes	*Obstetrician/ gynecologist (OB/GYN)*	A specialist who diagnoses and treats problems of the female reproductive system
Cardiologist	A specialist in the diagnosis and treatment of heart and blood vessel disorders	*Oncologist*	A specialist who diagnoses and treats cancerous growths and tumors
Dermatologist	A specialist in the diagnosis and treatment of skin disorders	*Ophthalmologist*	A specialist who diagnoses, treats, and provides general care of eye disorders
Family practitioner	A physician who offers routine medical service for a variety of ailments	*Orthopedist/ orthopedic surgeon*	A specialist who diagnoses, treats, or provides surgical care for bone and joint injuries and problems
Endocrinologist	A specialist in the diagnosis and treatment of glandular disorders		
Exercise physiologist	A specialist in the effects of exercise on the function of body systems	*Otolaryngologist*	A specialist who specializes in ear, nose, and throat disorders
Gastroenterologist	A specialist who diagnoses and treats disorders of the stomach and intestinal tract	*Pathologist*	A specialist who examines body organs, tissues, cells, and fluids to determine disease states
Geneticist	A specialist who diagnoses and treats genetic diseases	*Pediatrician*	A physician who treats childhood diseases
Health educator	A specialist in the field of health education and health promotion who holds a degree in a health-related area	*Physical therapist*	A specialist who rehabilitates people after impairment due to injury or disease
		Physician assistant	Health care professional trained to assist physicians
Hematologist	A specialist who diagnoses and treats blood-related disorders	*Plastic surgeon*	A specialist who provides corrective surgery for irregularities of body or facial contours
Neurologist	A specialist who diagnoses and treats diseases of the brain, nervous system, and spinal cord	*Psychiatrist*	A physician who diagnoses and treats mental and emotional disorders
Neurosurgeon	A specialist who is similar to a neurologist but who specializes in surgery	*Pulmonary specialist*	A specialist who diagnoses and treats disorders of the respiratory system
Nurse practitioner	Nurse specialist with additional training in a specified area, such as OB/GYN	*Urologist*	A specialist who diagnoses and treats disorders of the urinary tract

Source: Rebecca J. Donatelle and Lorraine G. Davis, *Access to Health,* 5th ed., p. 605 (Table 24.1). Copyright © 1998 by Allyn & Bacon. Reprinted by permission of Allyn & Bacon.

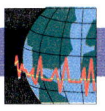

CULTURAL VIEW

The Chinese Tradition of Acupuncture

Since at least the second century B.C., Chinese doctors have been sticking thin needles into the skin of the ailing. Acupuncture is based on the concept that within the body there are numerous channels called meridians. When energy is blocked along any of the meridians, an excess of energy results in some channels and a deficiency occurs in others. Over time, these imbalances can lead to illness. Acupuncture is a way of restoring balance by triggering shifts of energy with hair-thin, disposable needles inserted into the body. These needles are inserted in some of the 361 classical acupuncture points.

Why this has the power to heal is a mystery, which is one reason why the U.S. medical establishment has viewed it skeptically—at least until relatively recently. There is a growing contingent of U.S. physicians who swear by it. Frustrated by the limitations of Western medicine, which treats body parts separately, more than 3,000 physicians use acupuncture, which treats the whole body, the mind, and the emotions. In addition, there are some 7,000 practicing acupuncturists who are not physicians. The number of acupuncturists is likely to increase after an expert panel convened by the National Institutes of Health found "clear evidence" in 1997 that acupuncture is effective treatment for certain types of ailments.

With findings based on well-conducted studies, the panel reported that acupuncture could cut by 50 percent the number and severity of episodes of nausea and vomiting caused by cancer chemotherapy drugs, surgical anesthesia, or morning sickness during pregnancy. The panel found that using acupuncture to reduce pain following dental surgery had even more dramatic results: patients who received acupuncture before the removal of impacted molars had an average of only seventeen minutes of post-surgical pain, in contrast to ninety-four minutes for patients treated with conventional pain drugs. The experts also found evidence—although not as strong—that acupuncture is effective for treating menstrual cramps, drug addiction, stroke, headache, and even tennis elbow.

Acupuncture is already being used in about one thousand drug addiction treatment facilities, where clinicians have found it has a calming effect on drug addicts and reduces their craving for drugs. This might be due to a release of endorphins as part of the acupuncture process. Endorphins are pain-relieving substances produced by the body.

Acupuncture is also gaining popularity with patients. An estimated 15 million Americans have tried it at least once. Many states have accredited licensure programs for acupuncturists, and some insurance companies pay for treatment. If you are interested in receiving acupuncture treatment, be sure to inquire about the acupuncturist's training and whether he or she has a license to practice.

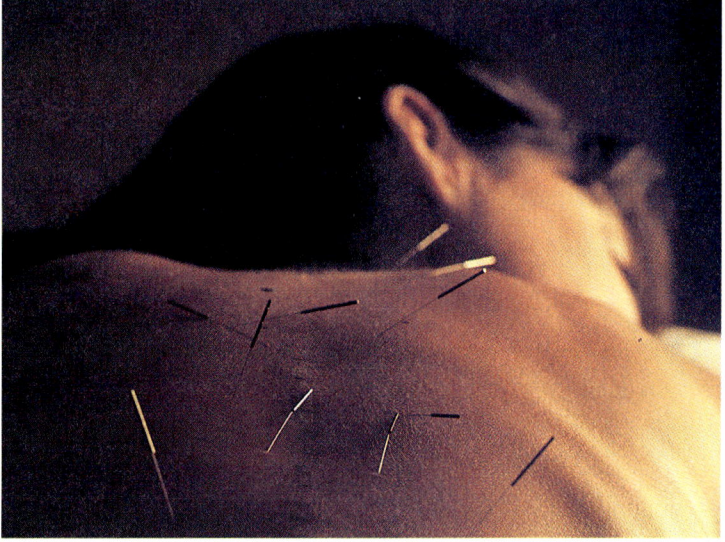

Acupuncturists relieve pain by inserting special needles at key points in the body. (Source: © Tony Stone Images/Kindra Clineff)

physical therapies involving electric current, ultrasound, and light therapy; therapeutic counseling; and pharmacology. Naturopathy is based on the healing power of nature. The FDA lists nine herbs that can cause serious problems, including kidney failure and stroke: chaparral, comfrey, germander, jin bu huan, lobelia, magnolia, ma huang, stephania, and yohimbe. A well-trained naturopath will steer you away from risky botanicals.

Far from being off beat, many of the alternative treatments have become mainstream and licensed practitioners are covered under a growing number of insurance plans. One national HMO began covering them when it found that one third of its members had used some form of alternative medicine in the last two years.

At some point—or at several points in your life, depending on how often you move and other lifestyle circumstances—you will be in a position to need a new physician or want to try an alternative therapy. Here are some options you should consider when choosing a new health care practitioner:

- Ask your current physician for a recommendation. Contrary to what you think, this will not preclude you from getting a recommendation for an alternative practitioner. A national survey found that 60 percent of physicians had at some time referred patients to practitioners of alternative medicine.
- Ask the student health service or human resources director where you work for the names of physicians other students or employees like—or dislike.
- If you know a nurse, ask which physicians he or she recommends seeing—or avoiding. Nurses know more about good and bad health care practitioners than many other health professionals.
- Find out about your new doctor's training and experience. Ask if he or she is board certified. Although all physicians must be licensed to practice

> Most physicians consider any of the following an emergency and reason to go immediately to the emergency room of the nearest hospital:
>
> abdominal pain (severe)
> animal bites
> bleeding (severe, uncontrollable)
> broken bones
> bullet or stab wounds
> burns (severe)
> chest pains (severe)
> choking (or difficulty breathing)
> convulsions
> diarrhea (prolonged)
> drug overdose
> eye injuries or sudden loss of vision
> head injury
> heat stroke (dehydration)
> hypothermia (dangerously low body temperature)
> inhalation of gaseous fumes
> inhalation of smoke
> insect stings resulting in shortness of breath
> poisoning
> slurred speech (or loss of speech)
> snake bites
> temperature over 103° F
> unconsciousness
> vomiting (prolonged)

Figure 21.2 What is Considered an Emergency?

medicine, some are also board certified. This means the doctor has completed several years of training in a specialty and has passed an exam.

When You Go to the Hospital

Medical facilities provide a range of care, including primary, secondary, and tertiary care. **Primary care** is provided as **outpatient care** by a physician in the office or at an emergency room in a hospital or clinic.

Secondary care is usually provided as **inpatient care** in your local community hospital. Uncomplicated surgery is an example of secondary care. The three most often performed surgeries today are childbirth by cesarean section, gallbladder removal, and hysterectomy. An alternative to hospitalization for minor procedures is treatment in a special facility within the hospital or in a freestanding facility, where surgery is performed without the patient staying overnight.

Tertiary care, which is often provided at hospitals affiliated with medical schools or regional referral centers, includes special procedures, such as open-heart surgery, kidney dialysis, and other sophisticated treatments.

When selecting a hospital for primary emergency care, look for the best one near where you live with good access to secondary care in case additional care is needed (see Figure 21.2). In contrast, you might want to go to a tertiary care facility some distance from your home, perhaps in a different city. There are special centers for liver or heart transplants. Also, for example, some facilities specialize in treating breast cancer; others are best for lung disease. The selection of a tertiary care hospital is usually made by you in conjunction with your physician.

Unless it is a medical emergency, most health plans have to give advance approval, or **preadmission certification,** for you to go to the hospital. Otherwise, the cost of your hospital care may not be covered. (You will learn more about what is and what is not covered in health plans in the following section.) Most plans also establish how long you can stay in the hospital for each condition. Many procedures that were once done in the hospital (e.g., tonsillectomy) are now done on an outpatient basis.

Paying for Health Care

Traditionally, most people have had access to the health care system through their private health insurance plans, which are either provided by their employers, offered through their colleges or through a professional association to which they or their parents belong, or purchased individually. There are also public federal programs that provide insurance and/or access to health care. For example, people over age sixty-five are covered by Medicare, and low-income and disabled persons meeting certain qualifications are covered by Medicaid. In addition, there are some people who are **uninsured** (have no health insurance) and some who are **underinsured** (have policies that do not meet their needs or that place them at significant financial risk).

Many employers provide health insurance benefits to workers and their families as part of an employment package. Usually, employers pay most of the cost of the monthly or quarterly premium and employees pay the rest. Full-time students up to age twenty-three or twenty-five (depending on the plan) can be classified as "over-age" dependents and may remain on their families' insurance plan (see the Healthwise Consumer box).

Shopping for health insurance is complicated because so many different options are available. Choosing a plan can be a costly decision if you select the wrong one. Because your health care needs change, you might want to adjust your health insurance plan over time. For example, having a pregnancy-related

primary care Routine medical care provided by a physician in the office or at an emergency room in a hospital or clinic.

outpatient care Care provided in a physician's or other health practitioner's office, in an emergency room in a hospital, or in a specialized ambulatory clinic; does not involve hospitalization or overnight stays.

secondary care Care involving surgery and nonroutine medical treatment, usually delivered in a hospital.

inpatient care Health care provided in a hospital.

tertiary care Special medical procedures, such as open-heart surgery and transplants, performed mostly at hospitals affiliated with medical schools or at large regional hospitals.

preadmission certification Approval from a health plan of the need for inpatient hospital care prior to the actual admission.

uninsured Having no health insurance.

underinsured Having limited health insurance that compromises one's access to health care services and places one at significant financial risk.

HEALTHWISE CONSUMER

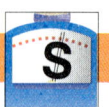

Covering College Students

Who covers college students for health care when they crash their bikes, twist their knees playing ultimate Frisbee, or come down with a serious illness? In some cases, the answer is no one. More than a quarter of all Americans aged eighteen to twenty-four—and a fifth of people aged twenty-five to thirty-four—have no insurance.

If you do not have access to health insurance through your parents, there are several affordable options:

- Most colleges and universities offer a student health plan. If you have school insurance, make sure it covers the summer months as well.
- When you graduate and do not go directly to a job that provides health insurance, see if the alumni association has a health plan. Often association plans have good rates.
- Some insurance companies provide short-term coverage, from three months up to one year. This is a good option if you think you are likely to be enrolled in an employer's plan soon.

Most colleges and universities also provide some care through the student health service. Typical services include distributing cold medication, treating minor injuries, and providing health education on everything from alcohol abuse and AIDS to hypertension and weight loss. Students should not rely on the college health service for their primary source of care. Most of the services are not set up to do this, and they are not accredited by any national body.

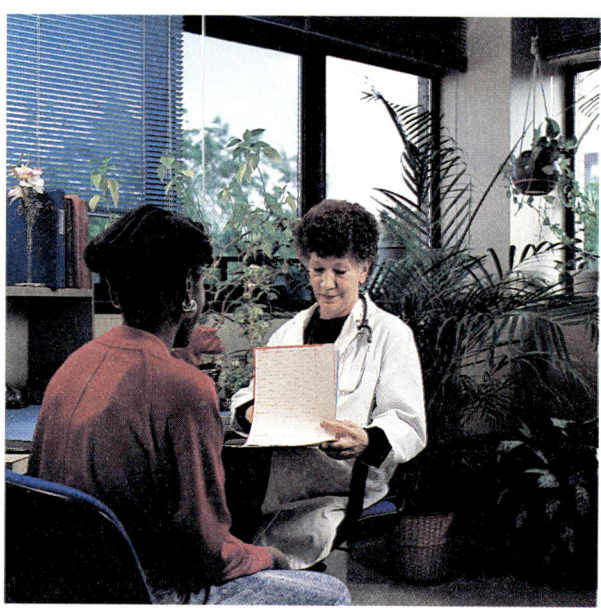

Having a physician who knows you and your health status is important. Your student health center can be a beneficial resource, but you still need a primary care physician. (Source: FPG International.© Jeff Kaufman)

benefit is important during the years that you might want to have a family, but it is no longer necessary later in life.

Critical Thinking Question

A growing concern among the general public is emergency admission of uninsured patients. Do you think all hospitals should be required to accept uninsured patients in emergency situations? If hospitals must accept uninsured patients, who will pay for the treatment? What are possible options for making sure the ill receive proper care?

Health Insurance Terms

There are many terms that are useful to know before you shop for health insurance. The following are key terms that you are likely to see when you review different policies.

COINSURANCE Percentages of covered benefits that the insured person and the insurance company each pay. The most common coinsurance plan is one in which the insured person pays 20 percent of the expenses and the insurance company pays 80 percent.

COORDINATION OF BENEFITS Limiting benefits to no more than 100 percent of allowable medical expenses in cases in which two or more insurers cover the same person. This can occur when both a husband and wife receive family health insurance through their respective employers.

COPAYMENT A cost-sharing arrangement in which a person in a health plan pays a specified charge for a specified service, such as $10 for an office visit or $2 for a prescription drug.

DEDUCTIBLE A set dollar amount of covered expenses that an individual must pay before reimbursement for expenses may begin. These usually range from $0 to $250 for group insurance, but can go as high as $1,000.

MAXIMUM OUT-OF-POCKET EXPENSE The maximum amount that an insured person must pay during a designated period for expenses covered by the plan. This typically ranges from $500 to $1,000 a year.

MAXIMUM POLICY LIMIT The total benefits that a policy will pay within a particular period of time, usually either the life of the policy or a calendar year. Common policy limits are $250,000 to $500,000 within a one-year period.

PREEXISTING CONDITIONS A limit on coverage for a specific condition if an insured person has previously been treated for that condition. Preexisting conditions are usually covered after twelve months. If you have been insured for at least twelve months and switch plans, any preexisting conditions will be covered under the new plan.

SPECIFIED MEDICAL LIMITATION A dollar limit placed on treatment of certain medical conditions or types of treatment, such as home health care and hospice care.

Traditional Indemnity Plans

The traditional way to get health insurance coverage is through an **indemnity plan,** in which you pay for most of your medical bills and then file a claim to be reimbursed. This is also called **fee-for-service.** This approach gives you the greatest amount of flexibility in choosing physicians, hospitals, and other health-related services. But it is also the most costly.

In addition to monthly premiums, indemnity plans have a deductible that you must pay for physician services before the insurer will reimburse for claims. Once that deductible amount is reached, most insurers reimburse only up to a certain amount for legitimate claims. In most plans, there is a coinsurance, with insurers paying a larger part of the bill (usually 80 percent) and the insureds paying a smaller part (usually 20 percent).

Fee-for-service plans can also place limits on the extent of coverage for all people insured under a plan, as well as on individual people applying for coverage if they have a preexisting condition. For example, if a person has been seek-

indemnity (fee-for-service) plan
Insurance coverage in which a person pays for most of his or her medical bills and then files a claim to be reimbursed.

HERE'S LOOKING AT YOU

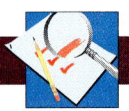

What Is Your Best Health Insurance Buy?

What should you look for when you are in the market to enroll in a health plan? For some people, cost is most important. For others, having access to certain services is number one on the list. Here are two worksheets for you to use to compare up to three different health plans in terms of how much they will cost you and what services you will get.

Look at your medical and insurance records from last year as a guide to what services you might use this year. Add up the actual costs to you, including premiums. Estimate what you might spend on your health care in terms of deductibles, coinsurance, and/or copayments, and services that are not covered by the health plan.

Worksheet A

	Plan #1	Plan #2	Plan #3

What is your monthly premium?
   Individual
   Family			

Multiply by 12 for annual cost			

What is your deductible, if there is one?
   Individual
   Family			

What is your coinsurance rate or copayment, if there is one? (Note if there is a higher rate for special services, such as outpatient mental health care.)			
Are there any annual limits for days or services covered and amount spent on you?			
What is the maximum you will have to pay out-of-pocket each year?			
What is the lifetime limit, if any, that you will be reimbursed?			
Based on last year's experience, estimate how much your health care will cost, including the premium, deductible, coinsurance, and/or copayment.			

HealthLinks

National Committee for Quality Assurance
www.ncqa.org/

The NCQA assesses and reports on the quality of managed care plans, including health maintenance organizations (HMOs).

ing medical treatment for a knee injury just prior to joining a new plan, the new health insurer can refuse to pay for any treatment for up to twelve months.

Managed Care Plans

Managed care plans have agreements with certain physicians, hospitals, and health care providers to give a range of services to plan members at a reduced cost. This limits your freedom to choose physicians in exchange for lower costs and less paperwork than in a fee-for-service plan. Managed care has been around for decades but began to become popular starting in the late 1980s as a way to contain health care costs. There are three basic types of managed care plans: health maintenance organizations, point-of-service plans, and preferred provider organizations.

Worksheet B

Service	Plan #1	Plan #2	Plan #3
Hospital care			
Surgery (inpatient and outpatient)			
Office visits to your doctor			
Maternity care			
Well-baby care			
Immunizations			
Mammograms			
Medical tests, X rays			
Mental health care			
Dental care, braces, and cleaning			
Vision care, eyeglasses, and exams			
Prescription drugs			
Home health care			
Nursing home care			
Services you need that are excluded			
Preexisting conditions that you have that will not be covered ever			
Preexisting conditions that you have that will be covered after a waiting period			
Other issues that are important to you: Choice of doctors; Convenient location of doctors and hospitals; Ease of getting an appointment; Minimal paperwork; Waiting period before coverage begins; Total estimated yearly cost to you (figure from Worksheet A)			

Source: National Institutes of Health, Agency for Health Care Policy and Research

HEALTH MAINTENANCE ORGANIZATIONS Health maintenance organizations (**HMOs**) offer a defined set of benefits according to a predetermined monthly premium. There are only limited or sometimes no costs beyond the monthly premium. A visit to the physician's office, for example, can cost only $10 a visit, in contrast to seventy-five dollars under a fee-for-service plan.

When you join an HMO, you will be assigned to a family physician or internist who acts as the gatekeeper to all other health services provided by the HMO. You may be given a choice of several physicians, all contract employees of the HMO. If you want to see a dermatologist or a cardiologist in the HMO, you would first have to see your assigned or chosen family physician, who would determine whether it was necessary for you to see that specialist. This approach holds down costs, but it also severely limits flexibility and choice of physicians

health maintenance organizations (HMOs) Prepaid plans that offer a defined set of benefits according to a predetermined monthly premium.

and hospitals. Some HMOs are beginning to allow members enrolled in the plan to contact certain specialists in the plan without seeing the primary care physician first. If you choose to see a physician outside the HMO, you have to pay 100 percent of the cost.

On the plus side, HMOs tend to offer one-stop shopping. Often, you will be able to get all your outpatient medical needs tended to in one treatment center. HMOs are also not permitted to add a waiting period for people who have pre-existing conditions.

POINT-OF-SERVICE PLANS One of the fastest growing type of HMO is a **point-of-service plan (POS),** which is an indemnity-type of option. In this plan, if you need to see a specialist, your primary care doctor makes the referral to someone in the plan, just as in a traditional HMO. Members can refer themselves to a physician outside the plan and still get some coverage—although they have to pay a coinsurance for it. A POS option costs more money than an HMO but less than fee-for-service.

PREFERRED PROVIDER ORGANIZATIONS Another popular option is a hybrid form of insurance that merges the best features of traditional indemnity insurance and HMOs. Under a **preferred provider organization (PPO),** you pay monthly premiums and have deductibles and copayments just as you would in an indemnity plan, but the copayment is lower.

In a PPO, you can choose your own physicians and kinds of services you want as long as they come from a list of preferred physicians and facilities. If you use these preferred providers, your share of the copayment drops to 10 percent, and in some cases it might be eliminated entirely. You have to use these preferred providers because they have agreed to treat all participants in the PPO at a discounted rate. This discount contributes to keeping your copayment lower than it would be in a traditional indemnity plan. If you go outside the network, your copayment can rise to 50 percent, depending on the type of service sought.

HEALTH SKILLS

Asking Questions about a Health Plan

Regardless of the type of health insurance you choose, you should ask a number of questions before agreeing to participate in a plan:

- What type of coverage do you need? What services are you and/or members of your family most likely to need in the coming years? Will the plan cover them? You may have heard stories about someone who contracted a major illness and then found out that his or her insurance did not provide coverage for it. The only way to avoid such situations is to be informed in advance.
- How do you feel about having limits placed on your choice of physicians or hospitals, and how important is the cost of services to you? Managed care plans limit your choice. Fee-for-service plans do not place limits but will cost you more money.
- What is the plan's policy on special areas of coverage such as maternity, laboratory charges, and prescription fees? Maternity coverage is often incomplete. Some policies offer full coverage if the employee gets pregnant and virtually none if a male employee's wife or dependent child gets pregnant.
- When does coverage take effect? This may seem like a simple question, but some employers require that you work for three to six months before you can be covered under their plan. Timing can also be critical when pregnancy is concerned, particularly if conception occurred before the insurance took effect.

- Overall, does this plan meet your needs? Are other policyholders satisfied with the extent of coverage? If it is a managed care plan, how long do you have to wait to see a physician? Are there physicians and hospitals in the plan that are convenient to where you live or work? How much paperwork is involved?

Don't choose an insurance carrier or plan just because it is the cheapest available. As with most consumer decisions, it is usually wise to shop around. To help you make the right decision, fill in the worksheets in the Here's Looking at You box.

Drugs as Medicine

Of all consumer issues, the purchase and use of drugs present one of the most important challenges. Each year, Americans take more than $20 billion worth of drugs in search of either getting well or staying well. About half of this money goes for **prescription drugs,** which are ordered specifically for you by your physician and filled by a registered pharmacist; the other half is for **over-the-counter (OTC) drugs,** a vast assortment of medicines, ranging from aspirin to wart removers, that you can buy without a prescription.

What is the difference between these two types of drugs? Prescription drugs are defined primarily as those unsafe for use except under professional supervision. They can include drugs that are habit forming or unsafe because of their toxicity. OTC drugs are considered safe for consumers to use if they follow the directions and warnings on the drug's labels. Sometimes, a stronger version of a drug can be obtained only by prescription even though a weaker version is available without a prescription. This is the case with ibuprofen, a popular pain reliever used for headaches, arthritic and joint aches, and soft tissue injuries.

Some drugs are available only under their original brand names. This is especially true of drugs developed by a single pharmaceutical company and still protected by a seventeen-year, exclusive patent. Most drugs on the market however, are also available as less expensive, generic drugs. Generic drugs have the same active chemical ingredients as their brand name counterparts, but some generic drugs are absorbed at different paces and may not be as effective as their brand name counterparts.

Critical Thinking Question

The *Healthy People 2000* objectives include the following: "Increase to at least 75 percent the proportion of people who receive useful information verbally and in writing for new prescriptions from prescribers or dispensers." FDA surveys show that 24 percent of respondents in 1992 said they had been given written information about their prescription drugs. By 1996, that proportion had risen to 67 percent. What might be the benefit to public health of this increase? Who should be responsible for providing information about prescription drugs? What is the consumer's responsibility concerning information about prescription drugs?

point-of-service (POS) plans HMOs having an indemnity-type option that lets members get care from physicians and other providers outside the plan's network.

preferred provider organization (PPOs) A hybrid form of insurance that merges features of traditional fee-for-service insurance and prepaid plans.

prescription drugs Drugs ordered specifically for a person by his or her physician and filled by a registered pharmacist.

over-the-counter (OTC) drugs Drugs that can be purchased without a prescription.

The Correct Way to Take Medications

When you have a prescription or buy an OTC drug, do you know when to take it? How many times a day? For how long? To make the most of your health care dollar, use prescription drugs as directed. For example, you might feel better after you start a seven- to ten-day course of antibiotics, but you still need to take the drug for the full specified period of time to actually cure the illness because the drug needs time to get rid of all the infectious agents, not just the ones causing the worst symptoms. Similarly, medicines may need to be taken several times throughout the day at specific intervals in order to keep the right amount of the drug in your bloodstream at all times. Too much could cause an adverse reaction; too little might not be effective.

Sometimes, a prescription reads "take on an empty stomach—one hour before or two hours after meals." In this case, food in the stomach slows down the absorption of the drug and makes it less effective. Other drugs need to be taken with meals because the food helps the body absorb them better.

The correct time of day to take drugs also varies. It may be best to take a diuretic—a medicine that increases urination—no later than 6 P.M. unless your physician says otherwise, so that you won't have to go to the bathroom several times during the night. But it may be better to take a drug that causes drowsiness, such as an antihistamine, in the evening so that it does not interfere with your daily activities.

Directions for taking drugs are important and you should discuss them with your physician and/or pharmacist. However, most of us don't do this. According to an FDA survey, fewer than 4 percent of patients say they asked questions about their prescriptions when they were in their physicians' offices. Although physicians took this as a sign that their patients were clear about how and when to take their medication, the fact is that about half of all prescription drugs are taken improperly. Patients on long-term medications often stop taking them, and each year, more than 230 million prescriptions written by physicians for their patients are not taken at all.

Because of the many problems associated with taking drugs—and with not taking them correctly—it is important to keep your pharmacist informed about which drugs you take. The pharmacist has a record of all prescribed drugs filled in a particular store (or sometimes in a chain of pharmacies) but does not know which OTC drugs you take unless you inform him or her. With this information, the pharmacist is in a good position to alert you to any possible problems. For this reason, it is recommended that you use the same pharmacy each time you get a prescription drug filled.

The National Council on Patient Information and Education suggests that patients ask these five questions when given a new medication:

1. What is the name of the drug and what is it supposed to do?
2. How and when do I take it, and when do I stop taking it?
3. What food, drinks, other drugs, or activities should I avoid while taking the drug?
4. What are the side effects, and what should I do if they occur?
5. Is there any written information available about the drug?

In addition, the council advises patients to tell their physicians and pharmacists what other drugs—both prescription and nonprescription—they are taking, the names of any drugs they are allergic to, and, for women, whether they are pregnant or plan to become pregnant. The Developing Health Skills box provides some additional hints for reading your prescriptions.

Sources of Health Information

You can get health information on many of the topics covered in *HealthStyles* from your student health service. In addition, thousands of toll-free numbers

DEVELOPING HEALTH SKILLS

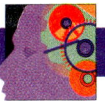

How to Read a Prescription

It might look incomprehensible to you, but what your physician writes on the prescription that you give to a pharmacist is very important information. The series of abbreviations translates into instructions for the precise kind of medicine you need and how often and when you should take it. Ask your pharmacist to explain any term, abbreviation, or instruction you do not fully understand.

Here are some of "instructions" that physicians write to pharmacists:

ac	before meals	hs	before bedtime	qid	four times a day
ad lib	as desired	mg	milligram	s	without
bid	twice a day	ml	milliliter	sig ut dict	take as directed
c	with	noct	at night	stat	at once
cap	capsule	pc	after meals	tid	three times a day
cc	cubic centimeter	po	by mouth	top	apply topically
ext	for external use	prn	as needed	x	times
gtt	drops	qd	once a day		

have been established to offer free medical information ranging from referrals to local physicians to practical information on specific diseases. For example, if you are having a diabetic friend to dinner, a call to the American Diabetes Association's 800 number could help you know what foods you can safely serve. *Health Hotlines* is a compilation of organizations' addresses and telephone numbers prepared by the National Library of Medicine. You can find listings selected from it at the end of each chapter of *HealthStyles*.

Health information—from the most recently published federal health statistics to the location of support groups for people who have migraine headaches—is also available on the Internet. This relatively new source of information is proving useful in helping consumers make decisions related to their health. Many health organizations have developed their own home pages or sites on the World Wide Web as a means of communicating with their members and others interested in their issues. For example, the full text of *Health Hotlines* is available through the National Library of Medicine Website.

The problem with the Internet, however, is that your computer cannot tell you what information is accurate and what information is bogus. Currently, much of the information on the Web is subjective, inaccurate, and out of date. At the same time, the most up-to-date information can also be found on the Web. So even though the Internet and the Web have provided access to massive amounts of information, the consumer still must decide about the credibility of each source, the accuracy of each bit of information, and the extent to which the information is up-to-date.

There is no absolute way to assure that all information found on the Web is accurate, unbiased, and up-to-date. But here are some good ideas for checking Web sources that you use:

- *Trust well-known organizations to provide comprehensive information.* For example, the American Cancer Society and the American Lung Association are

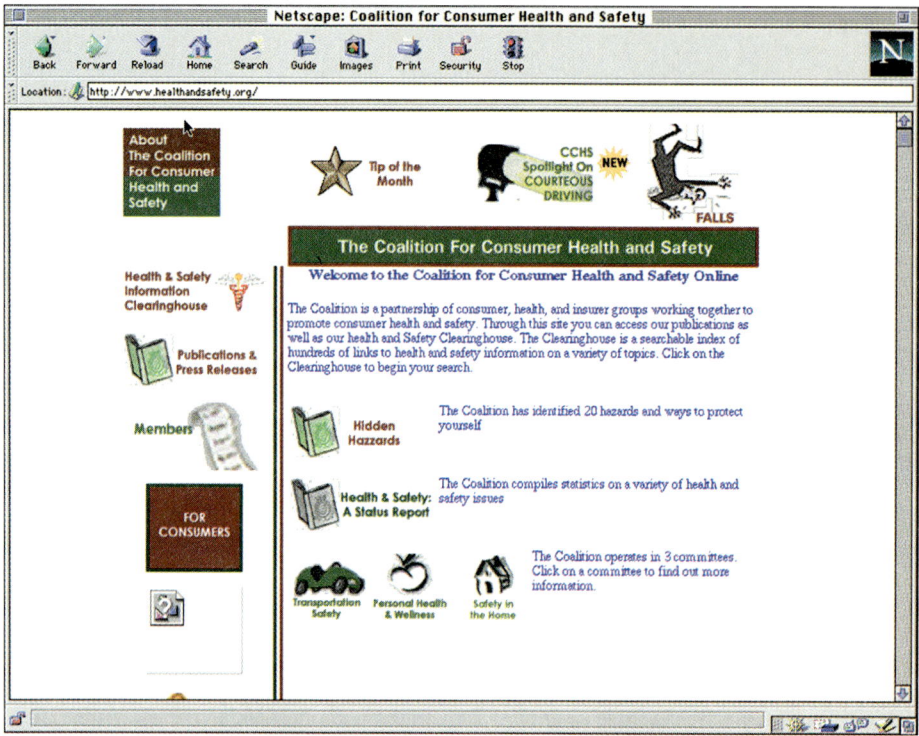

Health information is available on the Internet. This home page will lead you to health and safety information.

more likely to provide high-quality information than a website named Bill's Cancer Experience. Federal offices such as the Centers for Disease Control and Prevention (CDC) and the Office of Disease Prevention and Health Promotion in the Department of Health and Human Services are excellent sources of objective information, as are respected medical schools and universities. It is a good idea to compare information that can be found in websites of advocacy organizations such as Greenpeace with that which can be found in the more objective voluntary organizations or government offices. (Even some of the most well-known organizations produce biased information, so be careful.)

- *Always compare sources.* It is not a good idea to look in only one place for information. Even when you find information quickly, it is a good idea to compare that information with other sources. The best information found on the Web is usually cited in or linked to several locations. Be cautious with information that is not duplicated in trusted sources.
- *Distrust extremes in data.* Good science involves sharing information, so when a website is found that claims to be the only source of a certain "fact," it is a good idea to distrust that fact.

You can surf the Internet for health information by using the addresses provided in each chapter of *HealthStyles*. You may also want to use one of the numerous search engines, such as Alta Vista (altavista.digital.com) or Yahoo (www.yahoo.com), that serve as card catalogs for millions of Web pages worldwide. Two medicine-specific search engines are Achoo (www.achoo.com) and HealthAtoZ (www.Healthatoz.com). More than 9 million college students use the Internet regularly for information as well as for fun. Now you can log on for your health.

Key Concepts

1. Americans spend more money on health care than do people in any other country. In 1995, nearly $1 trillion was spent on health in the United States.
2. Consumers need accurate and unbiased information to make good health care decisions.
3. Quackery refers to a health claim made for a product or method that cannot be justified by scientifically derived evidence. It costs American consumers several billion dollars a year in useless tests and treatments.
4. It is estimated that nearly 50 percent of patients in legitimate cancer therapy also try unproven treatments.
5. Other vulnerable targets for quackery products are people seeking quick weight loss, larger breasts, hair restoration, and removal of wrinkles.
6. Most Americans get access to the health care system through their health insurance plans.
7. The traditional way to get health insurance coverage is through an indemnity plan in which you choose your own physicians, pay most of your medical bills, and file a claim to be reimbursed.
8. When you join a health maintenance organization (HMO), you will be assigned to a family physician or internist who will act as the gatekeeper to all other health services provided by the HMO.
9. About 50 percent of all prescription drugs are taken incorrectly, and more than 230 million prescriptions that are written by physicians for their patients are not taken at all. To get the most out of your health care dollar, use prescription drugs as directed.
10. A vast amount of health information is available on the Internet. This information can be useful in helping consumers make better health care decisions, but as with all information, it is important to make sure that it is accurate, unbiased, and up-to-date.

Review Questions

1. Explain the importance of information to wise consumer decision making and describe how information can be incomplete or biased.
2. List five advertising techniques used to promote health products and services.
3. Explain the meaning of health fraud and list five ways to spot it when it occurs.
4. List four rights you have as a consumer of health-related products and services.
5. Describe how to file a consumer complaint.
6. Explain how to go about selecting a physician. Include in your response seven optional approaches to this task.
7. Differentiate between the insured, the uninsured, and the underinsured.
8. Explain the difference between traditional indemnity plans, health maintenance organizations, and preferred provider organizations.
9. Differentiate between prescription and over-the-counter drugs and briefly describe how each should be taken.
10. Explain how you would go about finding additional information about health products or services. Include in your explanation the use of hot lines and the Internet.

Selected Bibliography

"Finding Medical Help Online." *Consumer Reports* (February 1997): 27–32.
Health Hotlines. Bethesda, MD: National Library of Medicine, 1996.
"How Is Your Doctor Treating You?" *Consumer Reports* (February 1995): 81–88.
Vickery, D., and J.F. Fries. *Take Care of Yourself: The Consumer's Guide to Medical Care.* Boston: Addison-Wesley, 1990.

HealthLinks: Web Sites for Understanding Health Care

You can access better health as it relates to this chapter by checking out some of the following sites on the Internet. These and sites identified within the chapter can be accessed directly when you visit the *HealthStyles* Web Site located on the Allyn and Bacon homepage at **http://www.abacon.com.**

Consumer Product Safety Commission
www.cpsc.gov
CPSC is an independent federal regulatory agency that focuses on reducing the risk of injury or death from consumer products, from automatic-drip coffee makers to toys to lawn mowers. Visitors can use the Web Site to report unsafe products or call the CPSC toll-free hot line at (800) 638-2772 or (800) 638-8270 for the hearing and speech impaired.

Electronic Policy Network
tap.epn.org/idea/health.html
As part of the Electronic Policy Network, the Health Policy page contains a "virtual" magazine of articles for all age groups containing timely information and ideas about national policy and politics as they relate to health care.

Institute of Medicine
www.iom.edu
The Institute of Medicine is dedicated to the advancement of scientific knowledge and the health and well-being of all people of this nation and the world. It provides objective, timely, and authoritative information to government, the professions, and the public through its elected membership and access to the best expertise.

National Library of Medicine
www.nlm.nih.gov
This Web site contains every significant program of the National Library of Medicine, from medical history to biotechnology.

Health Hotlines: Making Health Care Decisions

American Academy of Family Physicians
(800) 274-2237
8880 Ward Parkway
Kansas City, MO 64114-2797

American Academy of Medical Acupuncture
(800) 521-2262
5820 Wilshire Boulevard, Suite 500
Los Angeles, CA 90036

American Board of Medical Specialties
(800) 776-2378
47 Perimeter Center East, Suite 500
Atlanta, GA 30346

Department of Health and Human Services, Inspector General's Hotline
(800) 368-5779
P.O. Box 23489
Washington, DC 20026

Medic Alert Foundation International
(800) ID-ALERT (432-5378) (outside California)
(800) 344-3227 (within California)
2323 Colorado
Turlock, CA 95381-1009

National Fraud Information Center
National Consumers League
(800) 876-7060
815 15th Street NW
Washington, DC 20005

People's Medical Society
(800) 624-8773
462 Walnut Street
Allentown, PA 18102

Glossary

abortion The termination of pregnancy.
absolute strength The total force that an individual can exert when flexing muscles; usually measured in pounds.
abstinence The choice of not consuming alcoholic beverages in any form (see also sexual abstinance).
acceptable risk A circumstance in which the benefits outweigh the risks; when the likelihood of ill effects is very small.
acceptance The stage of dying in which the person understands that death is inevitable.
achievable age The age to which a person could live under ideal conditions.
acid rain Precipitation having a higher than normal level of acid due to the combination of sulfur oxides and moisture in the air.
acquaintance rape Sexual assault committed by a person known to the victim.
acquired immune deficiency syndrome (AIDS) A combination of symptoms caused by the human immunodeficiency virus (HIV).
active euthanasia Direct action taken to bring about death, such as taking a dying person off life supports.
active immunity The body's development of its own resistance to disease.
acute stage The stage at which symptoms of a disease are fully developed.
acyclovir A drug used to relieve the symptoms of genital herpes infection.
addiction A strong desire or need to continue using tobacco, alcohol, or another drug.
adipose tissue Tissue in which fat from food is stored in the body.
adiposity A surplus of body fat.
advance medical directive A person's written declaration about what should happen if he or she becomes unable to make decisions about his or her own medical care.
aerobic To be "with oxygen"; a process of energy production through which carbohydrates, fats, and proteins are used to produce energy and carbon dioxide and water are given off as by-products.
aerobic capacity The largest volume of oxygen that your body can consume in one minute; also called maximal oxygen uptake, or VO_2 max.
affective disorder A condition in which moods or emotions become extreme and interfere with daily life.
ageism The term used to describe prejudice and discrimination against the elderly based on misconceptions regarding age.
air bags Safety devices located behind the steering wheel and/or the dashboard that automatically inflate on impact during a frontal or side crash.
air pollution The contamination of air by waste products.

alarm reaction The first stage of the general adaptation syndrome; the body mobilizes its forces to meet a threatening situation.
alcohol abuse A pattern of pathological use of alcohol that results in impaired social or occupational functioning.
alcohol addiction Extensive dependence on alcohol; this dependence is so acute that the acquisition and use of alcohol becomes the focus of everyday life.
alcohol dependence When a person is so physically attached to alcohol that he or she cannot live comfortably without it.
alcoholic Someone who suffers from alcoholism and who has lost control over his or her drinking.
Alcoholics Anonymous A member organization of recovering alcoholics who provide social support for avoiding the use of alcohol.
alcoholism A progressive disease related to the uncontrolled use of alcohol that interferes with the drinker's health and social functioning.
allergen A substance that is perceived by the body as an irritant; induces an allergic or hypersensitive state or reaction.
allergy The result of the body's overzealous response to an allergen.
alveoli The balloon-like air sacs at the end of the bronchioles of the lung.
Alzheimer's disease A degenerative disorder that causes dementia in middle to late life.
amenorrhea An abnormal absence or suppression of menstruation.
amino acids A class of organic compounds that are the building blocks of proteins.
amnesia Partial or total loss of memory.
amniocentesis Means of testing amniotic fluid to indicate the presence or absence of certain genetic conditions, such as Down syndrome, in a fetus.
anaerobic To be "without oxygen"; the process of energy production in which surges of energy are needed for a brief amount of time.
androgens Male sex hormones.
anger The stage of dying in which the person is angry at almost anything.
angina pectoris Chest pain; a symptom of a condition in which the heart does not get as much blood as it needs.
anorexia nervosa An eating disorder characterized by starvation behavior brought on by a preoccupation with thinness.
antibiotic A chemical substance that destroys or inhibits the growth of bacteria.
antibodies Specific proteins that are produced principally in the blood in response to foreign substances in the body.

antigens Foreign substances in the body that cause the production of antibodies.
anxiety A state of apprehension or tension, often accompanied by physiological signs.
arrhythmia An erratic heartbeat.
artificial insemination Introduction of semen into the vagina by artificial means, using a syringe.
asthma A breathing disorder that causes wheezing, coughing, and difficulty in breathing.
asymptomatic carrier A person who has a disease but no symptoms.
asymptomatic period A period in which a disease exists without any outward signs or clinical symptoms.
atherosclerosis Hardening of the arteries due to a buildup of fatty plaque.
auscultation Listening to the sounds made by various body structures.
autoimmune disease A disease in which antibodies attack the body's own cells as if they were an invading infection.
autopsy A surgical examination of the body to determine the cause of death.
bacteria Single-celled, plant-like microbes that act to produce symptoms of infection.
bacterial pneumonia Pneumonia that develops as a result of invasion of the lungs by bacteria.
balanced diet An eating pattern that includes a variety of foods in amounts that result in health enhancement.
bargaining The stage of dying in which the person bargains for more time.
barrier methods Methods of contraception that physically separate the sperm from the egg; include condoms and diaphragms.
basal cell A small, round cell in the lower part (base) of the epidermis.
basal metabolic rate The speed with which the body expends calories on basic functions at a resting state.
baseline data Information about health that must be evaluated or interpreted in order to determine health status.
battery Any illegal beating or touching of another person.
behavior modification Therapy designed to change the learned behavior of an individual.
benign tumor A tumor that is usually harmless and does not invade other cells or spread to other parts of the body.
benzene A chemical that can cause leukemia in humans.
bereaved Survivors of a recently deceased person who experience a sense of loss and grief.
bereavement The period during which a sense of loss is felt owing to the death of a loved one.
binge drinking Having five drinks in a row for men or four in a row for women.

binge eating Eating excessively; consuming greater than the normal amount of food usually taken in at one sitting.

binge eating disorder An eating disorder characterized by periods of uncontrolled eating.

bioelectrical impedance A test that uses a weak electrical current to measure the body's fat content.

biopsy The removal of bits of living tissue and fluid from the body for diagnostic examination.

birth control Prevention of pregnancy for the purpose of family planning.

birth control pill A pill, consisting of chemicals similar to hormones normally produced in a woman's body, that prevents pregnancy.

bisexual A person who has a sexual attraction to people of both sexes.

blackout A temporary form of amnesia in which the individual appears to be conscious of what he or she is doing but later cannot remember much if any of what happened.

blood alcohol concentration (BAC) A measure of the amount of alcohol in the blood.

body mass index (BMI) A numerical representation of the relationship of height and weight that correlates positively with measures of body composition such as underwater weighing and the pinch test.

bradycardia Abnormally slow beating of the heart.

brain dead A state that occurs when there is no longer brain activity.

breast self-examination (BSE) An examination done by a woman to herself to identify abnormal breast tissue.

breech presentation Positioning of the baby's feet or bottom first in the birth canal.

bulimia An eating disorder characterized by the extreme behavior of binge eating and vomiting.

burnout The emotional exhaustion caused by the stresses of work and other responsibilities.

calculus Dental plaque that has hardened on tooth surfaces; also called tartar.

calorie A unit measuring the energy produced by food when oxidized in the body.

cannabis Marijuana, hashish, ganga; the dried flowering tops of the hemp plant, *Cannabis sativa*.

carbohydrate Nutrients made of sugars and starches; the body's primary source of energy.

carbon monoxide A colorless, odorless, poisonous gas that is produced by the incomplete burning of carbon in fuels.

carcinogen A cancer-causing agent or factor.

cardiopulmonary resuscitation (CPR) A combination of mouth-to-mouth breathing and chest compression used during cardiac arrest to keep blood flowing to the heart muscle and brain; an emergency procedure.

cardiovascular disease Disease of the heart and blood vessels.

cataracts Clouding of the lens of the eye.

cerebellum The portion of the brain that contributes to the control of movement.

cerebrum The part of the brain responsible for reasoning and inhibitions.

cervix The opening of the uterus into the vagina.

cesarean section Removal of the baby through an incision in the abdominal wall rather than through the birth canal.

chain of infection A metaphor for infectious disease transmission in which each link in the chain represents a single factor necessary for disease to spread.

chancre A painless, round sore with raised edges indicative of syphilis.

child abuse Any intentional physical, sexual, or psychological assault on a child.

child-resistant packaging Product packaging designed to discourage or prevent children from gaining access to the contents.

chlamydia A common bacterial STD, which, if untreated, can cause serious, painful infections of the urinary tract in men and infection of the reproductive organs in women.

chlorofluorocarbons (CFCs) Compounds used as aerosol spray propellants and refrigerants that contribute to the depletion of the ozone layer.

cholesterol A white, crystalline substance found especially in animal fats, blood, nerve tissue, and bile; in excessive amounts, a factor in atherosclerosis.

chorionic villus sampling (CVS) A technique in which the chorionic villi, hairlike projections on a membrane surrounding the interior of the uterus, are tested to determine the presence or absence of certain genetic conditions.

chronic bronchitis A condition in which the bronchial tubes become inflamed as a result of irritation.

chronic fatigue syndrome A group of symptoms that result in a prolonged state of fatigue.

chronological age A number representing the number of years since birth.

cirrhosis of the liver A disease in which scar tissue replaces normal liver tissue and interferes with the liver's ability to function.

cochlea The inner ear.

codependency A relationship in which one person contributes to another person's dysfunctional behavior by accepting it or masking it from others.

colon cancer Cancer of the large bowel.

columbarium A special vault for urns containing ashes of cremated bodies.

commitment The cognitive component of love characterized by a desire to maintain a highly valued relationship, even when self-sacrifice is required to do so.

complementary protein relationship The idea that two or more foods, none of which when taken alone would provide a complete protein, can be combined at a meal resulting in a complete protein.

complete protein A protein containing all nine essential amino acids.

complex carbohydrate A basic nutritional component made of long chains of simple sugars that are slowly broken down in the body.

conception The union of sperm and egg.

concordance rate The extent to which a trait is found in both members of a twin pair.

conditioning period The period of exercise during which a training effect is reached and maintained.

conflict resolution A process of negotiation between two individuals, facilitated by a third party, with the goal of resolving differences.

contraception The intentional prevention of conception.

contraimplantation Preventing implantation of the fertilized egg.

contraindications Circumstances that make use of a pharmaceutical or medical product inadvisable.

controlled substance A chemical that has been identified through legal review as a threat to an individual and/or to society.

convalescence A state characterized by a decline in the severity of disease symptoms.

cool-down period The period of exercise in which the intensity of exercise is reduced to allow the body to recover partially from the conditioning period.

coping An adaptation to stress.

coping skills Strategies used to deal constructively with stressors.

crack babies Babies born addicted to crack cocaine.

cremation The burning of a dead body into ashes.

crowning The point of labor at which the cervix is completely effaced and dilated to ten centimeters and the baby's head can be seen.

date rape Unwanted sexual contact that is committed on or by a date.

defense mechanisms Coping strategies by which people defend themselves against negative emotions.

dehydration An abnormal loss of water.

dementia Mental confusion and loss of brain function that can be caused by disease or old age.

denial The stage of dying in which the person does not believe that death is going to happen to him or her.

dental caries Tooth decay.

dental plaque Noncalcified accumulation of microorganisms that attach to the teeth.

dependence A condition in which a person

is so physically and/or psychologically attached to a drug that he or she cannot live without it.

depressant A drug that slows down the body's functions and movements.

depression A mental disorder marked by sadness, anxiety, fatigue, underactivity, sleeplessness, and reduced ability to function and relate to others: the stage of dying in which anger is replaced with a sense of loss.

dermatitis A skin disorder in which an area of skin may become red, swollen, hot, and itchy.

designer drug A drug that looks like a drug already on the market but has something altered in its molecular structure so that it is a "new" drug and not explicitly banned.

detoxification The process of removing all alcohol or drugs from an individual's body.

detoxification program A treatment program that involves a gradual but complete withdrawal from an abused drug.

diagnosis A physician's opinion of the nature or cause of a disease based on observation and laboratory tests.

diaphragm A soft rubber cup that covers the entrance to the uterus.

diastolic pressure The pressure measured in the arteries when the heart relaxes.

dietary fiber Food that cannot be broken down by digestive enzymes. It passes down the intestinal tract and contributes to more rapid movement of wastes through the intestines.

dilation Opening of the cervix either for examination or for delivery of a baby.

dilation and evacuation A method of abortion performed in the second trimester in which the cervix is dilated and medical instruments are used to remove the contents of the uterus.

disordered thinking Disconnected or incoherent thought processes and speech.

distress The type of stress that brings about negative mental or physical responses, also known as bad stress.

diuretic A medication that promotes the excretion of excess body fluids and salt in the urine.

domestic violence A range of abusive behaviors perpetrated by one person against another within the domestic sphere.

drug A chemical substance that causes a change in the body's functioning, including physiological and psychological activity.

drug abuse The intentional and chronic misuse of a chemical substance.

drug dependent A drug user who relies on the use of a drug to carry out normal day-to-day activities; dependence may be physical or psychological.

drug interaction An adverse effect on the body that occurs when a drug is taken at the same time as food, vitamins, or another medication.

drug misuse The use of a prescribed medication without consulting a physician.

drug use The use of a chemical substance for the purpose intended to bring about a change in the way the body functions.

dual-career families Families in which both parents pursue their careers.

durable power of attorney for health care A document that identifies a representative to speak for a person about his or her health care if the person is unable to do so.

dysfunction The inability to function properly.

dysorganization Pain or difficulty in the process of organization or living.

dyspareunia Painful intercourse.

effacement The thinning of the cervix during the process of childbirth.

elective abortion Abortion that is medically induced.

electrocardiogram (ECG) A screening procedure used to detect heart disease; a graphic record of the heart's action obtained from an instrument that records heart activity.

electroencephalogram (EEG) A device that measures brain activity.

embalming The use of chemicals, internally and externally, to temporarily preserve the body for open casket viewing and/or transportation.

emotional abuse Depriving a child or close relative of love and affection; belittling or degrading another person.

emphysema A disease of the lungs, particularly the small air sacs, in which the lungs lose their ability to expand as a result of an accumulation of fluid in the tissue.

empty calories High caloric foods that contain sugar but few nutrients.

endemic The persistent presence of a disease in a population.

endorphin A hormone produced in the brain that helps give a sense of pleasure and satisfaction.

endurance The ability to exercise vigorously at a sustained level for a period of time.

epidemic The occurrence of disease in a given population at a greater prevalence than would normally be expected.

epidemiologist A person who studies disease in a population.

epidemiology The study of epidemics and the disease process in a population, including factors related to the presence of a disease or health condition.

episiotomy The small incision made between the opening of the vagina and the anus to ensure easier passage of the baby's head through the birth canal and to prevent tearing of the tissue.

eradication The removal of a disease by the elimination of all reservoirs of the disease-causing pathogen.

erogenous zones Those areas of the body especially susceptible to sexual arousal such as the penis, vagina, and nipples.

estrogens Female sex hormones.

eustress The type of stress that is a healthy part of daily living; it can result in the ability to relax and enjoy a feeling of peacefulness and calm.

excitement The period during which the body initially responds to sexual stimulation; includes erection of the penis in men and vaginal lubrication and clitoral erection in women.

exercise Bodily movement undertaken to improve or maintain one or more of the components of physical fitness.

exercise duration The length of time a person exercises.

exercise frequency How often an exercise is done.

exercise intensity The degree of energy that is exerted during exercise.

exhaustion The final stage of the general adaptation syndrome; it occurs when the body does not have a chance to restore itself to a state of equilibrium.

extended family Family members connected by blood, marriage, or adoption, who live in a location outside of one home.

fad diets Diets that are popular for brief periods of time then lose popularity. The loss of popularity usually results when the effectiveness of a fad diet is questioned.

false negative A test result that indicates no evidence of disease when the disease is present.

false positive A test result that indicates some type of medical condition when none exists.

family planning A process of establishing the preferred number and spacing of children in one's family and choosing the means by which this is achieved.

fasting Refraining from eating food of any type for a period of time.

fat-soluble vitamins Those vitamins that are transported and stored by the body's fat cells; examples are vitamins A, D, E, and K.

female condom Lines the inside of the vagina and covers the cervix; acts to prevent pregnancy and sexually transmitted diseases.

female orgasmic disorder Persistent or recurrent delay in, or absence of, orgasm in a female following a normal sexual excitement phase.

fetal alcohol effect (FAE) Impairment of fetal development linked to the mother's use of alcohol during pregnancy; may include some of the attributes of fetal alcohol syndrome.

fetal alcohol syndrome (FAS) A birth defect caused by alcohol consumption during pregnancy that is characterized by mental retardation, poor motor coordination, hyperactivity in childhood, facial deformities, and other abnormalities.

fever Above-normal body temperature.

fiber A complex carbohydrate that is indigestible by humans.
fibrillation Irregular convulsive movement of the heart muscle.
fight-or-flight reaction The body's reaction to stress in which it becomes physically ready to resist or fight a stressor or to run from it.
flame-retardant materials Substances designed to resist or retard burning.
flexibility The range of movement an individual can achieve around a joint or group of joints.
fluoride A trace mineral used to help prevent dental caries.
food additive Any substance used in producing, processing, treating, packaging, transporting, or storing food to enhance food, enrich food, or lengthen its grocery store shelf life.
foreplay Sexual pleasuring.
functional age A number representing the ability to function; a tool for comparing actual age with ability to function.
fungal pneumonia Inflammation of the lungs caused by a fungus.
fungi Single-celled or multicelled plant-like organisms that usually grow on the surface of the skin.
gang rape A rape committed by a group.
gateway drugs Drugs such as tobacco, alcohol, and marijuana that most users of illicit drugs have tried before their first use of cocaine, heroin, or other illicit drugs.
gay A homosexual orientation; a homosexual man or woman.
gender identity A sense of comfort with one's gender; an acceptance of one's maleness or femaleness.
general adaptation syndrome (GAS) The theory proposed by Hans Selye in which there are three distinct phases to the body's reaction to stress: alarm reaction, resistance, and exhaustion.
generativity A concern for family and society.
gerontologists Specialists who study the social, biological, behavioral, and psychological aspects of aging.
gingivitis A condition in which the gums are red, tender, and swollen.
global warming The gradual rise in the average temperature of the earth.
grief A deep sadness caused by a loss.
hallucination The sensation of seeing or hearing things that are not present.
hallucinogen A drug that causes a great change in perception.
hangover A condition caused by excess alcohol consumption and characterized by nausea, upset stomach, anxiety, and a headache.
hazardous waste Waste that is flammable, explosive, corrosive, or toxic.
health A state of complete physical, mental, and social well-being; not merely the absence of disease or infirmity.
health assessment An analysis of a broad range of factors affecting an individual's health.
health attitude A behavioral intention concerning health, usually expressed in positive or negative terms.
health behavior Actions and habits that may lead either to enhancement and protection of a person's health status or to its decline.
health belief A health-related concept thought to be true whether supported by evidence or not.
health history A history of the patient's health as well as of the health of his or her family.
health knowledge The accumulation of factual information that influences health decision making.
health literacy The capacity of an individual to get, interpret, and understand basic health information and services and the competence to use such information and services in ways that are health enhancing.
health maintenance organizations (HMOs) Prepaid plans that offer a defined set of benefits according to a predetermined monthly premium.
health momentum A perception of movement toward or away from good health that results from decisions and health behaviors of the past.
health risk The likelihood of developing a certain disease or health condition.
health risk appraisal A survey instrument that is based on questions about a person's history, lifestyle, and medical status for the purpose of determining his or her likelihood of developing a health problem.
health risk assessment An assessment to determine the risk for contracting a disease.
health skills Abilities that influence health development, health status, and health maintenance.
health style The sum of health knowledge, health skills, and health behavior. Health style is most easily observed in personal health decisions.
health value Something of importance that is related to health.
heart attack (myocardial infarction) A condition that occurs when the blood supply to part of the heart muscle (the myocardium) is severely reduced or stopped. Normally circulating blood brings oxygen and other nutrients to the heart.
heart rate The number of heartbeats per minute.
heart transplant A surgical procedure in which a normally functioning heart from a person who has recently died is implanted into a person with a diseased heart.
helper T-cells White blood cells that are needed by the body's immune system to fight a variety of disease-causing organisms.
hemiplegia The loss of sensory and motor function on one side of the body.
hepatitis An inflammation of the liver, usually caused by a virus.
hepatitis A A form of hepatitis transmitted in human wastes and contaminated food and water.
hepatitis B A form of hepatitis transmitted by blood and sexual contact.
hepatitis C A form of hepatitis, previously known as non-A, non-B hepatitis, that resembles other forms of hepatitis but cannot be classified as either.
herd immunity The vaccination of a large proportion of a population against a particular disease to significantly reduce the chances of spread of infection.
herpes simplex type 2 A virus usually transmitted by sexual contact and causing open sores on the genitals.
heterosexual A person who has a sexual attraction to people of a different sex.
high density lipoprotein (HDL) A fatty substance that is the type of cholesterol that is considered good and that prevents atherosclerosis.
holistic health The concept of health involving physical, mental, emotional, social, spiritual, and environmental aspects of an individual as well as of the community in which he or she lives.
homicide The killing of one human being by another.
homosexual A person who has a sexual attraction to people of the same sex.
hospice A specialized health care program, usually for the last weeks or months of life, emphasizing the management of pain and other symptoms associated with terminal illness, in contrast to treatment.
host susceptibility The ease with which a person is exposed to and becomes infected by a pathogen.
human chorionic gonadotropin (HCG) A hormone secreted from placental cells; a pregnancy test looks for the presence of this hormone.
human immunodeficiency virus (HIV) The virus that causes AIDS.
human papilloma virus (HPV) The agent responsible for an STD characterized by warts, usually on the genitalia; also called genital warts.
hydrocarbons A chemical compound made up of hydrogen and carbon; the major chemical ingredient of many fuels.
hypertension A chronic disease better known as high blood pressure.
hypertension High blood pressure.
hypoglycemia Low blood sugar.
hypothermia Loss of body temperature to subnormal levels; can result in mental confusion, unconsciousness, and death.
hypothyroidism Not enough thyroid activity.
illness behavior Action taken by a person who has reason to believe that he or she is not well.
immune deficiency disease Any of a variety

of diseases or syndromes that compromise the immune system.

immunity The body's ability to destroy pathogens that it has once encountered, before they are able to cause disease.

impact The stage of bereavement in which loved ones react with shock, disbelief, and denial.

impotence Persistent or recurrent inability to attain erection or to maintain it until completion of the sexual activity.

in vitro fertilization A procedure in which the sperm and egg from a man and a woman are combined in a glass container and a fertilized embryo is implanted into the woman.

incidence data Data that provide a precise count of disease cases.

incomplete protein A protein in which one or more of the essential amino acids is missing.

incontinent Unable to control one's bowels or release of urine.

incubation period The period of time following exposure to an infectious disease before symptoms appear.

indemnity (fee-for-service) plan Insurance coverage in which a person pays for most of his or her medical bills and then files a claim to be reimbursed.

indoor pollution The contamination of indoor air by waste products or natural pollutants.

induction The method of abortion in which labor is artificially induced.

infectious disease Also known as *communicable* or *contagious* disease. A disease caused by pathogens, such as bacteria or viruses, that spread from someone who is infected to someone who is not yet infected.

infertility The inability of a couple to conceive after one year of intercourse without contraception.

inflammation The body's response to injury; it fights infection and promotes healing.

influenza A severe viral infection involving the respiratory tract.

inhalant A chemical that is inhaled through the nostrils to cause a quick rush to the brain; abused inhalants include airplane glue, paint thinner, and butyl nitrite.

inhibited sexual desire Persistent or recurrent deficient (or absent) sexual fantasies and desire for sexual activity.

inhibitions Self-imposed controls on emotions and behavior intended to assure socially acceptable interactions with others.

initiator A carcinogen that starts cell damage that leads to cancer.

inpatient care Health care provided in a hospital.

intentional injuries Injuries that result from planned events associated with suicide, homicide, and assault.

intercourse Sexual behavior involving penetration, usually of the penis of a man into the vagina of a woman; a description of a variety of sexual behaviors, including anal, vaginal, and oral stimulation and/or penetration.

interferon A chemical substance produced by white blood cells that "interferes" with growth of a virus and also inhibits the virus's ability to infect cells; also made synthetically.

interpersonal skills The techniques involved in relating to other people.

intimacy The emotional component of love characterized by a desire to be close, to interact at the intellectual level, to share feelings, and to acknowledge each other's desires.

intoxicated Consuming enough alcohol to experience its effect. Usually indicated by a high blood alcohol concentration, delayed muscle coordination, and impaired judgment.

intrauterine device (IUD) A small plastic birth control device that is inserted into the uterus by a physician.

isokinetic exercise An exercise in which there are slow-moving contractions throughout a full range of movement against a constant resistance.

isometric exercise An exercise involving the contraction of muscles performed against an immovable object.

isotonic exercise An exercise involving the contraction of muscles against a movable resistance.

Kaposi's sarcoma A rare, deadly cancer characterized by reddish-purple blotches on the skin; one of the symptoms of AIDS.

keratosis A rough patch or horny growth of the skin.

ketosis An accumulation of chemical compounds called ketones in the blood.

labor The process of childbirth from the initial contractions of the uterus to the delivery of the baby and the placenta.

laboratory tests Procedures that involve the examination of blood, tissue, and other biologic materials for the diagnosis, prevention, or treatment of disease.

lactovegetarians Vegetarians whose diet includes dairy products but no other animal products.

landfills An area where trash and other wastes are deposited and covered with soil.

late syphilis A disease characterized by generalized infection that can produce heart failure, blindness, loss of muscle control, brain damage, and death.

lead A metal found in exhausts, emissions, and paint.

lesbian A homosexual woman.

lesions A change in tissue, or sores.

leukoplakia White patches on the oral mucosa that may transform into a malignancy.

libido The biological urge or appetite for sexual activity; also called sex drive.

life expectancy The average number of years of life remaining at any given point.

living–dying interval The time between the diagnosis of a terminal condition and death.

living will A will that stipulates which medical treatments are and are not to be used in the final days of life.

low birthweight babies Babies born weighing less than 2,500 grams, or five pounds eight ounces.

low density lipoprotein (LDL) A fatty substance that is the type of cholesterol that is considered bad and that promotes atherosclerosis.

lumpectomy The surgical removal of only the cancerous lump from the breast.

Lyme disease A bacterial infection transmitted by deer tick bites.

main effect The desired (intended) physical or mental response of the body to a drug; sometimes called the primary effect.

mainstream smoke The smoke inhaled and exhaled by the smoker.

maintenance program A treatment program that involves providing a less dangerous drug to prevent withdrawal symptoms.

major depression Depression that is extreme, more intense, and longer lasting and that usually interferes with daily life; often characterized as a mood or affective disorder.

male condom A thin rubber sheath for the penis that collects semen ejaculated during sexual intercourse; acts to prevent pregnancy and sexually transmitted diseases.

malignant tumor A cancerous tumor that spreads to nearby tissues and organs, crowding out healthy cells and replacing them with cancer cells.

mammography A screening technique used to detect breast cancer.

manic-depressive illness A form of depression characterized by cycles of manic highs and depressive lows; also called bipolar disorder.

marital rape A rape that occurs when a spouse forces unwanted sexual contact on his or her spouse or estranged spouse.

masturbation Sexual self-stimulation.

maximal heart rate The maximum number of beats per minute that should be reached during exercise; usually equal to 220 minus the person's age.

medical assessment An evaluation conducted by a medical professional that focuses on identification of the presence or absence of a disease.

medulla The part of the brain that controls breathing.

melanin Brownish-black skin pigment.

melanoma A skin cancer that often starts as a mole-like growth and grows in size and changes color; the most serious of the various types of skin cancer.

meningitis An inflammation of the

membranes surrounding the spinal cord and brain.

mental health A state of emotional and social well-being; a state in which an individual is capable of healthy interaction with his or her environment and of enduring the hard times of life, with resilience.

mental illness A disorder or problem of the mind that prevents a person from being productive, adjusting to life, or getting along with other people.

metastasize To spread to other parts of the body through the bloodstream or lymph system.

minor depression An emotional state in which a person's normal feelings of sadness, guilt, and hopelessness are exaggerated.

miscarriage Spontaneous abortion.

MMR vaccine A vaccine that provides immunity to measles, mumps, and rubella.

modified radical mastectomy A selective removal of the breast and surrounding tissue.

mononucleosis A disease of unknown cause; symptoms include fever, headache, nausea, extreme fatigue, and swollen spleen and lymph nodes.

monounsaturated fat The type of fat that has one hydrogen available to bond and is liquid at room temperature; usually comes from plant or fish sources.

morbidity data A statistical measurement of the proportion of a specific population affected by a disease or sickness over a specific period of time.

morning-after pill A form of hormonal contraception used within the first seventy-two hours after unprotected sexual intercourse; generally considered an emergency method of birth control that prevents implantation.

mortality data The number of deaths by disease or sickness in a given population over a specific period of time.

mourning Expressing grief at someone's death.

mucous membranes The moist, protective lining that covers some of the openings to the body and the air passages.

multiple hazards Simultaneous exposure to more than one health threat.

mutagen An agent that causes hereditary changes on the cellular level that may be passed from one generation to another.

mycoplasma A tiny microorganism and causative agent of many diseases of the joints and lungs.

myocardial infarction Damage of heart tissue caused by an interruption of blood supply to the heart that can result in death.

myotonia Muscle tension in response to sexual stimulation.

narcotic A drug that reduces pain and induces sleep.

natural childbirth Delivery of a baby "naturally," without the aid of drugs.

Neisseria gonorrhoeae The bacterium that causes gonorrhea.

neurons The basic cells of the nervous system.

neuroses Cognitive distortions or unsatisfactory ways of reacting to life situations.

neurotic To display a neurosis.

neurotransmitters Chemicals that facilitate the passage of impulses in the brain.

nicotine The ingredient in tobacco smoke that causes addiction.

nicotine addiction The state of being physically and emotionally dependent on nicotine.

nicotine replacement Therapy in which a person who smokes gets nicotine by means other than tobacco.

nitrogen oxides Poisonous gases that are produced when fuel is burned at very high temperatures.

nonpoint source pollutant Nonpoint source pollutants enter a body of water as runoff or seepage.

non-REM sleep Sleep during which the eyes are relaxed and not moving; the period of sleep associated with cell regeneration.

nonspecific defense mechanisms The body's various barriers to all disease; as opposed to those defense mechanisms intended to prevent one particular disease.

nosocomial infection A hospital-acquired disease; most are caused by bacteria.

nuclear family The immediate family; parents and/or guardians and their children, usually living together.

nurse-midwife Registered nurse who has completed advanced training in gynecology and obstetrics.

nutrients The basic chemical compounds that make up food.

obesity An excessive amount of body weight relative to body fat.

occasional drinker A person who drinks an alcoholic beverage every now and then but seldom consumes enough alcohol to become intoxicated.

opportunistic diseases Diseases common to individuals infected with HIV that under normal conditions would be defeated by the body's immune system.

orgasm The climax phase of sexual excitement.

osteoporosis A disorder in which bone density decreases, making the bones more likely to break.

outercourse Mutual masturbation; when two people manually stimulate one another's genitals to achieve sexual pleasure.

outpatient care Care provided in a physician's or other health practitioner's office, in an emergency room in a hospital, or in a specialized ambulatory clinic; does not involve hospitalization or overnight stays.

over-the-counter (OTC) drugs Drugs that can be purchased without a prescription.

overdose A serious reaction to an excessive amount of a drug that can result in coma or death.

overmedication Consuming a high dose of medication, or combination of medications, resulting in symptoms (side effects) that compromise accurate medical care.

overweight An excess of body weight relative to a specified standard for height and age.

ovolactovegetarians Vegetarians whose diet includes eggs as well as dairy products.

ozone A poisonous form of oxygen that chemically reacts with a variety of substances.

ozone layer A region of the stratosphere, which filters out ultraviolet rays from the sun.

palpation Touching body parts with the hands.

pandemic The occurrence of a disease that affects virtually an entire population or the entire world.

Pap smear A test for identifying cervical cancer that involves scraping and analyzing cells from the cervix.

parasitic worms Multicelled animals that release toxins inside the body, feed on blood, and compete with the host for food.

Parkinson's disease A serious illness marked by progressive loss of normal muscle function; over time, the muscles become stiff, causing shaky movements.

partial mastectomy The surgical removal of only the part of the breast containing the cancerous lump.

particulates A tiny pollutant in the air such as dust, soot, and mold spores.

passion The motivational component of love characterized by a desire to give and to receive sexual pleasure and to achieve sexual gratification.

passive euthanasia Indirect action taken to bring about death, such as withholding something needed by a dying person to sustain life.

passive immunity Resistance to disease that initially comes from an external source.

passive seat belts Seat belts that automatically place a shoulder restraint around the driver and the front seat passenger upon their entering the car.

passive smoking Inhaling tobacco smoke from the environment, as a result of someone else smoking.

pathogen A microorganism, such as a bacterium, virus, protozoan, parasitic worm, fungus, or rickettsia, that causes disease.

patient package insert An information sheet, required by the FDA, that, among other things, warns the consumer of possible contraindications for use of a drug or medical product.

pelvic inflammatory disease (PID) An

infection in the pelvic area usually involving the uterus, fallopian tubes, and/or ovaries; half the cases are caused by chlamydia.

perchloroethylene (PCE) A suspected carcinogen used in dry cleaning.

periodontitis Degeneration of the gum tissue that holds the teeth in place; also called pyorrhea.

periodontal disease Gum disease.

personality hardiness A state of resiliency due to clear self-concept.

phagocytes White blood cells that attack and consume foreign cells.

phobia An unreasonable fear of some object or situation.

physical abuse The infliction of physical injury that causes substantial harm over a period of time.

physical examination An examination by a physician that involves inspection, auscultation, and palpation of the body.

physical fitness How efficiently the body works as measured by strength, flexibility, and endurance.

physical neglect A deprivation of the basic necessities of life, including food, clothing, sanitary living conditions, and medical care.

physician-assisted suicide A form of active euthanasia in which the patient is allowed to bring about his or her own death by self-administering a lethal drug provided by the physician.

pinch test A test that uses special skin-fold calipers to pinch layers of fat at specific body sites; a measure of body fat.

placenta The structure that develops from the wall of the uterus and serves as an organ of interchange between the mother and the fetus.

plaque A deposit of fatty material in a blood vessel wall.

plateau The stage of sexual stimulation just prior to orgasm consisting of increasing and decreasing sexual stimulation.

pneumonia An inflammation of the lung tissue.

Pneumocystis carinii **pneumonia** A rare form of pneumonia that is often present in persons living with AIDS.

point-of-service (POS) plans HMOs having an indemnity-type option that lets members get care from physicians and other providers outside the plan's network.

point source pollutant Point source pollutants enter a body of water at a specific point.

polyunsaturated fat The type of fat that has several hydrogens available to bind and is soft at room temperature; usually comes from plant or fish sources.

portal of exit The means by which the pathogen moves out of the source into a new host.

preadmission certification Approval from a health plan of the need for inpatient hospital care prior to the actual admission.

preconception care Health-promoting action taken prior to conception for the purpose of reducing health risks to mother and child.

precycling The practice of choosing products that have the potential for reuse, using packaging that can be used for other purposes, or choosing packaging that has already been recycled.

preferred provider organization (PPOs) A hybrid form of insurance that merges features of traditional fee-for-service insurance and prepaid plans.

premature death Years of potential life lost; usually measured in terms of years of potential life lost before age 65.

premature ejaculation Persistent or recurrent ejaculation occurring after minimal sexual stimulation or before, on, or shortly after penetration and before the person wishes it.

premenstrual dysphoric disorder A form of depression occurring just prior to menstruation and characterized by fatigue, irritability, mood swings, and physical symptoms such as abdominal bloating, swollen hands or feet, headaches, and tender breasts; a severe form of premenstrual syndrome.

premenstrual syndrome A combination of emotional and physical features which occur before menstruation; characterized by mood changes, discomfort, swelling and tenderness in the breasts, a bloated feeling, headache, and fatigue.

prenatal care Health-promoting action taken after conception and before birth for the purpose of reducing health risks to mother and child; medical care during pregnancy.

presbyopia A difficulty in reading materials at close range; common in older persons.

prescription drugs Drugs ordered specifically for a person by his or her physician and filled by a registered pharmacist.

prevalence data Data concerning the existing cases of a specific disease at a certain point in time in a population.

prevention Taking health-promoting action to reduce the risk of disease or injury.

preventive behavior Action taken by a person who is essentially healthy in order to remain healthy.

primary care Routine medical care provided by a physician in the office or at an emergency room in a hospital or clinic.

primary health assessment Procedures, usually including identification of risk factors, designed to measure a state of well-being in order to prevent disease.

primary stressor Something that initiates the stress response.

primary syphilis Characterized by painless sores, called chancres, at the site of the infection.

prion A mutated, three-dimensional protein that changes the shape of surrounding prions, causing pockets of diseased and dying brain cells.

problem drinker A person who uses alcohol in a manner that causes physical, psychological, or social harm to the drinker and/or others.

pro-choice A political position that supports the idea that a woman has the right to choose whether or not she wishes to continue a pregnancy.

prodromal stage A highly contagious period in a disease in which some symptoms may be apparent but the infected person does not feel ill.

Prohibition A period of time in U.S. history when the manufacture, sale, or transport of intoxicating liquors was prohibited by law.

pro-life A political position that supports the idea that a pregnant woman must carry the pregnancy to term because the developing fetus is a human being and has a right to live.

promoter A carcinogen that helps cancer to grow.

proof The percentage of pure alcohol in a beverage; the percentage of alcohol is half the proof.

prostate-specific antigen (PSA) test A blood test that can identify signs of prostate cancer.

protein A group of complex compounds containing amino acids that are essential for growth and repair of tissue.

protozoa Single-celled parasites that produce toxins and release enzymes that interrupt the body's ability to function normally.

protozoal vaginitis A condition transmitted sexually and characterized by a foul or fishy odor, accompanied by itching, burning sensations and pain in the vaginal area.

psychological abuse Acts that lead to mental anguish, such as threats insults, and unreasonable demands and that damage the victim's self-esteem over time.

psychological age A number representing a perceived age (how old you feel).

psychoneuroimmunology The study of how the brain affects the immune system.

psychoses Mental disorders that can result in a loss of touch with reality.

pulse The palpable flow of blood in the arteries caused by the regular contraction of the heart.

purging To self-induce vomiting and/or to otherwise rid the body of excessive food; often done after binges by a bulimic person.

pyrogen A chemical that signals the brain to raise body temperature.

quackery A health claim made for a product or service that cannot be justified by scientifically derived evidence.

quadriplegia Total paralysis of the body from the neck down, affecting arms and legs.

quickening Fetal movements felt by the mother.

radical mastectomy The complete surgical removal of the breast and surrounding tissue, particularly the lymph nodes.

rape An act of violence in which a person is forced to engage in unwanted sexual intercourse.

rape trauma syndrome A group of symptoms, such as anxiety, sleeplessness, eating disorders, nightmares, guilt, and low self-esteem, that can strike after the occurrence of rape.

rapid eye movement (REM) sleep Sleep during which the eyes flicker back and forth behind closed eyelids; the period of sleep associated with dreaming.

receptor site The location in the body at which a drug triggers a response.

recoil The stage of bereavement in which the bereaved superficially carry on and try to return to normal.

recommended dietary allowances (RDAs) Guidelines for the average amounts of some of the essential nutrients to be consumed by healthy individuals over a period of time.

recovery A period in which infection is successfully defeated and the body returns to its healthy state; also the stage of bereavement in which the bereaved begin to show signs of returning to a more normal life.

refractory period The recovery period experienced by most men after orgasm; during this period a man does not respond to sexual stimulation.

relative strength A measure of strength determined by dividing absolute strength by body weight.

reservoir of the pathogen A place (either a human or an animal) where a pathogen resides.

resistance The capacity of the immune system to fight the invasion of an organism; also the second stage of the general adaptation syndrome; the body relaxes and returns to its normal state after the immediate threat has disappeared.

resolution The stage of sexual response following orgasm in which physiological responses reverse and a sense of relaxation overcomes the body.

resting heart rate The number of heartbeats per minute in a resting state.

Reye's syndrome A condition characterized by neurological disorders and swelling of the brain; may result in significant permanent brain damage.

rhythm method The method of contraception that relies on knowing when a woman ovulates and then calculating when her fertile and infertile periods occur.

rickettsia A rod-shaped microorganism that is transmitted by vectors and causes a variety of diseases, such as typhus.

risk age The age to which a person will probably live given the individual's current risks.

risk factor A condition or habit that puts a person in danger of negative health occurrences.

risk-taking behavior Actions that intentionally place an individual at risk for personal injury.

runner's high The feeling of euphoria due to an increase in the production of the hormone endorphin during or following exercise.

sadistic rape A rape that involves torture or mutilation of the victim.

safer sex A pattern of responsible sexual behavior characterized by reduced risk for disease.

saturated fat The type of fat that has all hydrogen sites occupied and is usually solid at room temperature; usually comes from animal sources and is thought to encourage plaque build-up.

schizophrenia A complex mental illness in which an individual has a distorted view of reality.

screening Analysis of risk factors done on a person thought to be well for the purpose of preventing disease or making an early diagnosis.

seasonal affective disorder A form of depression brought on by lack of sufficient daylight.

secondary care Care involving surgery and nonroutine medical treatment, usually delivered in a hospital.

secondary health assessment Procedures designed to measure the extent of an illness in order to diagnose and treat it.

secondary infection An infection that occurs in conjunction with, or as a result of, another infection but arises from a different pathogen.

secondary stressor An additional stressor that continues the stress response.

secondary syphilis A highly contagious disease characterized by a general rash on the body, sore throat, fever, and pains in the joints and muscles.

self-actualization The ability to seek the highest and most idealistic state that can lead to a person's fullest possible development.

self-assessment An evaluation of health status based on data collected on oneself by oneself.

self-concept A person's view of himself or herself gained through an assessment of strengths and weaknesses.

self-efficacy A person's belief that he or she is capable of accomplishing a task or series of tasks under certain conditions.

self-esteem How a person values himself or herself.

sensate focus A therapeutic technique in which a couple is taught the nonverbal communication of touching in order to help alleviate difficulty having sexual intercourse or performance anxiety.

serotonin A neurotransmitter associated with the regulation of aggression, mood, and memory.

set point A particular weight at which a person's body functions normally.

sex drive The biological urge or appetite for sexual activity; also called libido.

sex role Overt behaviors that disclose ourselves as male or female to others.

sexual abstinence A behavioral choice not to engage in vaginal intercourse.

sexual abuse A criminal offense in which a person is used for sexual purposes.

sexual dysfunctions Disorders that interfere with the ability to enjoy a healthy sexual experience.

sexual orientation A person's enduring attraction to individuals of a particular gender.

sexual revolution A period of time (thought to begin in the 1960s) characterized by a significant liberalization of sexual behavior and attitudes.

sexuality A collection of qualities that makes up a person's sexual attitudes and behaviors and influences his or her relationships with others.

sexually transmitted diseases (STDs) Infectious diseases and syndromes that are spread primarily through sexual activity.

shock A condition of reduced circulation to the vital organs.

sick-role behavior Action taken by a person who has been diagnosed as sick.

side effect An unwanted or even dangerous physical or mental effect caused by a drug or medicine.

sidestream smoke The smoke originating from the burning end of the cigarette between puffs, that adversely affects the health of individuals nearby.

sigmoidoscopy A screening procedure in which a physician uses a hollow lighted tube to inspect the rectum and lower colon.

simple carbohydrate A basic nutritional compound made of short chains of simple sugars that are broken down quickly in the body.

single-parent family A family in which only one parent lives in the home and takes care of the children.

situational abstinence The choice not to consume alcoholic beverages in situations in which the consumption of alcohol would present a health risk.

smog A brownish haze that forms when hydrocarbons react with nitric acid in the presence of sunlight.

smoke detectors Smoke-sensitive devices designed to alert occupants of a room or space in the event of a fire.

smokeless tobacco Tobacco products that are chewed, placed in the mouth, and/or sniffed through the nose.

smoking cessation The process of breaking a smoking habit; stopping the use of tobacco.

social drinker A person who drinks regularly in social settings but seldom

consumes enough alcohol to become intoxicated.

sonogram A diagnostic tool that allows the physician indirectly to see the developing fetus and its individual organ systems.

spermicide An acidic substance that kills sperm.

spouse abuse Any intentional physical, sexual, or psychological assault by a spouse.

squamous cell A flat cell that makes up most of the epidermis.

staging The use of drugs in a predictable progression beginning with gateway drugs, such as tobacco and alcohol, and progressing to hard drugs, such as crack cocaine and heroin.

starches White, tasteless substances found in potatoes, rice, corn, wheat, and other vegetable products.

sterilization A form of birth control in which steps are taken to permanently end fertility.

stimulant A drug that speeds up the body's functions and movements.

strength The extent to which an individual is capable of exerting force in one effort, as needed.

stress A reaction of the body and mind to the mental and emotional strain placed upon them.

stress electrocardiogram (ECG) A maximal exercise tolerance test using a treadmill to produce an elevated heart rate in order to reveal how the heart performs under pressure and high-intensity exercise.

stress inoculation A cognitive-behavioral stress management program involving education, rehearsal, and application of stress-management techniques.

stress response A series of events, caused by stressors, within the body that involves chemicals, hormones, and neural impulses.

stressor A specific event that disrupts equilibrium and initiates complex biochemical responses.

stressor identification The recognition of stress in order to begin effective management.

stroke A clot or break in a blood vessel in the brain that disrupts blood flow to the brain.

suicidologist A person who studies suicide.

sulfur oxides Acrid poisonous gases produced when fuel containing sulfur is burned.

synergistic effect Occurs when two or more substances present at the same time result in a total effect much greater than the sum of the effects of each substance.

syphilis A bacterial STD that spreads through the bloodstream and causes a systemic infection.

systemic infection An infection affecting the body as a whole.

systolic pressure The pressure measured in the arteries when the heart contracts.

tachycardia Excessively rapid beating of the heart.

tar The most carcinogenic substance in cigarettes; the gummy mixture left over from burning.

target heart rate range Heart activity high enough to bring about a training effect and low enough to be safe.

temporary threshold shift (TTS) Temporary hearing loss usually caused by a sudden loud noise.

teratogen An agent that causes birth defects.

tertiary care Special medical procedures, such as open-heart surgery and transplants, performed mostly at hospitals affiliated with medical schools or at large regional hospitals.

thalamus The part of the brain that plays a part in controlling the senses.

thalidomide A drug taken as a sedative in the early 1960s and subsequently found to cause severe deformities in the extremities of developing fetuses; in late 1990s used to treat certain cancers and AIDS.

thanatology The study of death and the psychological and social problems associated with it.

therapeutic community A residential treatment center where people who abuse drugs can live and learn to adjust to drug-free lives.

tight building syndrome Characterized by unhealthy indoor air that results from a lack of circulating air or a lack of ventilation.

tolerance The progressive change in the body's reaction to a drug, causing an individual to need more and more of the drug to achieve the same effect.

toxic chemical A chemical that is poisonous; exposure can cause bodily reactions ranging from watery eyes to unconsciousness and death.

toxin A poisonous substance produced by a microorganism; can cause certain infectious diseases.

trace minerals Minerals that are essential for proper growth and functioning but are needed in very small amounts.

training effect Health benefits, most notably increased heart efficiency, produced by exercising for a sufficient duration and intensity.

transdermal nicotine patch A form of nicotine replacement that, when applied to the skin, releases nicotine into the system at a constant rate.

transient ischemic attack (TIA) A stroke that causes minimal damage but signals the possibility of a more severe stroke.

trauma A wound or injury, whether intentional or unintentional.

trichloroethylene (TCE) A suspected carcinogen used as a degreaser in machine shops.

trichomoniasis A protozoal vaginitis transmitted primarily through sexual means.

tubal ligation A surgical procedure in which the fallopian tubes are cut and tied in order to prevent the passage of the egg and the subsequent union of sperm and egg.

tuberculosis An airborne bacterial disease spread by inhaling germs called tubercle bacilli; symptoms include fever, wasting, and cheesy formations in the lungs.

tumor A mass of tissue that accumulates in the body.

Type A personality A person who is excessively competitive, aggressive, driven, and impatient.

Type B personality A person who is more relaxed and patient than one who has a Type A personality.

underinsured Having limited health insurance that compromises one's access to health care services and places one at significant financial risk.

underwater weighing A test of body fat that weighs a person underwater to determine body composition.

underweight Less body weight relative to a specified standard for height and age.

uninsured Having no health insurance.

unintentional injuries Injuries that are caused by unplanned events, such as automobile crashes, falls, poisonings, fires, and drownings.

vacuum aspiration A method of abortion performed in the first trimester that involves dilation of the cervix and removal of the contents of the uterus by suction.

vaginismus Recurrent or persistent involuntary spasm of the musculature of the outer third of the vagina that interferes with sexual intercourse.

vaginitis A vaginal infection usually caused by yeast or protozoa.

vagus nerve The nerve that runs between the posterior part of the brain stem and the stomach and gives your brain the message that you are full.

vasectomy Surgically cutting and tying the vas deferens of the man, thus preventing the passage of sperm.

vasocongestion The pooling of blood in tissues during sexual excitement; also called tumescence.

vegan Vegetarians who do not eat any food of animal origin.

vegetarian A person who follows a diet consisting of no meat, chicken, or fish; all nutrition is obtained from vegetables, fruits, grains. Some vegetarians eat dairy products.

violence The use of force with the intent to harm oneself or another person.

virulence The strength of pathogens present during disease transmission.

virus A chain of nucleic acid surrounded by a protein coat that invades cells and uses the cells' reproductive capabilities.

warm-up period The period of exercise in which the body becomes prepared for exertion.

water-soluble vitamins Those vitamins not

stored in the body, with excesses excreted in the urine; examples are B-complex vitamins, and vitamin C.

wellness A description of health that includes the human potential for a high level of well-being while taking into consideration environmental and personal limitations.

withdrawal A group of symptoms that occur when a person stops taking a drug; also the method of contraception in which the man withdraws his penis from the vagina before ejaculation.

withdrawal symptoms Symptoms ranging from mild discomfort to very traumatic events when a drug is not present in the body.

yeast infection A condition characterized by itching; burning during urination; a white, thick, odorless discharge; painful intercourse; and general discomfort. Caused by *Candida*.

yo-yo dieting Going on and off diets.

Index

Boldface numbers indicate pages on which key terms are defined.

A

Abortion, 467–470
　spontaneous, 467
Absolute strength, **162**
Abstinence
　alcohol, **220**, 221–222, 224
　drug, 256–260
　sexual, **413**
　　and STDs, 399–400
　situational, **224**
　total, **224**
Acceptable risk, **529**
Acceptance, stage of dying, **514**, 515
Accidents. *See also* Injuries; Motor vehicle accidents
　alcohol-related, 215–216
　falls, 304, 487–488, 496–497
　fires, 305
　fireworks-related, 307
　in the home, 303–308
　motorcycle, 299–301
　poisoning, 307–308
　preventing, 308–309
　responding to, 310–311
　water-related, 302–303, 306
Accutane, 451
Achievable age, 34–**35**
Acid rain, **532**–533
Acquaintance rape, 283–284
Acquired immune deficiency syndrome. *See* AIDS
Active euthanasia, **508**
Active immunity, **359**
Acupuncture, 565, 567
Acute stage, of infection, 364, **365**
Acyclovir, **393**
Addiction, **183**
　alcohol, **213**. *See also* Alcohol abuse; Alcoholism
　caffeine, 234
　drug, 183, **240**. *See also* Drug use and abuse
　nicotine, 183, 184–185
Adipose tissue, **139**
Adiposity, **127**
Adolescence. *See* Teenagers
Adoption, 448
Adults
　alcohol consumption, 207–208
　nutrition, 115
　perception of death, 513
　sexuality, 410
Advance medical directives, **511**–512
Advertising
　cigarette, 182
　fraudulent, 562–563
　health care, 561–563
　obesity and, 136
Aerobic, **162**, 163
Aerobic capacity, **162**, 163–164
Affective disorders, **62**
African Americans
　AIDS incidence, 387–388
　cocaine use, 252
　heart disease, 323, 323*t*
　mortality data, 323*t*
　prostate cancer, 334, 338
　smoking, 180, 180*t*
　violent crime and, 265, 266*f*, 267, 269, 269*f*
Agammaglobulinemia, 362
Age
　accidental injury and, 292
　achievable, 34–**35**
　chronological, **478**
　crime victimization and, 265, 266*f*, 267
　drunk driving and, 297
　functional, **478**
　infertility and, 448
　measuring, 478
　psychological, **478**
Ageism, **478**, 479
Aging, 476–501. *See also* Elderly
　alcohol consumption and, 208
　biological changes, 485–495
　exercise and, 161–162
　health problems, preventable, 495–497
　and mental ability, 489–490, 493
　misconceptions about, 479
　psychology of, 480–482
　quiz, 492–494
　styles of, 480–482
　theories of, 477–478
　weight gain and, 139–140
AIDS, 363, 366*t*, **386**–391, 396*t*
　awareness campaigns, 382
　cancer and, 333
　demographics, 387–388, 388*f*
　in drug users, 252–253
　prevention, 354–355
　and psychoneuroimmunology, 363
　stress and, 82
　tests, 390–391
　treatment, 390
Air bags, 297
Air pollution, **530**–536, 531*t*, 549*t*
　indoor, 547–551, 548*f*, 549*t*
Air quality, 532
Alarm reaction, 75–76
Alcohol abuse, 211–218. *See also* Alcohol consumption; Alcoholism
　addiction, 212, **213**
　avoiding, 224–227
　binge drinking, 208, 215, 236*t*
　and cancer, 332
　defined, 218
　dependence, 211–212, **213**
　poisoning, 215
Alcohol consumption, 18, 206–229. *See also* Alcohol abuse; Alcoholism
　abstinence, 208–209, 221–222, 224
　bicycling accidents and, 302
　calories, 212*t*
　as cause of death, 206, 215–217
　central nervous system effects, 213–214, 241*f*
　control of access to alcohol, 223–224
　crime and, 271–272
　as cultural tradition, 211
　demographics, 207–209, 236*t*
　drownings and, 302
　drug interactions, 226, 242
　with food and other drink, 225–226
　in France, 213
　health effects, 212–217
　limiting, 226–227
　moderate, 212–213
　motor vehicle accidents and, 215–217, 216*f*, 291–292, 297
　motorcycle accidents and, 300
　pace, 224–225
　policies to limit, 223–224
　during pregnancy, 214–215, 451
　reasons, 209–212
　violence and, 271
Alcoholic, **208**, 219
Alcoholics Anonymous (AA), **220**, 221
Alcoholism, **218**–222. *See also* Alcohol abuse; Alcohol consumption
　abstinence vs. moderation, 221–222
　causes, 220–221
　as disease, 218
　environment and, 220
　heredity and, 219–220
　self-assessment test, 219
　treatment, 220–222, 255
　in women, 208
Allergens, **355**, 362
Allergy, **362**
　smoking and, 191
　total allergy syndrome, 550–551
Alternative medicine, 565–568
　for cancer, 341–342
　practitioners, 565–568
Alveoli, **532**, 533
Alzheimer's disease, **490**–495
Amenorrhea, 128, **129**, 450
American Cancer Society, 577–578
American Lung Association, 577–578
American Medical Association, on physician-assisted suicide, 510
Amino acids, **98**, 99
Amnesia, **214**
Amniocentesis, **452**
Amphetamines, 243, 245*t*
Anabolic steroids, **244**
Anaerobic, **164**, 165
Anatomy, reproductive
　female, 433–438, 434*f*–435*f*
　male, 430*f*, 430–433, 432*f*
　test, 438–439
Androgens, 411–412, 430
Anger, 51
　stage of dying, **514**, 515
Angina pectoris, 128, **129**, **188**, 189, **326**
Anorexia nervosa, 128, **129**, 141–143, 159
Antibiotics, **355**
Antibodies, **359**
Antigens, **359**
Anxiety, 58, **59**, 59*f*
Areola, 434
Arrhythmia, **326**
Art therapy, for cancer, 342
Arteries, hardening of. *See* Atherosclerosis
Arteriosclerosis. *See* Atherosclerosis
Artificial heart, 328
Artificial insemination, 448, **449**
Asbestos, 549*t*
Aspirin
　and heart disease, 327–328
　and influenza, 375
Assertiveness
　to avoid alcohol abuse, 226–227
　to avoid drugs, 258
　to avoid tobacco use, 184
Asthma, 320*t*, **530**–531
Asymptomatic carrier, 382, **383**
Asymptomatic period, 319
Atherosclerosis, **100**, 101, **188**, **325**–326
Athletes. *See also* Exercise
　dietary needs, 112
　eating disorders, 143
　elderly, 498
　health problems, 159
　steroid use, 244, 251
　women, 157–159
　young, 159
Athlete's foot, 366*t*
Auscultation, 36–37
Autoimmune diseases, **362**
Automobiles. *See* Motor vehicle accidents; Motor vehicle pollution
Autopsy, **519**–520
AZT (azidothymidine), 390

B

Bacteria, **355**
　diseases caused by, 357*t*
　　new, 373*t*, 374
　　STDs, 393–395
Bacterial pneumonia, **368**–369
Balanced diet, 144–**145**
Baldness, 486
Barbiturates, 243, 246*t*
Bargaining, **514**, 515
Barrier methods, of contraception, 464–465
Basal cell, **335**
Basal metabolic rate, **139**
Baseline data, **25**
Battery, **274**, 275, 277
Beer
　calories, 212*t*
　pregnancy and, 215
Behavior modification, for smoking cessation, **196**, 197
Benign tumor, **330**
Benzene, **530**, 531
Bereaved, **516**, 517
Bereavement, 517–518, **520**, 520–523
BHA (butylated hydroxyanisole), 108–109
BHT (butylated hydroxytoluene), 108–109
Bicycling
　helmet use, 300–302
　in Holland, 536
　safety issues, 301–302
Binge drinker, **208**
Binge drinking, 208, 215, 236*t*
Binge eating, **141**–142
Binge eating disorder, 142–143
Bioelectrical impedance, **131**
Biology, and sexuality, 411
Biopsy, **319**
Birth control, **458**–459. *See also* Contraception
Birth control pills, **460**–461
　and rise of STDs, 383
Birth defects, 451, 530
　alcohol-related, 214–215, 451
　prevention, 449
　rubella-related, 371
　STD-related, 393–395
Birthing centers, 455
Bisexuals, **412**–413
Blackout, **214**
Blindness, in infants, 393–394
Blood alcohol concentration (BAC), 216, **217**
　in drunk drivers, 225*t*, 297
Blood cholesterol. *See* Cholesterol
Blood pressure. *See also* Hypertension
　diastolic, **326**, 327
　systolic, **326**, 327
Body fat, **131**, 139
　and aging, 486
　measuring, 131

Body image, test, 136
Body mass index (BMI), 130f, **131**
Body shape, cultural perspectives on, 132
Bone loss. *See* Osteoporosis
Bradycardia, **326**
Brain
 and Alzheimer's disease, 491
 drug and alcohol effects, 241f, 241–242
 prion-related infections, 356
Brain dead, 506, **507**
Breast cancer, 334
 as cause of death, 323, 323f, 331t
 incidence, 331t
 risk factors, 320t, 332–333
 screening, 337–338
 self-examination, 338, **339**, 339f, 340
 treatment, 339
Breast self-examination (BSE), 338, **339**, 339f, 340
Breasts, 433–434, 435f
Breech presentation, **457**
Bronchitis, chronic, 190, **191**
Bubonic plague, 352
Buddhists, death traditions, 509
Buildings, pollution inside, 547–551
Bulimia, 128, **129**, 141–142
Burial, 508–509
Burnout, 78, **79**
Burns, 305–307
 first-aid for, 305
Butter-margarine question, 101

C
Caffeine, 234
 sources, 235t
Calcium, 104–105
 foods with, 104f
Calculus, **344**
Calories, **137**
 in alcoholic and carbonated drinks, 212t
 exercise and, 140, 256t
 low-fat diet and, 138
 required, 139
 weight gain and, 137–139
Camel cigarettes, 182
Campylobacter jejuni, 374
Canada, gun control in, 270
Cancer, 330–341. *See also specific types of cancer*
 carcinogens, **184**, **330**, **332**, **529**
 death rates, 331t, 333t
 demographics, 330, 331t, 333t
 exercise and, 157–158
 forms, 331t, 333–336
 pain, 346
 pesticides and, 539
 risk factors, 332–333
 screening, 336–339
 self-tests, 338–339
 smokeless tobacco and, 194
 smoking and, 186–188, 189f, 193
 smoking cessation and, 188f–189f
 treatments, 339–342
 quack, 563
 viruses as causes, 372
Cannabis, **239**, **244**, 250t. *See also* Marijuana
Carbohydrates, 97–99
 weight gain and, 137–139
Carbon monoxide, **532**, 549t
 pregnancy and, 191
 smoking and, **184**, 185, 192
Carcinogens, **184**, **330**, **332**, **529**
Cardiopulmonary resuscitation (CPR), **310**, **311**, **328**
Cardiovascular disease, **322**–**328**. *See also* Heart disease
 forms, 325–327
 risk factors, 324–325
Cataracts, **488**
Centers for Disease Control (CDC), 578
Central nervous system, effect of alcohol, 213–214, 241f, 241–242
Cerebellum, **213**
Cerebrum, **213**
Cervical cancer, 372
 and genital warts, 391
 risk factors, 320t
 screening, 337
Cervical os, 436
Cervix, 436, **455**
Cesarean section, **457**
CFCs (chlorofluorocarbons), 534, **535**
Chain of infection, 353f, 353–355
Chancre, **394**
Check-ups, cancer-related, 338–339
Chemical sensitivity, multiple, 550–551
Chemotherapy, 339–341
Chewing tobacco, 193
Chicken pox, 366t
Child abuse, 273, 276–278, **277**, 279f
 as crime risk factor, 265–266
 emotional, 276, **277**
 physical neglect as, 276–**277**, 279f
 reporting, 278
 sexual, **277**–279, 279f
 signs, 279f
Childbirth, 454–458
 natural, **455**
Child-proof packaging, **307**
Children. *See also* Child abuse; Teenagers
 alcohol abuse risk factors, 227
 of alcoholics, 221
 bicycle accidents, 300
 childhood diseases, 371
 drug use risk factors, 237
 falls, 304
 flu treatments, 368
 lead poisoning, 533
 nutrition, 114
 perception of death, 512
 pertussis, 361
 poisoning, 307
 sexuality, 410
 skin cancer, 336–337
 smoking and, 181–182, 193
 television violence and, 272–273
Child-resistant packaging, **307**
China
 acupuncture in, 567
 elderly in, 479t
Chlamydia, 393–394, 396t
Chlamydia pneumoniae virus, 372
Chlorinated dioxins, 545
Chlorine, in water supply, 537
Chlorofluorocarbons (CFCs), 534, **535**
Cholesterol, **100**–**102**
 atherosclerosis and, 101, 325
 exercise and, 157
 heart disease and, 100–101, 324–325
Chorionic villus sampling (CVS), 452–453
Christians, death traditions, 508–509
Chromosomes, 411, 411f
Chronic bronchitis, 190, **191**
Chronic diseases, 316–349
 behavioral causes, 319–322, 320t–321t
 characteristics, 318–322
 demographics, 317, 317f
 versus infectious disease, 318
 living with, 344–346
 risk factors for, 320t–321t
Chronic fatigue syndrome, **368**, 369–370
Chronic illness, 318, **319**
Chronic obstructive pulmonary disease, 188f
Chronological age, **478**
Cigarettes. *See also* Smoking; Tobacco
 advertising, 182
 house fires and, 305
 low-yield, 192
 marijuana and, 236–237
Cigars, 193
Circulatory diseases, smoking-related, 191
Circumcision, 431
Cirrhosis of the liver, **214**
 risk factors for, 320t
Cities
 air pollution and, 531–532
 crime and, 267
Clitoris, 434
Cocaine, 236t, 242–243, 245t
 effect on fetus, 253
Cochlea, 546, **547**
Codeine, 243, 248t
Codependency, **220**, 221
Coffee, 234, 235t
Cognitive therapy, as cancer treatment, 341
Cognitive-behavioral skills, to manage stress, 90–91
Cohabitation, 444
Coinsurance, 571
Coitus, 418
Colds, 364–365, 366t
College students
 accidental injuries, 290, 291f
 alcohol consumption, 208–210, 215, 236t
 date rape, 283, 284f
 drug use, 236t, 237–238
 drunk driving, 297
 eating styles, 112, 119
 experience of death, 504, 513
 health insurance, 569–570
 STDs, 380–381, 393
 stressors, 82–84
Colon cancer, **98**
Colorectal cancers, 331t, 333t, 334–335, 338
Colorings, artificial, 108–109
Columbarium, **520**
Commitment, **415**
Common cold, 364–365, 366t
Communicable diseases. *See* Infectious diseases
Communication
 about sex, 413–414
 nonverbal, 414
 to reduce stress, 87
 saying no, 414
Companionate love, 415–416
Complaints, about health care, filing, 564
Complementary protein relationship, **100**
Complete protein, **100**
Complex carbohydrate, **97**
Compost, 544
Conception, 448, **449**, 450
Concordance rate, **220**
Conditioning period, **169**

Condoms
 female, 464, **465**
 male, 464, **465**
 proper use of, 398, 464
 and STD prevention, 385, 461–462
Conflict resolution, **274**–275
Consumer issues
 fad diets, **145**
 food shopping, 120–121
 health care choices, 559–579
Consumer Product Safety Commission, 308, 564
Consumer Reports, 560f, 561
Contagious diseases. *See* Infectious diseases
Contraception, 458–467, **459**
 decisions about, 466–468, 470–471
 emergency, 466–467
 failure rates, 461t
 methods, 459–467, 465t
Contraimplantation, **465**
Contraindications, 560, **561**
Controlled substances, 238, **239**
Convalescence, from infection, 364, **365**
Cool-down period, **169**
Coordination of benefits, 571
Copayment, 571
Coping, **84**, 85
Coping skills, **86**–87
Copulation, 418
Coronary angioplasty, **328**, 329f
Coronary artery bypass, **328**, 329f
Corpus luteum, 437
Counselors, mental health, 68
Cowper's glands, 433
CPR. *See* Cardiopulmonary resuscitation
Crabs, 396t, 399
Crack, 246t, 253
Crack babies, **450**, 451
Cremaster muscle, 430–431
Cremation, 509, **520**
Crime, 264–287
 avoiding, 268
 costs, 265
 times and places, 267
 victims, 266f, 266–268
Crime tax, 265
Criminals, 265–267
Criteria pollutants, 530, 531t
Crowning, **455**
Cruzan, Nancy, 507
Cryptorchidism, 431
Cryptosporidium, 537
Cultural perspectives
 acupuncture, 567
 aging, 479t, 480–481
 bicycling versus cars, 536
 body weight, 132
 death, 508–509, 520
 gun control, 270–271
 smoking cessation, 196
 wine intake, 213
Culture
 alcohol consumption and, 211
 guns and, 270–271
 obesity and, 136
 sexual values and, 408

D
Dancers, eating disorders, 143
Date rape, **283**
Date-rape drug, 238
Death, 504–514, 522–525. *See also* Mortality
 advance medical directives and, 511–512
 behavioral causes, 14–15, 15t

biological definitions, 506–507
causes, 14t, 14–15
dealing with, 504–505
euthanasia debate, 507–510
legal definitions, 507
perceptions through life stages, 512–514
premature, **292**, 293–295
preparation, 522–523
religious definitions, 507
traditions surrounding, 508–509
Deductible, 571
Defense mechanisms, **84**, 85
against infection, 358–359
Dehydration, **106**, 107
Dementia, **63**, **490**
Denial, stage of dying, **514**, 515
Dental caries, **341**
fluoride and, 540
Dental disease, 320t, 341–345
Dental plaque, 343–344
Dependence
alcohol, 211–212, **213**
drug, **240**
Depo-Provera, 461
Depressants, **243**, 246t–247t
Depression, 60–64, **495**
and chronic disease, 345–346
in elderly, 493–495, **495**
major, **62**
minor, 60–61
as stage of dying, **514**, 515
and viral infection, 372
in women, 60–61
Dermatitis, **530**, 531
Designer drugs, **244**
Desire, sexual, **421**
inhibited, **422**
Detoxification
for alcoholism, **220**, 255
for drug addiction, **254**, 255
programs, **254**, 255
Diabetes
exercise and, 157
risk factors for, 321t
Diagnosis, 319
Diaphragm, **465**
Diastolic pressure, **326**, 327
Diet(s), 96–97. See also Eating patterns and styles; Nutrition; Weight loss
balanced, 144–**145**
calcium in, 104–105
cancer and, 332
fad, **145**
fast food, 113
French, 213
high-fiber, 98–99
high-protein, low-carbohydrate, 145
low-fat, 138
low-protein, high-carbohydrate, 145
protein-sparing, 145
questions to ask about, 146
salt in, 105–107, 106t
vegetarian, 113–119
water in, 107
yo-yo, **145**
Diet aids, 146–147
Dietary fiber, **98**, 99f
Digestive diseases, smoking-related, 191
Dilation, **455**
Dilation and evacuation, **470**
Dioxins, 545
Disability, living with, 344–346
Disease(s). See also Chronic

diseases; Infectious diseases
dental, 341–344
opportunistic, **386**, 387
Disordered thinking, 64, **65**
Distress, **77**
Disulfiram, 220–221
Diuretic, **142**
Diving, 303
Divorce, 444
Domestic partnership, 447
Domestic violence, **272**, 273–276, 277f
Dosage, of disease agent, 358, **359**
Double standard, sexual, 408
Drinking. See Alcohol consumption
Drinks, carbonated
caffeine in, 235t
calories in, 212t
Drowning, 302–303
Drug(s), 232–236. See also Drug use and abuse; Medication(s); *specific drugs*
absorbed, 243
availability, 238
caffeine content, 235t
defined, **233**, 235–236
dependent, **240**
designer, **244**
effects
on body, 240–242
on brain, 241f
on fetus, 253–254
emergency room mentions of, 252f
gateway, **236**, **237**
generic, 575
inhaled, 242–244
injected, 243
interaction, **42**, **240**, 241–242
with alcohol, 226, 242
legality issues, 238–239
over-the-counter, 233, 235t, **575**
prescription, 233–234, 235t, **575**
smoked, 243
swallowed, 243
trafficking, 254
types, 242–252, 245t–250t
Drug addiction, 183, **240**
Drug dependent, **240**
Drug misuse, **240**
Drug testing, 254
Drug use and abuse, 236–242, **240**. See also Drug(s); Medication(s)
abstinence strategies, 256–260
AIDS and, 252–253
among college students, 236t, 237–238
among elderly, 495–496
crime and, 266, 271–272
demographics, 236–240
impact, 252–254
methods, 242–243
motivations, 244–251
during pregnancy, 253–254, 451
progression into, 236
reasons, 237–239
solutions, 257
treatment, 254–256
in workplace, 254
Drunk driving, 217, 223, 226–227
accidents, 215–217, 216f, 291–292
blood alcohol concentrations, 225t, 297
demographics, 297
Dual-career families, 443
Durable power of attorney for health care, **511**–512
Dying, 514–517, 523–525

attitudes of elderly, 513
stages of, 514–515
Dysfunction, 58, **59**, 59f
Dysorganization, 58–**59**
Dyspareunia, **424**

E
Eating disorders, 128–129, 141–143
athletes and, 143, 159
symptoms, 142
Eating patterns and styles, 96–97, 112–113. See also Diet(s); Food; Nutrition
age-related, 114–115
bad habits, 119
changing, 119, 144–145
culture and, 112–113
in the home, 112–113
obesity and, 135–137
ECG. See Electrocardiogram
Ecstasy (drug), 244
Education
crime and, 266
smoking and, 179–180, 180t
EEG. See Electroencephalogram
Effacement, **455**
Ejaculation, 430, 432–433
premature, **422**, 423
Elderly, 477–501
alcohol consumption, 208
Alzheimer's disease, 490–495
attitudes toward death, 513
bone loss in, 486–488
caring for parent, 482–484, 484t, 496
as crime victims, 267
demographics, 478–479
depression, 493–495
exercise, 159–160, 498
falls, 304, 487–488, 496–497
health status, 478, 485
healthy aging, 497–498
hearing loss, 488
in Japan, 379t, 480–481
living arrangements, 478, 479t
memory loss, 485, 489–490
mental abilities, 489–490, 493
misconceptions about, 479
nutrition, 112, 115
quality of life near death, 513–514
sex life, 479, 488–489, 494
suicide, 65, 495
vision loss, 487–488
Elective abortions, **467**
Electrocardiogram (ECG), **325**
Electroencephalogram (EEG), 506, **507**
E-mail, harassing, 280
Embalming, **520**
Emergencies, 568f. See also Accidents
responding to, 310–311
Emergency room episodes, drug-related, 252f
Emotional abuse, of children, 276, **277**
Emotional skills, 8–9f
Emotions, 51–52
management, 87
Emphysema, 190, **191**
Employment, crime and, 266
Empty calories, **98**
Empty love, 417
Endemic, **26**, 27
Endometrium, 436
Endorphins, 160–**161**
Endurance, **162**, 163
Energy

body's use of, 139–140
from carbohydrates, 97
Entry into new host, pathogen's, 354
Environment
attitudes toward, 551–552
greenhouse effect and, 534, 535f
Environmental ethics, 551–552
continuum of, 552f
Environmental factors, in alcoholism, 220
Environmental health hazards, 528–553
airborne, 530–536, 531t, 549t
automobiles as, 535
criteria pollutants, 531t
global warming, 534–535
indoor, 547f, 547–551, 549t, **550**
injuries caused by, 292
multiple, 529
noise, 545–547, 546t
ozone layer depletion, 534
precycling and recycling, 540–544
solid waste, 540–544
synergistic effects of, 531
toxic waste, 544–545
waterborne, 536–540
Epidemic, **26**, 27
Epidemiologists, **26**, 27
Epidemiology, **26**, 27
Epididymis, 432
Episiotomy, **457**
Epstein-Barr virus, 369, 372
Eradication, 354–**355**
Erection, 431
Erickson's life cycle of developmental tasks, 482, 483t
Erogenous zones, **418**
Estrogen replacement therapy, 487
Estrogens, **157**–158, 411–412
heart disease and, 323–324
Ethics, environmental, 551–552
Ethnicity
crime and, 266f
drunk driving and, 297
smoking and, 180, 180t
Eustress, 77–**79**
Euthanasia, 507–512
active, **508**
passive, **508**
Excitement, sexual, 420–**421**
Exercise, 18, **157**
adherence, 172–173
aerobic, 163–165
anaerobic, 165
caloric expenditures, 156t
duration, **164**, 165
for elderly, 480–482, 498
frequency, **164**, 165
health benefits, 155–162
injuries, 169–172, 170f
intensity, **164**, 165–167
isokinetic, **162**, 163
isometric, **162**, 163
isotonic, **162**, 163
mental, 489–491, 494
moderate, examples, 153f
nonparticipation, reasons, 155f
participation, 153–155, 154t
personal program, 167–173
phases, 168–169
during pregnancy, 452
psychological benefits, 160–162
to reduce stress, 88–89, 141
safety precautions, 169–172
stretching, 164
weight and, 140–141
weight-bearing, 159–160

Exhaustion, **77**
Extended family, 442–**443**

F
Fad diets, **145**
Fallopian tubes, 433, 435
  chlamydia infection, 393–394
Falls, 304, 487–488, 496–497
False negative, **26**
False positive, **26**
Family(ies), 442–444, 445f
  alcohol abuse risk factors and, 227
  of alcoholics, 221
  as crime risk factor, 265–266
  deciding to have children, 446–447
  domestic partnership laws, 447
  drug use risk factors and, 237
  dual-career, **443**
  with elderly parents, 482–484, 484t
  extended, 442–**443**
  health histories, 37, 38f
  homicide and, 269–270
  in Japan, 480–481
  nontraditional, 447
  nuclear, 442, **443**
  sex roles, 410
  single-parent, **443**
  smoking and, 181
  violence in, 273–280
  weight and, 134–136
  without children, 444
Family planning, 446–447, 458, **459**, 470–471
Fast food, 113
  sandwich guide, 118f
Fasting, total, **146**
Fat-free food, 120
Fats, dietary, 18, 97, 100–102, 112f, 114, 139
  in butter and margarine, 101
  in ethnic foods, 116–117
  food labeling of, 120
  monounsaturated, **100**
  polyunsaturated, **100**
  saturated, **100**
  weight gain and, 137–139
Fat-soluble vitamins, **102**
Fatuous love, 415
FDA Consumer, 561
Fear, 51
Federal Trade Commission, 564
Fee-for-service plan, **571**
Female condoms, 464, **465**
Female orgasmic disorder, **424**
Fen/phen, 146–147
Festive malaise, 80
Fetal alcohol effect (FAE), **214**
Fetal alcohol syndrome (FAS), **214**, 215
Fever, **36**
  exercise and, 160
Fiber, **98**
  sources, 99f
Fibrillation, **326**
Fight-or-flight reaction, **84**, 85
Fiji, smoking cessation in, 196
Fimbriae, 435
Fires, in the home, 305–306
Fireworks, 307
First aid
  burns, 305
  for exercise injuries, 170
  poisoning, 307–308
  recommendations, 310–311
Fitness, 162–165. *See also* Exercise

  components, 162–165
  exercise and, 165–167
  personal program, 167–173
  physical, 162f
Fitness triangle, 162f
Flame-resistant materials, 306–**307**
Flavorings, artificial, 108
Flexibility, **162**, 163
  assessment, 164
Flu vaccine, 365
Fluoride, **538**
  in water supply, 539–540
Follicles, 435
Follicle-stimulating hormone (FSH), 436
Follicular phase, 437
Food. *See also* Diet(s); Eating patterns and styles; Nutrition
  additives, **106**, 107–109
  cancer and, 332
  contaminated, 357, 374
  ethnic, fat in, 116–117
  fast, 113, 118f
  ingredient labels, 120–121
  and food intake, 138
  nutrients, **97**–107
  organically grown, 120
  preparation, 121, 144
  processed, 109, 120
  selection, 120–121
  serving sizes, 111
  shopping, 120–121
  snacks, 119
  vitamin-enriched, 120
Food groups, 109–110
Food Guide Pyramid, 110–111, 112f
Food labels, 120f, 120–121
Food poisoning, 374
Foreplay, **418**
Formaldehyde, 549t
Framingham Heart Study, 324
France, alcohol consumption and diet in, 213
Frustration, 51
Functional age, **478**
Funerals, 508, **520**
Fungal pneumonia, **368**, 369
Fungi, **355**
  diseases caused by, 357t

G
Gang rape, **283**
Gasoline, 533
Gateway drugs, 236, **237**
Gays, 412–**413**
  violence against, 267
Gender identity, **406**–407
General adaptation syndrome (GAS), **75**, 75f
Generativity, **482**
Generic drugs, 575
Genetics. *See also* Heredity
  of sex identity, 411, 411f
Genital herpes, 382, 392–393, 397t
Genital warts, 391–392, 396t
Genogram, 38f
German measles, 366t, 371
Geronotologists, **477**
Giardiasis, 355
Gingivitis, **343**
Girls, steroid abuse, 251
Glans clitoris, 434
Glans penis, 430f, 431
Global warming, 534–**535**
Gonorrhea, 394, 397t
Great Lakes, pollution, 538
Greenhouse effect, 534, 535f
Greenhouse gases, 534

Grief, **520**–522
  helping friends in, 522
Groningen, Holland, 536
Group therapy, 67f
Gum disease, 341, 343–344
Gun ownership, 269–270
  homicide and, 269–271, 271f
  outside U.S., 270–271

H
Habits, 13–14
  eating, 119
  healthy, developing, 42
Hair, aging and, 486
Hallucinations, 64, **65**
Hallucinogens, **244**, 247t–248t
Hand washing, 358
Hangover, **214**
Hantavirus pulmonary syndrome (HPS), 374
Harvard Medical School Letter, 561
Hashish, 250t
Hashish oil, 250t
Hazardous wastes, **545**
Head injuries, bicycle-related, 300–301
Headaches, noise-related, 546
Health, 3–5
  attaining, 5–11
  defined by WHO, 3
  mental. *See* Mental health
  as personal responsibility, 18
Health and wellness continuum, 4f–5f
Health assessment, **25**–45
  community, 27–28
  medical, 37–41
  national program, 29–30, 31t
  personal, 32–43
  primary, **25**
  problems, 26–27
  secondary, **25**
  self-observation, 36–37
Health attitude, **12**
Health behavior, **10**–11
  changing after assessment, 43
  theories about changing, 34–36
Health belief, **12**–13
Health care, 558–581
  advertising, 561–562
  consumer rights, 563–564
  costs, 558–559, 559t
    smoking-related, 186t
  decision-making, 559–561
  filing complaints, 564
  fraud, 562–563
  information, 559–564, 576–581
  insurance, 569–575
  patient involvement, 560f
Health care practitioners
  alternative, 565–568
  getting information from, 563–564
  mental health, 67–69
  physicians, 565–569, 566t
Health history, 36–37
Health information, sources, 576–581
Health insurance, 569–575
  indemnity plans, 571
  managed care plans, 572–574
  questions to ask, 574–575
  terms, 571
  worksheet, 572–573
Health knowledge, 6–**7**
Health literacy, **7**
Health maintenance organizations (HMOs), 572–574, **573**
Health momentum, **12**, 13

Health records, 42
Health risk appraisal, 34–**35**
Health risk assessment, 32–**33**
Health risks, 33–34
Health skills, **8**–10
  typology, 9f
Health style, **10**, 11f
  common sense and, 18
  defined, 12
  personal, 12–14
Health value, **10**, 12
Healthy People 2000, 29–30, 31t
Hearing loss
  in elderly, 488
  noise-induced, 546t, 546–547
Heart
  aging and, 485
  artificial, 328
  exercise and, 156–157
Heart attacks, **326**
  ethnicity and, 323
  overweight and, 128
  smoking and, 189
  warning signs, 326
Heart disease, 322–325. *See also* Cardiovascular disease
  cholesterol and, 100–101, 324–325
  demographics, 322–323
  diagnosis, 325
  forms, 325–327
  prevention, 321t, 327–328
  risk factors, 321t, 324–325
  smoking and, 188–190
  smoking cessation and, 188f, 190
  treatment, 328
  viruses as causes, 372
  wine and, 213
Heart rate, **164**
  exercise and, 165–167
  maximal, 166–**167**
  resting, 166, **167**
  smoking and, 183
  target range, **167**
Heart transplant, **328**
Height-weight tables, 129t
  limitations of, 129–131
Helmets, 300–301
Helper T-cells, **386**, 387
Hemiplegia, **326**–327
Hepatitis, **370**
Hepatitis A, **370**
Hepatitis B, **370**, 372, 392, **393**
Hepatitis C, **370**, 372
Herbal medicine, 565–568
Herd immunity, **361**
Heredity
  and alcoholism, 219–220
  and cancer, 332–333
  and mutagens, 530
  and obesity, 134–135
  and osteoporosis, 488
Heroin, 240, 243–244, 248t, 271
Herpes, 392–393, 397t
  viruses, 372
Herpes simplex type 2, 392, **393**, 397t
Heterosexuals, 412–413
Hierarchy of human needs, 57f
High blood pressure. *See* Hypertension
High density lipoproteins (HDLs), 100–102, **175**
Hindus, death traditions, 509
Hip fractures, 496
Hispanic Americans
  as crime victims, 266f
  drunk driving, 297
  as homicide victims, 269f

HIV. See Human immunodeficiency virus (HIV)
HMOs. See Health maintenance organizations (HMOs)
Hodgkin's disease, 331t, 339
Holidays, stress of, 80
Holistic health, 3–4, 4f
Holland, bicycling in, 536
Holmes-Rahe Social Readjustment Rating Scale (SRRS), 77
Home
   accidents, 303–308
      eating patterns and styles, 112–113
      and obesity, 135–137
   homicides, 269–270
   pollution, 547–551, 548f, 549t
   safety checklist, 309
Homicide, 268–273, **269**
   alcohol and, 215, 271–272
   drugs and, 271–272
   guns and, 269–271, 271f
   in the home, 269–270
   minorities as victims, 269f
   times, 267
Homosexuals, 412–**413**, 447
Hormone replacement therapy (HRT), 487
Hormones
   production, 434
   and sex characteristics, 411–412
Hospice, 514, 515–517, 516t
Hospital care, 569
Hospital stays
   infections acquired during, **370**, 371–373
   weight and, 128
Host susceptibility, 354, **355**
Hostility, 51
Human chorionic gonadotropin (HCG), **450**
Human immunodeficiency virus (HIV), 386–391. See also AIDS
   effect on fetus, 253
   psychoneuroimmunology and, 363
   testing for, 390–391
   transmission, 388–390
Human papilloma virus (HPV), **391**–392, 396t
Hydrocarbons, **532**, 533
Hymen, 434
Hypertension, 105–**106**, **157**, **322**, 327
   exercise and, 157
   heart disease and, 323–324
   risk factors, 327
   salt and, 105–106
Hypnosis, for cancer, 342
Hypoglycemia, **490**
Hypothermia, **36**, **169**, 170, 302–**303**
Hypothyroidism, **133**

I
Illness behavior, 10–**11**
Imagery, as cancer treatment, 341–342
Immune deficiency diseases, **362**–363
Immune system, 359–363
   aging and, 485
   disorders, 362–363
   exercise and, 160
   stress and, 81–82
Immunity, **359**–362
   active, **359**
   boosting, 363
   herd, **361**
   passive, **359**
   vaccinations for, 360
Immunization, 354, 360–361. See also Vaccine(s)
Impact, stage of grief, **520**
Impotence, **422**, 423–424
In vitro fertilization, 448, **449**
Incidence data, **26**, 27
Income, crime and, 266f, 266–267
Incomplete protein, **100**
Incontinence, **490**
Incubation, **362**, 363
Incubation period, 382, **383**
Indemnity plan, **571**
Indoor pollution, 547–551, 548f, 549t, **550**
Induction, **470**
Infants
   blindness, 393–394
   HIV transmission to, 389
   low birthweight, 188f, 214, 450–451
   and maternal drug use, 253
   and maternal STD infection, 393–395
   nutrition, 114
   parental smoking and, 191, 193
Infatuation, 417
Infection. See also Infectious diseases
   chain of, 353f, 353–355
   exercise and, 160
   nosocomial (hospital-acquired), **370**, 371–373
   secondary, 355
   systemic, 393
Infectious diseases, 352–377
   bodily defenses against, 358–359
   causes, 355–356
   versus chronic diseases, 318
   emerging, 373–374
   eradication, 354–355
   hand washing and, 358
   immunity and, 359–363
   incidence trends, 368t
   new, 373t, 374
   prevention, 354, 374–375
   reemerging, 373–374
   sexually transmitted. See Sexually transmitted diseases (STDs)
   stages, 363f, 363–364
   transmission, 353f, 353–358
   types
      by cause, 357t
      common, 364–374, 366t–367t
Infertility, 448, **449**
   chlamydia and, 393–394
   smoking and, 190
Inflammation, **359**
Influenza, 365–368, 367t, 375
Information, in health care choices, 560–564, 576–578
Inhalants, 242–243, **244**
Inhibited sexual desire, **422**
Inhibitions, **214**
Initiator, **330**
Injuries. See also Accidents
   athletic, 159
   at-risk person, profile, 292–293
   bicycle, 300–302
   causes, 291–292
   costs, 293–296, 295f
   diving-related, 303
   exercise, 169–172, 170f
   fall-related, 304
   fire-related, 305–306
   fireworks-related, 307
   in the home, 303–308
   intentional, **291**
   motorcycle, 300–301
   prevention, 308–309
   responding to, 310–311
   risk factors for, 292–293
      test, 294
   scalding water, 306
   soft tissue, 159, 170
   work-related, 292–293, 293f
Inpatient care, **569**
Insects, infection-bearing, 354, **355**, 357
Intellectual skills, 8–9f
Intelligence, and aging, 489, 493
Intensive care units, infections acquired in, 371–373
Intentional injuries, **291**
Intercourse, **418**–419
   painful, 424
Interferon, **355**, 359
Internet, as health information source, 577–578
Interpersonal skills, 88, **89**
Interstitial cells, 431
Intimacy, **415**
Intoxicated, **210**
Intrauterine device (IUD), **465**
Isokinetic exercise, **162**, 163
Isolation, 87
Isometric exercise, **162**, 163
Isotonic exercise, **162**, 163
IUD, **465**

J
Japan
   elderly, 479t, 480–481
   gun control, 270–271
Jews, death and mourning traditions, 508–509
Jobs, high-risk, 292–293, 293f
Joints, exercise and, 169

K
Kaposi's sarcoma, 333, 372, **386**, 387
Kenya, 105
Keratosis, **337**
Ketosis, **145**
Kevorkian, Jack, 508
Kissing, and HIV transmission, 390
Kübler-Ross, Elizabeth, 514–515

L
Labels, food, 120f, 120–121
Labia majora, 434
Labia minora, 434
Labor, **455**–458, 456f–457f
Laboratory tests, 40
   errors in, 26
Lactovegetarians, **118**
Landfills, **540**
Late syphilis, **394**, 395
Laws
   on alcohol, 223, 226–227
   drugs taken during pregnancy and, 253–254
   on guns, 270–271
   on tobacco use, 198–199
Lead, **532**, 533
Learning
   elderly and, 489, 493
   as health skill, 9–10
Legionnaire's disease, 368
Lesbians, 412–**413**
Lesions, **393**
Leukoplakia, **193**
Libido, **418**
Lice, pubic, 396t, 399
Life expectancy, 28, 28f, **29**, 319
Life stages
   Erickson's developmental tasks, 482, 483t
   perception of death in, 482, 483t
Lifestyle
   and cancer risk, 339
   and chronic disease, 319–322
Light food, 120
Liking, 416
Liquor, calories in, 212t
Liver
   alcohol and, 214
   cirrhosis of, **214**, 320t
   hepatitis and, 370–372
Liver cancer, 372
Living, health skills in, 8–9
Living together, 444, 447
Living will, **511**, 511f
Living-dying interval, **514**
Love, 52, 414–417, 416f
Love Canal, 545
Low birthweight babies, **450**–451
   alcohol and, 214
   smoking cessation and, 188f
Low density lipoproteins (LDLs), **100**–101, **157**
Low-fat food, 120, 138
Low-yield cigarettes, 192
LSD (lysergic acid diethylamide), 243–244, 247t
Lumpectomy, **339**
Lung(s)
   aging and, 485
   air pollution and, 532–534
   disease risk factors, 321t
   smoking and, 190
Lung cancer, 334
   as cause of death, 323, 323f, 331t
   from cigar and pipe smoking, 193
   risk factors for, 321t
   risks from smoking, 189f, 332
   smoking and, 186–188, 332
   smoking cessation and, 188f–189f
Luo people, 105
Luteal phase, 437–438
Luteinizing hormone (LH), 437
Lyme disease, **370**, 371
Lymph node cancer, 339. See also Hodgkin's disease

M
Main effect, of drug, **240**
Mainstream smoke, 192, **193**
Maintenance program, **254**, 255
Major depression, **62**
Male condom, 464, **465**
Malignant tumor, **330**
Mammography, **337**
Managed care plans, 572
Manic-depressive illness, 62–**63**
Margarine, versus butter, 101
Marijuana, 244, 250t
   as medicine, 239
   risk factors for use, 236–238
Marital rape, **284**
Marriage(s), 444–449
   among elderly, 478
   without children, 444
Maslow's hierarchy of human needs, 57f
Mastectomy
   modified radical, **339**
   partial, **339**
   radical, **339**
Masters and Johnson, sexual response model, 420f, 420–421
Masturbation, **418**
Maximal heart rate, 166–**167**

Maximum out-of-pocket expense, 571
Maximum policy limit, 571
Means of transmission, 354, 356–357
Measles, 367t, 371
   German, 366t, 371
   vaccinations, 360
Medical assessment, 32–**33**, 37–41
Medication(s)
   abuse among elderly, 495–496
   advertising, 561–563
   for alcoholism, 220–221
   caffeine content, 235t
   correct use, 575–576
   filing complaints about, 564
   fraudulent claims, 562–563
   for genital herpes, 393
   heart disease, 327–328
   for HIV, 390
   for infections, 355
   marijuana as, 239
   over-the-counter, 233, 235t, **575**
   patient information, 560–561, 563–564, 576–579
   during pregnancy, 451
   prescription, 233–234, 235t, **575**
   sharing, 495–496
Meditation, 90
   for cancer, 342
Medulla, **213**
Meiosis, 431
Melanin, **332**
Melanoma, 331t, 333t, **335**, 336, **529**
Memory improvement, 490–491
Memory loss, in elderly, 485, 489–490, 494
Men
   alcohol consumption, 207–208
   cancer incidence, 331t, 333t, 334, 336, 338
   chlamydia and, 393
   crime and, 265–266
   domestic abuse and, 273–276
   exercise and, 157
   gonorrhea and, 394
   reproductive system, 430–433, 432f
   sexual dysfunction, 422–424
   smoking and, 179, 180t, 189f
   steroid use, 251
   unintentional injury and, 292
   violence and, 265–266
Menarche, 436
Meningitis, 392, **393**
Menopause, 436
Menstrual phase, 436
Menstruation, 436–438, 437f
   cessation, 128
   exercise and, 158–159
   irregular, 158
   low body weight and, 128
Mental ability, of elderly, 489–490, 493
Mental dysorganization, 58–64, 59f
Mental health, 48–71
   exercise and, 160–162
   resources, 67–68
   when to seek help, 68–69
Mental health practitioners, 67–69
Mental illness, 49. See also Depression; Mental dysorganization
   viruses as causes, 372
Meperidine, 249t
Mescaline, 244, 247t
Metabolism, weight and, 140
Metastasize, **330**
Methadone, 248t, 255

Methamphetamines, 245t
Methaqualone, 246t
Milwaukee, *Cryptosporidium* outbreak in, 537
Mind-body treatments
   for boosting immunity, 363
   for cancer, 341–342
Mineral(s), 103–104, 108
   deficiency, age-related, 114–115
Minor depression, 60–61
Minorities
   cocaine use, 252
   drunk driving, 297
   homicides, 269f
   smoking, 180, 180t
Miscarriage, **467**
MMR vaccine, **370**, 371
Mnemonics, 490
Moderation Management (MM), 220–221
Modified radical mastectomy, **339**
Mononucleosis, 367t, **368**, 369
Monounsaturated fat, **100**
Mons veneris, 434
Morbidity data, 28–**29**
Mormons, 29
Morning-after pill, 466, **467**
Morphine, 243, 249t
Mortality
   changes in, 319
   data, 28–**29**
Mothers Against Drunk Driving (MADD), 217, 226
Motor skills, 8–9f
Motor vehicle accidents, 291–292, 296–301
   air bags and, 298–299
   alcohol-related, 215–217, 216f, 291–292
   causes and risk factors, 291–293
   deaths, 296, 298f
   motorcycle, 299–301
   prevention, 296–301
   rate, 296
   seat belts and, 296–298, 298f
Motor vehicle pollution, 535
Motorcycles, 299–301
   helmets, 300–301
Mourning, **520**
   traditions, 508–509
MTV (Music Television) network, 382
Mucous membranes, 358, **359**
Multiple chemical sensitivity, 550–551
Multiple hazards, **529**
Multiple partners, and STDs, 383
Mumps, 371
Muscle(s)
   effect of aging on, 486
   progressive relaxation, 89–90
Mushrooms (hallucinogenic), 244, 247t–248t
Muslims, death traditions, 509
Mutagens, **529**
Mycoplasmas, **368**, 369
Myocardial infarction, **188**, **326**
Myometrium, 436
Myotonia, **418**, 419–420

N
Narcotics, **243**–244, 248t–249t
Native Americans
   alcohol consumption, 211
   death traditions, 509
   injury risk, 292
Natural childbirth, **455**
Naturopaths, 565–568

Needle exchange programs, 253
Needs hierarchy, 57f
Neisseria gonorrhoeae, **394**
Neurons, **488**
Neuroses, 58, **59**
Neurotic, 58, **59**
Neurotransmitters, **488**, 489
Nicotine, **183**, 184–185
   addiction, **183**, 184–185
   pregnancy and, 191
Nicotine gum, 198
Nicotine nasal spray, 198
Nicotine patch, transdermal, **198**
Nicotine replacement therapy, **196**, 197–198
Nipple, 434
Nitrates, 108–109
Nitrites, 108–109
Nitrogen oxides, **532**, 533, 549t
Noise pollution, 545–547, 546t
Nonpoint source pollutants, **538**
Nonprescription drugs. See Over-the-counter (OTC) drugs
Nonspecific defense mechanisms, 358, **359**
Non-REM sleep, 54
Nonverbal communication, 414
Norplant, 461, 464
Northern Ireland, gun control, 270–271
Nosocomial infections, **370**, 371–373
Notice to Health Care Providers card, 512, 512f
Nuclear family, 442, **443**
Nurse-midwife, **455**
Nursing homes, 478, 479t, 494–495
Nutrients, **97**–108
Nutrition, 97–107. See also Diet(s); Eating patterns and styles; Food
   age-related, 114–115
   artificial ingredients and, 107–109
   knowledge test, 110–111
   label information, 121
   recommendations, 103t, 109–111, 112f
   in sandwiches, 118f
   of young athletes, 159

O
Obesity, 114, **127**–128. See also Weight gain
   causes, 133–137
   fat and, 139
   heart disease and, 324
   hypertension and, 324
Occasional drinker, **210**
Occupational carcinogens, 332
Occupational Safety and Health Administration (OSHA), 308
Office of Disease Prevention and Health Promotion, 578
On Death and Dying (Kübler-Ross), 515
Opium, 243, 249t
Opportunistic diseases, **386**, 387
Organ donation, 518–519
   uniform donor card, 517f
Organically grown food, 120
Orgasm, **421**, 424, 430
Osteoarthritis, 169
Osteoporosis, 105, 486–488
   calcium and, 104–105
   prevention, 158–160
Outercourse, **418**
Out-of-pocket expense, maximum, 571
Outpatient care, **569**
Ova, 433

Ovaries, 433–434
Overdose, 242, **243**
Overmedication, **495**
Over-the-counter (OTC) drugs, 233, 235t, **575**
Overweight, **127**–128
Ovolactovegetarians, **118**
Ovulation, 435, 437
Ozone, **532**, 533–534
Ozone layer, 534, **535**

P
Pain, chronic, coping with, 345–346
Palpation, 36–37
Pandemic, 27
Pap smear, **337**
Papilloma virus, **391**–392, 396t
Parasitic worms, **355**
   diseases caused by, 357t
Parkinson's disease, **497**
Partial mastectomy, **339**
Particulates, **532**, 533
Passion, **415**
Passive euthanasia, **508**
Passive immunity, **359**
Passive seat belts, **297**
Passive smoking, 179, 192–**193**, 531
   avoiding, 184
Pathogen, 353
   reservoir of, 354, **355**
Patient package insert, 560, **561**
Patient Self-Determination Act, 511
Pauling, Linus, 365
PCBs (polychlorinated biphenyls), 545
PCP (phencyclidine), 244
Pelvic inflammatory disease (PID), **393**–394
Penis, 430f, 430–431
Perception, in coping, 86
Perchloroethylene (PCE), **538**
Perimetrium, 436
Periodontal disease, **341**, 343–344
Periodontitis, 343
Peripheral artery disease, 188f
Personality hardiness, **84**, 85
Pertussis, 361, 367t
Pesticides, 538–539, 549t
Peyote, 244, 247t
Phagocytes, 358–**359**
Phencyclidine, 247t
Phobias, 58–**59**
Physical abuse, **274**
Physical examination, 36–41
Physical fitness, **162**
Physical neglect, of children, 276–277
Physician-assisted suicide, **508**–510
Physicians, 565–569, 566t
Physician's Desk Reference, 561
Physiology, reproductive
   female, 433–438
   male, 430–433
   test, 438–439
Pinch test, **131**
Pipes, 193
Placenta, **450**
Plaque, **100**, 101, 319, 325
   dental, 343–344
Plateau, sexual, **421**
Pneumocystis carinii pneumonia, **386**, 387
Pneumonia, 368–369
   bacterial, 368–369
   fungal, 368, 369
Point-of-service plans (POS), 574, **575**
Point source pollutants, **538**

Poisoning, 307–308
  alcohol, 215
  food, 374
Polio, 360–361
Pollution, 529–551, 553–555. *See also* Environmental health hazards
  air, **530**–536, 531*t*, 532–535, 549*t*
  criteria pollutants, 530, 531*t*
  indoor, 547–551, 548*f*, 549*t*, **550**
  noise, 545–547, 546*t*
  solid waste, 540–544, 542*f*
  toxic waste, 544–545
  water, 536–540
Polychlorinated biphenyls (PCBs), 545
Polyunsaturated fat, **100**
Portal of exit, 354, **355**
POS. *See* Point-of-service plans (POS)
Pounds, calories and, 137–139
Poverty, crime and, 266–267
Power of attorney for health care, durable, **511**–512
PPOs. *See* Preferred provider organizations (PPOs)
Prayer, as cancer therapy, 342
Preadmission certification, **569**
Preconception care, 448–449
Precycling, **540**, 541
Preexisting conditions, 571
Preferred provider organizations (PPOs), 574, **575**
Pregnancy, 449–454
  alcohol and, 214–215
  childbirth preparation, 454–455
  chlamydia and, 393–394
  drug use during, 253–254
  fetal health tests, 452–453
  gonorrhea and, 394
  menstrual cycle, 436–438, 437*f*
  preconception care, 448–**449**
  prenatal care, **450**–452
  signs, 450
  smoking and, 190–191
  syphilis and, 395
  teen, 447
  tests, 450
  trimesters, 453*f*, 453–454
  tubal, 393–394
  unintended, 458, 458*t*
Premature death, **292**, 293–295
Premature ejaculation, **422**, 423
Premenstrual dysphoric disorder, **62**
Premenstrual syndrome, 62–**63**
Prenatal care, **450**–452
Prepuce, 431
Presbyopia, **488**
Prescription drugs, 233–234, 235*t*, **575**–576
Prescriptions, how to read, 577
Preservatives, 108
Prevalence data, **26**, 27
Prevention, 14–18, **15**
Preventive behavior, **10**–11
Primary care, **569**
Primary care physicians, 565
Primary health assessment, **25**
Primary stressor, **77**
Prions, **355**–356
  diseases caused by, 357*t*
Problem drinker, **218**–219
Processed food, 120
Processing aids, 108
Pro-choice, **470**
Prodromal stage, **362**, 363
Progesterone, 437–438
Progressive muscle relaxation, 89–90

Prohibition, 223
Pro-life, **470**
Promoter, **330**
Proof, 224
Prostate cancer, 331*t*, 334, 338–341
Prostate gland, 433
Prostate-specific antigen (PSA) test, 338, **339**
Protease inhibitors, and HIV, 390
Protein(s), **98**, 99–100
  complete, **100**
Protozoa, **355**
  diseases caused by, 357*t*
Protozoal vaginitis, 399
Prusiner, Stanley B., 355–356
Psilocybin (mushrooms), 244, 247*t*–248*t*
Psychiatric disorders. *See also* Mental dysorganization
  viruses and, 372
Psychiatrists, 67
Psychological abuse, **274**
Psychological adjustment, to chronic disease, 345–346
Psychological age, **478**
Psychologists, 67
Psychoneuroimmunology, **53**, **341**, 342
  and AIDS, 363
Psychoses, 64, **65**
Psychotherapy, for elderly, 493, 495
Psychotic disorders, 64
Puberty, 410
Pubic lice, 396*t*, 399
Pulse, 36–37, 166
Purging, **141**–142
Pyorrhea, 343
Pyrogen, **36**

Q
Quackery, **562**–563
Quadriplegia, **303**
Quarantine, 354
Quickening, **454**, **455**

R
Radiation
  as cancer cause, 332
  as cancer therapy, 339–341
Radical mastectomy, **339**
Radon, 548–549
Rape, **280**–284, 282*f*
  acquaintance, **283**–284
  aftermath, 284
  costs, 265
  times, 267
Rape trauma syndrome, 284*f*
Rapid eye movement (REM) sleep, **54**
"The Real World" documentary, 382
Receptor site, **240**
Recoil, stage of grief, **520**, 521
Recommended dietary allowances (RDAs), **109**
  for vitamins, 103*t*
Recovery
  from infection, 364, **365**
  stage of grief, **522**
Recreational accidents, 301–303
  prevention checklist, 309
Recycling, **542**–544
  quiz, 543
Red dye No. 2, 108–109
Reduced fat food, 120
Refractory period, **422**
Relationships
  of elderly, 488–489
  living together, 444, 447

  love and, 414–417
  marriage, 444–449
  sexual, 417–419
Relative strength, **162**
Relaxation, 89–90
  smoking and, 183
Relaxation therapy, as cancer treatment, 341–342
Religious perspectives
  on death, 507–509
  on sex, 409
REM sleep, **54**
Reproductive system, 429–439
  chlamydia and, 393
  defined, 429
  female, 433–438, 434*f*–435*f*, 437*f*
  male, 430*f*, 430–433, 432*f*
  test, 438–439
Reservoir of the pathogen, 354, **355**
Resistance, 358, **359**. *See also* Immunity
  to rape, 282–283
  to stress, **77**
  to violence, 268
Resolution, sexual, **421**
Resting heart rate, 166, **167**
Retirement communities, 478, 488
Reye's syndrome, **374**, 375
Rhythm method, **460**
Rickettsias, **355**
  diseases caused by, 357*t*
Rights, of health care consumers, 563–564
Risk age, 34–**35**
Risk factors, 32
  in family tree, 38*f*
Risk-taking behavior, **291**
Road rage, 292
Road safety, 296–301, 309
Robbery, 265, 267
Rock concerts, noise hazards at, 547
Roe v. Wade, 469
Rohypnol (date-rape drug), 283
Romantic love, 415
Roofies, 283
RU-486, 469–470
Rubella, 366*t*, 371
Rubeola, 367*t*
Runner's high, 160–**161**
Running shoes, 171
Rural areas, crime in, 267

S
Sadistic rape, **283**
Safe sex, 382, 385–387
  versus safer sex, 401
Safer sex, 18, **400**–401
Safety precautions, in exercise, 169–172
Salt, dietary, 105–107
  content in foods, 106*t*
Saturated fat, **100**
Scabies, 399
Schizophrenia, 64, **65**
Science, bogus, in health information, 561–563, 578
Screening, 337
Scrotum, 430, 430*f*
Seasonal affective disorder (SAD), 62–**63**
Seat belts, 296–298
  and crash death rate, 298*f*
  passive, 297
Secondary care, **569**
Secondary health assessment, **25**
Secondary infection, **355**
Secondary stressor, **77**
Secondary syphilis, **394**–395
Sedentary lifestyle, heart disease

  and, 324–325
Self-actualization, **54**, 58
Self-assessment, 32–**33**
  errors, 26
Self-concept, **54**–55
Self-efficacy, **54**, 57
Self-esteem, **54**–57
  drug abuse and, 256–257
  rating scale, 56
Self-observation, 36–37
Semen, 433
Seminal vesicle, 433
Seminiferous tubules, 431
Sensate focus, **424**–425
Serotonin, **65**
Set point, **135**
Sex, 417–419. *See also* Sexuality
  communication, 413–414
  dating and, 284*f*
  and elderly, 479, 488–489, 494
  origin of values regarding, 408–410
  physiological changes, 419–421
  psychological component, 421–422
  safe, 382, 385–387, 401
  safer, 18, **400**–401
  and STD prevention, 384–386
Sex characteristics, determination of, 411, 411*f*
Sex drive, **418**
Sex role, **406**–407
Sexual abstinence, **413**
  and STDs, 399–400
Sexual abuse, of children, **277**–279
Sexual dysfunctions, **422**–425
  therapies, 424–425
Sexual harassment, 278–280
Sexual orientation, **412**–413
Sexual response, 419–422
  four-stage model, 420*f*, 420–421
  healthy, 407
Sexual revolution, **408**
Sexuality, **406**–413
  anatomy and physiology, 429–439
  biology and, 411–412
  cultural attitudes, 408–409
  individual values, 409–410
  influences, 407*t*, 408–413
  religion and, 409
Sexually transmitted diseases (STDs), 380–403, **381**
  bacterial, 393–395
  incidence, 383*t*
  prevention, 383–387
  spread of, 382–383
  symptoms, 396*t*–397*t*, 399–400
  transmission cycle, 384*t*
  types, 396*t*–397*t*
  viral, 386–393
Shock, 310
Shoes, exercise, 169, 171
Shopping, food, 120–121
Sick building syndrome. *See* Tight building syndrome
Sick-role behavior, **10**–11
Side effects, drug, **240**
Sidestream smoke, **179**, 184, 192–193
Sigmoidoscopy, 338, **339**
Simple carbohydrate, **97**
Single-parent family, **443**
Situational abstinence, **224**
Skin
  aging and, 485–486
  pollution and, 531
  smoking and, 191
Skin cancer, 332, 335–337
  prevention, 337

Sleep, 52–54
  elderly and, 494–495
Sleep deprivation, 53
Smallpox, 352, 354, 362
Smog, **532,** 533
Smoke detectors, **305**–306
Smokeless tobacco, **193**–194
Smoking, 178–203. *See also* Smoking cessation; Tobacco
  as addiction, 183
  advertising and, 182
  and benzene exposure, 531
  cancer and, 186–188, 189*f*, 193, 332
  changing attitudes towards, 198–201
  cigar, 193
  demographics, 179–181, 180*t*, 236*t*
  effect on infants, 191, 193
  fires caused by, 305
  health care costs, 186*t*
  health impact, 18, 185–192
  heart disease and, 188–190, 324
  history, 200, 200*f*
  of illicit drugs, 243
  low-yield cigarettes, 192
  passive, 179, 184, 192–**193**
  physical effects, test, 187
  pipe, 193
  during pregnancy, 190–191, 450–452
  reasons for, 181–184
  related poor health habits, 13–14, 14*t*, 180–181
  relaxation and, 183
  stroke and, 190
Smoking cessation, 195–198, **196**
  checklist, 197
  in Fijian village, 196
  health benefits of, 188*f*–189*f*
  heart disease and, 190
  lung cancer and, 189*f*
  methods, 196–198
  physical problems, 195–196
  pregnancy and, 191
  stroke and, 190
  weight gain and, 195–196
  withdrawal symptoms, 195
Snuff, 193–194
Social drinker, **210**
  former alcoholic as, 221
Social skills, 8–9*f*
Social workers, 67–68
Sodium, dietary. *See* Salt
Solid waste, 540–544, 542*f*
Solitude, 55
Sonogram, **452**
Spanking, 277
Specialists, 565, 566*t*
Specified medical limitation, 571
Sperm, 430–433, 431*f*, 431–432
Spermatids, 431
Spermicide, **465**
Spontaneous abortion, 467
Sports. *See* Exercise
Spouse abuse, **272**
Squamous cell, **335**
Staging, 236, **237**
Stalking, electronic, 280
Starches, **98**
State health rankings, 6*f*–7*f*
STDs. *See* Sexually transmitted diseases (STDs)
Sterility. *See also* Infertility
  chlamydia-induced, 393–394
Sterilization, **465**
Steroids, anabolic, **244,** 251
Stimulants, **243,** 245*t*–246*t*
Strength, **162**–163
Stress, 74–93, **75**

adaptation, 85–91
behavioral effects, 81
coping with, 85–88
drugs and, 258–259
exercise and, 88–89, 141, 160
health effects, 81–82
immune system and, 81–82
positive and negative, 77
reactions to, 75–77
sources, 76*f. See also* Stressors
subjective effects, 81
Stress electrocardiogram, **325**
Stress inoculation, **89,** 90–91
Stress response, **75**
Stressors, **75**
  college-related, 82–84
  identification, **86**
  primary, **77**
  rating scale, 78–79
  secondary, **77**
  work-related, 84–85
Stretching exercises, 164
Stroke, **326**–327
  hypertension and, 324
  risk factors for, 321*t*
  smoking and, 190
  smoking cessation and, 188*f*
  women and, 323, 323*f*
Students Against Drunk Driving (SADD), 217
Substances, abused, 234–235. *See also* Drug(s)
Sugar, 97–98
Suicide, 64–66
  alcohol-related, 215
  elderly, 65, 495
  physician-assisted, **508**–510
  teen, 65
  warning signs, 66
Suicidologists, 64, **65**
Sulfites, 109
Sulfur oxides, **532**
Sun exposure
  skin cancer and, 332, 335–337
  vision loss and, 487
Sunburn, 336–337
Surrogate motherhood, 448
Sweden, elderly in, 479*t*
Swimming, risks, 302–303
Switzerland, gun control, 270
Symptomatic period, 319
Synergistic effect, **226,** 241–242, 531
Syphilis, 394–395, 397*t*
  late, **394**, 395
  secondary, 394
Systemic infection, **393**
Systolic pressure, **326,** 327

T
Tachycardia, **326**
T'ai chi, 88, 498
Tar, **184**, 185
Target heart rate range, **167**
Tartar, 344
Tea, caffeine in, 235*t*
Teenagers
  alcohol use, 209, 217, 223, 227
  as athletes, health problems, 143, 159
  chlamydia and, 393
  crime and, 265–267
  drug use risk factors, 237
  drunk driving and, 217, 223
  nutrition, 112, 115
  perception of death, 513
  pregnancy, 447
  sexuality, 410
  skin cancer risk, 336–337
  smokeless tobacco use, 194

smoking and, 179, 181–182, 199
steroid abuse, 251
suicide, 65
Television
  obesity and, 136–137
  violence on, 272–273
Temporary threshold shift (TTS), 546, **547**
Teratogens, **529**
Tertiary care, **569**
Testes, 431
Testicles, 430–431, 431*f*
Testicular cancer
  death rate, 331*t*
  self-test for, 338
Testosterone, 430
Tetrahydrocannabinol, 250*t*
Thalamus, **213**
Thalidomide, **450,** 451
Thanatology, **505**
Therapeutic communities, for drug abusers, **254**, 255–256
Tight building syndrome, **547**
Time management, 86*f*, 86–87
Tissue plasminogen activator, **157**
Tobacco, 178–203. *See also* Smoking; Smoking cessation
  addiction, 183
  changing attitudes toward, 198–201
  chewing, 193
  components, 184–185, 549*t*
  history and timeline, 200, 200*f*
  low-yield, 192
  smokeless, **193**–194
Tobacco companies
  advertising by, 182
  lawsuits against, 199
Tolerance, **218**
  alcohol, 218
  drug, 240
Tooth decay, 341, 343–344, 540
Total abstinence, **224**
Total allergy syndrome, 550–551
Total fasting, 146
Toxic chemicals, **545**
Toxic shock syndrome, **374,** 375
Toxic waste, 544–545
Toxin, **355**
Trace minerals, **102,** 103–104
Training effect, **167**
Tranquilizers, 243, 246*t*–247*t*
Transdermal nicotine patch, **198**
Transient ischemic attack (ITA), **326,** 327
Trauma, **291**
Trichinosis, 355
Trichloroethylene (TCE), **538**
Trichomoniasis, **399**
Tubal ligation, 466, **467**
Tubal pregnancy, 393–394
Tuberculosis, 370
  chain of infection, 353*f*
Tumor, **330**
  benign, **330**
  malignant, **330**
Type A personality, **79**
Type B personality, **79**

U
Ulcers, viruses as cause, 372
Underinsured, **569**
Underwater weighing, **131**
Underweight, 128, **129,** 141–143
Uniform donor card, 517*f*
Uninsured, **569**
Unintentional injuries, **291**
University of California at Berkeley Wellness Letter, 561

Upper respiratory infections, smoking-related, 191
Urethra, 431
U.S. Environmental Protection Agency (EPA), 530
Uterus, 433, 436

V
Vaccine(s), 360–361
  flu, 365
  hepatitis B, 392
  MMR, **370,** 371
Vacuum aspiration, **468,** 469
Vagina, 433
Vaginismus, **424**
Vaginitis, **394,** 395–399
Vagus nerve, 134, **135**
Vas deferens, 432–433
Vasectomy, 466, **467**
Vasocongestion, **418,** 419–420
Vectors, 354, **355,** 357
Vegans, 118
Vegetarians, **100,** 113–119
  balanced diet, 119
Victims
  crime, 266*f*, 266–268
  rape, 281
Violence, 264–287, **265**
  alcohol-related, 215, 271–272
  against children, 276–278, 279*f*
  costs, 265
  domestic, **272,** 273–278, 277*f*
  against domestic partner, 273–276
  drugs and, 271–272
  factors, 269–272
  prevention, 268
  reactions, 268
  television and, 272–273
  against women, 273–276, 277*f*, 280–284
Virulence, 358, **359**
Viruses, **355**
  cancer-causing, 333, 372
  Chlamydia pneumoniae, 372
  common cold, 365
  diseases caused by, 357*t*, 372
  Epstein-Barr, 369, 372
  and heart disease, 372
  hepatitis, 370–371
  herpes, 372, 392, **393,** 397*t*
  human papilloma, 391–392, 396*t*
  interferon and, 359
  newly identified, 373*t*, 374
  and psychiatric disorders, 372
  STD-causing, 386
  and ulcers, 372
Vision loss
  in elderly, 487–488
  smoking and, 191
Vitamin(s), 102–103, 103*t*
  as additives, 108
  overeating, 119
Vitamin deficiency, and age, 114–115
Vitamin-enriched food, 120
Vulva, 433

W
Wakes, 508
Walking, 166
Warm-up period, **168**–169
Waste
  hazardous, **545**
  solid, 540–544, 542*f*
  toxic, 544–545
Water, 107
  contaminated, 357, 536–537
  scalding, 306
Water pollution, 536–540

Weight, 126–149
 aging and, 486
 assessment, 128–133
 body fat and, **131**
 body mass and, 130f, 130–131
 changes, assessment, 37
 control, 143–147
 eating behavior and, 135–137
 height and, 129–131
Weight gain, 137–139. *See also* Obesity
 during pregnancy, 452
 smoking cessation and, 195–196
Weight loss, 143–147. *See also* Diet(s); Eating disorders
 diets and, 145
 drugs for, 146–147, 251
 fasting and, 146
Weight-bearing exercise, 159–160
Well-being, psychological, 49
 exercise and, 160–161
Wellness, 4–**5**
Wellness Inventory, 16–17
White Americans
 heart disease and, 323
 mortality data, 323t
White blood cells, 359
Whooping cough, 361, 367t
Wine
 calories, 212t
 heart disease and, 213
Withdrawal, **460**
 from drugs, **240**
Withdrawal symptoms
 alcohol, **218**
 caffeine, 234
 tobacco, **183**
Women. *See also* Pregnancy
 abused, 273–276, 277f
 AIDS, 387–388, 389f
 alcohol consumption, 207–208
 bone loss, 104–105, 158–160, 486–488
 cancer, 323, 323f, 330, 331t, 334, 336–338, 340
 crime and, 266, 266f
 depression, 60–61
 drunk driving, 297
 elderly, 158–160, 478, 486–488, 496
 exercise, 157–160
 heart disease, 323f, 323–324
 hip fractures, 496
 injuries, 292
 leading causes of death, 323f
 rape, 280–284
 reproductive system, 433–438
 sexual dysfunction, 424
 smoking, 179, 180t, 189–191
 STDs, 393–399
 steroids, 251–252
 vaginitis, 395–399
Working, health skills in, 10
Workplace
 air pollutants, 547–550, 549t
 drug use, 254
 injuries, 292–293, 293f
 stressors, 84–85
World Health Organization (WHO), 3
World Wide Web, as health information source, 577–578
Wrinkling, 485–486

Y
Yeast infection, **394**, 395–399, 397t
Yo-yo dieting, **145**

Z
Zamora, Pedro, 382

Contents Photo Credits
P. vii © Tony Stone Images/Brian Bailey; p. vii © Tony Stone Images/Phil Schofield; p. ix © Tony Stone Images/Peter Poulides; p. xi © Tony Stone Images/Lori Adamski Peek; p. xii © Stock, Boston; p. xiii © Tony Stone Images/Dugald Bremner.

Chapter Opener Photo Credits
P. 1 © Tony Stone Images/Brian Bailey; p. 22 © Tony Stone Images/David Hanover; p. 46 © Tony Stone Images/Ben Osborne; p. 72 © Tony Stone Images; p. 94 © Tony Stone Images/Phil Schofield; p. 124 © Tony Stone Images/Lori Adamski Peek; p. 150 © Tony Stone Images/Lori Adamski Peek; p. 176 The Image Works/© Bob Daemmrich; p. 204 Stock, Boston/© M. Grecco; p. 230 Stock, Boston/© Frank Siteman; p. 262 The Image Works/© T. Shumsky; p. 288 © Tony Stone Images/Donald Johnson; p. 314 Stock, Boston/© Keren Su; p. 350 Photo Researchers, Inc./Tektoff/Rhone-Merieux—CNRI Science Photo Library; p. 378 The Image Works/© Esbin/Anderson; p. 404 Image Works/ © Esbin/Anderson; p. 428 © Tony Stone Images/Lori Adamski Peek; p. 440 © Tony Stone Images/Lori Adamski Peek; p. 474 Stock, Boston/© Frank Siteman; The Image Works/© Bachmann; p. 526 © Tony Stone Images/ Dugald p. 556 © Tony Stone Images/Andy Whale.